AF383275

Hernias and
Surgery of the Abdominal Wall

Springer

*Paris
Berlin
Heidelberg
New York
Barcelona
Budapest
Hong Kong
London
Milan
Santa Clara
Singapore
Tokyo*

Hernias and Surgery of the abdominal wall

Edited by J. P. Chevrel

With the Collaboration of

P. Amid R. Bendavid M. Caix G. Champault J.L. Dumas J.B. Flament
Ph. Galinier A.E. Gilbert M.F. Graham J. Hureau S. Juskiewenski
D. Marchac C. Meyer J.P.H. Neidhardt J.P. Palot J. Pradel-Raynal
J. Rives R. Stoppa J. Taboury G.E. Wantz

Preface by Lloyd M. Nyhus and by G.E. Wantz

with 451 illustrations

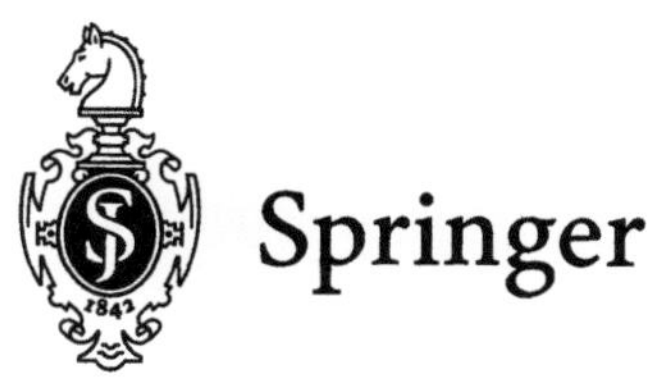 Springer

Professor J. P. Chevrel
Service de Chirurgie Générale et Digestive,
Hôpital Avicenne,
Université Paris 13, 125 Route de Stalingrad,
F-93009 Bobigny
France

Translation:
Dr. Elliot Goldstein, A. Marston, MA DM MCh FRCS

Revision:
A. Marston, MA DM MCh FRCS

Original French edition
Chirurgie des parois de l'abdomen
© Springer-Verlag Berlin Heidelberg New York Tokyo 1985
ISBN 978-3-642-48883-2   ISBN 978-3-642-48881-8 (eBook)
DOI 10.1007/978-3-642-48881-8

ISBN 978-3-642-48883-2

Cataloguing-in-Publication Data applied for
Die Deutsche Bibliotek = CIP Einheitsaufnahme
Hernias and surgery of the abdominal wall / ed. by J. P. Chevrel. With the collab. of P. Amid... Pref. by Lloyd M. Nyhus and
G. E. Wantz [Transl. Elliot Goldstein] - 2., rev. ed. - Berlin; Heidelberg; New York; Barcelona; Budapest; Hong Kong. Londres;
Milan; Paris; Santa Clara; Singapour; Tokyo : Springer, 1997
  1. Aufl. u.d.T.: Surgery of the abdominal wall
  Franz. Ausg. u.d.T.:Chirurgie des parois de l'abdomen

This work is subject to copyright. All rights are reserved, whether the whole or part of the material is concerned, specifically the rights of translation, reprinting, reuse of illustrations, recitation, broadcasting, reproduction on microfilm or in any other way, and storage in data banks. Duplication of this publication or parts thereof is permitted only under the provisions of the German Copyright Law of September 9, 1965, in its current version, and permission for use must always be obtained from Springer-Verlag. Violations are liable for prosecution under the German Copyright Law.

© Springer-Verlag Berlin Heidelberg 1998
Softcover reprint of the hardcover 2nd edition 1998

The use of general descriptive names, registered names, trademarks, etc. in this publication does not imply, even in the absence of a specific statement, that such names are exempt from the relevant protective laws and regulations and therefore free for general use.

Product liability: The publishers cannot guarantee the accuracy of any information about the application of operative techniques and medications contained in this book. In every individual case the user must check such information by consulting the relevant literature.

SPIN: 105 74 140   90/2918 - 5 4 3 2 1 0   Printed on acid-free paper

Foreword to the Second Edition

This book, written mostly by French surgeons and surgeon-anatomist is about the abdominal wall. There is nothing comparable to it nor is there any publication as comprehensive. It covers every aspect of the abdominal wall from anatomy and hernias to tumors, burst abdomens, and abdominal reconstruction in children and adults. Among the striking features of the book is unity even though it was written by multiple authors. The chapters do not overlap and flow smoothly from one to another in English, beautifully translated from French. For me reading it from cover to cover was a pleasure, yet my chief use of this book is to reference a subject, as the thumbed pages of my first edition attest. The second edition brings each chapter up to date and includes numerous new illustrations.

The illustrations of anatomy and operative procedures need special comment for they are especially elucidating, uniquely French, and for me an educational treat. Usually North American surgery treatises are illustrated by medical artists who draws what they see using line or halftone techniques. In this book, however, the illustrations are schematic and were initially prepared by the authors themselves. In France, not rarely, professors of surgery, and almost all professors of anatomy illustrate their lectures and surgical essays by drawing schematically on the blackboard or on paper. They are skilled at this and I have watched them with envy. The illustrations in this book are professional reproductions of the schematic drawings the authors used to illustrate their chapters and are exactly like those they use to teach anatomy and surgery to their students

As expected, considerable space is allocated to hernias of the abdominal wall. French surgeons have been the world leaders on this subject. The first edition of this book introduced to English speaking surgeons for the first time Fruchaud's myopectineal orifice, the anatomic area where all groin hernias originate, and the innovative and revolutionary surgical techniques for successfully repairing complex hernias of the groin and intimidating major incisional hernias. These techniques are now recognized worldwide as the preferred procedures for these very difficult problems.

The book's origins stem from the founding members of Groupe de Recherche et d'Étude de la Paroi Abdominale (GREPA). What started as a club of ten congenial French surgeons, interested chiefly in the anterior abdominal wall is now an international organization of surgeons of all disciplines who are united in solving the problems of every aspect of the abdominal wall. This book, conceived and edited by J.P. Chevrel, has, like GREPA, also grown and, as such, epitomizes this organization. The book is invaluable and will be a great help for medical students surgical residents and practicing surgeons.

George Wantz, M.D.

Clinical Professor of Surgery
The New York Hospital - Cornell Medical Centre, New York, NY

Foreword to the First Edition

The abdominal wall has always been of interest to surgeon-anatomists. It was recognized as a barrier, and volumes have been written demonstrating how to breach this wall. Similarly, great importance has been placed on the methods of repairing the abdominal wall, whether that repair is necessitated by a primary operative wound, a congenital failure, an acquired defect, or the ubiquitous iatrogenic problem, the postoperative abdominal wall hernia.

French surgeons have a long tradition of excellence in the field of human anatomy: the names of Paré, Bichat, Cloquet, and Fruchaud readily come to mind. It is not surprising then, that this comprehensive text on the subject of the abdominal wall and its defects emanates from France.

Although there are many interesting aspects to this presentation of abdominal wall problems, I find the review of prosthetic material and its use to be most unique. The synthetic meshes available today may well revolutionize our various approaches for repair of hernial defects. Considerable experience has evolved in the use of these prosthetic materials, particularly in the United Kingdom and Europe. I have been a proponent of prosthetic mesh for the cure of recurrent groin hernia during the past decade. According to the results reported in this book, the use of a prosthetic material in selected patients needing primary hernia repair seems indicated.

I would be remiss if the organization GREPA were not highlighted. It is common today to form clubs dedicated to the study of single organ systems, such as the pancreas or the esophagus. GREPA is a group dedicated to the study of problems relating to the abdominal wall and is another exemple of how concentrated attention given to a single subject can significantly advance our knowledge. Editor Chevrel and his colleagues can be proud of what has been accomplished by GREPA and the superb documentation of its efforts in this monograph.

Lloyd M. Nyhus

M. D., Dr. h. c., Warren H. Cole Professor and Head, Department of Surgery
University of Illinois
College of Medicine at Chicago, USA

Introduction to the First Edition

It has now been 8 years since the working group known as GREPA was formed (Groupe de Recherche et d'Étude de la Paroi Abdominale - Group for Research and Study of the Abdominal Wall). Its founding surgeons were initially united by a common desire to promote the study of the abdominal wall. Very quickly strong bonds of friendship developed among the founding members of GREPA.

Many talented surgeons were already distinguished for their work on the abdominal wall. However, it was our belief at that time that an up-to-date analysis of new techniques, modern prosthetic materials and certain little known surgical approaches would lead to improved results in surgery of the abdominal wall.

A few members of GREPA, who had previously done considerable work in the field of abdominal wall surgery, agreed to collate the fruits of their vast experience in this book. I am greatly indebted to them for their contribution; they have brought a certain distinction to this sometimes difficult and often underestimated field of surgery.

This book is divided into two parts.

The first part begins with the classical surgical anatomy of the abdominal wall and its weak points. This section is followed by a study of the electromyography and histoenzymology of the muscles, with special emphasis on recent findings. Part One concludes with the diagnostic features of ultrasonography and computerized tomography of the abdominal wall.

The second part of this book is devoted to the study of the abdominal wall according to the following outline:

- Surgical approaches
- Pre- and postoperative care
- Postoperative complications
- Closed trauma of the abdominal wall
- Defects of the abdominal wall: pathological, iatrogenic
- Hernias
- Pathology of the umbilicus
- Plasty of the abdominal wall
- Abdominal wall in infants and children

Each of the contributing authors has been asked to give the essential fruits of his experience. No attempt has been made to produce an encyclopedia of the abdominal wall or treatise of surgical technique. The modest aim of this book is to present a series of traditional and modern, or even still little known solutions to the pathological conditions involving the abdominal wall. It is hoped that these solutions will be of benefit to the experienced surgeon as well as the young surgical resident.

On behalf of the contributing authors, I would like to express our sincere gratitude to Doctor Götze who sponsored this book for publication by Springer-Verlag. We also thank Mrs. A. Travadel who designed the illustrations.

This book is dedicated to my four daughters.

Paris, October 1986   J. P. Chevrel

List of Co-authors

Parviz K. Amid, MD
Lichtenstein Hernia Institute Inc.
9201 Sunset Boulevard, Suite 505, Los Angeles, CA 90069, USA

Robert Bendavid, MD
Shouldice Hospital
7750 Bayview Avenue, Box 370, Thornhill, Ontario L3T 4A3, Canada

Pr Michel Caix
Le Picq, F-87510 Perilhac

Pr Gérard Champault
Service de Chirurgie Digestive, Hôpital Jean Verdier,
Avenue du 14 Juillet, F-93140 Bondy

Pr Jean-Paul Chevrel
Service de Chirurgie Générale et Digestive, Hôpital Avicenne,
125, route de Stalingrad, F-93009 Bobigny

Pr Jean-Bernard Flament
Service de Chirurgie Digestive, Hôpital Robert Debré
Avenue du Général Koenig, F-51092 Reims Cedex

Arthur I. Gilbert, MD, FACS
Hernia Institute of Florida
6250 Sunset Drive Nr 200, Miami, Florida 33143, USA

M. F. Graham, MD
Hernia Institute of Florida
6250 Sunset Drive Nr 200, Miami, Florida 33143, USA

Dr Jean-Luc Dumas
Département de Radiologie
Hôpital Avicenne,
125, route de Stalingrad, F-93009 Bobigny

Pr Jacques Hureau
85, Avenue Émile Thiébaut, F-78110 Le Vésinet

Pr Serge Juskiewenski
Service de Chirurgie Infantile et Néonatale, CHU Purpan,
Place du Dr. Baylac, F-31059 Toulouse Cedex

Pr Daniel Marchac
130, rue de la Pompe, F-75016 Paris

Pr Jean-Pierre Hanno Neidhardt
Service des Urgences Chirurgicales, Centre Hospitalier Lyon Sud,
Chemin du Grand Revoyet, F-69310 Pierre Bénite

Pr Jean-Pierre Palot
Service de Chirurgie Digestive, Hôpital Robert Debré
Avenue du Général Koenig, F-51092 Reims Cedex

Dr Jeanine Pradel-Raynal
59, Boulevard Lannes, F-75116 Paris

Pr Jean Rives
3 rue Dufrenoy, F-75016 Paris

Pr René Stoppa
77bis, rue Laurendeau, F-80090 Amiens

Dr Jacques Taboury
Service de Radiologie, Hôpital Saint Antoine
184 rue du faubourg Saint Antoine, F-75571 Paris Cedex 12

George E. Wantz, MD
517 E. 71 Street, New York, NY 10021, USA

Table of Contents

Chapter 2. Functional Anatomy of the Muscles of the Anterolateral Abdominal Wall: Electromyography and Histoenzymology - Relationship Between Abdominal Wall Activity and Intra-abdominal Pressure
M. Caix with the collaboration of G. Outrequin, B. Descottes, M. Kalfon, X. Pouget, and G. Catanzano

Part 2. Surgical Techniques

Chapter 4. Surgical Approaches to the Abdomen
J. P. Chevrel with the collaboration of G. Champault 65

Chapter 8. Defects of the Abdominal Wall
J. P. H. Neidhardt, J. P. Chevrel, J. B. Flament and J. Rives 111

Chapter 9. Hernia of the Abdominal Wall

R. Stoppa with the collaboration of P. Amid, R. Bendavid,
G. Champault, J. P. Chevrel, J. B. Flament, A. Gilbert,
C. Meyer, J. P. Palot, G. E. Wantz

Chapter 10. Pathology of the Umbilicus
G. Champault 279

Part 1. General

1 Surgical Anatomy of the Anterolateral and Posterior Abdominal Walls and Points of Weakness

J.P.H. Neidhardt

I. The Anterolateral Abdominal Wall

The term anterolateral abdominal wall refers to all of the layered structures covering the abdomen. This wall occupies a hexagonal area limited by the following structures: above, by the angle of the xiphoid process, chondrocostal margin, and cartilage of the two lowermost ribs; laterally, by the midaxillary line; below, by the anterior part of the pelvic skeleton and pubic symphysis.

This section deals successively with the following aspects of the anterolateral abdominal wall: the superficial layers (skin and areolar subcutaneous tissue); the myofascial layers constituting a bracelike complex originating from the oblique and transverse muscles and ensheathing the recti abdomini; the transverse fascia; the deep areolar adipose tissue (fascia propria). After the description of the surgical anatomy, the points of weakness of the anterolateral abdominal wall, viz, the umbilicus and linea alba, inguinofemoral region, and semilunar line (Spigelius line) are delineated.

A. Cutaneous and Subcutaneous Layer

The structure and organization of this layer have considerable influence on the planning of abdominal wall incision. Furthermore, its vascularization is a determining factor in the mobilization of surgical flaps, the possibility of mass closure to allow cutaneous cover of the viscera, and the removal of free flaps used in microsurgical grafting. Finally, knowledge of the innervation of this layer is of importance from the semiological standpoint, since referred visceral pain often projects to the cutaneous layer of the abdominal wall.

The skin is relatively mobile over the myofascial layers of the anterolateral abdominal wall, although its median area is stabilized by the umbilicus which acts like a central "thumbtack".

The loosely organized subcutaneous tissue forms a pad, which may be very thick, containing within it the superficial fascia. Regarding spatial organization, the major feature of this layer is the *elastic traction lines*. These lines run transversely across the anterolateral abdominal area. Their direction is practically horizontal in the supraumbilical region, but below they slant downward to outline an arc of increasing superior concavity as they progress towards the pubic region. In some subjects these traction lines form transverse abdominal creases, which may be highly visible, according to the degree of adiposity, and may even

lead to the formation of deep folds with accompanying superficial pathological changes.

Two of these transverse folds are of special importance: First, the transverse suprapubic fold, running just below the upper limit of the pubic hair in women, is the landmark for Pfannenstiel's incision. The second important subumbilical fold begins slightly below the anterior-superior iliac spine and slants downward half-way between the umbilicus and the pubis. This fold is the site of a "horizontalized" McBurney's incision, which is prone to very little distortion, thus yielding an aesthetic incisional scar.

Cutaneous incisions made perpendicular to these lines of traction show a tendency to spread apart. Oblique incisions require careful identification of the extremities and middle of the wound if one is to avoid an unattractive result.

B. Vascularization of the Cutaneous Layers of the Abdomen

1. Arterial Vascularization

The cutaneous layers of the abdominal wall are rich in arterial vessels, and thus the skin is "rooted" to the layer beneath it. Numerous arterial pedicles emerge from the anterior surface of the rectus sheath in the area of the oblique and transverse muscles and then ramify extensively under the integument. Some of these pedicles perforate the aponeurosis of the external oblique in the midaxillary line, while others emerge from the anterior lamina of the sheath of the rectus abdominis. These vessels are arranged in staggered fashion resulting from the regional metamerization. There are usually four supraumbilical and three subumbilical pedicles on each side. The umbilicus is surrounded by four highly anastomosed perforating arteries (periumbilical arterial circle).

The perforating arteries, arising deep in the cutaneous layers, are supplied by the lateral vessels of the abdominal wall, i.e., the lower intercostal and the lumbar arteries. These lateral vessels show many anastomoses with the deep circumflex iliac network.

In addition to these pedicles of deep origin, there are specific cutaneous arterial pedicles running upward from the inguinal region. The superficial epigastric and superficial circumflex iliac arteries, arising from the femoral artery, form a veritable vascular clamp encompassing a major part of the anterolateral abdominal wall. These two superficial arteries are highly anastomosed to one another and to the deep arterial network. The territory supplied by them extends a few centimeters lateral to the midline and ends about halfway between the umbilicus and the xiphoid process.

Accordingly, it is convenient for the surgeon to mobilize cutaneous flaps supplied by an inferior arterial pedicle. Flap mobilization which is extensive or which goes beyond the midline may compromise the blood supply from the perforating arteries and can lead to necrosis of the upper part of the flap. Nevertheless, it is theoretically possible to completely free all of the subumbilical skin from the underlying myofascial layer without compromising its vitality.

2. Venous Drainage

The system of venous drainage runs parallel to the arterial system. This venous network is a possible route of caval-caval anastomosis between the femoral and intercostal veins. In the region of the umbilicus, the venous system of the abdominal wall may communicate above with a patent ligamentum teres hepatis (Cruveilhier-Baumgarten syndrome) and below with the pelvic veins running along the allantoic sheath. (For further details, consult the section on the umbilical region)

3. Lymphatic Drainage

The system of lymphatic drainage is extremely diffuse, fanning out from the umbilicus. This system communicates with the deep hepatic and pelvic lymphatic networks. The lymphatic ducts of the abdominal wall run downward to the inguinal region, join the deep lymphatic trunks of the lumbar region laterally, and connect above with the intercostal and internal mammary systems. These different lymph vessels form a channel on each side and along the mamillary line. Primary cancer of the breast or of a supernumerary nipple may seed neoplastic nodes along this line.

C. Myofascial Layer

The organization of the myofascial layer of the abdominal wall is well known. The triple myofascial layer lies on either side of the two central paramedian pillars formed by the rectus muscles of the abdomen. The fibers of the three large muscles which make up this layer run obliquely to one another. These muscles are the external oblique, whose fibers slant mainly downward, forward, and inward; the internal oblique, whose fibers run in a direction opposite to those of the external oblique: and the transverse, whose fibers run horizontally.

These muscles are in reality myoaponeurotic systems comprising a muscle body extended by a wide fibrous sheet. The transverse displays two systems of aponeuroses, one anterior and the other posterior. These different aponeuroses are arranged in a spatially different manner in the upper two-thirds and lower third of the abdominal wall, and together they form the sheath of the rectus muscle.

1. Rectus Abdominis

The long rectus muscles of the abdomen run vertically from the anteroinferior thoracic skeleton to the pubic region. Each rectus is attached above by three digitations to the anterior part of the fifth rib, the sixth rib and its cartilage, and the seventh costal cartilage and xiphoid process. The body of the rectus is very broad above (mean width 10-12 cm at the level of the costal ridge and 5-8 cm near the umbilicus), but tapers downward to terminate in a fibrous tendon measuring 2-3 cm in width at the level of the pubis. The muscle displays considerable lateral protrusion, which may be visible through the skin. Conversely, in obese or anesthetized patients, identification of the rectus may be difficult, thus accounting for the fact that what is intended to be McBurney's incision is, in fact, often a pararectus incision.

Structure

The polygastric arrangement of the rectus is a reminder of the primitive metameric segmentation of the abdominal musculature. The muscle usually displays three fibrous intersections which are the equivalent of abdominal ribs, i.e., superior, middle, and inferior intersections, of which the latter lies at the level of the umbilicus. A fourth (subumbilical) intersection can be found in about 30% of subjects. These intersection fibrous bands are not complete in either the anteroposterior or the transverse direction and thus rarely extend fully across the muscle from its medial to lateral border.

A small arterial pedicle is almost always found below each of these fibrous intersections. It should be noted that section of one of the pedicles may sometimes lead to heavy bleeding. The lower part of the rectus extends down to the pubis as a single, much narrower unit. This should be taken into account when designing a flap to be taken from the anterior abdominal wall to avoid the flap's lateral extension completely beyond the rectus in the subumbilical region. (For example, Welti's procedure, described by Detrie, 1982; the reader should also consult the section on incisional hernia, page 145)

2. Oblique and Transversus Muscles

a) External Oblique

The fleshy body of this muscle is attached above to the lateral part of the thorax, i.e., the lateral surface of the lowest seven or eight ribs, via processes which interdigitate with those of the anterior serratus. The fibers of the muscle fan out in a downward direction. The entire length of the posterior part of the external oblique is composed of only fleshy muscle fibers inserting on the anterior end of the iliac crest and the anterior superior iliac spine. Conversely, all other parts of this muscle blend into its aponeurosis which spreads out in front of the rectus. Along the line extending from the xiphoid process to the pubic symphysis, the fibers of the muscle on one side interdigitate with those from the external oblique on the other side to form a herringbone pattern. This pattern shows progressive accentuation in the lower part of the muscle. The lower part of the aponeurosis of the external oblique forms an identifiable margin, even though it continues backward and downward to join the transverse fascia and femoral sheath. This lower border of the aponeurosis of the external oblique is referred to as the inguinal ligament. According to classical descriptions, this ligament is composed of separate fibers (stretching from the anterior-superior iliac spine to the pubic tubercle) around which are wound fibers originating from the external oblique. Many studies now shed doubt on this classical composition of the inguinal ligament.

The fibers of the aponeurosis of the external oblique separate from each other inferiorly and medially to form the opening of the superficial inguinal ring. Arcuate fibers close off the superior angle of this slit-like opening in the aponeurosis of the external oblique.

Action. The external oblique lowers the ribs (expiratory muscle), bringing the thorax closer to the pelvis. In case of unilateral contraction, the hemithorax on the opposite side is depressed and rotated towards the side of muscle contraction.

b) Internal Oblique

Owing to the direction of its fibers, which run opposite to those of the external oblique, the internal oblique has been likened to unsegmented internal intercostal muscles. Indeed, the muscle is inserted on the pelvic skeleton and stretches upward, forward, and medially to the thoracic border and linea alba. The aponeurotic fibers of the internal oblique are classically considered to be the major constituent of the sheath of the rectus.

The internal oblique inserts below on the following structures: the anterior two-thirds of the intermediate line of the iliac crest; the aponeurosis of the lumbosacral muscles; anteriorly, the anterior-superior iliac spine and classically along the lateral third of the inguinal ligament. The fleshy fibers of the muscle fan out in an upward direction. The posterior fascicles, composed only of fleshy muscle fibers over their entire length, insert on the cartilage of the lowest three ribs. The main part of the body of the muscle continues into its aponeurosis, which inserts on the linea alba. This aponeurosis, which blends into its homologs from the other flat abdominal muscles (i.e., the external oblique and the transverse) in the region of the linea alba, splits into two laminae (upper two-thirds of the aponeurosis) which pass around the anterior and posterior surfaces of the rectus. This classical conception of the rectus sheath has been contested by certain American authors, according to whom the posterior lamina of the sheath is derived essentially from the aponeurosis of the transverse.

At the level of the lower third of the rectus, the anterior passage of the aponeurotic system causes a rupture in the posterior wall of the fibrous rectus sheath referred to as the semicircular line of Douglas (arcuate line).

The innermost fibers of the internal oblique, originating from the anterior-superior iliac spine and lateral third of the inguinal ligament, run medially and slightly downward to fan out over the anterior surface of the rectus. These muscle fibers form the anterior part of the conjoint tendon (falx inguinalis or tendo conjunctivus). Two remarks should be made regarding this structure. First, the above-described fibers do not reinsert on the medial third of the inguinal ligament, thereby ensheathing the spermatic cord in a sort of hemisphincter, as is often described. Second, these fibers do not actually originate from the lateral third of the inguinal ligament, but rather are connected to the ligament via a relatively dense fibrous tissue. The fleshy fibers can be followed from the anterior-superior iliac spine along their initial course, parallel to what is to become the inguinal ligament.

The lower part of the internal oblique gives off fibers to the cremaster muscle which attaches to the fibrous part of the spermatic cord. In addition to this external part of the cremaster, medial fibers originating from the pubic tubercle can be seen to form the internal part of this muscle. All of the cremasteric fibers must be sectioned in order to gain proper access to the layer of the deep ring of the inguinal canal. In rare cases, the internal oblique appears to be traversed by the spermatic cord, but this arrangement is simply an exaggeration of the normal anatomy described above.

Action. The action of this muscle is comparable to that of the external oblique, although its unilateral contraction leads to rotation and lowering of the thorax on the side of the contraction.

c) Transversus Abdominis Muscle

Owing to the horizontal direction of its fibers, this muscle can be described from its posterior insertions to the linea alba in the midline. The transversus, from its cranial to caudal parts, is inserted posteriorly on the lower ribs, lumbar spine, and pelvic skeleton. The thoracic insertions of this muscle are on the medial surface of the cartilage of the lowest seven or eight ribs. The fascicles of the transverse interdigitate with the insertions of the diaphragm. Moreover, the transversus is the veritable antagonist of the diaphragm and the main expiratory muscle. The fleshy fibers of this muscle seem to emerge from within the thorax and to escape from the "hoodlike" xiphoid process.

In the lumbar region, the muscle is inserted on the tips of the costal processes of the lumbar vertebrae and, via its aponeurotic sheet, i.e., the posterior aponeurosis of the transversus, on the thoracolumbar fascia. The latter blends anteriorly into the parallel horizontal fibers of the muscle, which itself blends into the anterior aponeurosis of the transverse.

In the pelvic region, the transverse inserts on the anterior half of the medial edge (labium internum) of the iliac crest, the anterior superior iliac spine, and classically, the lateral third of the inguinal ligament (this insertion is similar to that of the internal oblique). In reality, these fibers of the transverse are attached to the iliac fascia behind the inguinal ligament and then run forward and inward and come to lie almost parallel to the deep surface of the internal oblique. These fibers constitute the herringbonelike muscle, erroneously termed the "conjoint tendon", and contribute to the formation of the cremaster.

The fleshy body of the transverse, except for its lowermost part, blends into the anterior aponeurosis of the muscle. The boundary between its muscular and fibrous parts is rather sinuous. Thus, the superior part of the muscle approaches the midline, while below, the muscle recedes posteriorly and laterally. In this way the upper fleshy part of the muscle lies beneath the rectus, whereas below it is clearly lateral to the rectus,

e.g., at the level of McBurney's incision. It is well known that subsequent to dissection of the internal oblique, the surgeon must look for the muscular part of the transverse in the area of the iliac spine in order to divide this muscle. Care should be taken not to overlook this muscle in the course of closure.

The aponeurosis of the transversus is the main constituent of the posterior lamina of the rectus sheath. Like all of this aponeurotic system, the lower third of the aponeurosis of the transverse lies in the anterior position and thus contributes to emphasizing the arcuate line.

Action. The basic function of the transversus is to ensure retention of the abdominal viscera. This muscle is very important in respiration, since it displaces or blocks the visceral mass under the diaphragm at the end of the initial stage of diaphragmatic inspiration. Disturbed mobility of the transversus is the main cause of respiratory insufficiency following laparotomy. Indeed, its powerful traction on the linea alba leads to considerable forces which tend to separate the margins of the laparotomy incision. This accounts for the greater incidence of respiratory disturbances and the higher frequency of wound dehiscence subsequent to vertical midline incision of the abdominal wall. Furthermore, the rapid retraction of the transversus explains the persistence of the dehiscence and the difficulties encountered in its treatment, even in the absence of loss of abdominal wall tissue. In such cases, the transverse muscles act mainly on the medial margin of the rectus muscles, thus transforming the latter into two separate fleshy columns displaying a spherical cross section. Anatomical reconstruction of the abdominal wall can only be achieved in these conditions by artificial means, e.g., Welti's procedure.

(1) Transversalis Fascia

This fibrous layer, whose surface is dull like frosted glass, lines the deep surface of the transverse and can be easily separated from the muscle over most of its surface. The transversalis fascia constitutes the anterolateral part of the fibrous layer which envelops the peritoneal serosa, similar to the envelopment of the pleural serosa by the endothoracic fascia. The transversalis fascia can no longer be individualized as a separate structure posteriorly, where it is in contact with the iliac fascia, and superiorly, where it lies under the diaphragm. Its mechanical resistance is very weak in the supraumbilical part of the anterolateral abdominal wall. However, below the umbilicus it takes on a certain structural consistency, which is reinforced in the inguinal region. At this level, the transversalis fascia displays the properties of a true aponeurosis, as pointed out long ago by Testut (1896), and tightly adheres to the posterior surface of the transverse, even seeming to extend the muscle downward. This fascia closes off the myopectineal orifice and inserts on the lower margin of the inguinal ligament, and laterally on the iliac fascia. Below the layer of the inguinal ligament it blends into the femoral sheath.

The importance of the transversalis fascia from the surgical standpoint has been largely debated. Although more or less ignored until recently by French surgeons, for many American surgeons it is the specific structure which must be sewn tight to ensure correction of direct inguinal hernia [McVay & Anson 1940].

(2) Fascia Propria

This areolar adipose layer of variable thickness, according to the individual, is often referred to as the subperitoneal fat, an inappropriate term when describing the anterior part of this fascia. It separates the transverse fascia from the peritoneum, except at the level of the umbilicus, where it is practically absent. The posterior part of the fascia propria is naturally thick where it fills in the angles of the posterior abdominal wall and surrounds the vascular and ureteral sheaths. The fascia propria also extends laterally where it is sometimes traversed by fibrous tracts which may limit or hinder surgical dissection of the peritoneum. It penetrates forward and downward between the bladder and the pubis into what is called Retzius's space (retropubic space) and laterally (in contact with the iliac fascia) invests Bogros's space (retroinguinal space). The fascia propria is a loosely organized and largely intercommunicating layer. Its structure thus accounts for the often widespread diffusion of subperitoneal cellulitis.

The fascia propria may also communicate with neighboring anatomical structures and spaces: above, the pleuroperitoneal hiatus of the diaphragm, bringing the fascia propria in contact with the subpleural tissue; the superficial layers of the lumbar region via posterior weak points (edema and posterior crepitation in cases of retroperitoneal cellulitis); toward the root of the lower limb via the infrapubic canal and greater sciatic notch (tumefaction of the root of the thigh, which is commonly mistaken for phlebitis in cases of deep pelvic cellulitis); downward and forward via the inguinal canal, leading to exteriorization of deep retroperitoneal hematoma, effusion, or emphysema.

3. Rectus Sheath
(Vagina Recti Abdominis)

This sheath truly exists only in the region of the upper two-thirds of the rectus muscles. This "borrowed" envelope tightly adheres to the muscles at the level of the fibrous intersections.

The anterior lamina of the rectus sheath (Fig. 1.1) is formed by the bracelike fibers of the oblique muscles, forming an overlapping herringbone pattern facing upward or downward at an angle of 90°-110°. This herringbone arrangement of the fibrous components of the sheath flattens out in the umbilical region, which probably accounts for the relative weakness of transverse sutures in this zone.

The posterior lamina of the sheath is derived mainly from the aponeurosis of the transverse. Neurovascular pedicles penetrate the rectus sheath through steplike openings in the posterior lamina. These narrow "buttonholes" in the posterior lamina may impinge on the nerves passing through them, thus leading to spontaneous pain syndromes via a phenomenon of entrapment. It should also be noted that transverse suture material often ruptures along this deep layer.

a) Arcuate Line
(Semicircular Line of Douglas)

The arcuate line lies roughly along the line joining the right and left anterior-superior iliac spines. It is sometimes a clearly defined, almost sharp structure. In other cases, it is marked by a progressive zone of transition where the resistant posterior lamina of the rectus sheath blends into the much weaker transverse fascia. This zone of transition is a weak area. However, since it is lined posteriorly by the umbilicoprevesical aponeurosis, which narrows upward, the zone of weakness lies at the most lateral part of the arcuate line. It is in this region that rare herniation, so-called Spigelian hernia (A. van der Spiegel) occurs.

b) Adhesion of the Rectus Abdominis
to the Laminae of its Sheath

The rectus can be mobilized within its sheath, except at the level of the fibrous intersections which adhere to the anterior lamina. Reconstructive procedures via freeing and turning down of the medial border of the rectus sheath (Welti's procedure) give more satisfactory results when performed at the level of the fibrous intersections than in the subumbilical region [Stoppa 1974]. Indeed, aponeurotic suturing at the subumbilical level must be done along a narrower band, owing to the subumbilical tapering of the rectus, which does

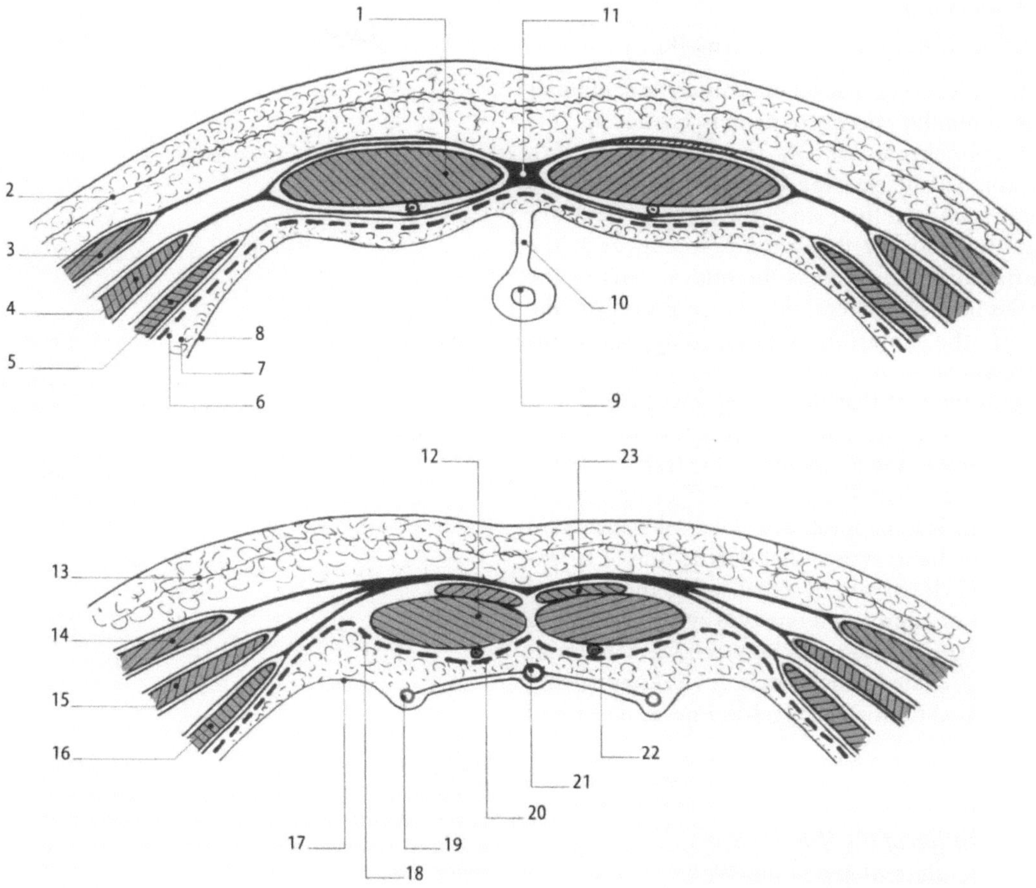

Fig. 1.1. Transverse section through the anterior abdominal wall: **a** made above the umbilicus; **b** made below the linea arcuata. *1* M. rectus abdominis; *2* fascia superficialis; *3* m. obliquus externus abdominis; *4* m. obliquus internus abdominis; *5* m. transversus abdominis; *6* fascia transversalis; *7* fascia propria; *8* peritoneum; *9* lig. teres hepatis; *10* lig. falciforme hepatis; *11* linea alba; *12* m. rectus abdominis; *13* fascia superficialis; *14* m. obliquus externus abdominis; *15* m. obliquus internus abdominis; *16* m. transversus abdominis; *17* peritoneum; *18* fascia transversalis; *19* chorda arteriae umbilicalis; *20* prevesical fascia; *21* chorda urachi; *22* arteria epigastrica inferior; *23* m. pyramidalis abdominis

not allow the muscle to be pulled as close to the midline as in the supraumbilical region. The adhesion of the rectus to the lateral margin of the sheath is very weak. Thus, the muscle can be freed easily and displaced medially. It should be noted that pararectus incisions may cause damage to the innervation of the rectus.

4. Linea Alba (see page 22)

The linea alba is a solid median raphe running vertically down the entire upper part of the abdominal wall. Midline incision at this level can and should allow the surgeon to dissect between the rectus muscles without opening their sheath. Below the umbilicus, and especially the arcuate line, the fibrous separation of the rectus muscles is less obvious. Indeed, the medial borders of the two rectus muscles are often in contact with each other and may even overlap slightly. Identification of the interstitium between the two muscles is further complicated inferiorly by the presence of the small pyramidal muscles (in 90% of subjects), extending from the pubis to the center of the subumbilical midline. Thus, the surgeon should always look for the interstitium at a more superior site where the rectus muscles separate around the umbilicus. Careful manipulation of retractors is necessary in order not to lose identification of the muscular fascicles. The umbilicus interrupts the linea alba at roughly its center, as is described further on.

5. Semilunar Line
   (Spigelius Line)

A. van der Spiegel (1578-1625) described the semilunar line as the boundary between the muscle body and the anterior aponeurosis of the transverse (Fig. 1.2). Indeed, in most subjects, the semilunar line describes a medially concave line, since the upper and lower parts of the body of the transverse approach the abdominal midline, whereas the middle part of the muscle lies in a more lateral position, especially in the region of the anterior-superior iliac spine, as described above.

Owing to the fact that the myoaponeurotic boundary between the internal and external oblique does not correspond to the boundary of the transverse, the use of the term "lateral linea alba" to designate the semilunar line is not appropriate. This zone resembles a laterorectus band rather than a true line. It is traversed by pedicles arranged stepwise and thus offers a limited route of approach if one is to avoid destructive maneuvers. The intersection between the semilunar line and the arcuate line is a point of weakness giving rise to so-called hernia of Spigelius line, as described further on.

D. *Vascularization of the Muscle Layers of the Anterolateral Abdominal Wall*

1. Arterial Vascularization

The general pattern of the arterial vascularization of the anterolateral abdominal wall is well known. The vertical arterial axis lying along the posterior surface of the rectus comprises the inferior and superior epigastric arteries (the latter a branch of the internal thoracic artery). This vertical axis is reinforced by the more or less metameric arrangement of the lateral pedicles originating from the intercostal and lumbar arteries. The inferior epigastric artery is the predominant, but not exclusive, source of vascular supply to the abdominal wall. Ligation of this artery can thus be done without any real danger (Fig. 1.1).

The inferior epigastric artery arises from the external iliac artery just behind the inguinal ligament. It runs upward and medially to pierce the transverse fascia and comes to lie anterior to the fascia. It is accompanied by a thickening of this fascia, classically referred to as Hesselbach's ligament (interfoveolar ligament). The artery then runs a variable course toward the lateral border of the rectus, which it crosses at a point 4-8 cm above the pubis. The inferior epigastric

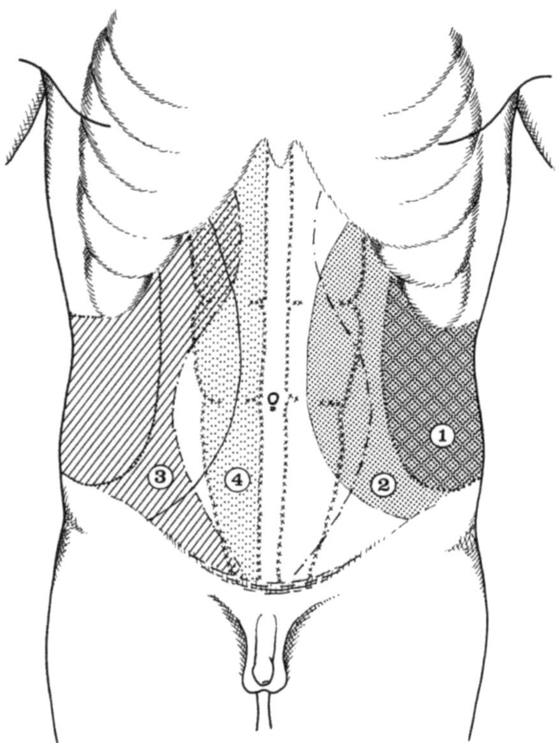

Fig. 1.2. Linea semilunaris. The myofascial boundary of the flat abdominal muscles (modified from Poirier & Charpy 1912). *1* M. obliquus externus abdominis; *2* m. obliquus internus abdominis; *3* m. transversus abdominis; *4* lateral margin of m. rectus abdominis

artery may be injured in the course of puncture of the iliac fossa, with low-lying appendicular or adnexal incisions, or during placement of supportive transparietal sutures. Such arterial injury may be dramatic, owing to the large diameter (equivalent to that of the radial artery) and high pressure of the inferior epigastric artery.

Posterior to the rectus, the artery divides into a descending branch, running toward the pubis, and an ascending branch, the larger of the two. The latter may persist as a single, dominant axis, which is split into numerous parallel ascending branches, or divide into two main branches running about 1 cm from the lateral and medial margins of the rectus.

Direct anastomosis between the inferior and superior epigastric arteries is relatively rare. The superior epigastric is an abdominal branch of the internal thoracic artery, descending via Larey's cleft (the sternocostal triangle), as described by Goinard and Curtillet (1929). A penicillate type of anastomosis [Salmon & Dor 1933] is the most frequent. Regardless of the anastomotic pattern, communication between the two arteries is well developed, since the opacification of one of them immediately leads to massive reflux of contrast material into the other.

The lateral arterial system is a reminder of the initial metameric arrangement of the arteries. These transverse arteries are supplied by the diaphragmatic branch of the internal thoracic artery, this branch being anastomosed to the termination of the lower intercostal arteries. Lower down, the lateral arterial supply is from the parietal branches of the lumbar arteries. The latter show many communications with the deep circumflex iliac artery, a branch of the external iliac artery. There are significant vertical anastomoses joining these metameric arteries to form a ladderlike system. Indeed, the opacification of the deep circumflex iliac artery leads to reflux attaining the thoracic level, even after the epigastric arteries have been ligated.

Accordingly, in the flanks there is a *parietal arterial plexus*, supplying the perforating branches, which, along with nerve filaments, enter the rectus sheath and anastomose to the vertical arterial axis.

The superficial perforating arteries, which were previously described in the section devoted to cutaneous vascularization, arise from the horizontal arterial system, their arrangement corresponding topographically to that of the latter. Nevertheless, these perforating arteries are also supplied by the vertical epigastric arterial axis. Accordingly, wide incisions for relaxation, including cutaneous detachment, should theoretically not compromise the cutaneous vascularization, providing that the epigastric arteries are left intact. As previously pointed out, the subcutaneous abdominal (superficial epigastric) and superficial circumflex iliac arteries form a veritable inferior cutaneous arterial pedicle.

At the level of the flat abdominal muscles, the arterial branches are found mainly in two layers, one on each side of the internal oblique. The richness of this vascular system implies that there is a risk of hemorrhage with all abdominal incisions other than those made along the midline. This is particularly true in the case of small "blind" flank incisions made in the area of the arterial plexus. Pronounced intra-abdominal bleeding may occur. In such cases the source of hemorrhage should be sought in depth, i.e., deep to the external oblique on both sides of the internal oblique. Application of superficial pressure is an inadequate therapeutic procedure, constituting a sort of plug which may actually promote the intra-abdominal bleeding.

Bilateral subcostal incision consistently leads to spurts of bleeding. The association of a midline and a pararectus incision and different extensions of a midline incision do not as a rule lead to disturbed parietal vitality. Nevertheless, in patients who have undergone multiple operations on the abdominal wall, numerous parietal islets isolated by lines of scar tissue (even old scars) may arise; neovascularization of such islets is often difficult to obtain. Likewise, the use of large, supportive, full-thickness (retention) sutures, often excessively tightened, can induce ischemic necrosis of the abdominal wall by causing interruption or excessive stricture of the longitudinal arterial axes. This situation is even further complicated when extensive counterincisions compromise any further lateral approaches. In sum, wound dehiscence is encouraged rather than prevented! Thus, so-called security procedures are valid only when the sutures are tightened moderately, and only when there is tension of the abdominal wall.

2. Venous Drainage

The system of venous drainage is patterned after that of the arterial vascularization. The inferior epigastric veins, two per artery of the same name, join together to form a short common terminal trunk drained by the external iliac vein.

The inferior epigastric veins run along the medial border of the artery for about 1 cm and then leave it to join the external iliac vein. The single terminal trunk of these veins, which can be used for chronic delivery of parenteral nutrition, almost always measures 3 cm in length. This venous trunk can be reached by the classical inguinal approach via the axilla of the spermatic cord, or by a vertical pararectus route exposing the origin of the venous trunk. The latter route allows catheterization of the vein at a safe distance from structures which might be injured.

3. Lymphatic Drainage

The upper part of the muscular abdominal wall is drained by the internal thoracic lymph nodes, while in the lower part drainage is via the external iliac nodes. Finally, lateral lymphatic drainage is via the lumbar nodes.

E. Innervation of the Anterolateral Abdominal Wall

The lower intercostal nerves and the nerves of the lumbar plexus supply the anterolateral abdominal wall.

1. Superficial Layers

The *dermatomes*, originating from the fifth through the 12th thoracic nerves, run like belts over the antero-lateral abdominal wall.

The dermatome corresponding to the tenth thoracic nerve runs at the level of the umbilicus (Fig. 1.3).

The two abdominogenital nerves (iliohypogastric and ilioinguinal nerves) supply sensory innervation to an oblique band of the abdominal wall comprising the lower part of the iliac fossa, the inguinal region, and part of the external genital organs (Fig. 1.4).

The genitofemoral nerve arises from the first and second lumbar nerves and contributes to the sensory innervation of the root of the external genital organs. It is also the motor nerve of the cremaster (Fig. 1.4).

The lateral cutaneous nerve of the thigh, originating from the second lumbar nerve, is not involved in the superficial innervation of the abdominal wall.

Owing to its course medial to the anterior-superior iliac spine, this nerve may be injured by certain incisions of the abdominal wall or when inserting drains in this region (Fig. 1.4) [Salama et al. 1982].

Superficial Projection of Visceral Sensitivity

According to the myelomere involved, pain from certain visceral structures may be referred to the anterior abdominal wall.

Table 1.1. indicates the myelomeres of the main abdominal viscera and their territories of possible abdominal wall projection.

Table 1.1. Referred pain from visceral myelomeres (posterior part of the intermediolateral region)

Myelomere		Peripheral projection
Heart	C8-T8	Left upper limb
Stomach	T6-T9	Epigastric region
Small bowel	T7-T10	Umbilicus
Kidney	T11-L1	Lumbar and inguino-hypogastric regions
Pelvic organs	T10-T12	Hypogastric region
Rectum	S2-S4	Perineum, external genital organs

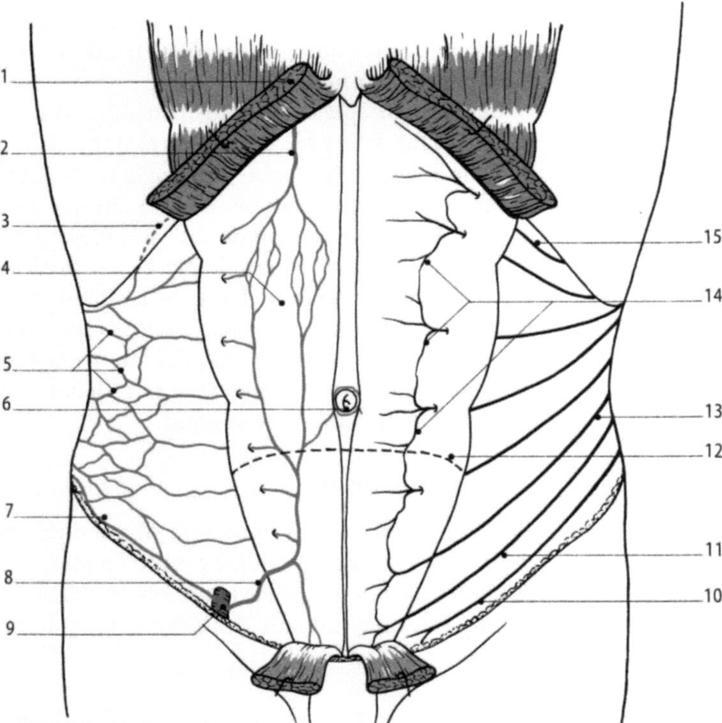

Fig. 1.3. Vascularization and inervation of the superficial layers of the anterior lateral abdominal wall. *1* M. rectus abdominis; *2* a. epigastrica superior; *3* a. musculophrenica; *4* posterior layer of the rectus sheath; *5* arterial plexus; *6* periumbilical vascular circle; *7* a. circumflexa ilium profonda; *8* a. epigastrica inferior; *9* a. iliaca externa; *10* n. ilioinguinalis; *11* n. iliohypogastricus; *12* projection of linea arcuata; *13* 12th intercostal n.; *14* nervous plexus of the rectus sheath; *15* 7th intercostal n.

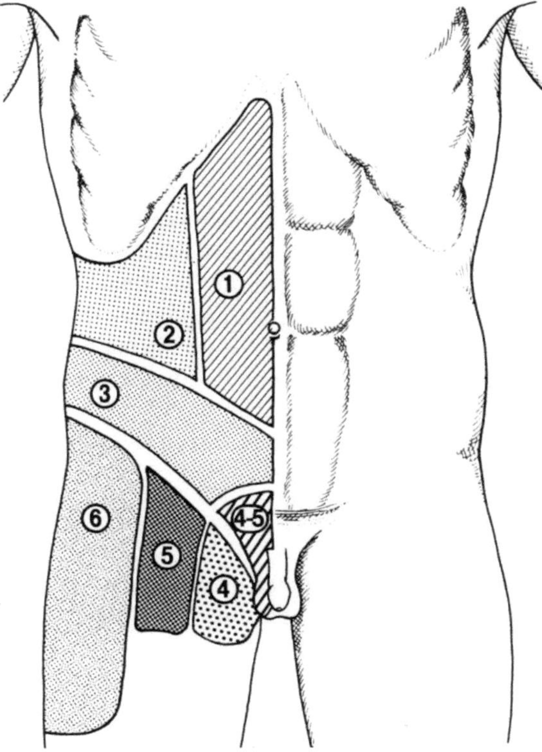

Fig. 1.4. Sensory territory of the anterior abdominal wall 1, 2: intercostal nerves. *1* Rami cutanei anteriores; *2* rami cutanei laterales; *3* n. iliohypogastricus; *4* n. ilioinguinalis; *5* n. genitofemoralis; *6* n. cutaneus femoris lateralis

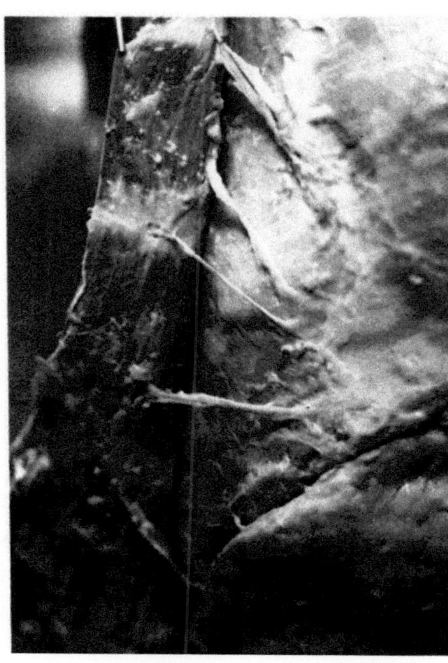

Fig. 1.5. Penetration of the m. rectus abdominis by the intercostal nerves (courtesy of Professor M. Caix, Limoges)

2. Deep Layers: Motor Innervation of the Parietal Muscles

The seventh through 12th intercostal nerves, along with the iliohypogastric and ilioinguinal nerves, supply the motor innervation of the anterolateral abdominal wall. The classical pattern of this motor innervation has been described by Hovelaque (1927). The seventh, eighth, and ninth intercostal nerves distribute to the supraumbilical part of the rectus. The tenth intercostal nerve runs toward the umbilicus along an imaginary line extending across the midline to the anterior-superior iliac spine on the opposite side. The 11th intercostal nerve passes below the umbilicus in the direction of the contralateral inguinal ligament. Finally, the 12th intercostal nerve runs in a very inferior position in the direction of the pubic tubercle on the opposite side (Fig. 1.5).

The motor branch of the iliohypogastric nerve reaches the inferior part of the rectus and the pyramidal, while that of the ilioinguinal nerve terminates in the flat abdominal muscles. The nerve trunks run first between the internal oblique and the transverse and then reach the rectus at a point slightly medial to its lateral margin (Fig. 1.5).

The seventh to 11th intercostal nerves display a recurrent course running upward along the deep surface of the common costal cartilage. These nerves divide into two branches beneath the rectus. One branch runs along the cartilaginous costal margin and terminates in the wall of the thorax. This branch innervates the internal intercostal. The other, inferior abdominal branch, traverses the cartilaginous costal margin and penetrates the posterior surface of the rectus. In the muscle this branch divides into a brush-like network of ascending and descending filaments overconnected to the homologous filaments of the different nerves supplying this muscle (Fig. 1.3).

These intercostal nerves are in a relatively protected position under the chondrocostal margin. A subcostal incision running two finger breadths below this ridge spares most of these nerves and their branches, thus accounting for the low incidence of paralysis of the rectus in this type of incision, whereas minor sensory disturbances are consistently reported below the inferior lip of the incisional scar. Conversely, the tenth intercostal nerve is almost always sacrificed in all subcostal incisions extending slightly downward and laterally.

The 11th and 12th intercostal nerves (the latter is more correctly referred to as the subcostal nerve) are often large trunks distributing especially to the flat abdominal muscles. They frequently run in a very inferior position, especially in elderly subjects whose lower ribs are in proximity to the iliac crest. Injury to these nerves usually arises in the course of longitudinal or oblique flank incisions, rather than in cases of subcostal incision. The iliohypogastric nerve contributes to the innervation of the lower part of the flat abdominal muscles, the rectus, and the pyramidal, whereas the ilioinguinal nerve does not usually apply the rectus. Finally, as described above, the genitofemoral nerve shows only a modest contribution to the abdominal wall innervation by its motor supply to the cremaster.

3. Neural Anastomoses
and Metamerization

The different neural metameres of the abdominal wall are largely anastomosed to one another in most cases (70% of subjects, according to Rousseau et al. 1982). Furthermore, within the rectus muscles, the myelomeres are not strictly separate, anastomoses being the general rule. Theoretically, the motor nerves originating from three successive spinal levels would have to be sectioned to produce paralytic incisional hernia of the corresponding rectus.

II. Weak Points
of the Anterolateral Abdominal Wall

Three weak points in the anterolateral abdominal wall are the umbilicus, the inguinal region, and the semilunar line.

A. Umbilicus

The umbilicus is a cicatricial structure lying slightly below the middle of the linea alba. According to classical descriptions [Testut 1896], it is located at the junction of the inferior 44/100 and superior 56/100 of the linea alba. This position corresponds to the junction of the wide upper and narrow lower parts of the linea alba, i.e., at the level of the third (usually the lowermost) fibrous intersection of the rectus muscles.

1. Outer Aspect

The umbilicus is a depression measuring 10-18 mm in diameter and slanting downward and backward to a depth which varies according to adiposity. It is limited superficially by a small fold, the deep part of which is more or less outlined by a groove corresponding to the zone of skin adhesion to the circumference of the fibrous umbilical ring. This zone of fixation is less pronounced in the upper part of the ring where the subcutaneous and preperitoneal adipoareolar tissues are in continuity. The fundus of the umbilicus resembles an irregular nipple, corresponding to the apex of the stellate umbilical cicatrix. The umbilicus may protrude anteriorly, or even be convex in cases of ascites or hernia.

2. Structure

The umbilicus is constituted by three structures: the umbilical ring, residual fibrous cords (ligamentum teres hepatis), and umbilical fascia.

a) Umbilical Ring

The umbilical ring is an orifice of the linea alba of variable shape and size. In most cases it resembles a transverse ovoid, but sometimes it is rectangular or circular. Its diameter varies from 2 to 8 mm. The umbilical ring displays thickened margins reinforced by arcuate fibers purported to be remnants of the so-called umbilical sphincter (Richet's sphincter). With advancing age the ring normally tends to close, giving way to a fibrous cicatrix in many elderly subjects (Fig. 1.6).

The area of the umbilical ring is partially occluded by four fibrous cords: the round ligament of the liver inserted into the superior pole of the annulus; the two umbilical arteries which converge upward and are occluded over their entire parietal course; and the urachus which bisects the angle formed by the umbilical arteries.

b) Round Ligament of the Liver

The round ligament of the liver usually divides into two cords inserting on either side of the superior pole of the umbilical ring, thus creating the so-called intervascular fossette. This ligament runs upward, backward, and to the right within the peritoneal cavity where it is invested by the peritoneum, i.e., the falciform ligament of the liver. The portion of the round ligament lying just above the umbilicus is most often very slender, about 3 mm in diameter. In this region it

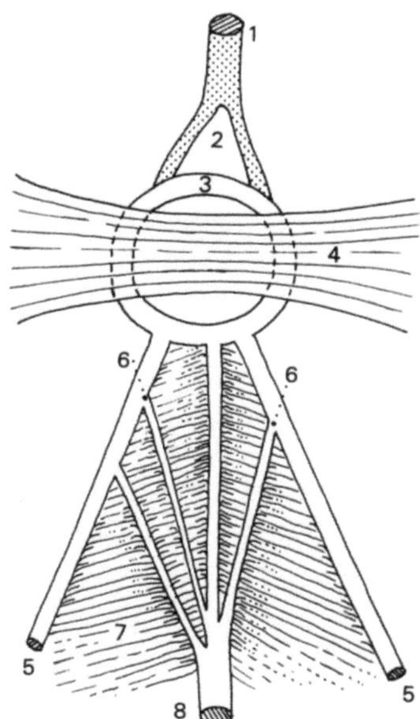

Fig. 1.6. Posterior view of the umbilical region. *1* Lig. teres hepatis; *2* intervascular fossa; *3* annulus umbilicalis; *4* fascia umbilicalis; *5* chorda art. umbilicalis; *6* subumbilical fibrous network; *7* umbilicoprevesical fascia; *8* chorda urachi

is surrounded by rather loose adipose tissue and thus can be easily approached by the extraperitoneal approach through a small vertical supraumbilical incision on the right side. Higher up the ligament is much thicker, but the extraperitoneal approach to it is difficult.

The round ligament of the liver is a vascular structure, and its lumen may become revascularized. [Chevrel et al. 1982]. Along its course are veins, arteries, and lymphatic ducts, anastomosing their respective-superficial and deep networks.

c) Umbilical Arteries

These two cordlike structures run up to and encroach upon the inferior part of the umbilical ring, which is narrowed in this region. The absence of one of the umbilical arteries may indicate the existence of a renal or genital malformation, usually on the same side as the missing artery.

The umbilical arteries add support to the prevesical fascia (umbilicoprevesical aponeurosis), a triangular fibrous sheet which runs downward to blend into the vesicopubic ligaments in the retropubic region and upward in contact with the umbilicus. The peritoneum adheres tightly to this fascia. The umbilical arteries also partially reinforce the abdominal wall at the site

where the posterior part of the rectus sheath is weakest.

d) Urachus

The urachus is a highly variable structure. It can be identified as a well-differentiated cord extending up to the inferior pole of the umbilical ring in only one-third of subjects. The urachus usually terminates a few centimeters below the umbilicus, where it gives rise to an insignificant filament or divides into several strands. The latter blend into the fibrous structures originating from the umbilical arteries, thereby forming a filamentous network of the umbilicus at the upper part of the umbilicovesical fascia. The umbilical arteries and urachus may sometimes fuse together to form a single fibrous cord attached to the inferior pole of the umbilical ring.

Full patency of the urachus, leading to urinary fistula, is a rare finding. Permeability of the lower part of the urachus is a potential cause of apical diverticula of the bladder. Patency of its upper portion leads to a pathological condition similar to pilonidal sinus. Finally, patency of its middle segment can lead to the development of small cysts of the urachus [Morin et al. 1968].

Histologically, the urachus is a canal composed of a fibrous adventitia, smooth muscle fibers running mainly lengthwise, and an epithelial lining, which may persist at some sites along the urachus in the adult. This epithelium takes on one of several aspects, i.e., poorly differentiated pavement (simple squamous), urothelial, or cylindrical (columnar) epithelium sometimes containing muciparous cells. Carcinoma is the most frequent type of malignant tumor of the urachus, although muciparous tumors may also be found.

e) Umbilical Fascia

This fibrous band, a condensation of the transverse fascia, was first described by Sachs in 1828. Present in about two-thirds of subjects, the umbilical fascia occludes the upper half of the umbilical ring at a site where this "fibrous trident" is lacking (Fig. 1.7).

In some cases the umbilical fascia is pulled away from the muscle wall by the posterior traction of the round ligament of the liver. This condition can lead to formation of Richet's "umbilical canal", which runs downward and forward and may be the site of indirect hernia.

The umbilical fascia may cover the entire umbilical ring. However, in most cases it is a differentiated structure only below the ring. In these conditions the peri-

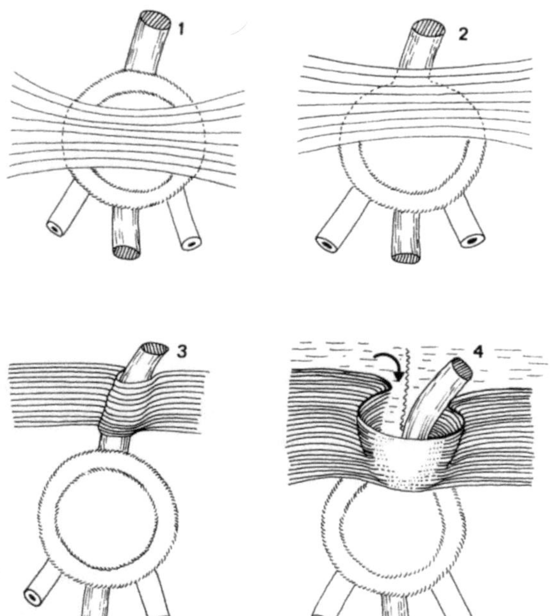

Fig. 1.7. Relations of the fascia umbilicalis and anulus umbilicalis (from Sachs & Richet; in Poirier & Charpy 1912). *1* Classical pattern; *2* most frequent pattern; *3* fascia umbilicalis and annulus umbilicalis independent; *4* formation of Richet's umbilical canal (*arrow* indicates course of potential superior hernia)

toneum is practically in contact with the skin of the umbilicus, thus predisposing to direct umbilical hernia.

f) Umbilical Peritoneum

The umbilical peritoneum, tightly adherent to the umbilical ring, overlies the convergent fibrous structures in this region. The peritoneum adheres loosely to the ring only in its superior part. The umbilical peritoneum extends several centimeters laterally and downward, this accounting for the fact that it is poorly adapted to layer-by-layer reconstruction of the abdominal wall in the periumbilical region. If cases of very tight peritoneal adhesion to the urachus and umbilicoprevesical fascia, cysts of the urachus may be complicated by peritonitis. Extraperitoneal excision of the cysts cannot always be achieved in such cases.

3. Vascularization and Innervation of the Umbilical Region

a) Arteries

The vessels of the umbilical region form a twin periumbilical arterial circle. The more superficial of these arterial networks, lying near the umbilical cicatrix, is formed by richly anastomotic arterial branches emanating from the anterior lamina of the rectus sheath.

The deep arterial circle, lying along the fibrous ring of the umbilicus, is supplied by two ascending branches of the inferior epigastric artery. This arterial circle communicates with the vascular network running along the round ligament of the liver and thus extends in depth.

Since it is vascularized from all sides by the superficial arterial circle and in depth by the deep arterial circle, the umbilicus is not prone to necrosis when it is either detached from the underlying layers or isolated by a circular incision leaving its connections to the fibrous ring intact.

b) Veins

The venous drainage shows a pattern similar to that of the arterial vascularization. The superficial periumbilical venous circle drains into the subcutaneous

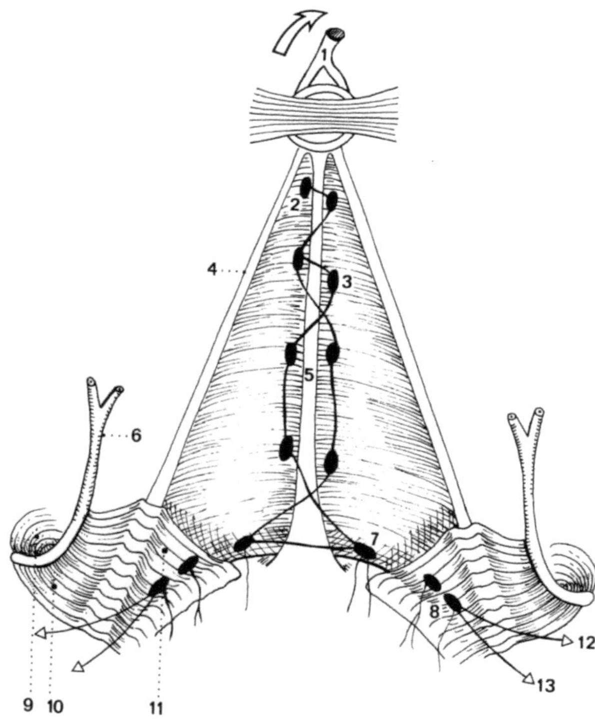

Fig. 1.8. Lymphatic drainage of the anterior abdominal wall (adapted from Heise 1954). *1* Lig. teres hepatis: communication with the lymphatic network of liver; *2* nodi umbilicalis; *3* periurachus lymphatic network; *4* chorda art. umbilicalis; *5* chorda urachi; *6* a. epig. inferior; *7* nodi praevesicales; *8* nodi paravesicales; *9* fovea inguinalis lateralis; *10* fovea inguinalis medialis; *11* fovea supravesicalis; *12* communication with external inguinal nodes; *13* communication with internal and common iliac nodes

abdominal network. The deep venous circle, similar to its arterial homologue, communicates with the veins of the round ligament of the liver.

c) Lymph Vessels

Once again, superficial and deep periumbilical networks can be identified. The superficial lymphatic network, running along the subcutaneous abdominal veins, drains into the upper two groups of inguinal nodes (Fig. 1.8). The organization of the deep lymphatic network accounts for the diffusion of malignant tumors of the sheath of the urachus. This deep network runs downward along the inferior epigastric vessels to the external iliac nodes, along the urachus to the pelvic nodes, and laterally along the transverse parietal vascular pedicles toward the lumbar region, lateral aortic ligaments, thoracic wall, and axilla. The deep lymphatic network is also drained toward the liver via the nodes of the round ligament of the liver.

In some cases a small lymph node can be found near the umbilicus. Invasion of the umbilicus should be sought in all cases of peritoneal carcinomatosis.

d) Nerves

The umbilicus constitutes the terminal territory of distribution of the 11th and 12th intercostal nerves. This region may be the site of referred pain originating from the myelomeres corresponding to certain visceral structures, i.e., pancreas, small bowel and bladder.

B. Inguinal Region

The inguinal region is a common site of hernia for three basic reasons. First, this area is a weak point framed by fibromuscular structures but occluded by a simple fibrous sheet, the transverse fascia, forming the myopectineal orifice. Second, the presence of the spermatic cord maintains an open sinuous channel, referred to as the inguinal canal, which is, however, not a true canal. Third, this region is frequently the site of congenital anomalies. Sliding indirect hernia of the funicular type should be considered either a congenital anomaly or a lesion initiated by a congenital disturbances.

These hernias are, of course, treated by resection of the sac. In both adults and children parietal repair is an accessory treatment. Many cases of recurrence are in fact due to the persistence of an unidentified hernial sac.

The inguinal region comprises three layers: outer, fascial, and deep myofascial.

1. Outer Layer

The hair-bearing skin of the inguinal region is marked by the flexion crease of the thigh, which does not spatially correspond to the inguinal ligament. The latter runs parallel to this line at a site lying about two finger breadths above it. In obese patients it is often useful to identify the bony landmarks of the inguinal ligament, i.e., the anterior-superior iliac spine and pubic tubercle.

The areolar subcutaneous tissue of the inguinal region is richly vascularized, sometimes being referred to as Thomson's "vascular layer". In addition to the veins and arteries, this tissue contains lymph vessels. The latter, which are invisible to the naked eye, may be seeded by infectious microbes during surgery, thus accounting for apparently idiopathic postoperative infection.

2. Aponeurosis of the External Oblique Muscle of the Abdomen

The superficial inguinal ring (annulus inguinalis superficialis) erroneously referred to as the external ring of the inguinal canal, is located above the pubic tubercle in the medial part of this fascial layer. In this region the spermatic cord lies in the highly vascular areolar subcutaneous tissue. Accordingly, care must be taken when dissection is done in this area.

Subsequent to incision made parallel to the fibers of the aponeurosis of the external oblique, the first step in the approach to this region is the debridement of the superficial inguinal ring. The latter can easily be identified by introducing a finger beneath the wound margins and sliding it along the deep surface of this aponeurosis.

3. Deep Myofascial Layer The Myopectineal Orifice

Deep to the aponeurosis of the external oblique, the transverse fascia, particularly thick in this region, can be seen to stretch across a framelike area formed by certain muscular and fibrous structures. The deep inguinal ring (annulus inguinalis profundus) is located at the superolateral part of this fibromuscular frame. The spermatic cord in males or the round ligament of the uterus in females runs obliquely downward and forward in contact with the transverse fascia (Fig. 1.9).

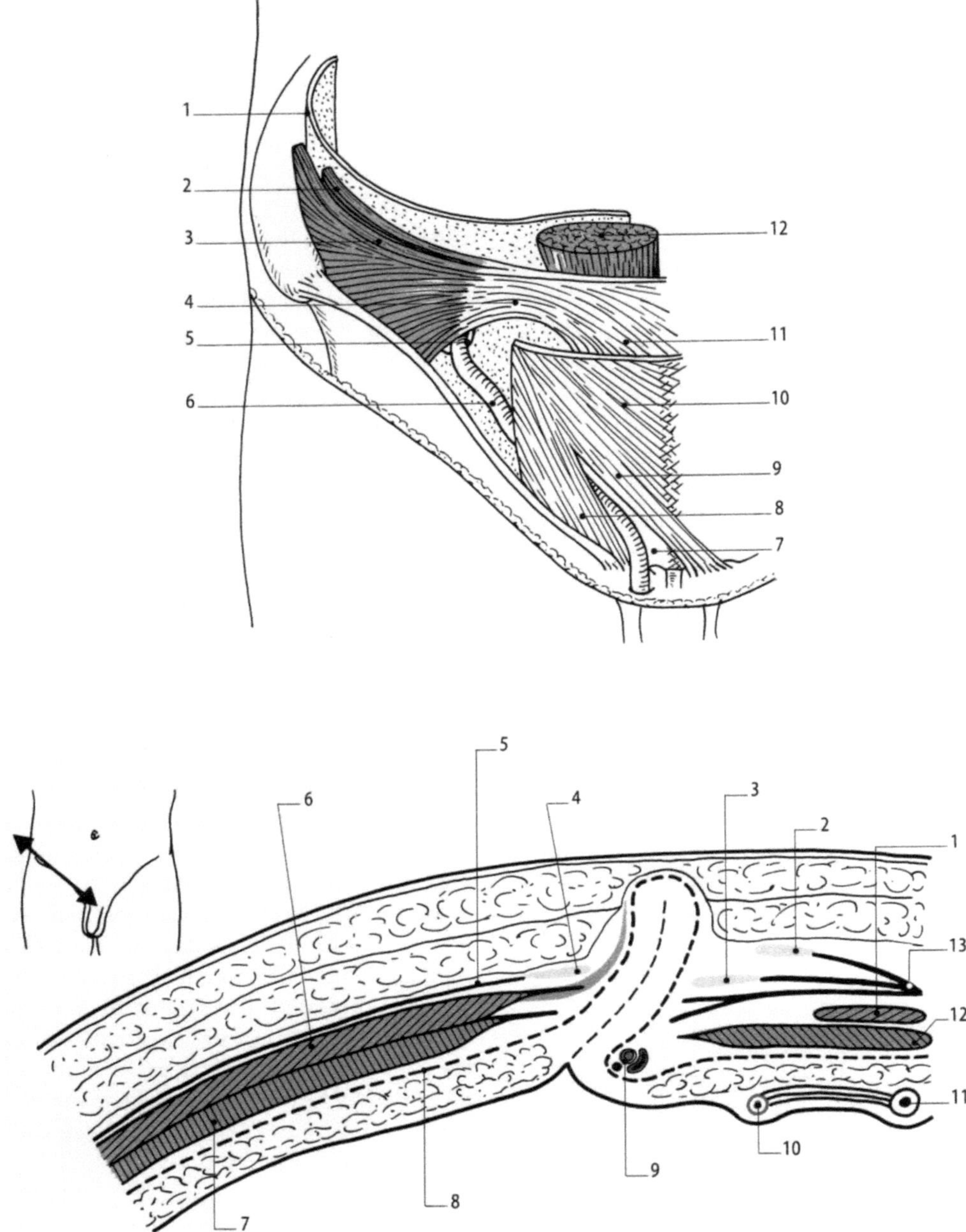

Fig. 1.9. a The meandre in the trajectory of the cord in the inguinal canal. *1* Fascia transversalis; *2* m. transversus abdominis; *3* m. obliquus internus abdominis; *4* falx inguinalis; *5* annulus inguinalis profundus; *6* spermatic cord (without m. cremaster); *7* annulus inguinalis superficialis; *8* crus laterale; *9* crus mediale; *10* aponeurosis of m. obliquus externus abdominis; *11* tendon conjunctivus; *12* m. rectus abdominis. **b** *1* m. pyramidalis abdominis; *2* crus mediale; *3* crus posterior; *4* crus laterale; *5* aponeurosis of m. obliquus externus abdominis; *6* m. obliquus internus abdominis; *7* m. transversus abdominis; *8* fascia transversalis; *9* a. epigastrica inferior; *10* a. ombilicalis; *11* urachus; *12* m. rectus abdominis; *13* linea alba

a) Components of the Fibromuscular Frame

(1) Medial Margin

The terminal part of the rectus and the overlying pyramidal form the medial boundary of the fibromuscular frame. The rectus terminates inferiorly on the surface extending from the pubic symphysis to the pubic tubercle. The anterior surface of the muscle is covered by a thick aponeurotic mantle, while its posterior surface is lined by only the transverse fascia. The lateral margin of the rectus sometimes presents a fibrous reinforcement which descends to the pubic tubercle and is referred to as Henle's ligament.

(2) Superior Margin

The superior boundary of the fibromuscular frame is formed by the so-called conjoint tendon (falx inguinalis), a twin muscular layer running roughly horizontally. It is formed by the overlapping of the internal oblique and transverse. As described previously, the muscle fibers of the conjoint tendon arise laterally, not from the inguinal ligament but rather from the iliac fascia of the psoas major and iliac muscles and from the anterior-superior iliac spine. These fibers initially run parallel to the inguinal ligament and are connected to it by fibrous bands. The fibers of the conjoint tendon then run upward and horizontally above the inguinal ligament, to terminate as a reinforcement of the prerectus aponeurotic layer. The layer of the internal oblique is superficial to that of the transverse and descends below the latter. The transverse can be exposed by applying traction to the aponeurosis which extends below the free margin of the muscle. This aponeurosis blends with the transverse fascia, thus accounting for the special mechanical resistance of the fascia in this region. The application of traction to this aponeurotic layer selectively pulls the transverse down toward the inguinal ligament.

(3) Inferior Margin

The lower boundary of the fibromuscular frame is a complex structure formed by two fibrous components. The latter are joined together medially but diverge as separate layers laterally, the angle of divergence being approximately 30°, thus forming an osteofibrous angle resembling a pair of geometric dividers. These two fibrous structures are the inguinal ligament and Cooper's ligament (pectineal ligament) lying posterior to and below the former. These two ligaments are partially connected by Gimbernat's ligament (lacunar ligament).

The *inguinal ligament* forms the reinforced inferior boundary of the aponeurosis of the external oblique. Opening of the aponeurosis, for example, in the approach to inguinal hernia, exposes this ligament as a whitish, ribbonlike structure which spreads out when the aponeurosis is pulled downward and laterally. The inferior margin of the inguinal ligament is not completely free, since it is in continuity with the fibrous structures blending above with the transverse fascia and below with the femoral sheath.

The question may be asked whether there is a truly individualized fibrous structure stretched between the anterior-superior iliac spine and pubic tubercle. The existence of the inguinal ligament (also referred to as the crural arcade in the French nomenclature) has been questioned by many authors. Nevertheless, posterior to the lower margin of the aponeurosis of the external oblique there is a fibrous structure sometimes called Thomson's band. The latter is attached medially near the pubic tubercle and runs laterally to the iliac fascia where it apparently divides into two layers. The deep layer runs behind the conjoint tendon and attaches to the iliac fascia. The very slender superficial layer continues in front of the conjoint tendon toward the anterior-superior iliac spine. The oblique fibers of the conjoint tendon seem to be attached to this superficial layer (Fig. 1.10).

In Bassini's operation the inguinal ligament is used at the inferior point to anchor the sutures, and it tends to tear in the direction of its fibers. Dissection around the inguinal ligament must be done with caution, owing to the very close proximity of certain blood vessels, especially the external iliac vein, which lies 4-5 cm lateral to the pubic tubercle. The points of entry and exit of each loop of suture material should differ slightly so that any excessive traction does not involve the same fibers, thus avoiding rupture of the aponeurosis.

The pectineal ligament (*Cooper's ligament*) is a very resistant, composite structure reinforcing the perioseum of the superior pubic ramus between the pubic tubercle and iliopectineal eminence. This ligament joins the inguinal ligament medially but diverges laterally from it when it runs in a much deeper position (Fig. 1.9). The angle between the two ligaments lies at the level of the upper end of the femoral infundibulum which is hidden under a loose diaphragm, the femoral septum, and bounded laterally by the external iliac vein. The femoral septum is the common site of crural hernia, for which a more proper term is femoral hernia.

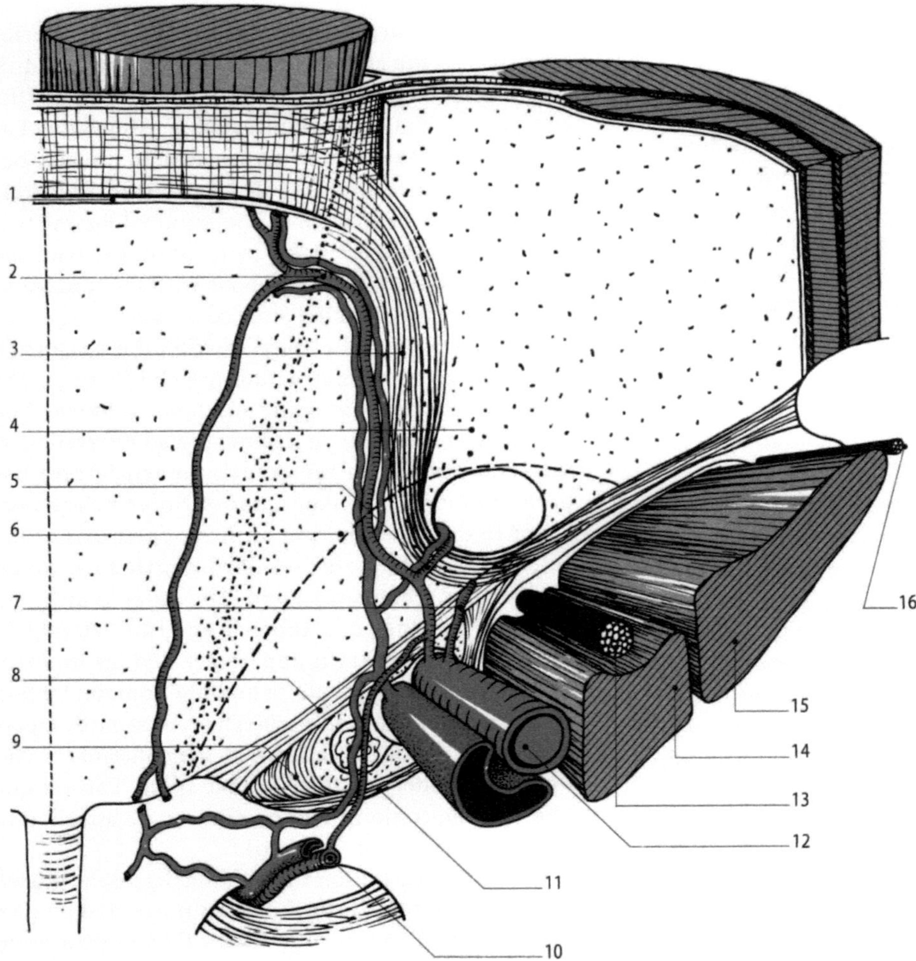

Fig. 1.10. Posterior view of the inguino-femoral region (peritoneum removed). *1* Linea arcuata; *2* a. epigastrica inferior; *3* lig. inter-foveolare; *4* fascia transversalis; *5* a. cremasterica; *6* projection of falx inguinalis; *7* a. circumflexa ilium profonda; *8* lig. inguinale; *9* lig. lacunare; *10* a. obturatoria; *11* lig. pectineale; *12* a. iliaca externa; *13* n. femoralis; *14* m. psoas major; *15* m. iliacus; *16* n. cutaneus femoris lateralis

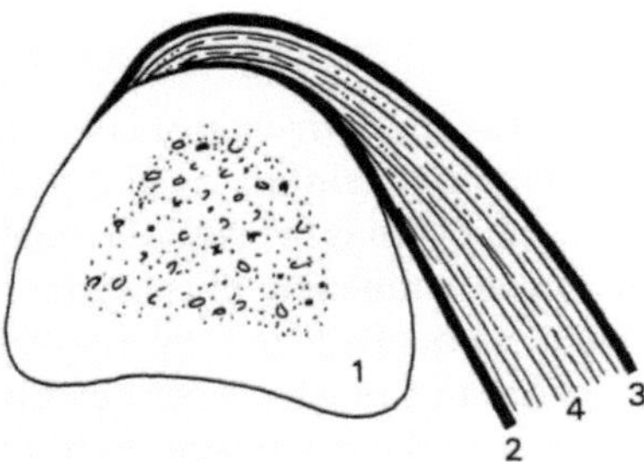

Fig. 1.11. Composition of Cooper's ligament (lig. pectineale). *1* Pecten ossis pubis; *2* deep fibrous layer: pubic periosteum reinforced by fibers from m. psoas minor; *3* superficial fibrous layer: aponeurosis m. pectineus; *4* fleshy fibers of m. pectineus

The pectineal ligament is a heterogeneous structure comprising three layers (Fig. 1.11). The deep layer is in continuity with the periosteum of the superior pubic ramus. The middle, muscular layer is formed by the uppermost fibers of the pectineal muscle inserted on the pubis. These fibers extend relatively far posteriorly. The superficial aponeurotic layer is very resistant, being formed by the overlapping of the vertical fibers of the aponeurosis of the pectineal muscle and transverse fibers running along the innominate line of the pelvis (arcuate line). Some of these fibers seem to emanate from the psoas minor.

The pectineal ligament displays an extreme degree of mechanical resistance. Although it is only a few millimeters thick, wires passed under the ligament in

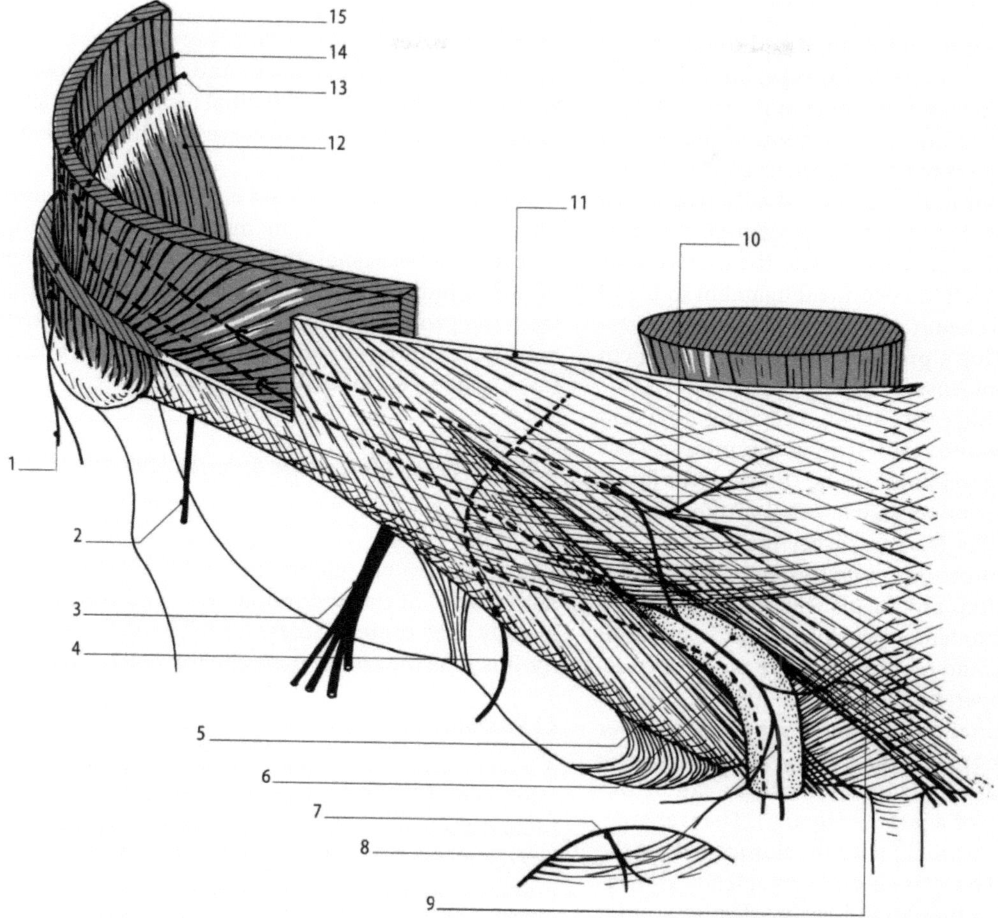

Fig. 1.12. Nerves of the inguino-femoral region. *1* Lateral cutaneous br. of n. iliohypogastricus; *2* n. cutaneus femoris lateralis ; *3* n. femoralis; *4* femoral br. of n. genitofemoralis; *5* spermatic chord; *6* genital br. of n. genitofemoralis; *7* n. obturatorius; *8* genital br. of nn. iliohypogastricus and ilioinguinalis; *9* pubic br. of n. iliohypogasricus; *10* anterior cutaneous br. of n. iliohypogastricus; *11* aponeurosis of m. obliquus externus abdominis ; *12* m. iliacus; *13* n. ilioinguinalis; *14* n. iliohypogastricus; *15* m. obliquus internus abdominis

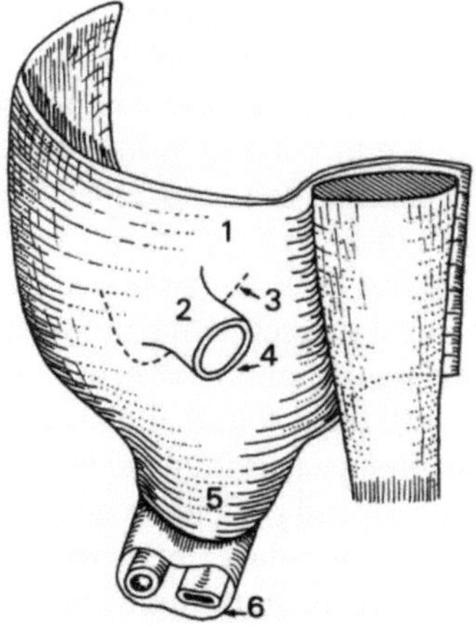

Fig. 1.13. The fascia transversalis in the anteroinferior part of the abdominal wall. *1* Fascia transversalis; *2* annulus inguinalis profundus; *3* lig. interfoveolare; *4* fascia spermatica interna; *5* prevascular extension of fascia transversalis; *6* sheath of femoral vessels

contact with the bone can be used to virtually lift up the whole body! In the treatment of hernia (McVay's or Goinard's operation) it is difficult to use the pectineal ligament for lateral support, since the ligament progressively descends in depth leading to a risk of compression of the external iliac vein.

The frame of the myopectineal orifice is closed by the lower part of the transversalis fascia (Fig. 1.12). The latter, which is rather weak elsewhere, constitutes a veritable aponeurosis in this region, where it extends under the inferior margin of the transverse. In this area the transversalis fascia presents arcuate reinforcements, as previously described by Testut (1896). Further support is added by Henle's ligament and Hesselbach's ligament (lig. intervofeolare), the latter acting as a fibrous reinforcement of the sheath of the inferior epigastric vessels. Laterally, the transversalis fascia adheres rather tightly to the iliac fascia and inferiorly, to the inguinal ligament and the pectineal ligament in the medial part of this region (Fig. 1.13). According to McVay and Anson (1940), the pectineal ligament is the true inferior insertion of the medial part of the transversalis fascia, whereas the areolar layer lying anterior to the fascia and adhering to the inguinal ligament should not be considered mechanically significant. At a more lateral site, the transversalis fascia separates from the pectineal ligament to blend with the femoral sheath anterior to the femoral vessels, thus delimiting a prevascular funnel about 3 cm long (the funnel of Anson and McVay).

According to this conception, direct inguinal and femoral hernia would result from a common mechanism, which is the weakness of the transversalis fascia medial to the inferior epigastric vessels. Anterior protrusion would thus lead to direct inguinal hernia, whereas inferior protrusion into the femoral infundibulum opening anterior to the plane of the transversalis fascia would lead to femoral hernia. Accordingly, both types of hernia would require the same mode of treatment - McVay's operation.

The deep inguinal ring is an opening in the upper lateral part of the transversalis fascia and resembles a veritable evagination of the fascia which can be likened to the lining of a jacket (Fig. 1.13). The transversalis fascia is in continuity with the fibrous coat of the spermatic cord. The latter is embryologically equivalent to the fascia, although it does not display similar mechanical properties. The deep inguinal ring is strengthened from below and medially by the passage of the inferior epigastric vessels and the reinforcement of Hesselbach's ligament (lig. interfoveolare). The latter has been considered a mechanically important structure. Tension on this ligament elevates and closes the deep inguinal ring, thus acting in opposition to the forces acting on the external inguinal fossa. The transversalis fascia, often disregarded by French surgeons, is considered by many North American authors to be the basic structure allowing closure of hernial orifices, either with retention sutures or by resection of part of the fascia. These maneuvers are the basis for McVay's or the Shouldice Hospital procedure (for more details, consult the section on hernia of the groin).

b) Umbilicoprevesical Fascia
and Inguinal Peritoneum

The ascending fibrous and vascular structures interposed between the transversalis fascia and peritoneum push up against the latter to form three inguinal depressions. From medial to lateral, these are: the internal inguinal fossa, lying between the urachus and

umbilical artery; the middle inguinal fossa, lying between the umbilical artery and inferior epigastric vessels; and the external inguinal fossa, located lateral to the umbilical vessels and corresponding to the deep inguinal ring.

The external inguinal fossa is a peritoneal infundibulum corresponding to the mouth of the embryonic vaginoperitoneal canal. This fossa is the natural course of sliding indirect hernia, whereas direct hernia results from the progressive dissension of the middle inguinal fossa. Sliding direct hernia via the supravesical fossa is an exceptional finding.

C. Other Weak Points of the Anterior Abdominal Wall

1. Linea Alba

The linea alba represents the site of insertion of the flat muscles of the abdominal wall, and the mist frequently used route of access for to the abdominal cavity. It is thus the commonest site for ventral hernia.

a) Radiological Study

A recent anatomico-radiological study [Rath et al. 1996] showed that the average length of the linea alba in 40 dissections was 29.11 cm (20-40). Its breadth is 1.72 cm above the umbilicus, 2.24 cm at the level of the umbilicus and 0.66 cm below it.

The results obtained from 40 tomodensitometric slices show that the in vivo values are somewhat different: the average breadth of the linea alba being 8.3 ± 5.63 above, 21.2 ± 8.07 at, and 9.3 ± 6.74 below, umbilical level. There is thus a considerable difference between the two studies at the supraumbilical level. Study of the frequency distribution of the breadth of the linea alba above the umbilicus on TDM cuts reveals two peaks, the first at between 5 and 6 mm, the second between 12 and 14 mm, corresponding to subjects ages less than or more than 50 years, respectively. The breadth of the linea increases significantly with age ($p = 0.005$). At umbilical level, the peak occurs at between 17 and 19 mm, most subjects being between 13 and 23 mm, and without significant increase with age. These results coincide with those found at dissection. Below the umbilicus, the first peak is found at between 5 and 6 mm and there is a second peak between 10 and 11 mm, revealing a significant enlargement with age ($p = 0.003$) the first peak corresponding to subjects less than 40 and the second to the older group. The only significant difference related to sex appears in the supraumbilical region, where males have a linea alba which is on average 4.2 mm wider than in females.

There is thus a clear change in dimension of the linea alba at around the 45th year, whereafter it enlarges both above and below the umbilicus. Values for the breadth of the linea alba which can be considered normal are as follows:

Above the umbilicus:	$\leq$ 45 years: 5-6 mm
	$\geq$ 45 years: 12-14 mm
At the level of the umbilicus:	19-23 mm
Below the umbilicus:	$\leq$ 45 years: 5-6 mm
	$\geq$ 45 years: 9-11 mm

Knowledge of these anatomical facts in regard to the linea alba enables one to define diastasis of the rectus muscles in terms of age. Below 45, any gap between the two upper rectus muscles of greater than 10 mm would be considered diastatic, as would one of 27 mm at umbilical level and 15 mm below. For subjects more than 45 years of age, the values would be 15, 27 and 14 mm respectively.

b) Functional Study

Two types of force act on the linea alba, in both normal and pathological conditions. These are the intra-abdominal pressure and the lateral traction of the broad muscles. It is the latter that determine the elasticity and degree of deformation of the tissues. Awareness of the normal parameters of the linea alba can establish an objective baseline for evaluation of the different prosthetic materials used in repair of ventral hernias.

Two types of test have been used in a recent study of the linea alba [Rath et al. 1996] a *bursting strain* test, which reproduces the action of the intra-abdominal pressure on the wall, and a *dynamometric* test which provides data on elastic and plastic deformation and the point of rupture produced by linear traction.

Busting strain tests show that the umbilical region seems the most resistant to pressure exerted from within: 6.715 kg/cm² on average (2.7-10.2). The resistance are more or less the same for the supraumbilical and infraumbilical portions of the linea alba (5.868-6.01 kg/cm² respectively). The difference between the three regions is not significant.

The *constraint* or force exercised by each section unit, measures the resistance of the tissues to linear traction, calculated with a dynamometer. For the supraumbilical linea alba, the mean constraint is 0.367 kgf/mm² (0.109-0.698), but this difference does not reach significance.

Deformation expresses the percentage elongation of the specimen at the moment of rupture produced by linear traction. The linea alba is slightly more deformable above than below the umbilicus (45.57% and 31.55% respectively).

Another value measured by the dynamometer is the *coefficient of elasticity*. The greater the value of this, the better the material can withstand a force without deformation. The mean coefficient of elasticity of the linea alba is slightly higher below than above the umbilicus: 2.429 kgf/mm² and 1.151 kgf/mm² respectively (p = 0.05). This may be explained bearing in mind the Law of Laplace, which states that, for a given radius, the pressure and elasticity of a sphere vary proportionally. In fact there exists a gradient of intra-abdominal pressure which decreases from below upwards, so that elasticity is proportionally raised below the umbilicus.

2. Semilunar Line

Hernia of this region is an exceptional finding, since the myofascial boundaries of the flat abdominal muscles do not lie over one another. The zone of weakness corresponds to the intersection of the semilunar line with the arcuate line. The passage in this area of the inferior epigastric vessels running along the posterior surface of the rectus contributes to the weakness of this region where the rare, so-called Spigelian hernia

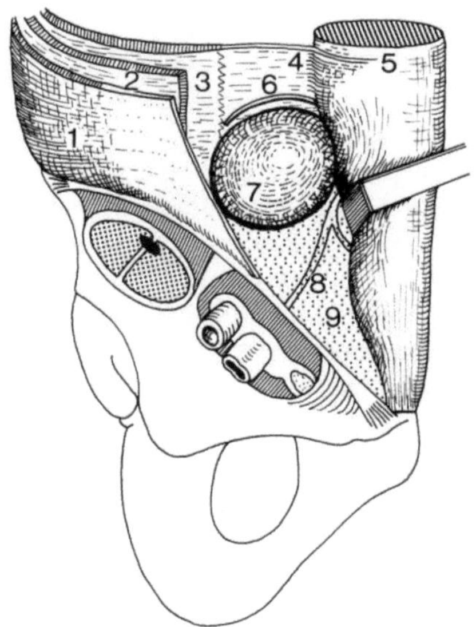

Fig. 1.14. Hernia of the linea semilunaris (Spigelian hernia). *1* M. obliquus externus abdominis; *2* m. obliquus internus abdominis; *3* m. transversus abdominis; *4* lamina posterior vaginae m. recti; *5* m. rectus abdominis; *6* linea arcuata; *7* hernial sac between the linea arcuata and a. epigastrica inferior, normally covered by the m. rectus abdominis; *8* a. epigastrica inferior; *9* fascia transversalis

arises (although Spiegel never described such a hernia). This type of hernia is found in the triangle bounded laterally by the semilunar line, superiorly by the lateral part of the arcuate line, and inferiorly and medially by the oblique course of the inferior epigastric vessels. Hernia may also develop with a twin sac lying above and below the inferior epigastric vessels, the latter separating the two hernial sacs like a bridle (Fig. 1.14).

When poorly limited inferiorly, hernia of the semilunar line would be a special subtype of direct hernia. The sac of Spigelian hernia develops beneath the rectus. Thus, this type of hernia remains intraparietal over a long period of time prior to its exteriorization along the lateral margin of the rectus and subsequent protrusion beneath the skin. Diagnosis may be difficult for quite some time and grasping of the filled hernia sac may be problematic.

Spigelian hernia, related to a rupture in the resistance of the posterior lamina of the rectus sheath, is difficult to manage. Treatment consists of retrorectus placement of a large flap derived from the anterior fibrous covering of the rectus, followed by suturing of the flap to the arcuate line above and to the strong part of the transverse fascia, or even the inguinal ligament, below.

III. The Posterior Abdominal Wall

The posterior abdominal wall, forming the backdrop of the abdomen, is described below from front to back, i.e., from deep to superficial layers. Less of a "surgical" structure than the anterior abdominal wall, it shows significant direct relations to the three main retroperitoneal sheaths, i.e., the central vascular sheath and lateral adrenorenoureteral sheaths. The posterior abdominal wall is in contact with the lumbar neural ganglia and contains within its muscles the lumbar plexus and an entire vascular network.

The classical zones of posterior weakness are Grynfelt's lumbar quadrangle (tetragonum lumbale, see Fig. 1.16) and Petit's lumbar triangle (trigonum lumbale, see Fig. 1.17), although lumbar hernia rarely occurs at these sites. Parietal weakness of the posterior abdominal wall is most often of postoperative or traumatic origin.

A. Deep Layer

The deep layer of the posterior abdominal wall comprises, in the midline, the lumbosacral spine flanked laterally by the iliopsoas and quadratus lumborum which mask the lumbar intertransverse muscles.

1. Median Spinal Axis

The lumbar spine, markedly convex anteriorly, is entirely covered by a fibrous coat consisting of the anterior longitudinal ligament, which terminates at the level of the second sacral vertebra, and the diaphragmatic crura. The right crus, the larger, lies over the bodies of L-2 and L-3 and the neighboring intervertebral disks. The left crus is usually smaller, lying over the body of L-2 and the neighboring intervertebral disks. From their insertions on the spine, the diaphragmatic crura run forward to form the aortic hiatus. Fleshy fibers arise from the upper margin of the fibrous arch of the hiatus. In this way, the diaphragmatic crura constitute the classical "fibrous bed" of the aorta in front of the lumbar spine. The flared part of the right crus penetrates between the aorta and the inferior vena cava. Although the latter is displaced slightly to the right, its close proximity should be kept in mind in the course of surgical repair of hiatal hernia. The first two intercostal arteries on the right and left sides pierce the fleshy part of the diaphragmatic crura as they run tangential to the bodies of the vertebrae.

The promontory of the sacrum protrudes into the space between the common iliac vessels like a bracket above the pelvis. The pelvic viscera are suspended from the promontory, via the thick fibrous coat covering it and the L-5–S-1 intervertebral space. The middle sacral vessels run anteriorly over the promontory. The danger point formed by the left common iliac vein, running obliquely across this region, should be kept in mind.

The sacrum, forming the posterior wall of the pelvis, contains the cavum durale down to the level of S-2. The vegetative nerves distributing to the sphincters and genital organs emerge through the third and fourth anterior sacral foramina. The position of these nerves should be borne in mind when using the transsacral approach to the rectum. Resection via the fourth sacral foramina can be done, whereas in the course of a more superior route it is imperative to preserve at least one of the third sacral foramina. The boundary between the sigmoid colon and rectum classically lies at the level of the anterior part of S-2–S-3.

The median osteofibrous spinal axis is extended laterally in cruciform fashion by the posterior part of the iliac crests. The latter seem to divide the muscles into two steplike layers. The upper layer is formed by the greater psoas lying medially and the quadratus lum-

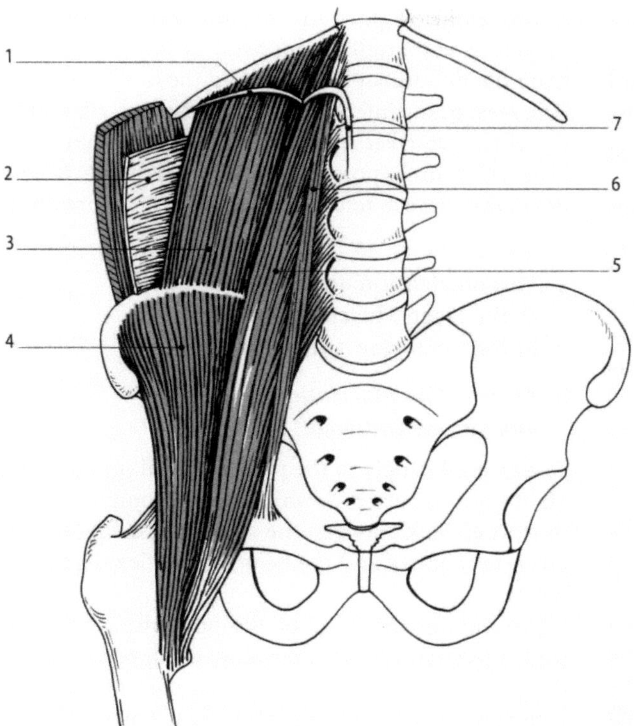

Fig. 1.15. Iliopsoas and quadratus lumborum muscles. *1* Lig. arcuatum laterale; *2* aponeurosis posterior m. transversus abdominis; *3* m. quadratus lumborum; *4* m. iliacus; *5* m. psoas major; *6* m. psoas minor; *7* lig. arcuatum mediale

borum laterally. The lower layer consists of the greater psoas flanked by the iliacus. The iliac crest thus resembles a very thick intersection reinforced by the iliolumbar ligament, which runs behind the greater psoas and spreads out on the anteromedial lip of the bony crest.

2. Lateral Spinal Muscles

a) Iliopsoas Muscles

The *psoas major* is a voluminous muscle extending from the 12th thoracic vertebra to the lesser trochanter. It flanks the lumbar spine and then runs along the innominate line of the iliac bone to leave the abdominal region via the muscular lacuna beneath the inguinal ligament.

The psoas major is a truly hollow muscle comprising two layers, anterior (corporeal) and posterior (costiform). These two layers are joined together laterally. The space between them contains the lumbar plexus, the ramifications of the lumbar arteries, the lumbar veins and their longitudinal anastomosis, and the ascending lumbar vein (Fig. 1.15).

The anterior corporeal layer of the muscle is attached to the spine from the 12th thoracic to the fourth lumbar vertebrae The insertions are mainly on the intervertebral disks rather than on the vertebral bodies themselves. These stepwise insertions are joined to one another by fibrous arches. The latter, arranged in opposition to the concavity of the lateral surfaces of the bodies of the vertebrae, form buttonholelike openings for the passage of the lumbar vascular pedicles and sympathetic communicating branches. On the right, these arcuate fibers are most often covered anteriorly by the right margin of the inferior vena cava. Owing to this arrangement, surgical identification of the sympathetic ganglia may be dangerous. Furthermore, the very short lumbar veins are also hidden and thus may be injured, especially when inserting a clamp. It has been proposed that the exposure of the posterior surface of the inferior vena cava be limited to the region of the intervertebral disks. However, owing to the variability of the metamerization of the lumbar veins, this procedure is not entirely free of risk.

The posterior costiform layer of the greater psoas inserts on the anterior surface of the transverse processes of all five lumbar vertebrae.

The greater psoas is thus well formed in the upper lumbar region. It leaves the diaphragm by passing under the medial arcuate ligament, sometimes referred to as the arch of the psoas. The iliac fascia is attached to the inferior margin of this ligament and lines the psoas major. An abscess originating from the 12th thoracic vertebra can thus travel downward along the fascia.

The *psoas minor* arises from vertical fascicles inserted on the 12th thoracic and first lumbar vertebrae. This muscle runs along the medial boundary of the psoas major to attach to the innominate line and iliopectineal eminence. The psoas minor is an occasional muscle (present in less than 50% of subjects). Its lowermost fibers may be seen to extend down to pectineal ligament. Finally, it is also attached to the deep surface of the iliac fascia and thus acts to stretch this fascia.

The iliacus originates from the greater part of the internal iliac fossa and stretches downward to the level of the anterior-inferior iliac spine. The muscle fibers, grouped together along the lateral margin of the psoas major, form, along with the latter, a groove for the femoral nerve. The iliacus fibers then wind around the terminal tendon of the psoas major and finally pass anterior to the latter to insert on the lesser trochanter and below; i.e., these fibers extend below the femoral insertion of the psoas major.

The *iliacus fascia* is a fibrous sheath common to the greater psoas and iliac muscles. It is relatively thin in its upper part, but becomes much thicker at the level of the iliac crest, where it ensheaths the intramuscular structures down to the lesser trochanter. Deep to the inguinal ligament the iliacus fascia is reinforced, thereby forming the iliopectineal arch, which separates the vascular and muscular lacunae. The iliac fascia can be stretched only slightly. This finding accounts for the rapidly compressive nature of hemorrhagic effusion originating from the rich vascular network within the psoas major. This type of hematoma occurs frequently in patients taking anticoagulants and it may lead to severe damage of the lumbar plexus.

b) Quadratus Lumborum Muscle

This muscle extends behind and lateral to the psoas major in the space bounded by the 12th rib, the tips of the transverse processes of the lumbar vertebrae, and the posterior part of the iliac crest. The muscle body, resembling a rectangle rather than a square, is composed of interlacing multidirectional fibers originating from the different bony margins listed above (Fig. 1.15).

The anterior part of the quadratus lumborum muscle is essentially composed of fibers extending from the iliolumbar ligament and the deep part of the iliac crest to the inferior margin of the 12th rib and the tip of the transverse processes of the lumbar vertebrae. The thinner posterior layer of the muscle extends down the 12th rib to the lumbar transverse processes.

3. Vascularization and Innervation of the Deep Muscle Layer of the Posterior Abdominal Wall

a) Arterial Vascularization and Venous Drainage

The arterial supply to the posterior abdominal wall is via the lumbar arteries, which form a complex anastomotic network between the 12th intercostal (subcostal) artery above and the deep circumflex iliac artery below.

The venous drainage of the posterior abdominal wall is particularly well developed, especially within the psoas major, where the veins communicate via conjugate vessels with the intraspinal venous plexuses and via the arches of the psoas with the inferior vena cava. The ascending lumbar vein is one of the roots of the azygos system. The venous network of the posterior abdominal wall (iliolumbar, lumbar, and ascending lumbar veins) is able to shunt most of the caval blood after a subrenal ligation of the inferior vena cava.

b) Lymphatic Network

The upper part of the posterior abdominal wall is drained by the lateral caval and lateral aortic lymph nodes. The transdiaphragmatic lymphatic channels form a direct communication between the retroperitoneal region and the subpleural space. This accounts for the rapid thoracic and mediastinal extension of certain pathological processes involving the retroperitoneal region, e.g., pancreatitis.

c) Innervation

The posterior abdominal wall is innervated via the lumbar plexus. The psoas major receives branches at different levels from the first through fourth lumbar nerves, and the psoas minor receives branches from the first and second lumbar nerves. Filaments arising from the femoral nerve supply the iliacus. The motor innervation of the quadratus lumborum is via the 12th intercostal nerve and branches from the first three lumbar spinal roots.

4. Site of Emergence of the Terminal Branches of the Lumbar Plexus in Relation to the Iliopsoas Muscle

The iliohypogastric and ilioinguinal nerves emerge from the lateral margin of the greater psoas at the level of the L-1–L-2 intervertebral disk and then run along the anterior surface of the quadratus lumborum posterior to the kidney. These nerves follow the iliac crest to finally enter the inguinal region.

The lateral femoral cutaneous nerve exits from the anterior surface of the psoas major at the level of the lower end of the third lumbar vertebra or the L-3–L-4 intervertebral disk. It runs obliquely outward and downward to cross over the lateral margin of the psoas major at the level of the L-4–L-5 intervertebral disk and then runs along the surface of the iliac bone to finally enter the muscular lacuna medial to the anterior-superior iliac spine.

The genitofemoral nerve appears on the anterior surface of the psoas major at a point slightly medial and inferior to the lateral femoral cutaneous nerve (L-4–L-5 intervertebral disk). It then descends parallel to the fibers of the psoas major just behind the inguinal ligament when it divides into terminal branches.

The femoral nerve leaves the lateral margin of the psoas major, becoming visible in the groove between the latter and the iliacus at the level of the sacral promontory. This nerve divides just below the inguinal ligament.

The obturator nerve emerges from the medial border of the psoas major at about the same level as the preceding nerve, i.e., at the site where the medial margin of this muscle crosses over the ala of the sacrum (the fossette of Cuneo and Marcille). In this region it is accompanied by the fifth lumbar nerve root, which receives the first sacral nerve root to form the lumbosacral trunk.

5. Action of the Deep Muscles of the Posterior Abdominal Wall

The iliopsoas, inserted on the pelvis and spine, acts mainly to flex and laterally rotate the thigh (psoitis posture) and thus is very important for walking. Acting on the axial skeleton, the psoas major resembles a polyarticular muscle, leading to lateral flexion and slight rotation of the spine on the side opposite the muscle. When both psoas major act simultaneously with the subject supine, they elevate the upper and lower parts of the trunk.

The psoas minor, which flexes the lumbar spine with respect to the pelvis, is a tensor muscle of the iliac fascia.

The quadratus lumborum acts as a lateral brace of the lumbar spine by pulling the iliac crest and the 12th rib closer to one another. This muscle can also be considered to depress the 12th rib, and thus acts as an accessory expiratory muscle.

B. Superficial Layer of the Posterior Abdominal Wall

Two layers of flat muscles and aponeuroses lie posterior to the deep muscle layer and extend laterally to blend into the anterolateral abdominal wall. From anterior to posterior, the first of these layers is that of the posterior aponeurosis of the transverse. This aponeurosis, lying posterior to the quadratus lumborum, is attached to the tips of the transverse processes of the lumbar vertebrae. Framed by muscle bodies, this aponeurotic layer constitutes a zone of weakness, the classical Grynfelt's lumbar quadrangle (Fig. 1.16). The

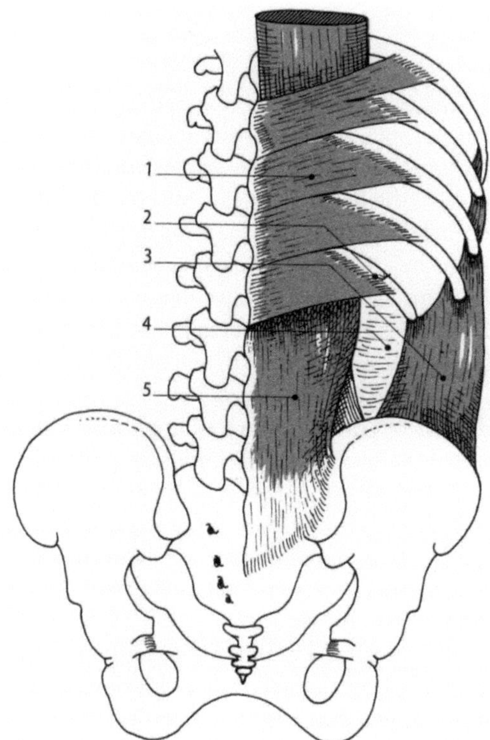

Fig. 1.16. Limits of the lumbar quadrangle (tetragonum lumbale). *1* M. serratus posterior-inferior; *2* 12th rib; *3* m. obliquus internus abdominis; *4* lumbar quadrangle (aponeurosis m. transversus abdominis); *5* m. erector spinae

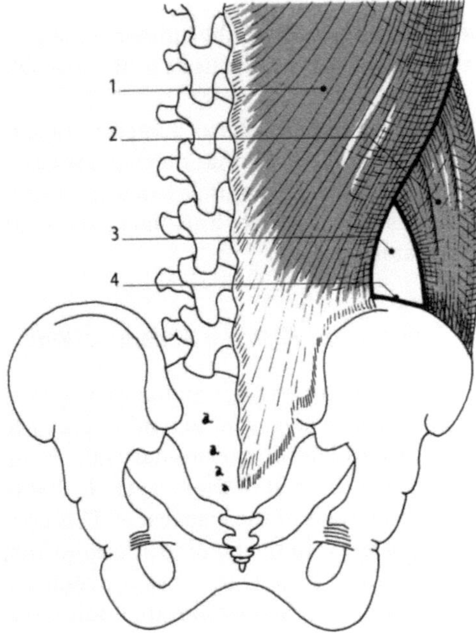

Fig. 1.17. Limits of the lumbar triangle (trigonum lumbale). *1* M. latissimus dorsi; *2* m. obliquus externus abdominis; *3* trigonum lumbale; *4* crista iliaca

medial boundary of this area is formed by the erector muscles of the spine inserted on the posterior part of the iliac crest, the posterior iliac spines and the posterior surface of the sacrum. These muscles spread out from their origin toward the ribs. This muscular mass is enveloped in a very resistant aponeurosis, which, along with the arches of the lumbar vertebrae and posterior surface of the transverse processes, forms a veritable osteofibrous canal (thoracolumbar fascia) through which the muscles pass.

The inferior lateral boundary of the lumbar quadrangle is formed by the internal oblique, which runs upward and forward to make an acute angle with the mass of spinal muscles. Moreover, the internal oblique is inserted on the thoracolumbar fascia and the posterior part of the iliac crest and extends up to the inferior margin of the 12th rib.

The superior medial boundary of the lumbar quadrangle is formed by the serratus posterior inferior. This muscle, extending over the mass of the spinal muscles, is attached via its inferior digitation to the inferior edge of the 12th rib.

Finally, a short part of the inferior margin of the 12th rib forms the superior lateral boundary of Grynfelt's lumbar quadrangle.

This muscular layer is lined posteriorly by a layer containing the superficial weak area of the region, i.e., Petit's lumbar triangle. The lumbar triangle is bounded by the following structures (Fig. 1.17): below, by the posterior part of the iliac crest; laterally and anteriorly, by the posterior margin of the external oblique running downward and forward, the anterior part of this muscle being entirely composed of fleshy fibers from the 12th rib to the iliac crest; and medially, by the lateral margin of the latissimus dorsi, which runs upward and laterally. The latter muscle originates from a large aponeurotic sheet attached to the spinous processes of the thoracic and lumbar vertebrae, the sacral crest, and the posterior iliac spine. This fibrous sheet continues medially with the thoracolumbar fascia and is often described as the superficial lamina of the latter.

Lumbar hernia in the area of the lumbar quadrangle (usually the upper part), which may enter into Petit's lumbar triangle, is a rare finding. In such cases the neck of the hernial sac is narrow, and treatment can thus be achieved with relative ease. Conversely, postoperative incisional hernia in this region is far more problematic. Hernia also sometimes occurs following closed trauma which causes destruction or detachment of the muscles in this region.

Significant tissue loss, often accompanied by paralysis of the abdominal strap resulting from motor nerve injury, requires the use of foreign or autoplastic material to achieve repair, i.e., large flaps of fascia lata cut in the external iliac fossa and reflected upward onto the iliac crest, as in Koontz's operation.

References

Arregui ME (1997) Surgical anatomy of the preperitoneal fasciae and posterior transversalis fasciae in the inguinal region. Hernia 1: 101-110

Chevrel JP (1994) Anatomie clinique. Le tronc. Springer Verlag, Paris

Chevrel JP, Salama J, Kemeny JL (1982) Etude anatomo-chirurgicale de la perméabilité du ligament rond du foie. Anat Clin 4: 285-287

Detrie P (1982) Nouveau traité de technique chirurgicale, vol IX. Masson, Paris

Goinard P, Curtillet E (1929) Le système artériel de la paroi abdominale antérieure. Travaux laboratoire d'anatomie, Faculté de médecine, Alger: 11-18

Heise G (1954) Probleme der Frühzystektomie mit klinischen, tierexperimentellen und anatomischen Studien. Wiss Z Univ, Halle-Wittenberg 3: 999-1048

Hovelaque A (1927) Anatomie des nerfs crâniens et rachidiens et du système grand sympathique. Doin, Paris

McVay CB (1984) Anson & McVay's surgical anatomy, 6th edn. W B Saunders, Philadelphia

McVay CB, Anson BJ (1940) Aponeurotic and fascial continuities in the abdomen, pelvis, and thigh. Anat Rec 76: 213-231

Morin A, Neidhardt JH, Spay G (1968) Les kystes suppurés de l'ouraque. Lyon Med 219: 1481-1509

Neidhart JPH (1994) Les muscles de l'abdomen. In: Chevrel JP (ed) Le Tronc: anatomie clinique. Springer-Verlag, Paris, pp 93-122

Pans A, Pierard GE, Albert A, Desaive C (1997) Biomechanical assessment of the tranversalis fascia and rectus abdominis aponeurosis in inguinal herniation. Preliminary results. Hernia 1: 27-30

Paturet G (1951) Aponévroses de l'abdomen. In: Traité d'anatomie humaine. Masson, Paris, pp 903-914

Poirier P, Charpy A (1912) Traité d'anatomie humaine, T II. Masson, Paris, pp 302-310

Poirier P, Charpy A (1912) Aponévroses de l'abdomen. In: Traité d'anatomie humaine. Masson, Paris, pp 336-380

Rath AM, Attali P, Dumas JL, Goldlust D, Zhang J, Chevrel JP (1996) The abdominal linea alba: an anatomo-radiologic and biomechanical study. Surg Radiol Anat 18: 281-288

Read RC (1992) Cooper's posterior lamina of transversalis fascia. Surg Gynecol Obstet 174: 426-434

Richet JL (1877) Traité pratique d'anatomie médico-chirurgicale Lauwereyns, Paris pp 741-758

Rousseau D, Descottes B, Kalfon M, Pouget X, Caix M (1982) Description et déductions fonctionnelles de l'innervation des muscles et du péritoine de la paroi antéro-latérale de l'abdomen. GREPA 4. Lab Bruneau, Paris, pp 11-12

Rouvière H (1939) Anatomie générale: origine des formes et des structures anatomiques. Masson, Paris, pp 63-76

Rouvière H (1939) Anatomie humaine. Masson, Paris, pp 80-84

Salama J, Sarfati E, Chevrel JP (1982) Les nerfs de la région inguinale. GREPA 4. Lab Bruneau, Paris, pp 7-10

Salmon M, Dor J (1933) Artères des muscles, des membres et du tronc. Masson, Paris

Skandalakis JE, Colborn GL, Skandalakis LJ (1997) The embryology of the inguino-femoral area: an overview. Hernia 1: 45-54

Skandalakis LJ, Colborn GL (1994) Surgical anatomy of the abdominal wall. In: Bendavid R (ed)Prosthesis and abdominal wall hernias. R G Landes, Austin pp 34-58

Skandalakis JE, Gray SW, Skandalakis LJ, et al (1989) Surgical anatomy of the inguinal area. World J Surg 13: 490-498

Stoppa R (1974) Les plasties de la paroi abdominale. Table ronde. Actual Chir, Masson, Paris, pp 662-736

Testut L (1896) Traité d'anatomie humaine. Doin, Paris

2 Functional Anatomy of the Muscles of the Anterolateral Abdominal Wall: Electromyography and Histoenzymology

Relationship Between Abdominal Wall Activity and Intra-abdominal Pressure

M. Caix *with the collaboration of* G. Outrequin,
B. Descottes, M. Kalfon, X. Pouget, and G. Catanzano

The descriptive anatomy and pathology of the abdominal wall are well known to surgeons and specialists in functional rehabilitation. Conversely, few studies have been devoted to the anatomophysiological features of the parietal muscles, and little progress has been made regarding the functional anatomy of the recti abdomini and flat abdominal muscles (the transverse and internal and external obliques).

The aim of the studies described below was to achieve a better understanding of parietal function. This work was based on detailed study of the structure of the parietal muscles by microscopic analysis of their constituent fibers, coupled with detailed analysis of their function using quantitative electromyography. Intra-abdominal pressure was then investigated in operated patients. As the reader progresses through this chapter, the classical and still valid notion of the correlations between structure and function should become apparent.

(ATPase and oxidative enzymes) and physiological properties, as shown in table 2.1.

The enzymatic and physiological differences of the three categories raise the question of their functional differences. This question has been summarized by Mayer (1973) in the following way:

The physiological properties of the motor units are correlated with their histochemical characteristics in such a way that the phasic motor units with a fast contraction time are formed of fibers rich in glycolytic activity, whereas the tonic motor fibers with a slow contraction time are formed of fibers rich in oxidative activity.

Based on these introductory notions, functional investigation of the abdominal musculature was carried out, beginning with the study of the enzymes of the muscles of the anterolateral abdominal wall.

I. Detailed Study of Structure: Histochemical Analysis of the Fibers of the Abdominal Wall

Histological analysis of normal muscle fibers examined under the light microscope does not allow the demonstration of any particular function of the fibers. Conversely, histochemical investigation reveals three categories of striated muscle fibers, which can be differentiated on the basis of their enzymatic apparatus

A. Material and Methods

In the course of abdominal surgery, biopsy specimens of muscle fibers were taken from the rectus, external oblique, internal oblique, and transverse muscles. Biopsy samples of the levator ani and one of the limb muscles (deltoid) were made for the purpose of comparison.

All muscle samples were subjected to histoenzymatic analysis for the determination of ATPase and oxi-

Table 2.1. Features of the three types of muscle fibers in the gastrocnemius and soleus of the cat [Engel et al. 1973]

	Types of muscle fibers	
	Type I or S (slow) 25%-40%	Type II or F (fast)
	rich in mitochondria (red muscle, slow)	rich in myofibrils (white muscle, fast)
Enzymatic apparatus		Type II A (FR) Type II B (FF)
Presence of ATPase and glycolytic enzymes	–	+ + + +
Presence of oxidative enzymes	+ +	+ –
Glycogen	–	+ + + + +
Estimated number of fibers per motor unit	Very few	Few Many
Physiological properties Sensitivity to fatigue Contraction time	Very resistant 58/110 ms (long)	Moderately res. Sensitive 30/55 ms 20/47 ms (intermediate) (short)

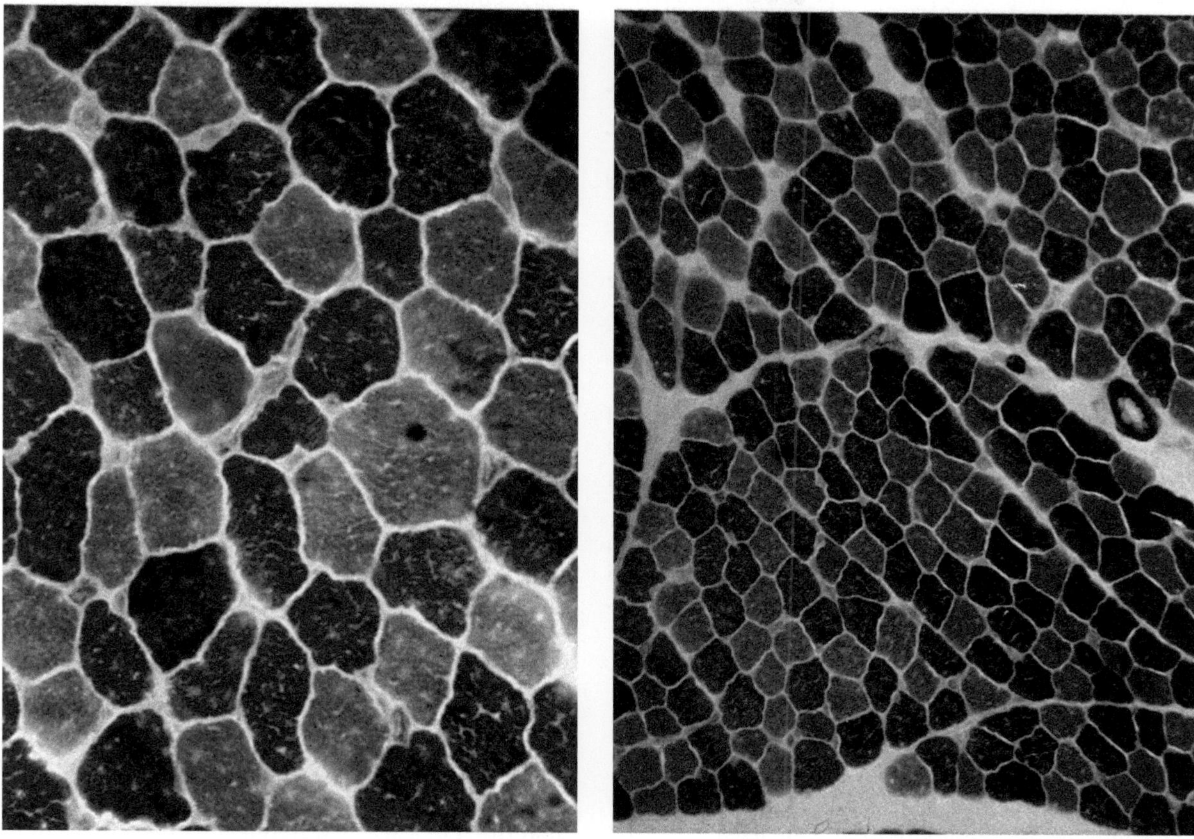

Fig. 2.1. Microscopic sections of the muscle fibers after histoenzymatic treatment. Type I fibers are darkly stained; type II fibers are lightly stained

dative enzymes. Subsequent to appropriate chemical treatment and preparation for microscopic examination, the fibers containing ATPase appear dark, those containing oxidative enzymes appear light, and a third category of fibers shows an intermediate degree of contrast (Fig. 2.1).

B. Results

In the long locomotor muscles of the limbs, one-third of the fibers are of the type I variety and two-thirds are of the type II variety [Dubowitz & Pearse 1960]. The abdominal wall muscles, on the other hand, display a clear predominance of type I fibers, as shown in table 2.2.

Several observations can be made regarding the results shown in this table: (a) type I (slow) fibers predominate over type II (fast) fibers in a proportion of 2/3-1/3 in all of the parietal muscles, except the exter-

Table 2.2. Mean percentages of type I and type II fibers in the muscles of the abdominal wall

	Fiber type				
	I (%)	II (%)	IIA (%)	IIB (%)	
Rectus	69	31	28	3	ATPase
abdominis	63	37			Glycerophosphate dehydrogenase
External	52	48			ATPase
oblique	54	46	40.9	5.1	Glycerophosphate dehydrogenase
Internal	64	36			ATPase
oblique	59	41	37.3	3.7	Glycerophosphate dehydrogenase
Transverse	68	32			ATPase
	60	40	37	3	Glycerophosphate dehydrogenase

Table 2.3. Percentages of type I and type II fibers in the levator ani and deltoid muscles

	Fiber type		
	I (%)	II (%)	
Levator ani	55	45	ATPase
	55	45	Glycerophosphate dehydrogenase
Deltoid	36	64	ATPase
	34	66	Glycerophosphate dehydrogenase

nal oblique, where the abundance of the two types of fibers is approximately equivalent; (b) type II B (fast fatigable) fibers are very scarce compared with type II A (fast resistant) fibers.

It is of some interest to compare these results with those of the histochemical analysis of the levator ani and deltoid (Table 2.3). It can be seen that the proportion of the two fiber types is quite different in the deltoid, i.e., two-thirds of the fibers are type II and one-third are type I.

C. Functional Deductions

The muscles of the abdominal wall have a special enzymatic apparatus with a predominance of type I (slow) and type II A (fast resistant) fibers. The type II B (fast fatigable) fibers are not absent, but their proportion is very small compared with the other fiber types. In sum, tonic and postural functions are the main attributes of the abdominal wall muscles.

II. Detailed Study of Function: Quantitative Kinesiological Electromyography of the Abdominal Wall Musculature

A. Principles of the Method

This technique involves global electromyography (EMG) using surface electrodes. Recordings are obtained during movement and then automatically analyzed in narrow frequency ranges.

1. Automatic Analysis of the Recordings

Such analysis is based on the method described by Willison (1963). For this purpose, the EMG apparatus (basic system: MS6 Medelec) is coupled to an additio-

nal module referred to as a potential analyzer (APA 62 Medelec). The automatic analysis is carried out over a predetermined time span of 1, 2, or 4 s. We selected an analysis time of l s, owing to the highly variable state of muscle capacity according to the subjects examined. The tracing obtained in the course of muscle contraction is instantaneously analyzed over a period of 1 s. The analyzer gives the following numerical data directly on the monitor screen or printout: (a) the cumulative sum of the signal amplitudes, expressed as the letter A (total amplitude); (b) the number of myoelectric signals, referred to as T (turns); (c) the mean signal amplitude, called M (mean amplitude).

2. Selection of Muscle Activities Within Narrow Frequency Spectra

The frequency range commonly used in clinical EMG is very large, i.e., 32 Hz to 3.2 kHz

Accordingly, many mixed signals are recorded with very different parameters of amplitude an frequency. However, the overall EMG pattern obtained allows interpretation of the recording.

By regulating a high-frequency and a low-frequency filter of the amplifiers of the EMG apparatus (amplifier AA6 III Medelec), the operator can vary the width of the frequency spectrum. Muscle activity can thus be quantified in a selected frequency range. Eight to ten frequency ranges were used in this study. Contraction of a given muscle was obtained for each frequency range and then analyzed:

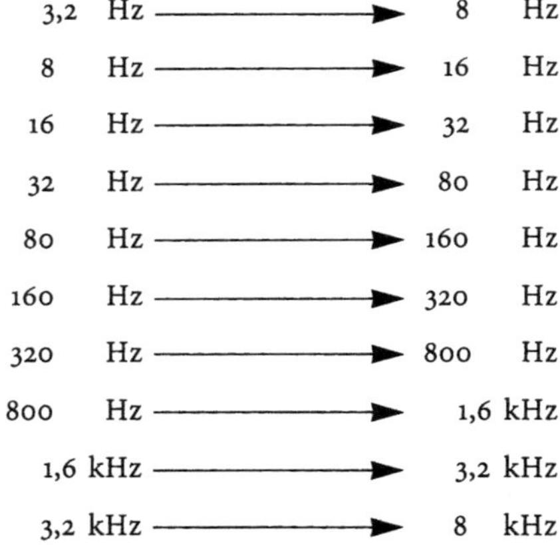

These different spectra cover the full frequency range used in clinical EMG, although the most significant values are obtained between 16 Hz and 3.2 kHz. In some muscles motor activity can be recorded up to a frequency of 8 kHz. Beyond this limit no coherent quantifiable activity is recorded.

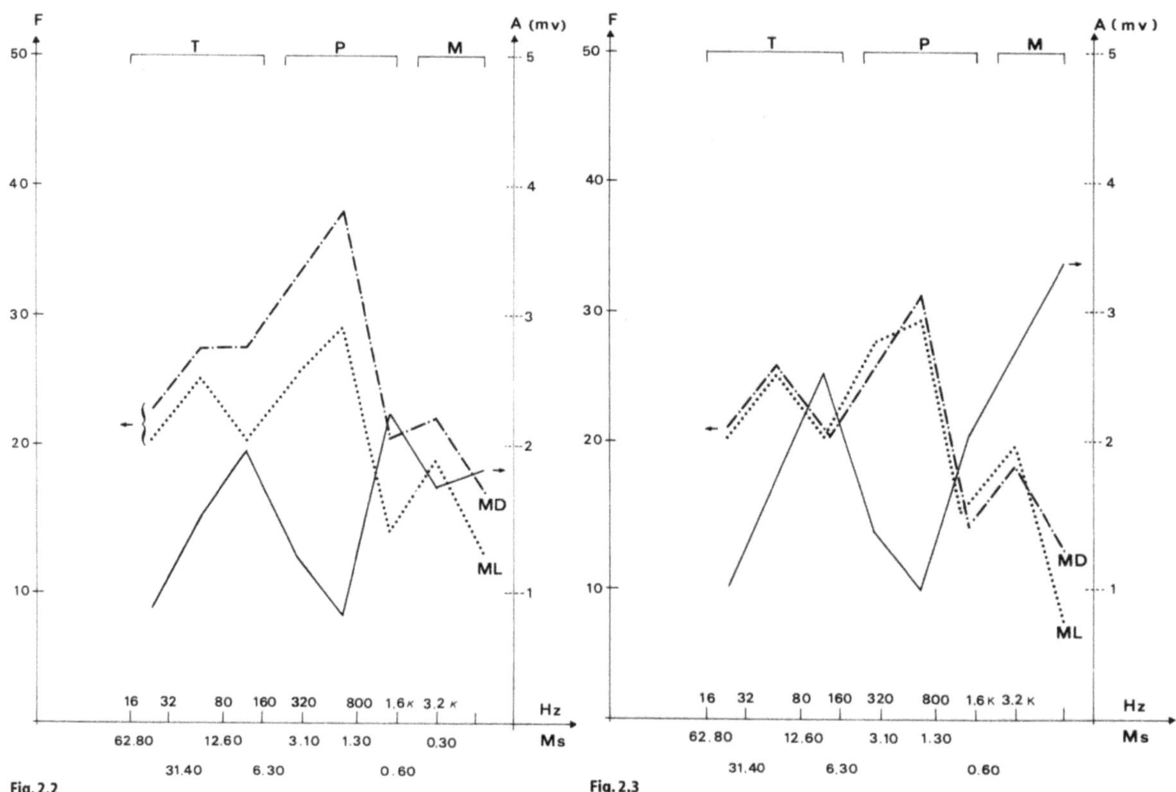

Fig. 2.2. Rectus and flat abdominal muscles. Note variation of frequency (*F*), in cycles/s, and amplitude (*A*), in millivolts, of the EMG signals as a function of signal width (*Ms*), in milliseconds. Mean values in 51 subjects. *MD* abdominal rectus; *ML* flat abdominal muscles: *T* tone; *P* posture; *M* movement; *Hz* frequency band; .... signal frequency in flat abdominal muscles (ordinate on *left*); _._._. signal frequency in rectus muscles (ordinate on *left*); __ signal amplitude as a function of signal width (ordinate on *right*)

Fig. 2.3. Rectus and flat abdominal muscles. Variation of frequency (*F*), in cycles/s, and amplitude (*A*) in millivolts, of EMG signals as a function of signal width (*Ms*) in milliseconds. Mean values in 35 men. Symbols as in legend to Fig. 2.2

B. Overall Results and Tentative Interpretation

The numerical data can be displayed graphically to show the number of signals per second (and their mean amplitude) in each frequency range explored. The graphic data in figures 2.2 and 2.3 give the results of the recordings of the rectus and flat abdominal muscles in two categories of subjects studied. Three types of motor activity were seen. The first arises in the 16 to 160 Hz range, the second in the 160 Hz to 1.6 kHz range, and the third in the 1.6-3.2 kHz range.

Another parameter given directly by the apparatus is the time constant of the signal, which is a function of the period and thus of the width of the signal. This constant is inversely proportional to the frequency[1].

The analysis of the different sectors of the full-frequency spectrum allows the classification of the signals as a function of their width, number, and amplitude. The latter two parameters are given directly by the automatic analysis.

Given the finding that the recorded signals display a different frequency, amplitude, and signal width, it can be concluded that these signals are produced by muscle fibers displaying different functions and physiological characteristics.

In an attempt to interpret these findings, we propose the hypothesis that the three categories of recorded motor activity correspond to the contraction of three functionally different populations of muscle fibers, as previously demonstrated by histochemical analysis:

---

[1] The time constant (τ) is a direct function of the signal period, according to the following formula: T (period) = $2\pi t$ and is inversely proportional to the frequency:

$$f \text{ (frequency in Hz)} = 1/T = 1/2\pi\tau$$

i.e., slow fibers, fast fibers resistant to fatigue (fast resistant fibers), and fast fatigable fibers. This hypothesis is based mainly on the notion of signal width.

Indeed, many studies have shown that there is a correlation between the histochemical structure of the motor units on the one hand, and their neurophysiological features on the other hand [Henneman & Olson 1965; Buchtal & Schmalbruck 1970; Sica et al. 1973; Warmolts & Engel 1973]. Burke (1973) stressed that the contraction time is one of the criteria for classification of the different types of motor units. Accordingly, it was postulated for the purpose of our study that the widest signals occurring in the low-frequency range corresponded to tonic activity, whereas the narrowest signals in the high-frequency range corresponded to phasic activity. Finally, the signals displaying an intermediate duration were considered to arise from postural activity of the muscle fibers.

An overall quantification of the results of this method allows the determination of the performance of the muscles of the abdominal wall with respect to the three modes of motor activity, i.e., tone, posture, and movement.

C. Results of the Method Applied to the Study of the Function of the Abdominal Wall Muscles

1. Technique

The activity of the parietal muscles was recorded using self-adhesive surface electrodes. For the recording of the activity of the rectus, the electrodes were placed in the paraumbilical region over a 10-cm-long area in the direction of the muscle fibers. The subject was requested to bend the trunk forward and to raise the shoulder and pelvic girdles and the lower limbs up to 30°.

The activity of the flat abdominal muscles was recorded by electrodes placed over the flanks between the 12th rib and the iliac crest. The electrodes were positioned in the direction of the fibers of the external oblique. The use of surface electrodes does not allow the identification of the activity of each of the flat abdominal muscles, and thus their overall activity is recorded. However, given these conditions, it is reasonable to assume that the activity of the external oblique contributes most to the EMG recording obtained. The recording of the flat abdominal muscles was performed while the subject turned the trunk contralaterally and at the same time elevated the shoulders, pelvis, and lower limbs.

The rectus and flat abdominal muscles were studied in 51 normal subjects. This heterogeneous population comprised the following subgroups: (a) according to sex: 35 men and 16 women; (b) according to the level of motor activity: 23 subjects not practicing sports and 28 athletic subjects (members of a sports club); (c) according to the ponderal index, which is an indicator of corpulence as a function of body weight and height, obtained by dividing the cube root of body weight by height: 16 lean subjects (ponderal index = 22-22.9); 20 average subjects (ponderal index = 23-23.9); 12 corpulent subjects (ponderal index = 24-24.9); three obese subjects (ponderal index = 25); (d) according to age: 14 subjects up to 20 years; 34 subjects between 21 and 50 years; three subjects over 50 years.

2. Comparative Performance of the Rectus and Flat Abdominal Muscles According to Study Subgroup

a) Assessment of Performance

The performance of a muscle can be estimated by the electrical potential produced in the course of a movement under a given load. The electrical potential is proportional to the load.

Electrical potential, expressed in millivolts, is given directly by the automatic analysis and appears on the monitor screen as the letter A, which corresponds to the total amplitude of the recording.

b) Results According to Subject Category

Once the zones of the frequency spectrum corresponding to tonic, postural, and phasic activity have been identified, it is possible to study the comparative performance of the abdominal muscles in each functional mode, i.e., tone, posture, and movement. The results of this study are expressed as histograms showing the

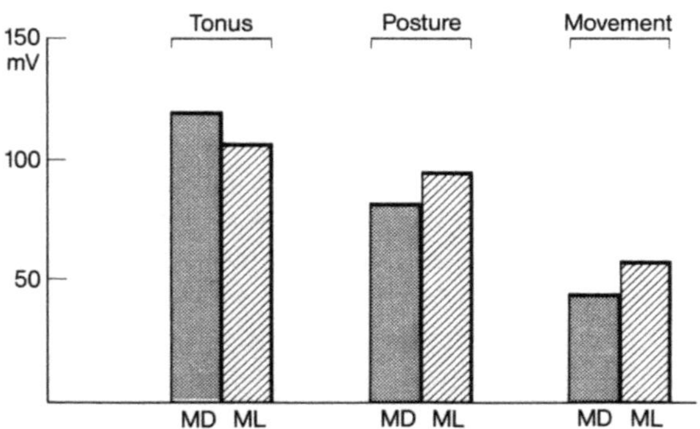

Fig. 2.4. Comparison of muscle activity in 51 subjects. *MD* m. rectus abdominis; *ML* flat abdominal muscles

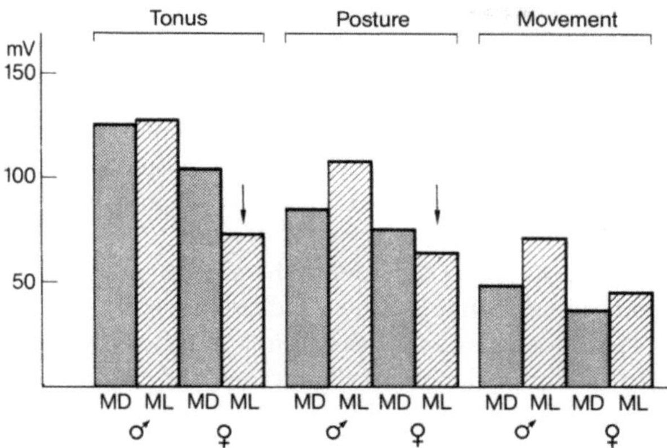

Fig. 2.5. Comparison of muscle activity in men and in women

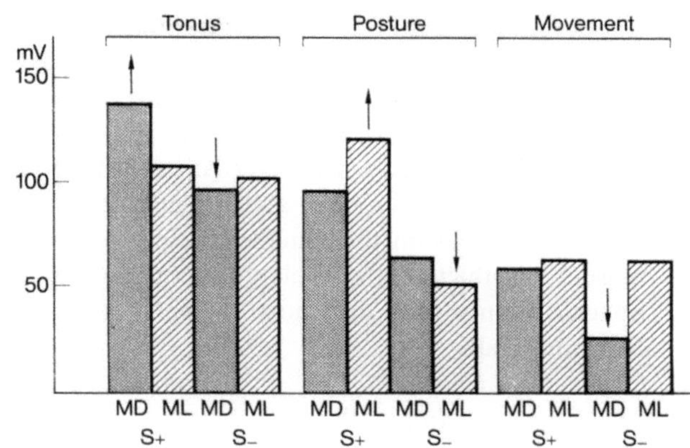

Fig. 2.6. Comparison of muscle activity in athletic and nonathletic subjects

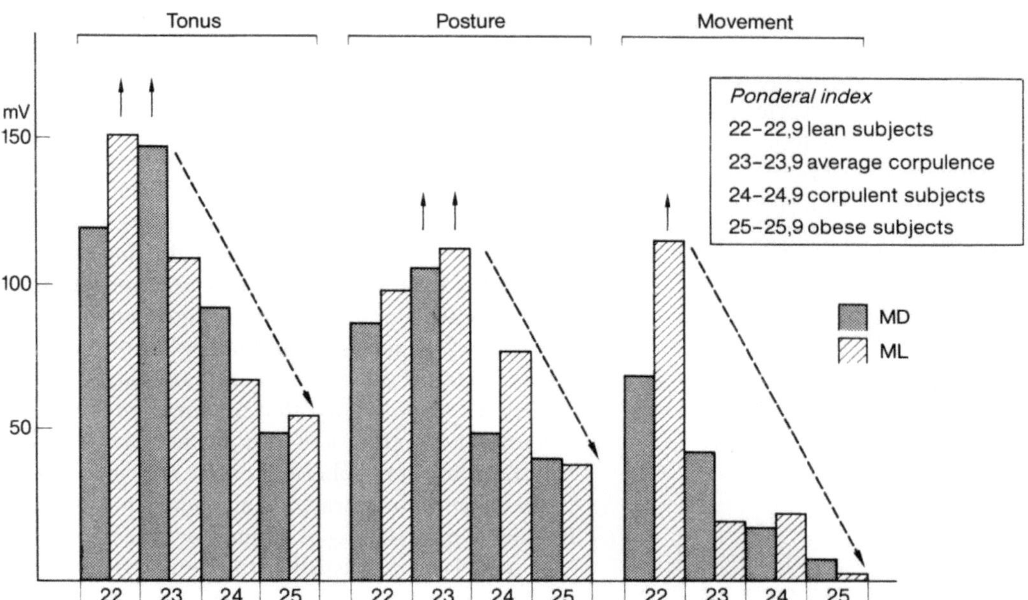

Fig. 2.7. Comparison of muscle activity according to the ponderal index. *MD* m. rectus abdominis; *ML* flat abdominal muscles

electrical potential, recorded in millivolts, during the contraction of the muscles in the different study groups.

The Whole Study Group. The histogram in figure 2.4 shows that tonic and postural activity predominate over phasic activity. Furthermore, it can be seen that the flat abdominal muscles show a much greater performance in posture and movement compared with the rectus, whereas the latter displays the most pronounced tonic activity.

Males versus Females. The overall muscular activity of the abdominal wall is greater in men than in women (Fig. 2.5). Comparative study of the different muscles in women shows that the activity of the flat abdominal muscles is significantly lower than that of the rectus muscles regarding tone and posture. Thus, the flat abdominal muscles are weakest (most vulnerable) in women.

Athletic versus Nonathletic Subjects. The overall muscular performance of the abdominal wall is greater in athletic than in nonathletic subjects (Fig. 2.6). The gain in performance owing to the practice of sports involves the tone of the rectus and the posture of the flat abdominal muscles. In nonathletic subjects the comparatively reduced performance involves the tone and movement of the rectus and the posture of the other muscles. In sum, the benefits obtained by sports (most of the athletic subjects played soccer and rugby) concern mainly tone and postural activity of the abdominal wall.

Subgroups According to Ponderal Index. As a general rule, muscular performance declines rapidly as the ponderal index increases toward obesity (Fig. 2.7). Regarding tone, the highest level of performance is seen in the flat abdominal muscles of lean subjects (thin-waisted subjects) and in the rectus muscles of average subjects. The subjects of average corpulence show the best results with respect to posture, whereas movement (phasic activity) is greatest in lean subjects (especially of the flat abdominal muscles). It can also be seen that the capacities of the abdominal wall of obese subjects are greatly reduced regarding tone and posture and are practically nil with respect to movement (especially the flat abdominal muscles).

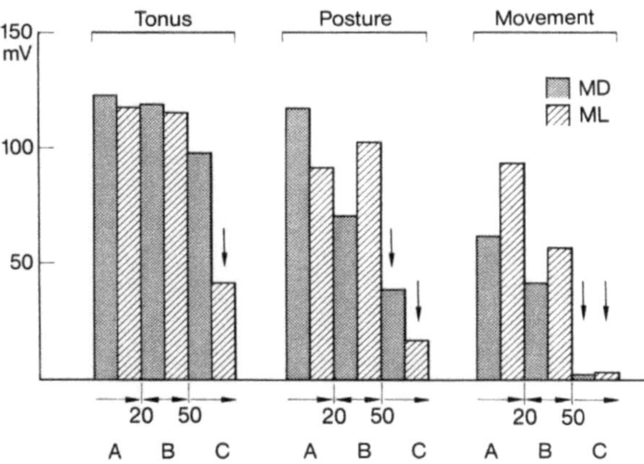

Fig. 2.8. Comparison of muscle activity according to age

Subgroups According to Age. Abdominal wall performance is markedly reduced in the over-50 age-group (Fig. 2.8). The decrease in tonic and postural activity involves the flat abdominal muscles, whose performance in movement is practically nil. It can thus be concluded that the flat abdominal muscles are weakest (most vulnerable) in this age group.

III. Study of Intra-abdominal Pressure in Operated Patients

The peritoneal cavity is a virtual space containing very little fluid and presents no exterior communications except, theoretically, the fallopian tubes in women. It is, in fact, a closed cavity.

Wildegas (1923) considered the abdomen, from the mechanical standpoint, a closed container formed by a rigid posterior wall - the spine - and flexible walls - the abdominal muscles, diaphragm, and pelvic floor. Thus, the infra-abdominal pressure can increase in only two conditions, i.e., contraction of the parietal muscles and acute distension of the abdominal viscera.

A. History

The first studies on this subject can be found in the lessons published by Paul Bert in 1870 on the comparative physiology of respiration. To achieve his measurements, Bert placed a small balloon in the ampulla of the rectum in dogs. Winckler et al. (1980) were the first to measure intra-abdominal pressure by installing a trocar in the peritoneal cavity of the dog and then connecting the instrument to a water manometer.

Two studies later became authoritative references on the subject of infra-abdominal pressure. Overholt (1931) installed intraperitoneal cannulas in dogs. Overholt's work showed that the mean pressure was low (about 8 cm H_2O), or even nil, and was less than the prevailing atmospheric pressure in some animals. It was also demonstrated that abdominal pressure fluctuated only slightly as a function of respiration.

In 1948, Drye published a study on intraperitoneal pressure in man. His investigations demonstrated a mean pressure of 8 cm H_2O. With the subject supine, no difference in pressure was found between the hypochondrium and the pouch of Douglas. Conversely, with the subject standing, pressure of the hydrostatic type was noted, i.e., increased pressure in the lowest regions. The effort of vomiting was found to markedly increase abdominal pressure to over 80 cm H_2O. Fluctuations of pressure related to respiration were small, as evidenced by a pressure increase of 3 cm H_2O on inspiration. In 1955, Campbell studied the function of the abdominal muscles in relation to intra-abdominal pressure and respiration.

In France, Barraya et al. (1978) investigated the drainage of the abdominal cavity. The results of this work confirmed those described above and added new

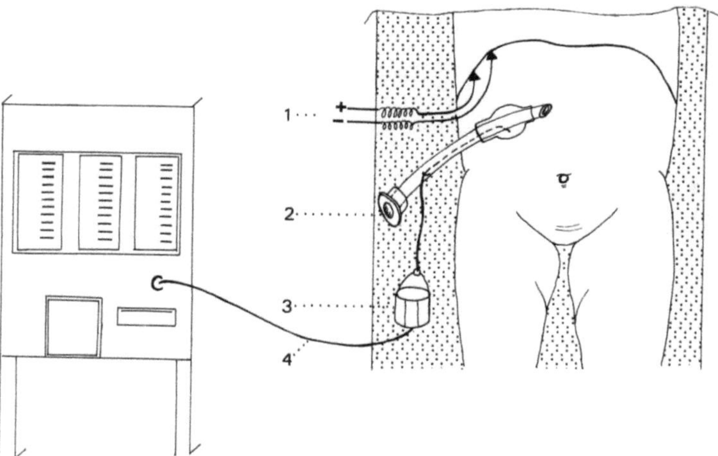

Fig. 2.9. Technique of measurement of intra-abdominal pressure and position of the EMG electrodes in the diaphragm. *1* Diaphragmatic electrodes; *2* intubation cannula with balloon; *3* Bentley pressure head; *4* recording apparatus

information on the circulation of the intraperitoneal fluid.

Delhez (1974) devoted an important chapter in his thesis to the electromyographic study of respiratory and abdominal muscular synergy. In a very interesting study, Grillner et al. (1977) investigated the role of the closed abdominal cavity acting as a pressure absorber in equilibrium with the spine. The following year, Diamant et al. (1978) studied the hemodynamic effects of increased intra-abdominal pressure. Finally, Flament and Clément (1979) described the fluctuations of abdominal pressure in relation to respiration.

B. Materials and Methods

Abdominal pressure was studied in 20 patients (12 men, 8 women) who had undergone abdominal surgery requiring tubular drainage. Owing to our reservations about placing pressure transducers directly in the human abdominal cavity, drainage and pressure recordings were achieved via low-pressure endotracheal cannulas of the type used in anesthesia. This type of cannula is sterile and atraumatic and has a lateral opening to assist drainage. Furthermore, the inner diameter is similar to that of the Silastic drainage tubes commonly used in abdominal surgery. The end of the cannula is fitted with a very malleable, low-pressure, inflatable balloon connected to a catheter. After installing the cannula, the balloon is inflated using a syringe, care being taken not to exceed 7 ml of air. Inflated in this way the balloon is not fully expan-

ded. Accordingly, its elasticity is nil and the pressure transmitted reflects the intra-abdominal pressure.

The balloon is then connected via a catheter to a pressure transducer (Bentley-Trantec model), which is in turn connected to an electronic pressure recorder (Philips model). The system must be calibrated prior to measurement with the zero setting corresponding to atmospheric pressure. The results obtained are thus given with respect to atmospheric pressure reference (Fig. 2.9).

In sum, intra-abdominal pressure acts on the balloon, which yields a measurement of this pressure. The recording device gives an instantaneous digital display of the intra-abdominal pressure (in mmHg) and a recording on millimetric paper. For each patient, 14 measurements were made in the subhepatic region, nine in the pouch of Douglas, and five in both regions simultaneously. For each recording, baseline pressure was first measured, followed by the pressure variations elicited by respiratory movements, speech, coughing, and efforts to defecate.

All measurements were made on the patient supine. Indeed, when the subject is standing the balloon in the pouch of Douglas is compressed by the weight of the abdominal viscera and thus no longer transmits the intra-abdominal pressure. In other terms, when the patient is standing, the pressure recorded in the pelvic region corresponds to the sum of the intra-abdominal pressure plus the weight of the viscera exerting a hydrostatic pressure. Pressure recordings were made every day from the first to fourth postoperative days, after which the drains were systematically removed.

C. Results

1. Baseline Pressure

a) First Postoperative Day

The mean pressure in the subhepatic region was 9.5 mmHg, but marked interindividual variability was noted (range: 7-21 mmHg). The mean pressure in the pouch of Douglas was 11 mmHg.

b) Fourth Postoperative Day

The mean pressure in the subhepatic region decreased to 7.8 mmHg, and little variability was seen according to subjects (range: 7-10 mmHg). In the pouch of Douglas the mean pressure was 9 mmHg.

2. Respiratory Modifications

Normal respiration modified the intra-abdominal pressure only slightly, the latter rising 1 mmHg on inspiration (Fig. 2.10). Deep inspiration led to a greater rise in pressure, although it did not exceed 4 mmHg (Fig. 2.11).

3. Effort of Defecation with Blocking of Expiration

The measurement of intra-abdominal pressure in the course of such effort showed a synchronous rise in the pressure of the hypochondrium and the pouch of Douglas, the pressure attaining 15 mmHg in both regions (Fig. 2.12). In normal subjects one would obviously expect an even greater pressure increase under these conditions.

4. Modulation of Abdominal Pressure by Speech

In contrast to breathing, speech led to more significant pressure fluctuations, especially in the course of loud speech (Fig. 2.13).

5. Effects of Coughing on Abdominal Pressure

Coughing was seen to be the factor leading to the greatest rise in intra-abdominal pressure. However, voluntary coughing was relatively unproductive and led to peak pressures of 30 mmHg on average, whereas productive, spontaneous coughing induced pronounced pressure increases with peak pressure often exceeding 80 mmHg (Fig. 2.14).

D. Comments

Resting baseline abdominal pressure was very low (about 8 mmHg) and relatively constant from patient to patient. These results are thus in agreement with classical data on this subject. In the supine position no significant pressure difference was seen in the different regions of the abdominal cavity. This result is logical, since the normal abdomen is not a compartmentalized structure.

Classical studies [Overholt 1931; Drye 1948] show that abdominal pressure in the standing position is of the hydrostatic type, i.e., pressure is greatest in the

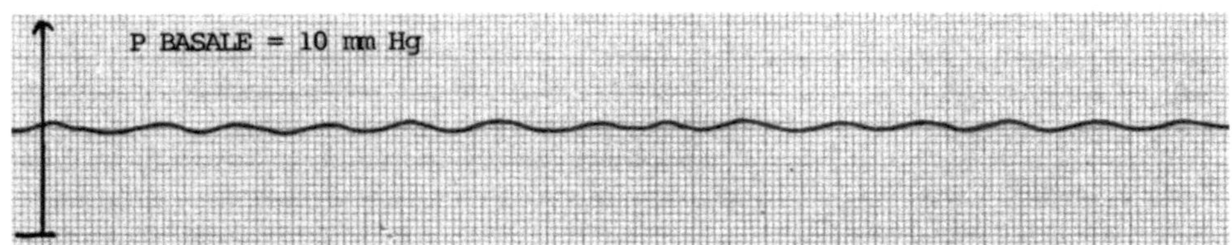

Fig. 2.10. Fluctuation of intra-abdominal pressure during normal respiration

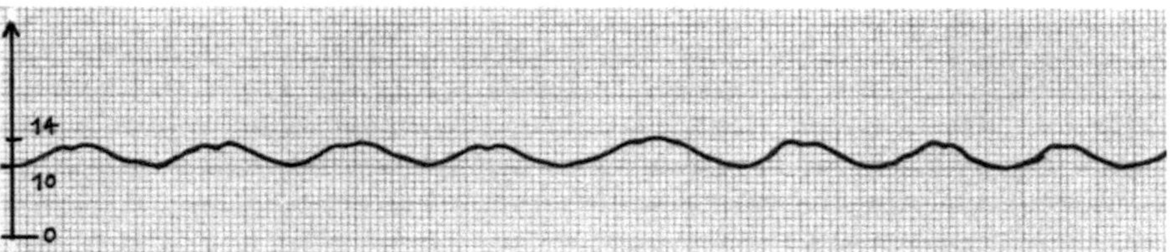

Fig. 2.11. Modification of intra-abdominal pressure during deep inspiration

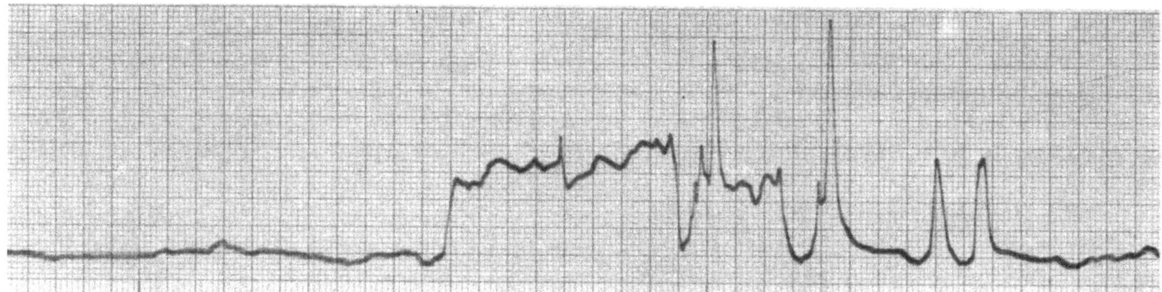

Fig. 2.12. Increased abdominal pressure during efforts to defecate, which led to two bouts of productive coughing

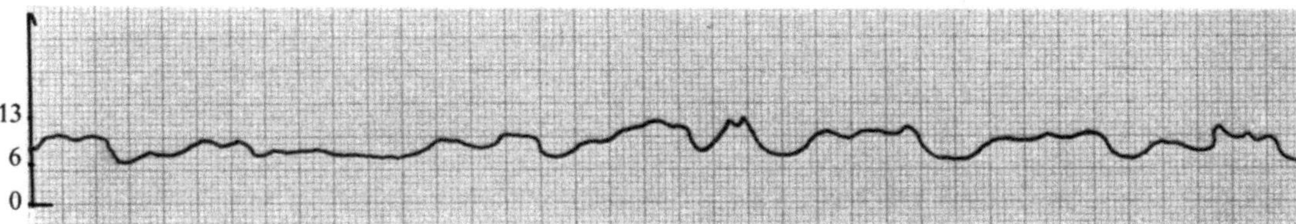

Fig. 2.13. Modulation of abdominal pressure during speech

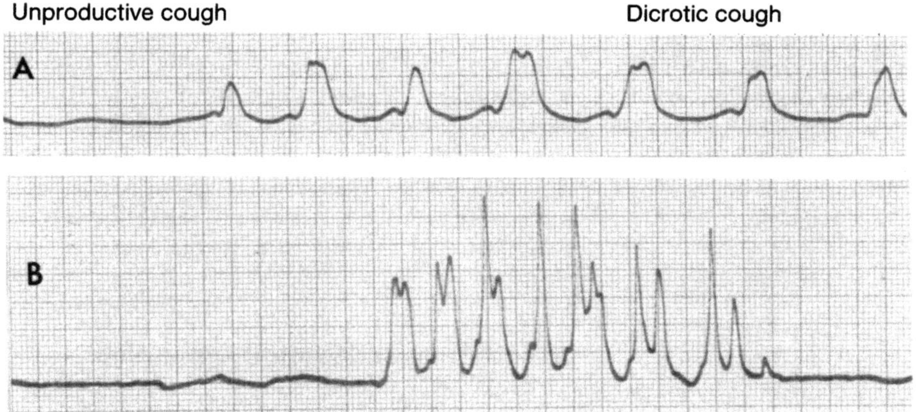

Fig. 2.14. Repercussions of coughing on abdominal pressure. *A* Voluntary cough; *B* spontaneous cough

lowermost regions of the abdomen. Under these conditions there is a threefold increase of the pressure in the pelvic region. With the subject upright, the pressure measured in the pouch of Douglas corresponds, in fact, to the weight of the abdominal and pelvic viscera. This pressure should be distinguished from the intraperitoneal pressure, as studied above, during effort and movement.

The use of the measurement technique described herein showed rather interesting results regarding the course of abdominal pressure in the postoperative period. Indeed, abdominal pressure was highest and more variable on the first postoperative day than on the fourth day, by which time pain had diminished and intestinal transit had been reestablished.

Normal respiration, related mainly to the action of the diaphragm, influences intraperitoneal pressure to a very slight extent. Special emphasis should be given to the role of the muscles of the anterolateral abdominal wall whose action to increase this pressure is required in speech, efforts to defecate, and especially in coughing. Indeed, the highest levels of peak pressure (above 80 mmHg) were found during productive coughing. The section below describes the cough mechanism, based on electromyography of the diaphragm and abdominal wall muscles.

IV. Correlation of the Activity of the Diaphragm and Abdominal Wall Muscles with Intra-abdominal Pressure

A. Material and Methods

In five patients the measurement of intra-abdominal pressure was associated with direct electromyographic recordings of the right diaphragmatic cupula. Wire EMG electrodes were implanted intraoperatively in the fibers of the diaphragm, thus allowing simultaneous measurement of diaphragmatic contraction and intra-abdominal pressure during normal respiration, forced inspiration, coughing, and efforts to defecate (Fig. 2.9). Finally, in a few operated patients surface electrodes were positioned on the abdominal wall to record the electrical activity of the abdominal muscles along with intra-abdominal pressure, as described above.

B. Results

1. With Normal Respiration

During normal respiration (Fig. 2.15) the EMG owed mainly the electrical activity of the diaphragm, whose potentials of motor activity are grouped together in phase with respiration. The activity of the abdominal muscles was very low and did not show any obvious rhythm with respect to normal respiration.

2. With Deep Inspiration

During deep inspiration (Fig. 2.16) pronounced diaphragmatic activity was evidenced as increased spatial and temporal recruitment accompanied by increased signal amplitude. The activity of the abdominal muscles was practically nil during the inspiratory phase but increased during expiration.

3. During Effort of Coughing

Mainly diaphragmatic activity was recorded during inspiration and until closure of the glottis (Fig. 2.17). However, when the glottis opened, allowing rapid expulsion of air under pressure, pronounced activity of the abdominal muscles was observed coupled with marked intermittent activity of the diaphragm in synchrony with the peaks of abdominal pressure increments up to 20 mmHg.

4. Infra-abdominal Pressure and Circulatory Physiology

Increased abdominal pressure contributes to the drainage of blood from the inferior vena cava to the right atrium and also induces a rise in capillary pressure. During walking and running, this phasic muscular activity acts like a pump to drive the abdominal venous blood upward against the forces of gravity, in harmony with the venous drainage of the lower limbs. At rest intra-abdominal pressure is obviously less than central venous pressure; if the opposite were true, the inferior vena cava would collapse.

In pathology, the severity of circulatory disturbances resulting from protracted occlusive syndromes is beginning to be understood. In such cases surgical decompression may be necessary, even in the absence of an identifiable mechanical obstacle. Indeed, this situation can be likened to a vicious circle, since venous compression can lead to circulatory and metabolic disturbances which increase the ileus.

V. Conclusions and Surgical Applications

The abdominal muscles exhibit mainly tone and postural functions, since they act as a retaining device for the abdominal viscera. The flat abdominal muscles are

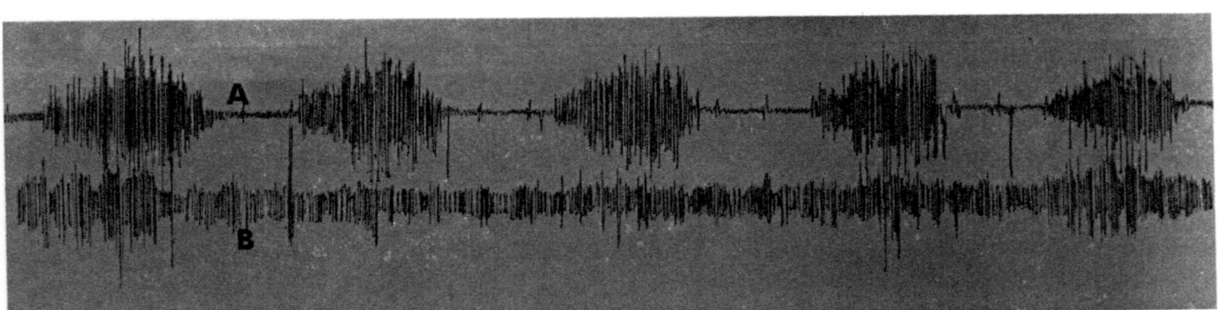

Fig. 2.15. Normal respiration: *above*, rhythmic activity of diaphragm; *below*, activity of abdominal wall muscles. *A* EMG of diaphragm, *B* EMG of flat abdominal muscles

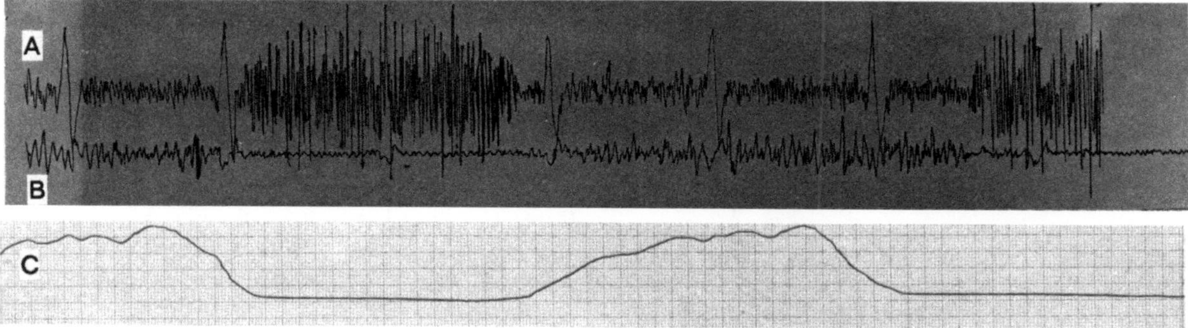

Fig. 2.16. Deep inspiration. *A* Diaphragm, *B* abdominal muscles, *C* abdominal pressure

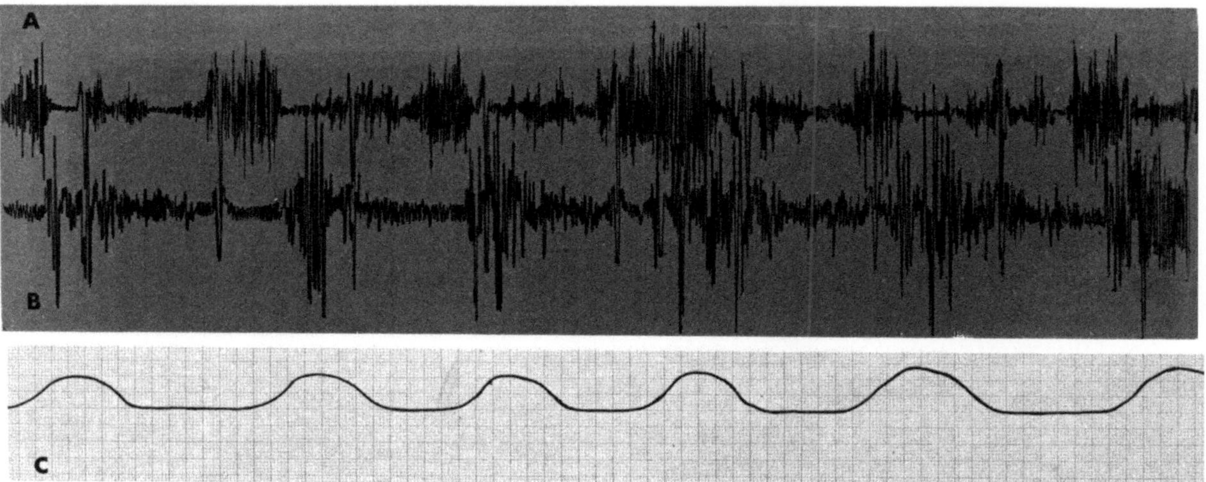

Fig. 2.17. Simultaneous recordings made during coughing efforts; *A* EMG of diaphragm; *B* EMG of flat abdominal muscles; *C* abdominal pressure

the most vulnerable, especially in women, and are the first to show signs of parietal deterioration related to age and obesity.

Infra-abdominal pressure at rest is low. It is slightly increased by deep respiration and markedly rises on coughing and efforts to defecate. Abdominal pressure is also higher in the very early postoperative period.

Surgical applications can be outlined on the basis of these conclusions. Prior to operation the surgeon should at least subjectively assess the quality of the abdominal musculature and establish the prognosis of the parietal repair. Surgical approaches to the abdominal wall are discussed elsewhere in this book. Nevertheless, it is reasonable to surmise from the above findings that transverse sections of the muscles, especially the flat abdominal muscles, will cause the greatest damage. Approaches based on muscular separation would thus seem preferable to the former, the operative field being enlarged by transaction of aponeurotic zones (linea alba, semilunar line, transverse

section of the posterior lamina of the rectus sheath with preservation of rectus continuity). At the end of the operation, a wise procedure may be to relieve the intravisceral hyperpressure by minimal enterostomy requiring only simple closure.

Finally, early postoperative rehabilitation of the respiratory apparatus and abdominal wall should be considered together. At this postoperative stage, electrical stimulation of motor activity of the abdominal wall leads to rapid recuperation of the natural muscle tone and to intraperitoneal "mixing", which promotes the resumption of intestinal transit.

References

Barraya L, Ndjaga MBA, Carles R (1978) Physiopathologie du péritoine, péritonisation drainage. Techniques chirurgicales Appareil digestif: 4303. Encycl Med Chir, Paris, 40070 1-16

Bert P (1870) Leçons sur la physiologie comparée de la respiration. Baillière, Paris, pp 338-346

Buchtal F, Schmalbruck H (1970) Contraction times and fiber types in intact human muscle. Acta Physiol Scand 79: 435-455

Burke RE (1973) On the central nervous system control of fast- and slow-twitch motor units. In: Desmedt JE (ed) New developments in electromyography and clinical neurophysiology, vol 3. Karger, Basel, pp 69-94

Campbell EJM (1955) The functions of the abdominal muscles in relation to the intra-abdominal pressures and the respiration. Arch Middx Hosp 5: 87-94

Delhez L (1974) Contribution électromyographique à l'étude de la mécanique et du contrôle nerveux des mouvements respiratoires de l'homme. Vaillant-Carmanne, Liege

Diamant M, Benumof JL, Saidman LJ (1978) Hemodynamics of increased intra-abdominal pressure. Anesthesiology 48: 23-27

Drye JC (1948) Intraperitoneal pressure in the human. Surg Gynecol Obstet 87: 472-475

Dubowitz V, Pearse AG (1960) A comparative histochemical study of oxidative enzyme and phosphorylase activity in skeletal muscle. Histochemie 2: 105-117

Engel WK, Burke RE, Tsairis P, Levine DN, Zajac III FE (1973) Direct correlation of physiological and histochemical characteristics in motor units of cat triceps surae muscle. In: Desmedt JE (ed) New developments in electromyography and clinical neurophysiology, vol I. Karger, Basel, pp 23-30

Flament JB, Clément C (1979) Les variations de la pression abdominale dans la région sous-diaphragmatique au cours de la respiration. Importance physiologique du cloisonnement anatomique. Nouvelle Presse Medicale 8: 612-613

Grillner S, Nilson J, Thorstensson A (1977) Intra-abdominal pressure changes during natural movements in man. Acta Physiol Scand 103: 275-283

Henneman E, Olson CB (1965) Observations between structure and function in the design of skeletal muscles. J Neurophysiol 28: 581-598

Mayer RF (1973) Observations on motor units in cat anterior tibial muscle. In: Desmedt JE (ed) New developments in electromyography and neurophysiology, vol 1, Karger, Basel, pp 31-34

Overholt R (1931) Intraperitoneal pressure. Arch Surg 22: 691-703

Pans A, Pierard GE, Albert A, Desaive C (1997) Biomechanical assessment of the transversalis fascia and rectus abdominis aponeurosis in inguinal herniation. Preliminary results. Hernia 1: 27-30

Sica REP, McComas AJ, Ferreira JCD (1978) Evaluation of an automated method for analysing the electromyogram. Can J Neurol Sci 5: 275-281

Warmolts JR, Engel WK (1973) Correlation of motor unit behavior with histochemical myofiber type in humans by open biopsy electromyography. In: Desmedt JE (ed) New developments in electromyography and clinical neurophysiology, vol 1. Karger, Basel, pp 35-40

Wildegas H (1923) Messen des intraperitonealen Druckes. Mitt Grenzgeb Med Chir 37: 308

Willison RG (1963) A method of measuring motor unit activity in human muscle. J Physiol 168: 35-36

Winckler K, Heriksen JH, Stage JG, Schlichting P (1980) Intraperitoneal pressure: ascitic fluid and splanchnic vascular pressures, and their role in prevention and formation of ascites. Scand J Clin Lab Invest 40: 493-502

3 Procedures for Investigation of the Abdominal Wall

J. Hureau
with the collaboration of
J. Taboury, J. Pradel-Raynal and J. L. Dumas

I. Echography of the Abdominal Wall

J. Taboury

In daily practice, study of the abdominal wall accounts for only a very small percentage of echographic procedures performed to investigate the abdomen.

Over a period of 8 years, during which more than 30,000 echography procedures were done in our busy, hospital practice, the study of the abdominal wall was requested by the departments of medicine or surgery (adults) only a few dozen times. This lack of demand is due to the easy clinical access to, and the apparent simplicity of the problems encountered in the pathology of the abdominal wall.

The section to follow presents an outline of the echographic features of the normal and pathological abdominal wall. From the practical standpoint, echography of the abdominal wall is of little diagnostic interest compared with clinical data (history of the disease, general history, physical examination). Regarding the assistance afforded by echography in certain cases of difficult diagnosis, e.g., hernia of the semilunar line, the number of published cases is too limited to allow conclusions about the real impact and reliability of this investigative procedure.

A. Technique of Echographic Investigation

The reduced thickness and peripheral localization of the constituent structures of the abdominal wall require that a special approach to echographic investigation be used.

The ultrasonic probes used in routine echography give little or no useful information in the first part of the ultrasonic spectrum (Fresnel's zone) when the probe is applied directly to the skin. Furthermore, the standard frequency of 3.5 MHz, used routinely, has been selected to allow the focalized ultrasonic beam to travel several tens of centimeters but with poor resolution, especially near the surface.

One technical modification for exploring the abdominal wall consists in placing a water bag between the skin and the probe head. In this way the surface planes (abdominal wall) lie at a distance where resolution of the ultrasonic beam is greatest (focal zone). However, the disadvantage remains regarding the use of a mean frequency of 3.5 MHz, which leads to poor resolution.

It is thus preferable, when studying the abdominal wall, to use small-diameter, high-frequency probes (5.7 or even 10 MHz), allowing better resolution with low penetration. This type of probe is placed directly on the skin or on a small interposed water bag, depending on the focal properties of the probe.

Under these technical conditions, an apparatus equipped with either manual or automatic scanning can be used (sectorial or rectangular field of exploration). The main advantage of the manual echograph is its large scanning field, whereas the automatic type of apparatus facilitates dynamic (muscle contraction) and static investigation (patient standing).

B. Echographic Anatomy of the Abdominal Wall

The anatomy of the abdominal wall [Bader & Mellière 1970] - more correctly its echographic representation - is highly variable [Morley & Barnett 1978], depending on the echographic technique used and especially the morphology of the subject under study (muscles more or less developed, fat more or less abundant; Figs. 3.1-3.4). The thinner the abdominal muscles (rectus, obliques and transverse), the less visible they are. Abundant fat yields echographic images of mediocre quality. The ideal subject for echographic investigation of the abdominal wall is a young, muscular man. Conversely, elderly, obese, multiparous women are poor study subjects.

1. Epidermis and Dermis

These superficial layers usually present as a single, homogeneous, echo-reflecting band (Fig. 3.1a).

2. Hypodermis

The thickness of the hypodermis varies considerably according to the amount of subcutaneous fat. The hypodermis is more or less visible in the form of a band of variable thickness and irregular contours. Its echostructure is less pronounced than that of the epidermis and dermis [Vincens & Bigot 1983]. The hypodermis displays a heterogeneous aspect owing to the lobulation of the adipose tissue (Fig. 3.1a, b).

3. Muscles of the Abdominal Wall

These muscles form two groups (Figs. 3.2 & 3.3). The rectus muscles run longitudinally on either side of the midline. The three *flat abdominal muscles* (external oblique, internal oblique, and transverse) can be seen to spread mainly over the flanks.

The echostructure of these muscles usually appears hypoechogenic and homogeneous, with fine internal

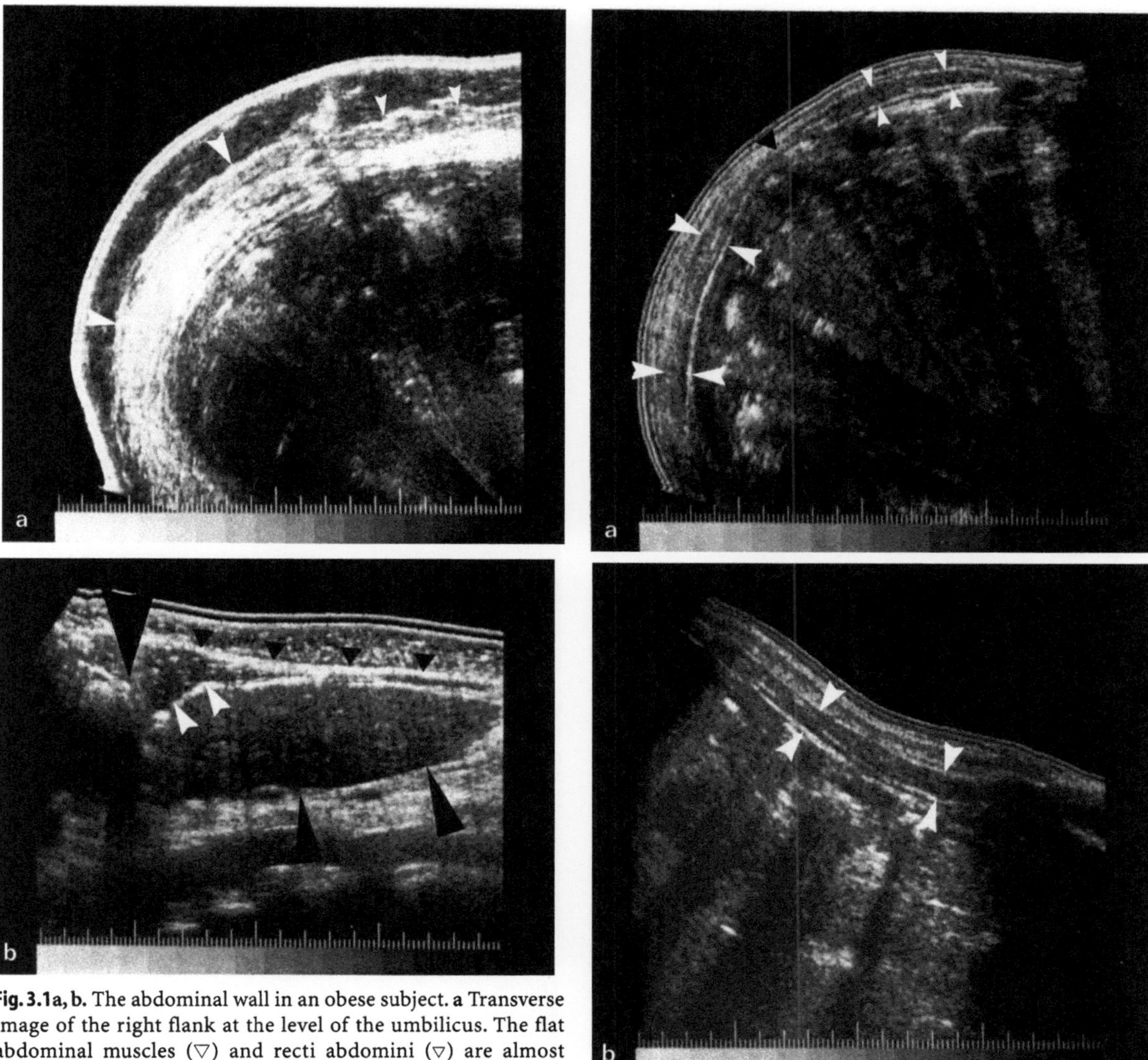

Fig. 3.1a, b. The abdominal wall in an obese subject. **a** Transverse image of the right flank at the level of the umbilicus. The flat abdominal muscles (▽) and recti abdomini (▽) are almost impossible to see since they are thin and hidden in the abundant areolar tissue and extraperitoneal subparietal and aponeurotic fat. The thick areolar hypodermic tissue is clearly visible between the cutaneous layer and myofascial structures.
b Longitudinal median xiphoumbilical image. The abundant extraperitoneal subparietal areolar tissue (▼) near the tip of the xiphoid process (△) should not be mistaken for a pathological collection of fluid. This subparietal tissue is limited anteriorly by the linea alba (▼) and posteriorly by the anterior surface of the left part of the liver (▲)

Fig. 3.2a, b. The normal abdominal wall. **a** Transverse imaging of the right hemiabdomen at the level of the umbilicus. The flat abdominal muscles (▽) are connected to the recti abdomini (△) by Spigelius' semilunar aponeurosis (▼). **b** Longitudinal imaging of the right loin region. The three flat abdominal muscles (▽) are separated medially from the abdominal viscera by a fine echogenic band corresponding to the peritoneum

parallel lines of greater echoreflection. The latter are visible only where the muscles are particularly well developed. These flat abdominal muscles display well defined contours, always bordered by a thin, highly echogenic line corresponding to their aponeurotic envelope.

In muscular subjects the rectus muscles are especially well developed at the level of and below the umbilicus. The three flat abdominal muscles, clearly visible in the flanks, can sometimes be distinguished as three different layers, separated by their aponeuroses (Fig. 3.3).

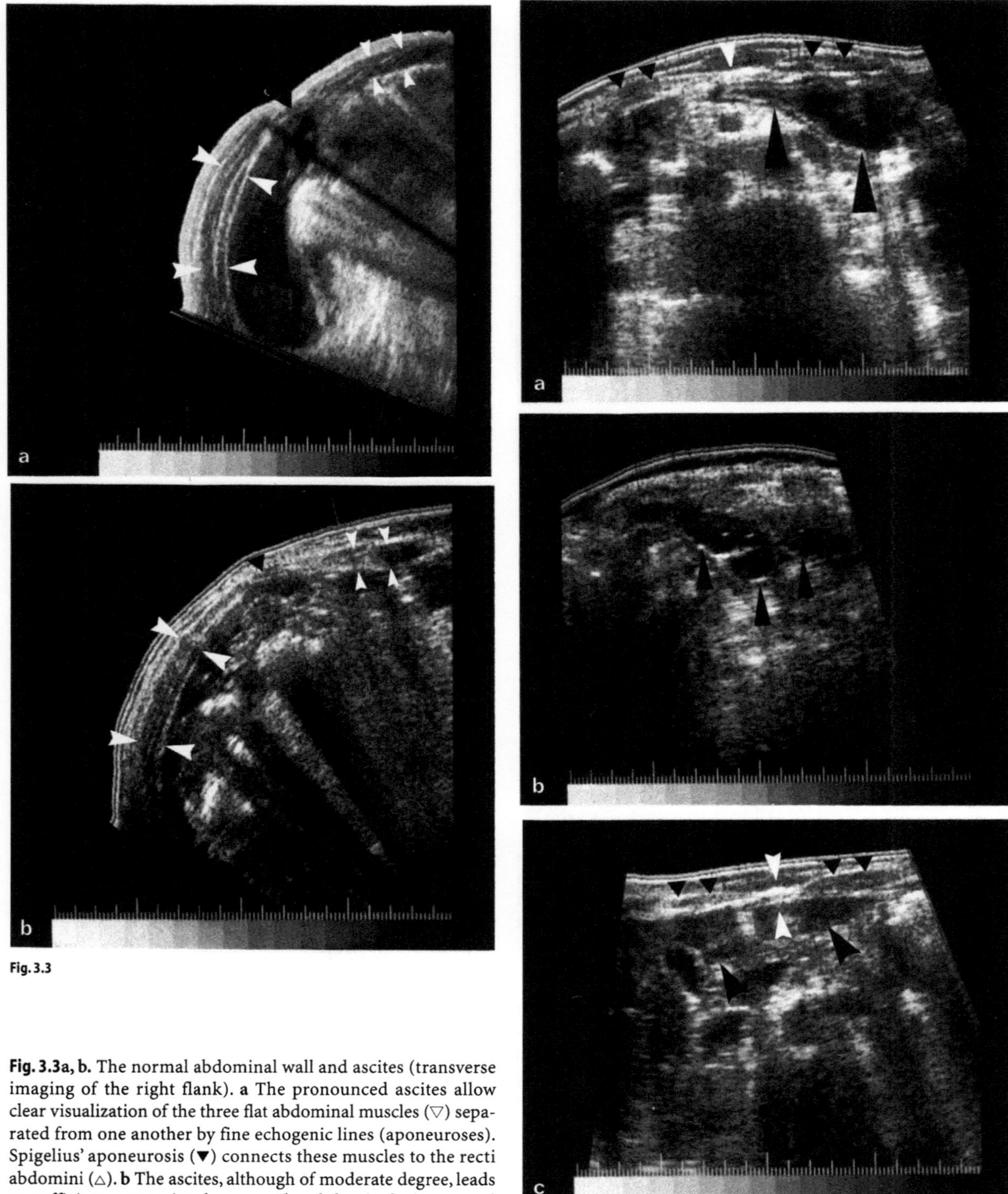

Fig. 3.3

Fig. 3.4

Fig. 3.3a, b. The normal abdominal wall and ascites (transverse imaging of the right flank). **a** The pronounced ascites allow clear visualization of the three flat abdominal muscles ($\triangledown$) separated from one another by fine echogenic lines (aponeuroses). Spigelius' aponeurosis ($\blacktriangledown$) connects these muscles to the recti abdomini ($\triangle$). **b** The ascites, although of moderate degree, leads to sufficient separation between the abdominal viscera and abdominal wall to clearly show the muscles and aponeuroses

Fig. 3.4a-c. The normal abdominal wall and its visceral relations. **a** Median transverse image of the subxiphoid region. The stomach, voluntarily filled with water ($\blacktriangle$), is clearly visible deep to the recti abdomini ($\blacktriangledown$) and linea alba ($\triangledown$). **b** Transverse image of the right paraumbilical region. The jejunum, containing water, can be seen deep to the abdominal wall ($\blacktriangle$). The flat abdominal muscles, thin in this region, are practically no longer visible. **c** Median transverse image of the subxiphoid region. The left part of the liver ($\blacktriangle$) is visible beneath the recti abdomini ($\blacktriangledown$) and the linea alba ($\triangledown$)

4. Sheaths and Aponeuroses

These structures form the envelopes of the rectus and flat abdominal muscles and determine their respective zones of insertion. The aponeuroses appear as fine echogenic lines around the muscle masses, or between them in the case of the three flat abdominal muscles (Fig. 3.3). These fibrous structures connect the muscles to one another and attach them to the skeleton. Two aponeurotic zones are particularly well evidenced on echography. The first of these is the linea alba, a thick aponeurotic layer uniting the rectus muscles on the midline and extending from the xiphoid process to the pubic symphysis (Fig. 3.4a-c). The second is the semilunar line (Spigelius line), connecting the flat abdominal muscles to the lateral margins of the recti (Figs. 3.2 & 3.3). The different ligaments, crura, and arches around the umbilicus and inguinal rings are not visible on echography.

5. Peritoneum

It would be more correct to refer here to the anatomical structure separating the deep aponeurosis of the abdominal muscles from the abdominal viscera. This structure varies considerably according to the region being investigated and the morphology of the subject. In echography, the term "peritoneum" designates the anatomical structure comprising, from its superficial to deep parts, the parietal fascia, the more or less loose areolar tissue, and the peritoneum. This structure is visible as a rather fine, echogenic band (Figs. 3.2 & 3.15d). In lean subjects it cannot be distinguished from the deep aponeuroses lining the recti and flat abdominal muscles. Conversely, in obese patients it appears separate from the deep aponeurosis owing to the abundant loose areolar tissue separating these two fascial layers.

Two zones (epigastric fossa and suprapubic region) display marked development of the extraperitoneal subparietal areolar tissue. These two areas form heterogeneous hypoechogenic zones, lying just posterior to the recti and linea alba, and thus should not be mistaken for a pathological collection of fluid in the subxiphoid or suprapubic space (Fig. 3.1b).

C. Echography of the Pathological Abdominal Wall

1. Parietal Collection of Fluid

The main indication for parietal investigation of the abdomen is fluid collection (Figs. 3.5 & 3.6). No special echographic features allow the different types of

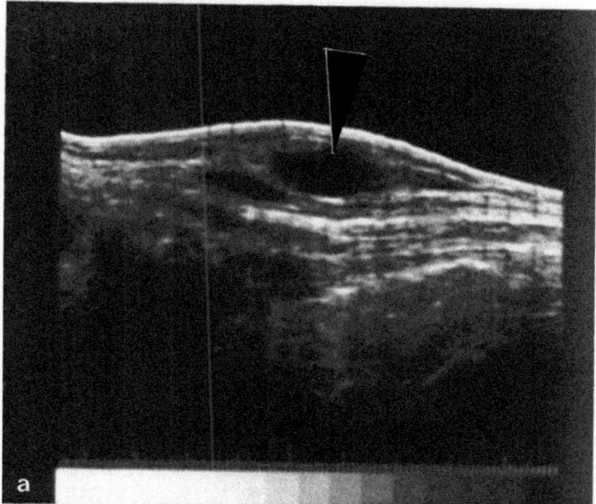

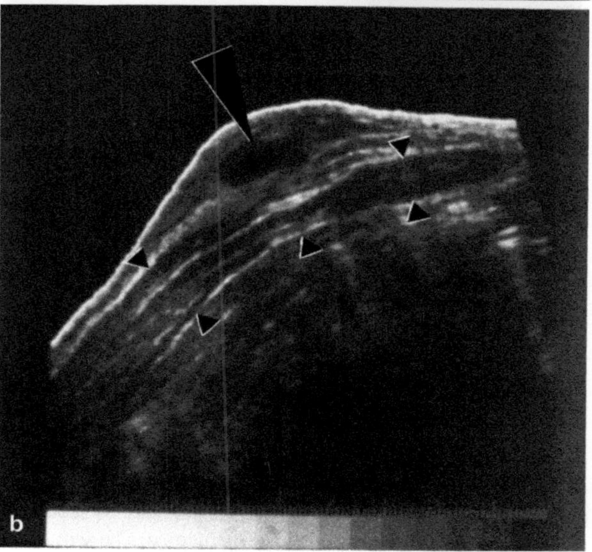

Fig. 3.5a, b. Subcutaneous parietal hematoma in a patient on anticoagulant therapy. **a** Longitudinal imaging showing the hematoma (▼). **b** Transverse imaging showing the hematoma (▼) facing the linea semilunaris (▼) joining together the flat abdominal and recti muscles (▼ ▲)

parietal fluid collections to be distinguished [Morley & Barnett 1978], i.e., an effusion of blood, an abscess, or a collection of serous fluid. These zones are more or less wide and anechogenic or weakly echogenic. As a function of their thickness (pus) or fluidity and coagulation or organization (hematoma), a given collection of fluid may change its echographic features with time (initially anechogenic to become progressively echogenic).

Echographic investigation may allow better identification of the site of puncture or incision of these

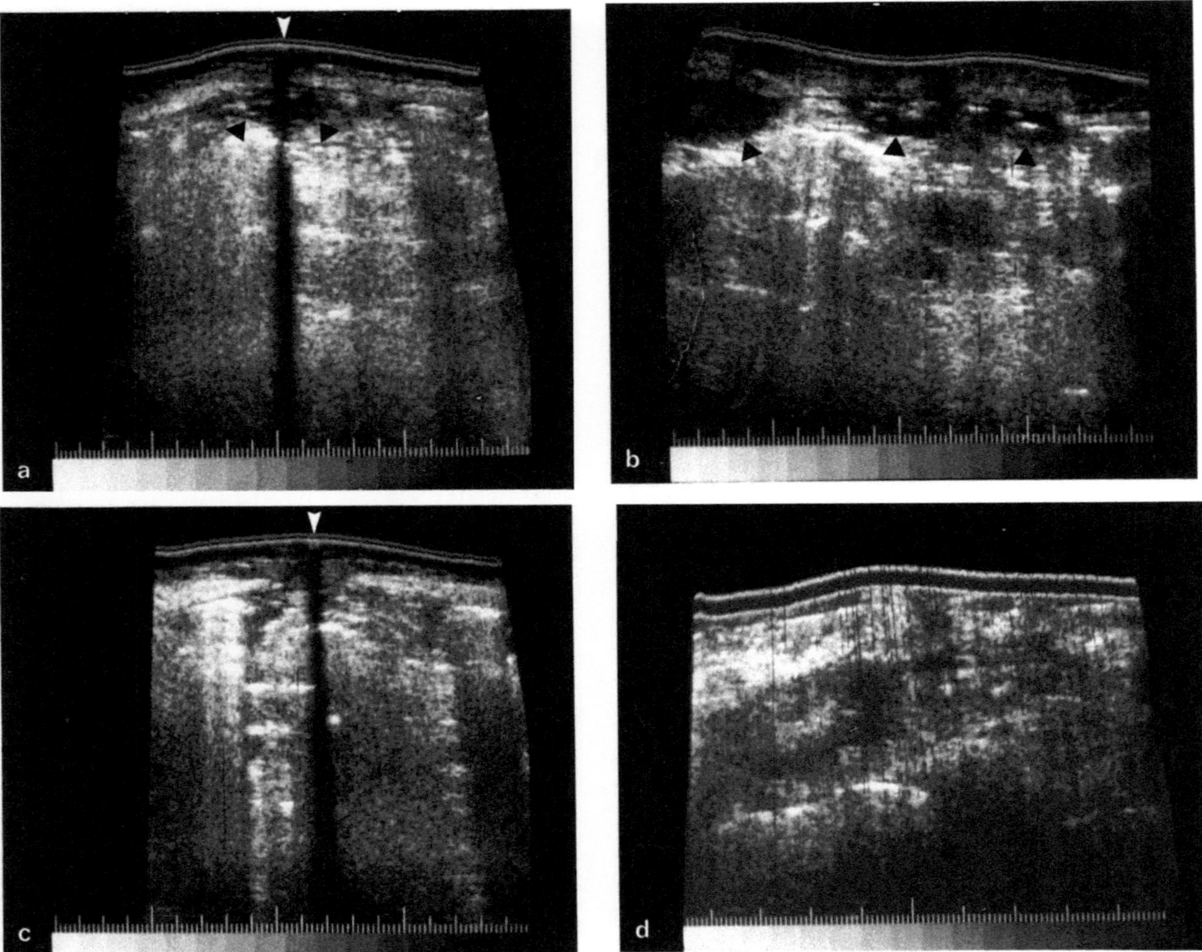

Fig. 3.6a-d. a and **b** Cicatrix with an infected subparietal extraperitoneal hematoma. The infected hematoma (▼) is clearly visible beneath the abdominal wall. **a** Median longitudinal image made along the cicatrix (▽). **b** Median transverse image showing the lesion (▲) deep to the abdominal wall. Note the well defined acoustic shadow of the cicatrix. **c** and **d** Normal cicatrix of the abdominal wall after spontaneous evacuation of the hematoma. **c** Longitudinal image: compare with a. **d** Transverse image: compare with **b**

lesions. In exceptional cases a foreign body may be seen (Fig. 3.7). In some patients echography may demonstrate subparietal or even intraperitoneal extension of fluid collection, as evidenced by the presence of a strangulated hourglass image at the aponeurotic and peritoneal sites of fluid expansion.

Two special cases merit emphasis. The first of these is a *midline parietal collection of fluid in the lower suprapubic region*. The exact site of the lesion is difficult to ascertain in cases where the recti and linea alba are not clearly visible. In these conditions the collected fluid lies in the subcutaneous region, the suprapubic space, or Retzius space. The second case is *parietal collection in the epigastric fossa*, which is difficult to differentiate from a subphrenic prehepatic abscess and

a subparietal extraperitoneal collection of fluid. Furthermore, it should be kept in mind that the normal image of the epigastric fossa may resemble a pathological collection of fluid (Fig. 3.1b).

2. Hernia

Although clinical diagnosis of hernia is usually achieved with ease, special echographic studies have been devoted to this subject [Spangen 1975; Morley & Barnett 1978; Deitch & Engel 1980]. Parietal hernia is probably the type of greatest interest for echography (hernia of the linea alba, umbilicus, semilunarline, lumbar quadrangle or triangle). Conversely, *orificial hernia* of the inguinal rings (direct or sliding indirect hernia) or the crural region is not a useful indication

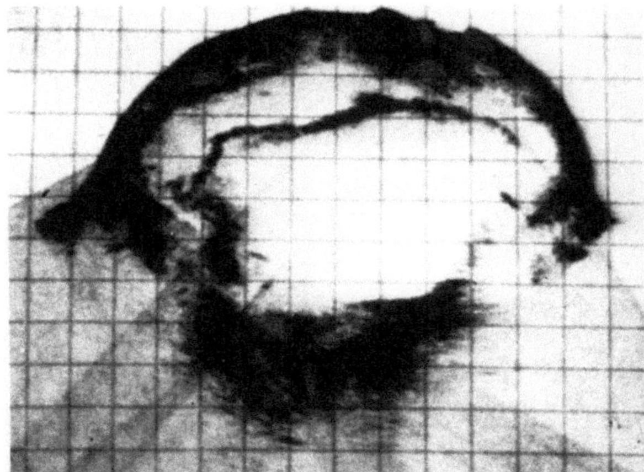

Fig. 3.7. Mersilene fragment floating in a sequestered fluid-filled cavity (Courtesy of J.B. Flament and J. Rives)

for echographic investigation. Echography may allow the identification of the presence of omentum or digestive viscera in the hernial sac, although clinical examination and, when necessary, standard and contrast roentgenograms are far superior diagnostic procedures.

Midline parietal hernia is far more frequent than paramedian parietal hernia. It is seen on echography as a localized deformity of the aponeurotic layers or even as an image of aponeurotic discontinuity with the presence of an abnormal mass [Deitch & Engel 1980]. Identification of the lesion is assisted by dynamic echography of muscle contraction or static investigation with the patient standing, except in cases of irreducible hernia. These midline lesions include umbilical hernia and hernia of the linea alba (Figs. 3.8 & 3.9).

Clinical diagnosis of paramedian parietal hernia (hernia of the semilunar line) is more problematic, since clinical examination is often negative. In such cases, echography may be of fundamental importance by demonstrating discontinuity of the deep aponeurotic layer and the presence of a mass between the transverse and oblique muscles [Deitch & Engel 1980]. We have not encountered any such cases in our experience.

3. Incisional Hernia

This type of lesion is not problematic with respect to diagnosis. Echography demonstrates a major hernial lesion with significant midline separation of the recti and disappearance of the linea alba or even the echographic "peritoneum" (Fig. 3.10).

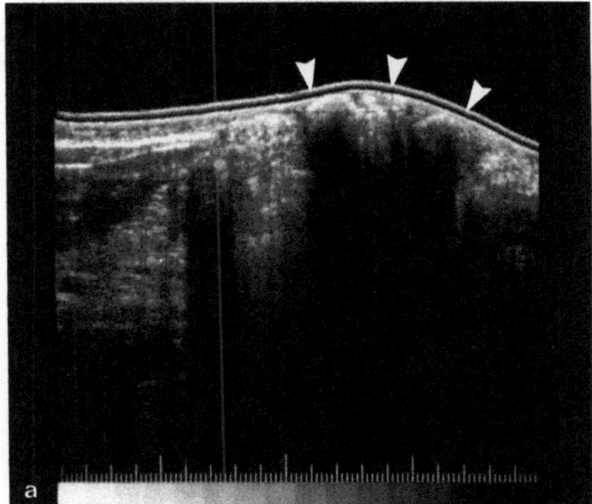

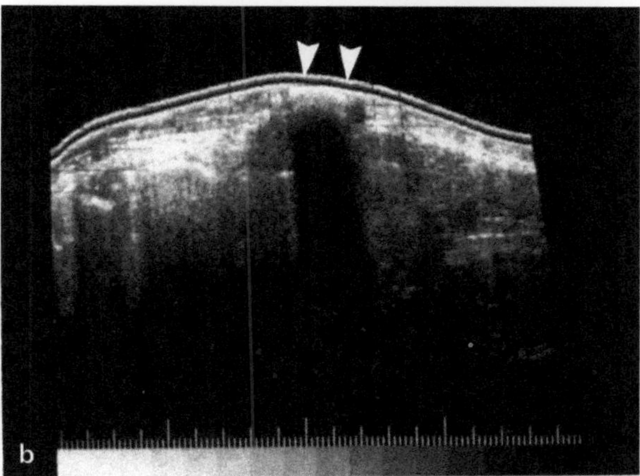

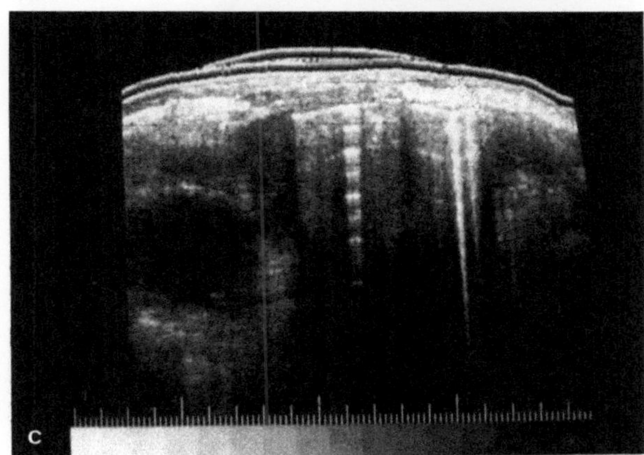

Fig. 3.8a–c. Umbilical hernia. Air-containing structures can be seen just beneath the skin near the umbilicus ($\bigtriangledown$). **a** Median longitudinal image. **b** Median transverse image. **c** Median transverse image of the subumbilical region. The visceral structures are separated from the skin by the components of the abdominal wall (muscles, aponeuroses), which is normal in this case

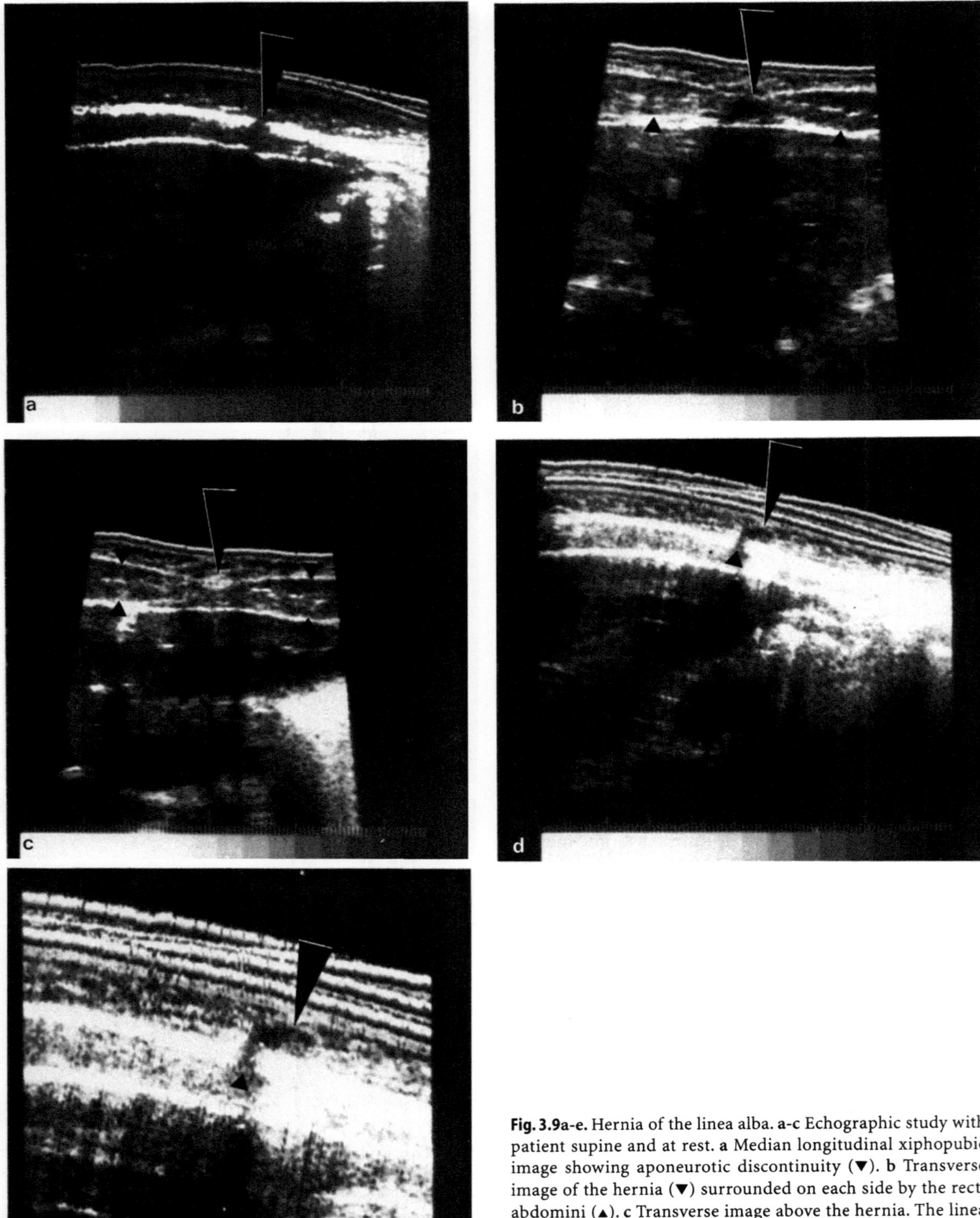

Fig. 3.9a-e. Hernia of the linea alba. **a-c** Echographic study with patient supine and at rest. **a** Median longitudinal xiphopubic image showing aponeurotic discontinuity (▼). **b** Transverse image of the hernia (▼) surrounded on each side by the recti abdomini (▲). **c** Transverse image above the hernia. The linea alba (▼) is intact between the recti abdomini (▲ ▼). **d** Echographic study during muscle contraction. Median longitudinal image. Note part of the subparietal extraperitoneal areolar tissue (▼) escaping through the hernial defect (▲). **e** Enlargement

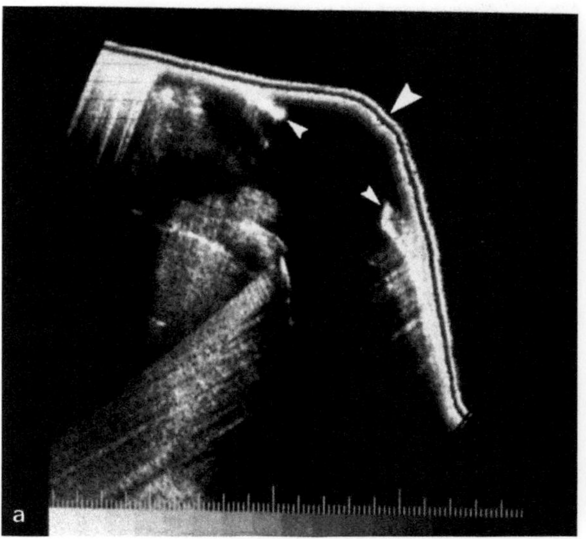 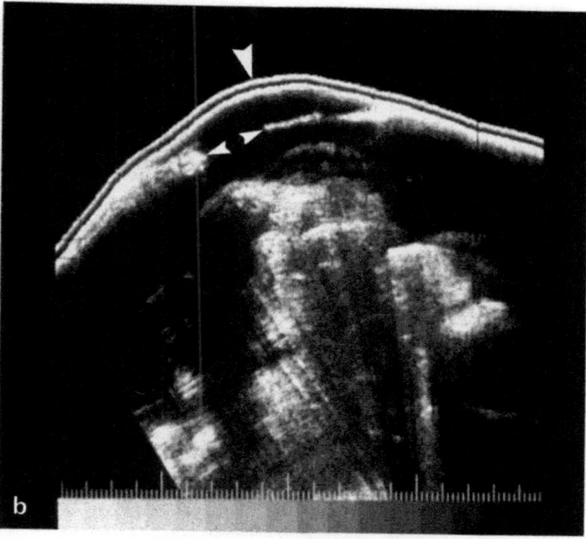

Fig. 3.10a, b. Wound dehiscence after treatment of umbilical hernia. The patient presented with alcoholic cirrhosis and pronounced ascites. The incisional hernia contains ascitic fluid, as evidenced by the obvious discontinuity of the linea alba and peritoneum (◁ ▷). a Median longitudinal image of the umbilicus. b Median transverse image of the umbilicus

4. Tumor

Regardless of their nature, all tumors seem to appear as a homogeneous hypoechogenic mass [Goldberg 1975; Hanson et al. 1983]. This accounts for the fact that in the absence of physical clinical data or information on disease course, a subcutaneous metastasis can be mistaken on echography for certain types of fluid collection, especially in the late postoperative period [Morley & Barnett 1978].

Differential diagnosis between malignant and benign tumors of the abdominal wall cannot be achieved by echography. The following types of tumor can be found: parietal metastasis (Fig. 3.11), sarcoma, benign rhabdomyoma, benign tumors of the aponeurosis, and subcutaneous lipoma. The latter is the only type of tumor displaying particular echogenic features that allow it to be distinguished from all other types of benign and malignant tumors of the abdominal wall [Goldberg 1975].

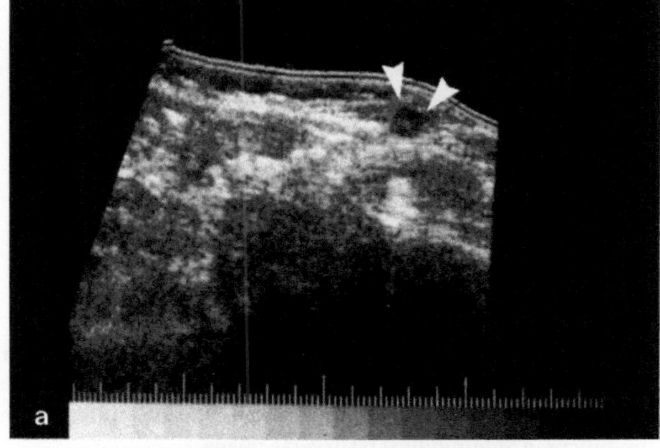

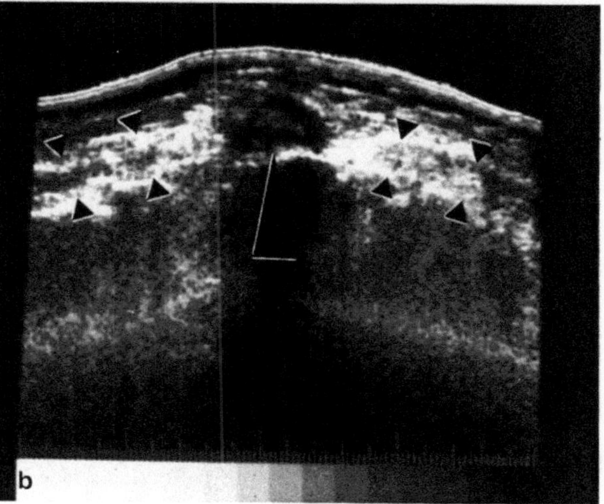

Fig. 3.11a, b. Parietal metastases. a Primary carcinoma of the breast (▽). b Primary adenocarcinoma of the colon (▲); the metastasis lies along the linea alba between the recti abdomini (▼▲)

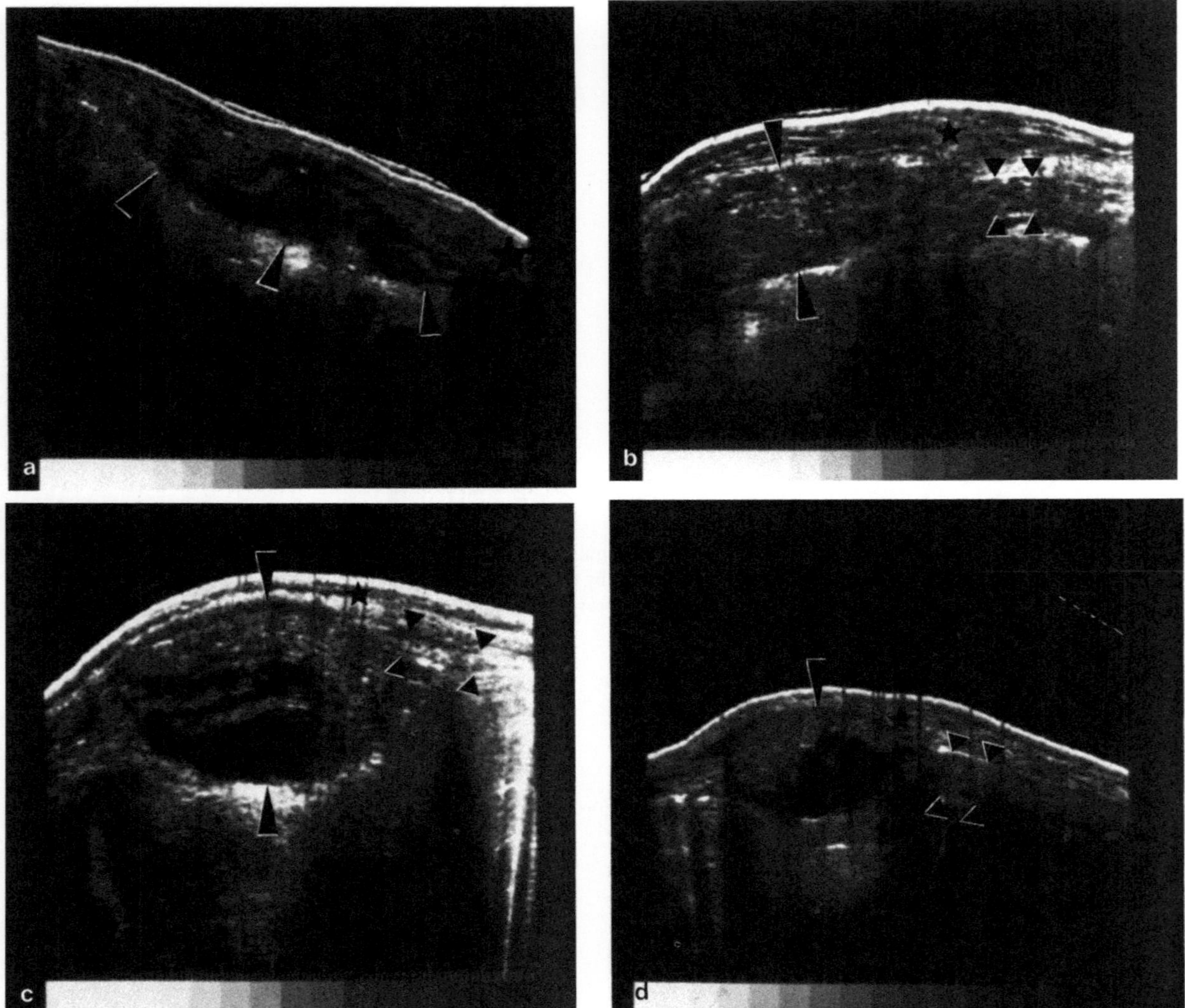

Fig. 3.12a-d. Hematoma of the rectus sheath on the right side (the patient was under anticoagulant therapy). **a** Right paramedian longitudinal image; note the spindle-like hematoma (▲) extending from the xiphoid process (∗) to the pubic symphysis (✳). **b** Subumbilical transverse image; hematoma (▼), midline (∗), normal left rectus abdominis (▼▲). **c** Transverse image through the umbilicus. **d** Subumbilical transverse image

5. Spontaneous Hematoma of the Rectus Sheath

We have encountered only one case of such spontaneous hematoma, and publications on this subject are rare [Morley & Barnett 1978; Deitch and Engel 1980]. The lesion can be evidenced on echography as an increase of the volume of one of the recti, especially in the subumbilical part of the muscle. The involved area is anechogenic when the hematoma initially forms and then modifies to become echogenic as the hematoma undergoes coagulation or organization (Fig. 3.12). The differential diagnosis is that of a fluid collection in the supravesical space or Retzius space.

6. Other Anomalies Seen on Echography

An *intraperitoneal effusion* is seen clearly separated from the abdominal wall by the echogenic line referred to as the peritoneum (Fig. 3.3).

In cases of *peritoneal carcinomatosis* or intraperitoneal space-occupying lesions, with or without free effusion, echography demonstrates the presence of poorly outlined tissue structures inserted directly on the echogenic "peritoneal" sheet. These solid lesions displace the highly echogenic and reflective air bubbles (contained within the intestines) from the abdominal wall. In cases where these intraperitoneal

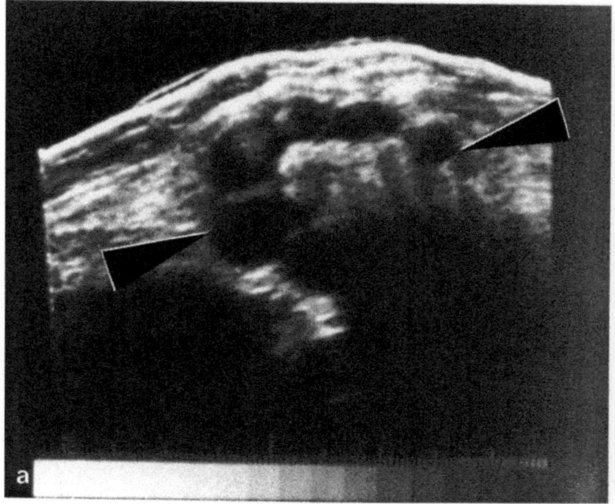

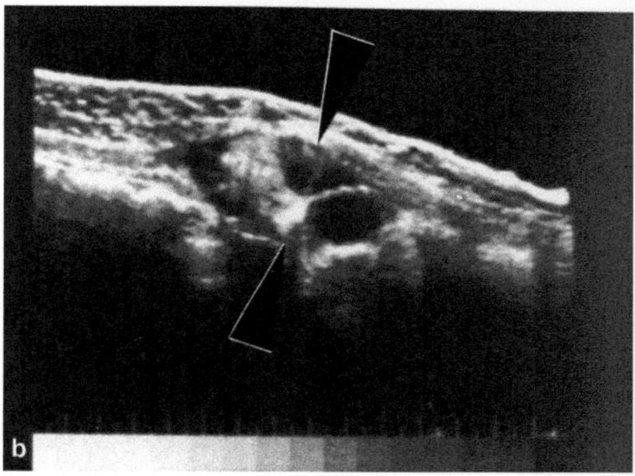

Fig. 3.13a, b. Ascites and peritoneal metastases from primary cancer of the ovary. The peritoneal metastases (▼) accompanied by ascites are clearly visible deep to the anterior abdominal wall (**a**) and near the diaphragm (**b**)

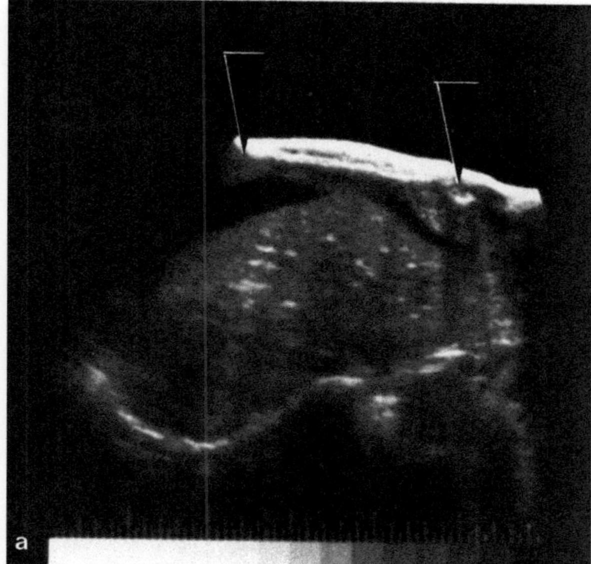

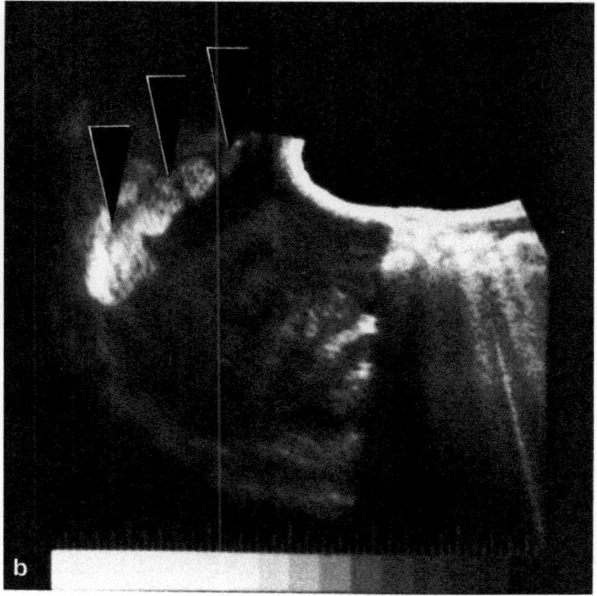

Fig. 3.14a, b. Large abdominopelvic tumor extending to the abdominal wall. The tumor (▼) can be seen to deform and interrupt the abdominal wall. **a** Subumbilical median transverse image; **b** subumbilical median longitudinal image

tumors are greatly developed, certain parts of the echogenic peritoneum may disappear (Figs. 3.13 & 3.14).

With persistence of the urachus, an expansion of the dome of the bladder can be seen between the peritoneal fasciae, posterior to the linea alba, running toward the umbilicus.

The umbilical vein and subparietal and periumbilical veins in Cruveilhier-Baumgarten syndrome lie between the peritoneal fasciae, just posterior to the muscles of the anterior abdominal wall. The intrahepatic origin of the umbilical vein can be identified in the recess of Rex. This vein then runs under the abdominal wall toward the umbilicus. In the region of the umbilicus several more or less sinuous veins, running in the lateral parietal or suprapubic direction, are seen posterior to the recti and linea alba (Fig. 3.15).

Lymphocele, hematoma, or urinoma may be seen on echography of a transplanted kidney.

Parietal hygroma, due to abnormal abdominal and thoracic lymphatic drainage, is not an indication for echography, as diagnosis can be easily made on the basis of clinical findings.

The *orifices*, especially in the inguinal and crural regions, may display adenopathy. Aside from adeno-

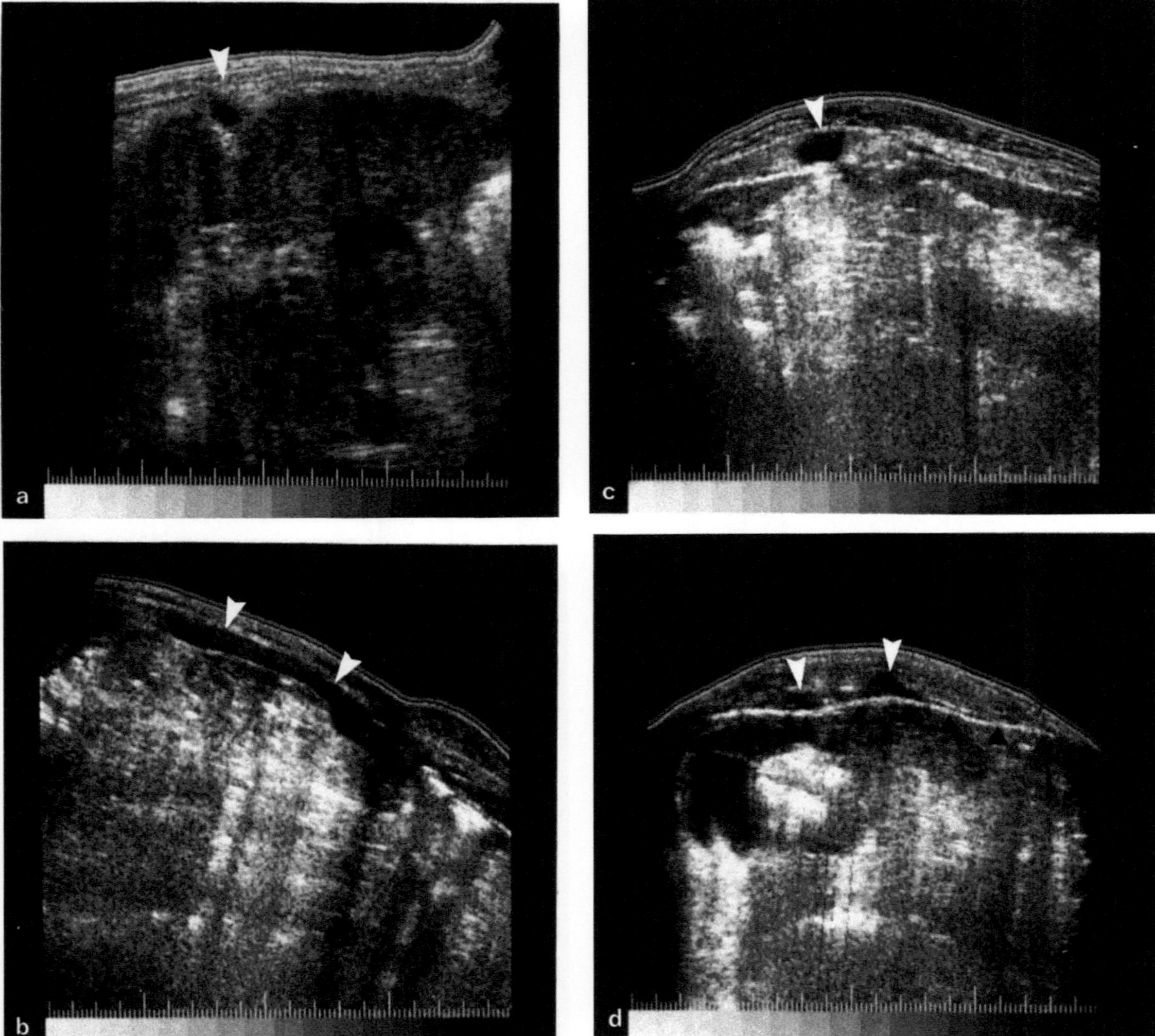

Fig. 3.15a-d. Cruveilhier-Baumgarten syndrome. **a** The umbilical vein ($\triangledown$) is visible near the falciform ligament between the third and fourth segments of the liver. **b** The umbilical vein ($\triangledown$) can be seen deep to the abdominal wall along the medial margin of the right rectus abdominis. **c** Right paramedian axial image along the umbilical vein. **d** Transverse image through the umbilicus. The umbilical vein ($\triangledown$) and a tributary ($\triangledown$) are visible deep to the recti abdomini and linea alba and anterior to the peritoneum. The latter appears as a highly echogenic posterior line separating the abdominal wall from the abdominal viscera ($\blacktriangle$)

megaly and aneurysm of the femoral artery, tumors or pathological fluid collection of the psoas may escape via the femoral ring. Adenomegaly, tumors of the spermatic cord, varicocele, or even a hypoplastic ectopic testicle may be seen in the region of the inguinal canal on echographic investigation in men.

Certain lesions of the digestive tract (tumor, marked parietal inflammatory lesions) are sometimes encountered in the course of abdominal exploration (known lesions or fortuitous discovery). Owing to their structure, these anomalies are easily identified as arising from the digestive tract and are seen on echography to be clearly separated from the parietal abdominal structures by the aponeuroses and "peritoneum" (Fig. 3.4).

7. Postoperative Investigation

Echography is of little value in the investigation of postoperative complications of the abdominal wall [Deitch & Engel 1980]. It is used in these conditions mainly to identify the existence of parietal fluid, collection (serous fluid, hematoma, or abscess), although the precise nature of the lesion cannot be detected. The only real value of echography is in cases where clinical examination is difficult or a suppurative postoperative lesion is suspected. Some authors have proposed that echography be used to demonstrate a possible recurrence of hernia.

8. Doppler Studies

Recently color Doppler flow ultrasound (US) was introduced in the assessment of the abdominal wall blood supply. The use of this method in the preoperative mapping of perforating arteries for transverse rectus abdominis myocutaneous flap reconstruction provides a rational basis for the procedure [Berg et al. 1994; Meunier et al. 1997].

D. Conclusion

Echographic study of the abdominal wall can be done in conditions where the appropriate apparatus is available and the morphology of the patient gives meaningful results. However, most types of parietal disease give such clear clinical signs that echography is not indicated or is even futile.

Diagnosis of hernia of the semilunar line (Spigelian hernia) might be the only meaningful indication for this investigative procedure. Indeed, according to certain authors, the echographic signs in such cases seem to be rather characteristic and thus of diagnostic significance, since the clinical signs are few or uncertain.

References

Bader JP, Mellière D (1970) Gastroentérologie. III. Parois abdominales. Cahiers intégrés de médecine n° 3. Masson, Paris

Berg WA, Chang BW, DeJong MR, Hamper UM (1994) Color Doppler flow mapping of abdominal wall perforating arteries for transverse rectus abdominis myocutaneous flap in breast reconstruction: method and preliminary results. Radiology 192: 447-450

Deitch EA, Engel JM (1980) Spigelian hernia: an ultrasonic diagnosis. Arch Surg 115: 93

Deitch EA, Engel JM (1980) Ultrasonic diagnosis of surgical diseases of the anterior abdominal wall. Surg Gynecol Obstet 151: 484-486

Goldberg BB (1975) Ultrasonic evaluation of superficial masses. J Clin Ultrasound 3: 91

Hanson RD, Unter TB, Haber K (1983) Ultrasonographic appearance of anterior abdominal wall desmoid tumors. J Ultrasound Med 2: 141-142

Meunier B, Watier E, Leveque J, Roche G, Rolland Y, Pailheret JP (1997) Preoperative color-doppler assessment of vascularization of the rectus abdominis: anatomic basis of breast reconstruction with a transverse rectus abdominis myocutaneous flap. A prospective study. SRA 19: 35-40

Morley P, Barnett E (1978) Gastrointestinal problems. Anterior abdominal wall. In: de Vlieger M et al. Handbook of clinical ultrasound. John Wiley & Sons, New York, pp 255-256

Spangen L (1975) Ultrasound as a diagnostic aid in ventral abdominal hernias. J Clin Ultrasound 3: 211

Vincens C, Bigot JM (1983) Etude échographique de la graisse. Cah Kinesither 100: 9-19

II. Computed Tomography of the Abdominal Wall

J. Hureau, J. Pradel-Raynal and J. L. Dumas

Computed tomography (CT) is a very satisfactory technique for studying the abdominal wall. Each axial cut shows the entire abdominal wall (anterolateral and posterior regions), with each of its layers and its relations to the abdominal viscera clearly visible. Lesions can be easily identified, owing to their different density compared with the adipose and myofascial layers [Fisch & Brodey 1981].

A. Computed Tomography of the Normal Abdominal Wall

The structures of the abdominal wall can be seen from the superficial to the deep layers. The skin appears fine, dense, and regular on CT. The subcutaneous tissue, composed of low-density fat, is of variable thickness. It is more developed in women than in men, as fat tends to accumulate within the abdominal cavity in the latter. The linea alba is easy to identify as a structure extending 3 cm lateral to the midline. The transverse section of the subcutaneous abdominal vessels is often seen.

The recti (of variable thickness) form the anterior median part of the myofascial layer, whereas the lateral part of this layer comprises the flat abdominal muscles (external and internal obliques and transverse). Each of these muscles can be identified easily because of the fatty layers separating them.

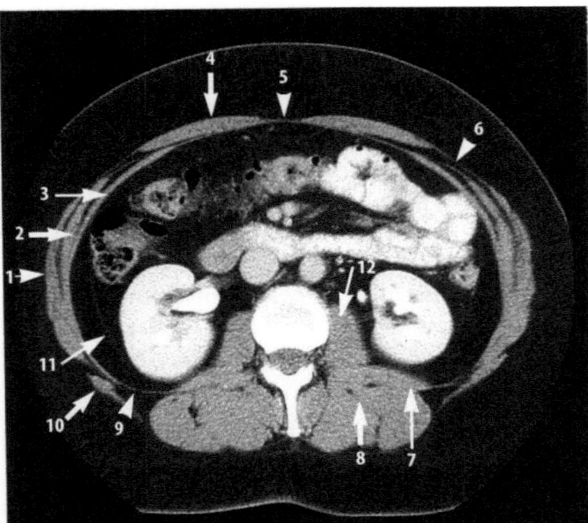

Fig. 3.16. Transverse CT section showing the structures of the abdominal wall at the subcostal level (L-2) in a fat subject. *1* External oblique muscle; *2* internal oblique m.; *3* transversus abdominis m.; *4* rectus abdominis m.; *5* linea alba; *6* aponeurosis; *7* quadratus lomborum m.; *8* erector spinae m.; *9* tendon of origin of transversus abdominis m.; *10* latissimus dorsi m.; *11* peritoneum; *12* psoas major m.

Posteriorly, the latissimus dorsi and quadratus lumborum are also clearly visible, the latter forming the posterolateral muscular wall of the renal fossa. In the median posterior region, the lumbar spine can be seen, flanked laterally by the right and left psoas muscles, which form the medial posterior wall of the renal fossa.

Behind, the spinal muscles occupy the spinal and retrotransverse gutters. The transverse fascia lines the full circumference of the abdominal cavity and blends posteriorly with the iliac fascia at the level of the psoas muscles.

The subperitoneal areolar tissue is a thin adipoareolar structure in the anterolateral region and forms a thicker layer in the anterior part of the abdominal wall. The normal parietal peritoneum, lining all parts of the abdominal cavity, is rarely identifiable on CT. Conversely, pathological conditions leading to thickening of the peritoneum render it visible. The fat within the abdominal cavity offers an ideal contrast with respect to the parietal myofascial layers. The bowel loops can be clearly distinguished from the adipose tissue, especially when the patient has been adequately prepared by repeated ingestion of diluted contrast material (e.g., Gastrografin) for 24 h prior to CT, allowing opacification of the bowel.

B. Computed Tomography of the Pathological Abdominal Wall

1. Tumor Masses

a) Benign Tumors

A desmoid tumor, arising from the intermuscular connective tissue, is clearly seen as a mass lesion, most often in the anterolateral parts of the abdominal wall. These dense, pebble-shaped tumors, displaying relatively well-defined contours, occupy and disrupt the muscular wall. They show little enhancement after intravenous injection of iodinated contrast material. Their shape and relations to the abdominal viscera, or even the bone, have been well studied with computed tomography. Lipomatous tumors, often arising from the fat of the rectus, are of special interest, since CT allows demonstration of the lesion and its anatomical relations. CT may even lead to histological diagnosis on the basis of the characteristic density of the fatty tissue (Fig. 3.17).

b) Malignant Tumors

Primary malignancies of the abdominal wall often arise from the muscle and include myxosarcomas or fibroreticulosarcomas and liposarcomas. They often involve the muscular or areolar fascial layers of the abdominal wall. The lesion and its origin can be identified on CT as a dense, often heterogeneous mass. Injection of contrast material may show the presence of hypodense zones within the tumor, suggestive of necrosis. The extension of the lesion and its invasive nature appear as dense stroma running through the subcutaneous areolar tissue with thickening and retraction of the cutaneous layers (Fig. 3.18). In some cases the tumor can be seen to invade the abdominal cavity. Tumors of the psoas major are among the most frequent, and sometimes involve the entire muscle and even its iliac bundle. The iliac fascia may constitute a temporary but veritable barrier to the anterior invasion of these tumors.

Metastatic lesions of the abdominal wall can result from any malignant tumor in the cutaneous and subcutaneous tissue. Cancer of the ovary is a particularly frequent primary origin of metastatic nodules (often multiple) involving the subcutaneous areolar tissue or subperitoneal fat of the abdominal wall (Fig. 3.19). These nodules usually measure 1.5-3.0 cm in diameter but may be much larger. They display well-defined contours and are of variable density. Cancer of the digestive tract, especially the colon, may also give rise to similar metastatic nodules (Fig. 3.20).

Parietal extension of primary intra-abdominal malignancy originating from the digestive tract, liver, or retroperitoneal structures is clearly shown on CT. Furthermore, this procedure allows assessment of the extent of the invasion of the abdominal wall. CT is also particularly useful for the screening or identification of recurrent malignancy in the renal fossa subsequent to ablation of a primary tumor of the kidney. This is practically the only investigative procedure allowing identification of a recurrence of malignancy and its frequent extension to the cutaneous layer of the abdominal wall (Fig. 3.21).

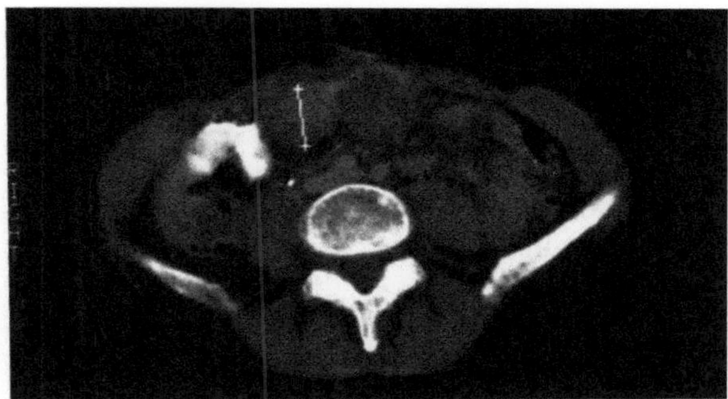

Fig. 3.19. Metastatic nodules originating from a primary ovarian malignancy

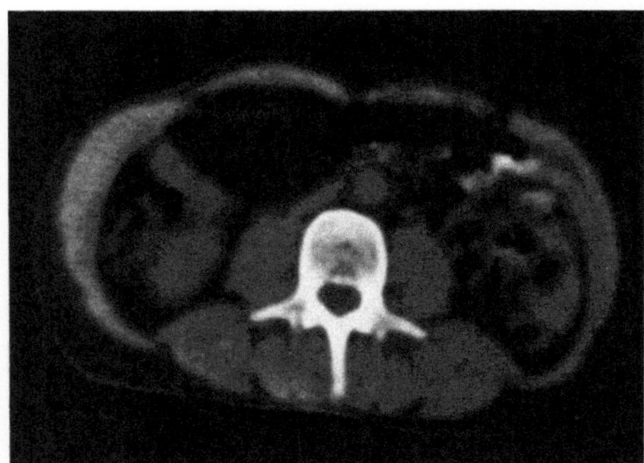

Fig. 3.17. Lipoma of the rectus abdominis. Note the fatty density in the rectus sheath

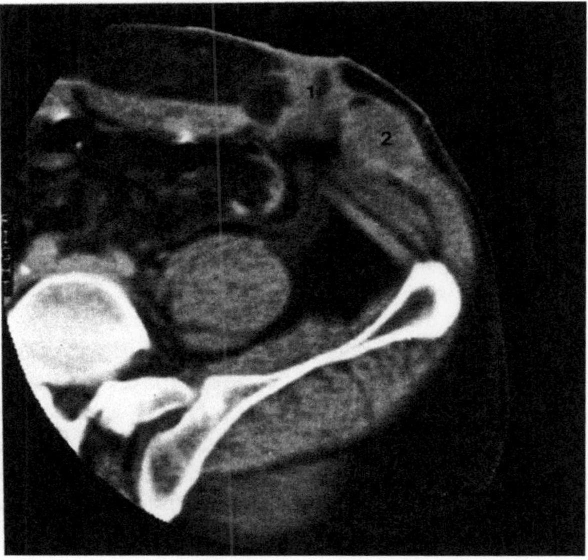

Fig. 3.20. Metastatic nodule from a primary rectosigmoid malignancy, arising from the artificial anus. *1* artificial anus; *2* metastatic nodule

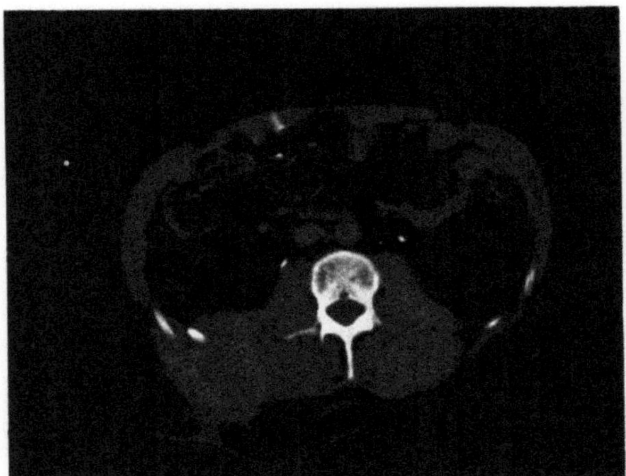

Fig. 3.18. Fibrosarcoma of the right posterior part of the myofascial layer of the abdominal wall. The lesion is evidenced as a heterogeneous density invading the areolar subcutaneous tissue and cutaneous layer

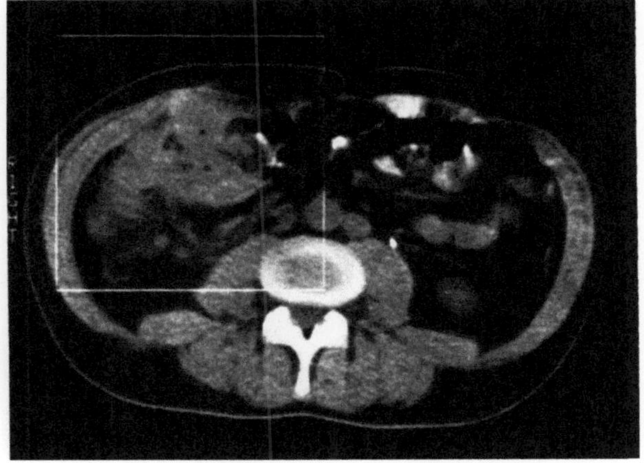

Fig. 3.21. Parietal extension of a primary malignancy of the cecum

2. Inflammatory Lesions

Postoperative abscess of the abdominal wall is in itself rarely a sufficient indication for CT. Nevertheless this technique clearly shows the lesion as a well-defined, hypodense image of the abdominal wall. A more interesting indication, which can be identified almost only on axial CT, is abscess of the psoas involving the sheath or muscle itself. In such cases, CT demonstrates a clearly outlined, hypodense lesion and allows determination of its origin (usually the vertebrae) and extent (sometimes down to the inguinal region) (Fig. 3.6). The distinction between abscess and hematoma is theoretically simple to achieve, since the latter contains fresh blood which is hyperdense. However, unless investigation is done during the first few days following the development of the lesion, differential diagnosis is not possible, since both types of lesions will show up as a nonspecific, low-density image. The involvement of the cutaneous layers of the abdominal wall by an underlying lesion can be detected by CT. This procedure may even lead to the diagnosis of an inflammatory lesion originating from the kidney. Indeed, an initial perirenal inflammatory process, after having destroyed the perirenal fascia and invaded the posterior perirenal spaces, may traverse the transverse fascia to finally invade the myofascial and cutaneous layers, i.e. phlegmon of the renal fossa extending to the abdominal wall.

Contribution of magnetic resonance imaging (MRI) in the diagnosis of cellulitis of the abdominal wall was

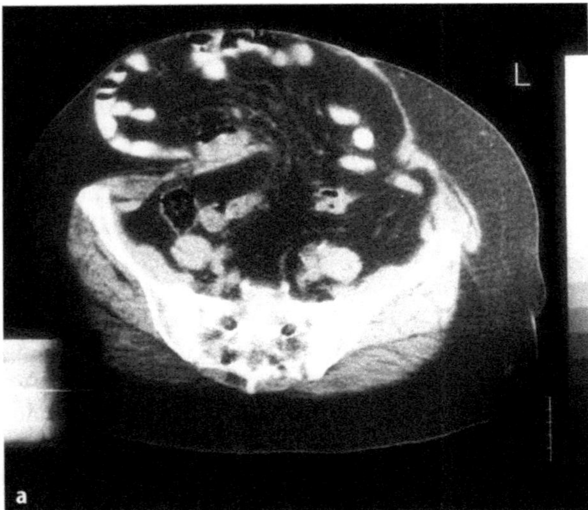

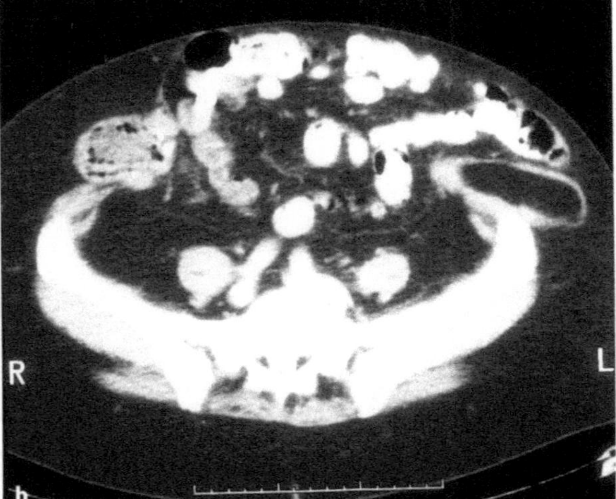

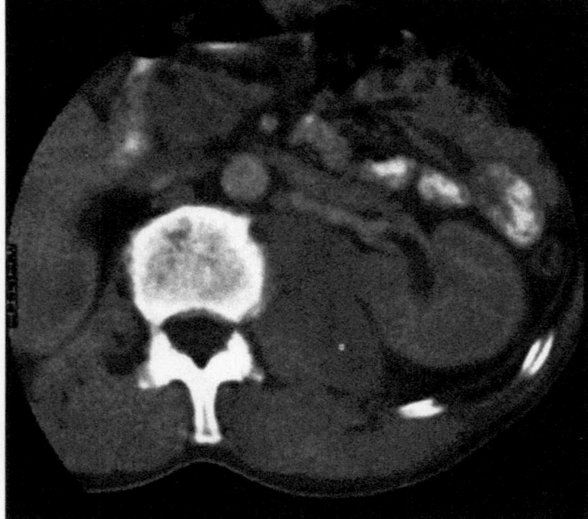

Fig. 3.22. Abscess of the left psoas muscle. Note the increased size of the muscle, displaying a hypodense area containing pus

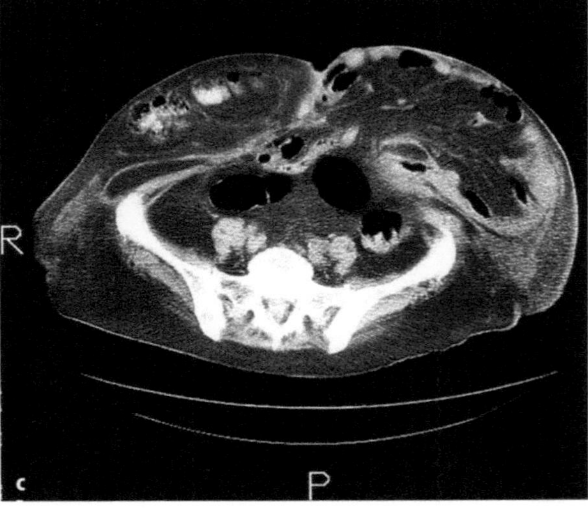

Fig. 3.23. CT scans of the abdominal wall before operating for incisional hernia (document of J.P. Chevrel)

reported [Rahmouni et al. 1994]. Linear streaks which were hypointense on T1-weighted images and hyperintense on T2-weighted images were present within the subcutaneous fat. In necrotizing infections the T2-weighted images were most striking as they showed the hyperintense signal abnormalities extending at the deep fasciae and within muscles.

3. Abdominal Wall Hernias

Computed tomography allows evaluation of suspected abdominal wall hernias and incisional hernias, and detection of those that are clinically occult [Miller et al. 1995]. CT shows the abdominal wall defects and the hernial contents, as well as signs of bowel ischemia (Fig. 3.23). Ventral hernias are well evaluated with CT which can be of useful adjunct in demonstrating the herniation site and the condition of bowel loops. Especially when the clinical diagnosis of incisional, Spigelian, or obturator hernias is difficult, CT becomes the initial modality of choice. The superior and inferior lumbar spaces as sites of lumbar hernias are also particularly well analyzed with CT. In major indirect inguinal hernias the CT preoperative recognition of organs incorporated into the hernia could be essential to avoid injury during surgical repair. Moreover, CT can demonstrate appendicitis, diverticulitis, and tumor of the herniated bowel loops. Nevertheless, herniography was found superior to cross-sectional imaging such as CT in the diagnosis of groin hernias because the patient is usually scanned in the supine position [Harisson et al. 1995]. Groin hernias containing only fat are also easily overlooked on CT scans. Classification of inguinal hernias as direct or indirect with CT alone can be difficult. As a general feature, one of the main advantage of CT is the ability to depict pathologic conditions other than hernias that may be responsible for the patient's symptoms.

C. Conclusion

Computed tomography is an important procedure in the investigation of the abdominal wall and allows the clear identification of the constituent structures.

In cases of a clinically identified abdominal tumor, CT can demonstrate the parietal origin of the lesion, its extension, and possibly its histological nature. The procedure also allows identification of parietal lesions not suspected on the basis of clinical data, e.g. metastases or invasion of the abdominal wall.

References

Fisch AE, Brodey PA (1981) Computed tomography of the anterior abdominal wall. J Comput Assist Tomogr 5: 128-133

Harrison LA, Keesling CA, Martin NL, Lee KR, Wetzel LH (1995) Abdominal wall hernias: review of herniography and correlation with cross-sectional imaging. Radiographics 15: 315-332

Kux M (1993) Etude échographique et TDM des grandes éventrations traitées par prothèse de Mersilène prépéritonéale. Monographie GREPA 15: 70-71

Miller PA, Mezwa DG, Feczko PJ, Jafri ZH, Madrazo BL (1995) Imaging of abdominal hernias. Radiographics 15: 333-347

Rahmouni A, Chosidow O, Mathieu D, Gueorguieva E, Jazaerli N, Radier C et al (1994) MR imaging in acute infectious cellulitis. Radiology 192: 493-496

Part 2. Surgical Techniques

4 Surgical Approaches to the Abdomen

J. P. Chevrel
with the collaboration of
G. Champault

All of the abdominal viscera can be approached through various incisions in the abdominal wall. However, in certain special cases, diaphragmatic incision plus thoracotomy or thoracolaparotomy may be required, although the indications for these relatively destructive incisions have greatly diminished over recent years. They have been replaced by large unilateral or bilateral subcostal incisions.

The abdomen can be opened via numerous incisions which, for the sake of simplicity, can be divided into three groups: anterior incisions, lateral and posterior incisions, and thoracoabdominal incisions. From the etymological standpoint, the term laparotomy refers to incision of the flank, whereas celiotomy should be used when referring to longitudinal midline incisions of the abdomen. However, it is customary to use the term laparotomy to describe any incision leading to opening of the abdominal cavity.

Carried out for more than 20 years by gynecologists, laparoscopy was initially introduced as a diagnostic method but has now become a therapeutic procedure.

Since the first operation by Mouret in 1987 and the publication by Dubois in 1990, its applications have progressively extended to include biliary and apendicular disease, gastro-esophageal reflux, colonic, splenic and esophageal disease, as well as hernias of the groin and linea alba. In this chapter we will review the traditional anterior incisions (vertical, transverse or oblique) lateral and posterior incisions, thoraco-abdominal incisions and the new possibilities offered by laparoscopic surgery.

I. Anterior Incisions

A. Longitudinal

Midline incisions are widely used, since they can be made rapidly, induce relatively little hemorrhage when strictly in the midline, can be extended lengthwise from the xiphoid process to the pubis, can be closed rapidly, and, in the absence of wound dehiscence (see Chap. 5, II, B.), allow solid closure of the abdominal wall (Fig. 4.1). Furthermore, this type of incision is often less noticeable than other types.

1. Supraumbilical Midline Laparotomy

This incision can be used to approach the supramesocolic region of the abdomen. The skin is usually incised from the tip of the xiphoid process to a point 1 cm above the umbilicus, but the incision may be extended downward to gain a few centimeters by skirting to the

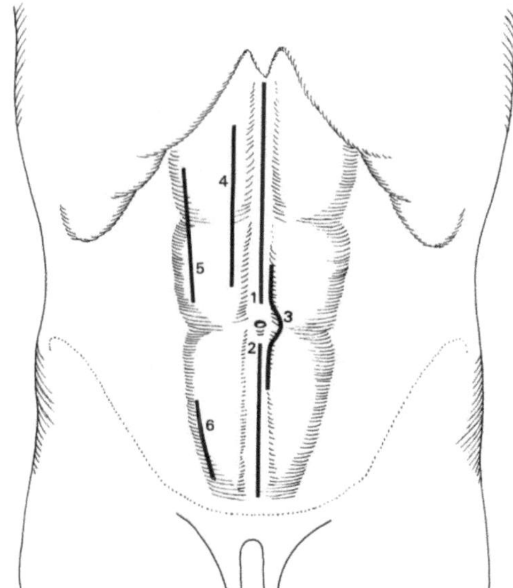

Fig. 4.1. Longitudinal incisions of the abdominal wall. *1* Midline supraumbilical; *2* midline subumbilical; *3* midline supra- and subumbilical; *4* transrectus (medial pararectus); *5* lateral pararectus; *6* Jalaguier's incision

left of the umbilicus. However, when possible it is recommended that the incision stop 1 cm above the umbilicus, since at this level the linea alba consists of strong overlapping fibers forming a herringbone pattern, whereas closer to the umbilicus on either side the fibers run horizontally. Sutures placed in the latter region may lead to small tears which contribute to future wound dehiscence. In this author's opinion, it is preferable to incise the subcutaneous fat with the diathermy scalpel to achieve good hemostasis. The procedure is completed with a few points of electrocoagulation. Conversely, the linea alba should be incised with the plain scalpel, since coagulation can alter the vascularization, which is already rather reduced in the midline. The midline is easy to identify when the incision is begun near the xiphoid process. It is preferable not to cut the bone, since this may lead to osteoma of the abdominal wall (see page 101).

The peritoneum is then opened with the diathermy scalpel, after which it is advisable immediately to divide the ligamentum teres flush with the liver, thereby allowing the falciform ligament to be cut in turn. These procedures are done so that adequate protection of the abdominal wall can be achieved by installing packs soaked in antiseptic solution (iodinated polyvidone), these being protected by a circular plastic field (wound protector).

Exposure of the operative field is achieved using retractors causing the least possible trauma. It is preferable to use wide retractors, e.g., Cresson's, Olivier's, or Toupet's retractor, rather than Gosset's retractor, as when used during a long operation the metal blades of the latter create two small vertical grooves which may cause ischemia and eventually postoperative incisional hernia. Closure can be done in many ways depending on the suture material used, the number of layers repaired, and the type of suture employed, i. e, interrupted or continuous. In cases where there are no factors suggesting a risk of wound dehiscence, we perform a two-layered closure. The deep peritoneal layer is repaired by everting the lips of the incisional wound in order to reduce visceral adhesion to a minimum. Polyglycolic acid sutures (0 or 00, according to brand) are used for this purpose. The linea alba is then closed as a separate layer by two continuous sutures using slow-absorbing material. One continuous suture is made in descending fashion and the other in the opposite direction to ensure solid closure at both ends of the wound. There is no significant difference in the incidence of wound dehiscence when continuous or interrupted sutures are used (see page 80) or when slow-absorbing or nonabsorbable material is employed (see page 81), or when closure is done with a single layer or with two layers.

Separate closure of the subcutaneous layer may be indicated in obese patients. The aim in such cases is to abolish the tunnel that forms between the two folds of adipose tissue, which may attain a thickness of 10 cm. The sutures should take up the full thickness of this tissue so that the wound margins are in close contact with each other. It is sometimes advisable to drain the wound using either capillary (horsehair) or suction drainage. The horsehair drain can be brought out at both ends of the incision. When a suction drain is used, it is recommended that the drain exit at a point about 10 cm from the operative wound in order to avoid retrograde contamination of the latter.

The skin is closed using simple interrupted or everting mattress sutures, according to the surgeon's preference. (Agraffes can also be used for this purpose, and when the clamps are loosened early, an aesthetic scar is obtained). It should be kept in mind that although continuous sutures can be made more quickly, they are less practical in cases where the wound has to be reopened to evacuate a localized hematoma or abscess of the abdominal wall.

2. Subumbilical Midline Laparatomy

This approach is used mainly in surgery of the pelvic viscera and terminal colon. With the surgeon usually on the patient's left side, the skin is incised from the upper margin of the pubic symphysis to the umbilicus and after around the left side of the latter. The midline is more difficult to identify here than in the supraumbilical region, since the space between the recti is very small or practically nonexistent below the arcuate line (line of Douglas). The midline is easier to identify at the upper end of the incision, just below the umbilicus. The incision is begun with the plain knife, although its lower half can be made using straight scissors. The latter should first be used closed to dissect between the aponeurotic layer and peritoneum down to the pubic symphysis. Such midline dissection facilitates the descending aponeurotic incision. The subsequent steps are identical to those for the midline supraumbilical incision. The surgeon should be careful to terminate the incision of the peritoneum on the upper margin of the pubic symphysis in order to avoid injury to a visceral structure. Repair of the abdominal wall is slightly different than with the supraumbilical approach, since the peritoneum cannot usually be identified separately near the umbilicus. Closure of the peritoneal layer is made in the caudocranial direction with the sutures taking up the transverse fascia and peritoneum. In the region where the linea alba can be identified above the arcuate line, closure is achieved downward as a single layer using interrupted or continuous full-thickness sutures. Below the arcuate line the premuscular fascial layer is closed anterior to the peritoneal layer in an upward direction, using a continuous suture with slow-absorbing material.

3. Combined Supra- and Subumbilical Midline Laparotomy

This type of approach is used in emergency surgery of the abdomen in cases lacking a clear preoperative diagnosis and when investigation of the entire abdominal cavity may be necessary. The length of the incision can vary, the maximum being from the xiphoid process, around the left of the umbilicus, and down to the pubis. Sternotomy can be done if necessary to extend the operative field into the thorax.

4. Paramedian Laparotomy

This approach is not commonly used in France, but the incidence of burst abdomen and incisional hernia does not seem to be any higher when this type of incision is used [Grenier et al. 1971].

a) Transrectus Incision

The skin is incised two finger breadths lateral to the midline. Subsequent to incision of the subjacent anterior lamina of the rectus sheath, the fibers of the rectus are separated longitudinally and then the posterior lamina of the rectus sheath and peritoneum are opened via a vertical incision. Closure is achieved in two layers. The simplest procedure is to use continuous sutures with slow-absorbing material. This incision can be made on the left side when nutrition is to be delivered by gastrostomy or jejunostomy.

b) Lateral Pararectus Incision

The skin is incised slightly medial to the lateral margin of the rectus. Subsequent to opening of the anterior lamina of the rectus sheath, the lateral edge of the rectus is reflected medially and then the posterior lamina of the sheath and the peritoneum are incised longitudinally. One of the commonest types of lateral pararectus incision is via Jalaguier's approach, i.e., subumbilical. Used for appendectomy, this approach carries the risk of injury to the epigastric vessels, although such damage is not of major severity. Conversely, when the incision is enlarged one or more intercostal nerves may be sectioned. Such denervation can lead to secondary, so-called paralytic incisional hernia. Accordingly, we have proscribed the use of this incision and prefer instead a transverse incision which can be easily enlarged laterally and superiorly. Furthermore, we prefer by far the subcostal approach to the biliary apparatus rather than the route via a superior lateral rectus incision.

c) Medial Pararectus Incision

Used to replace a midline supraumbilical approach, the medial pararectus incision is made one finger breadth lateral to the midline. This incision differs from the transrectus approach in that the medial edge of the rectus is displaced laterally. The posterior lamina of the rectus sheath and the peritoneum are then incised longitudinally at a distance from the midline. In our opinion, this approach offers no advantage with respect to midline laparotomy, which can be done more quickly, or to a transverse abdominal incision, which is just as solid on closure.

B. Transverse

The use of transverse incisions is currently on the increase in France in surgery of the intraperitoneal viscera and in retroperitoneal vascular or urological surgery. Transverse incisions (Fig. 4.2a) can be made at any level of the anterior abdominal wall. The fleshy fibers of one or both rectus muscles and the aponeu-

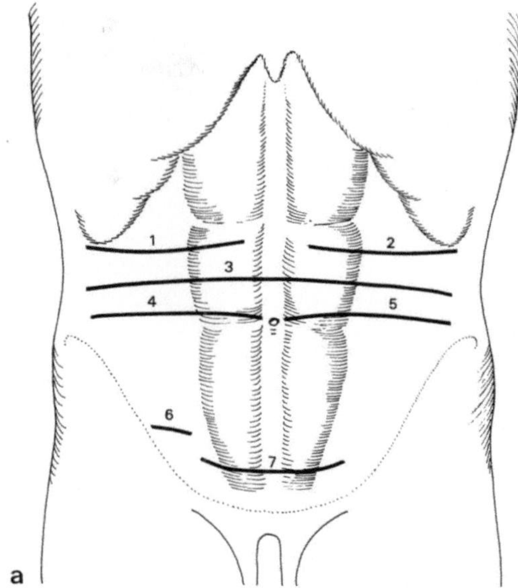

Fig. 4.2a-e. Transverse incisions of the abdominal wall. **a** *1* Right transverse subcostal (Bazy's incision); *2* left transverse subcostal; *3* transverse supraumbilical (Sprengel's incision); *4* right transverse paraumbilical; *5* left transverse paraumbilical; *6* right transverse iliac; *7* transverse suprapubic (Pfannenstiel's, Bardenheuer's, or Cherney's incision)

roses of the flat abdominal muscles (internal and external obliques and transverse) are usually sectioned laterally. However, to facilitate closure the transaction should be as limited as possible with regard to the fleshy fibers of the flat abdominal muscles. Scrupulous hemostasis is required. Closure is usually done as a two-layered procedure. The main advantage of the transverse incision would be a reduced risk of burst abdomen and incisional hernia, although the validity of this opinion is difficult to confirm and is even questioned by some authors [Greenall et al. 1980]. Described below in descending order are the different levels of transverse incision of the abdominal wall.

1. Right Transverse Subcostal

This incision is used in surgery of the biliary apparatus. Since it is made in a skin fold, an aesthetic scar is obtained in young women. However, exposure is reduced as compared with an oblique subcostal incision in tall slender subjects, since the right transverse subcostal incision is rather low in such people.

2. Left Transverse Subcostal

This incision can be used for splenectomy in young patients. However, we prefer an oblique subcostal

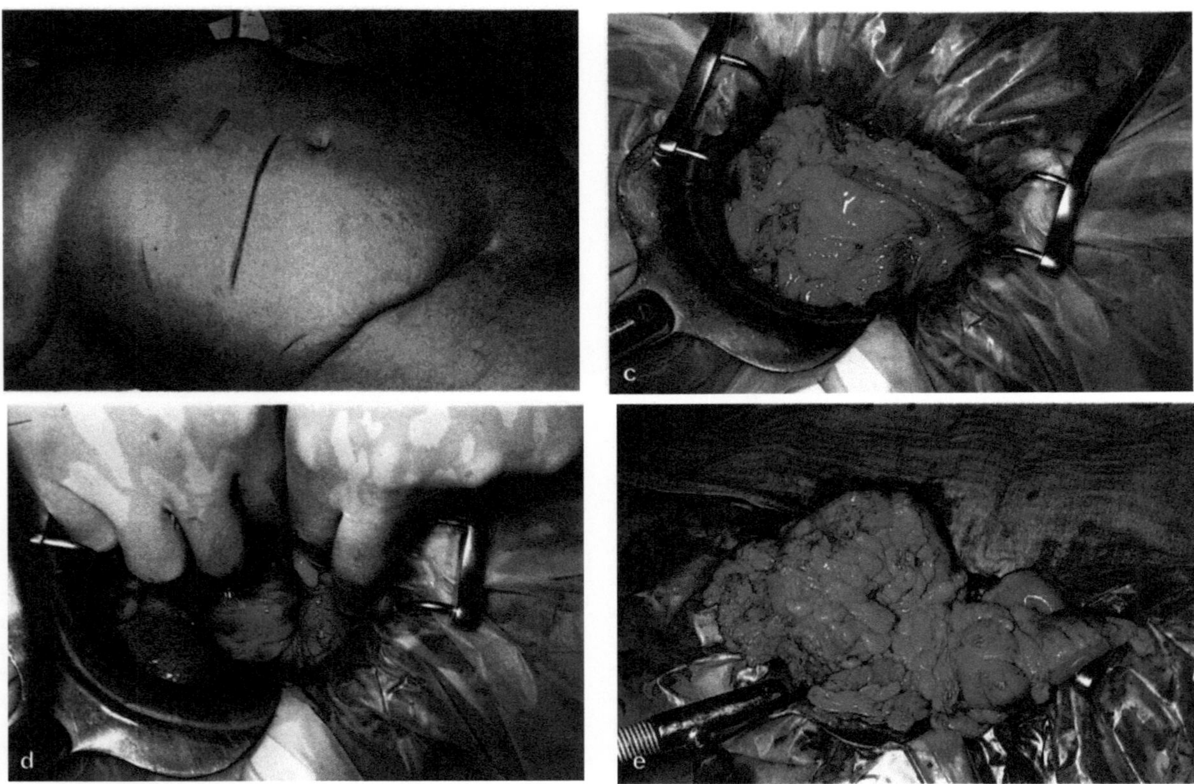

Fig. 4.2 b Approach via the right transverse paraumbilical incision. **c** Exposure of the cecum and appendix prior to dissection. **d** The retractor (Cresson's model) in the upper field gives good exposure of the hepatic flexure of the colon. **e** Subsequent to dissection the entire right colon can be easily mobilized through this incision

approach since, once again, this transverse incision offers less exposure of the operative field.

3. Bilateral Transverse Supraumbilical

This type of incision [Sprengel in Quenu & Perrotin 1960] can be made at different levels above the umbilicus, and according to the operation to be done, it can even be made in the subumbilical region. Widely used in surgery of the subrenal segment of the aorta, the bilateral transverse incision offers less exposure of the supramesocolic region than does an arcuate subcostal incision (Leclerc's incision; see page 73).

4. Right Paraumbilical

This incision is made one finger breadth above or below the umbilicus and affords excellent exposure for right colectomy (Fig. 4.2b). The rectus and aponeuroses of the flat abdominal muscles are sectioned whereas the fleshy fibers of the latter are left intact. Downward traction with a retractor allows easy mobi-

lization of the cecum (Fig. 4.2c). Similarly, upward traction can be used to easily free the hepatic flexure of the colon (Fig. 4.2d). This operation can be accomplished through an incision only 10 cm in length (Fig. 4.2e). Solid repair of the abdominal wall can be achieved after this approach, which in our opinion is far superior to a midline or oblique incision.

5. Left Transverse Paraumbilical

This approach can be used for left colectomy. The incision should be slightly longer than one on the right to facilitate the freeing up of the splenic flexure (which is deeper than the hepatic flexure) and to achieve anastomosis. In tall, slender subjects, a midline subumbilical incision extending above the umbilicus gives better exposure for a very low-situated anastomosis.

6. Transverse Incision of Right Iliac Fossa

When made over a few centimeters, this incision which can be used for appendectomy, gives a very aesthetic scar.

7. Pfannenstiel's Transverse Suprapubic

This aesthetic incision, allowing solid closure of the abdominal wall, is used in gynecological surgery. The skin is incised in an upwardly concave arc in the suprapubic fold, two finger breadths above the pubis, i.e., in the area of the pubic hair (Fig. 4.2a). The premuscular fascia is then incised transversely at a point one finger breadth above the skin wound, and thus the two incisions do not overlap. The fascial incision is extended to the lateral margin of the recti but not beyond to the aponeurosis of the internal oblique since this may lead to opening of the inguinal canal, thereby creating a zone of weakness (Fig. 4.3a). The upper part of the premuscular aponeurotic sheet is then freed from the fleshy muscle fibers of the recti, with thorough hemostasis of the small perforating vessels. The dissection should extended upward, prac-

tically to the level of the umbilicus. Next, the recti and small pyramidal muscles are separated in the midline, after which the transverse fascia and peritoneum are sectioned longitudinally (Fig. 4.3b). Closure is achieved as a three-layered procedure. The peritoneum and transverse fascia are closed using a continuous, slow-absorbing suture. Next, the recti are approximated in the midline by a few interrupted sutures. The third layer, i.e., the transverse aponeurosis, is repaired with a continuous suture (0 Vicryl). Since dissection of the aponeurosis may cause heavy bleeding it is advisable to install two suction drains (Jost-Redon model), one deep and one superficial to the aponeurosis.

Variations on Pfannenstiel's Incision

Bardenheuer's incision [described in Detrie 1982] is rather commonly used in the United States. It differs from Pfannenstiel's incision in that the recti are sectioned transversely. The transected muscle bodies are repaired with figure-of-eight sutures using slow-absorbing material.

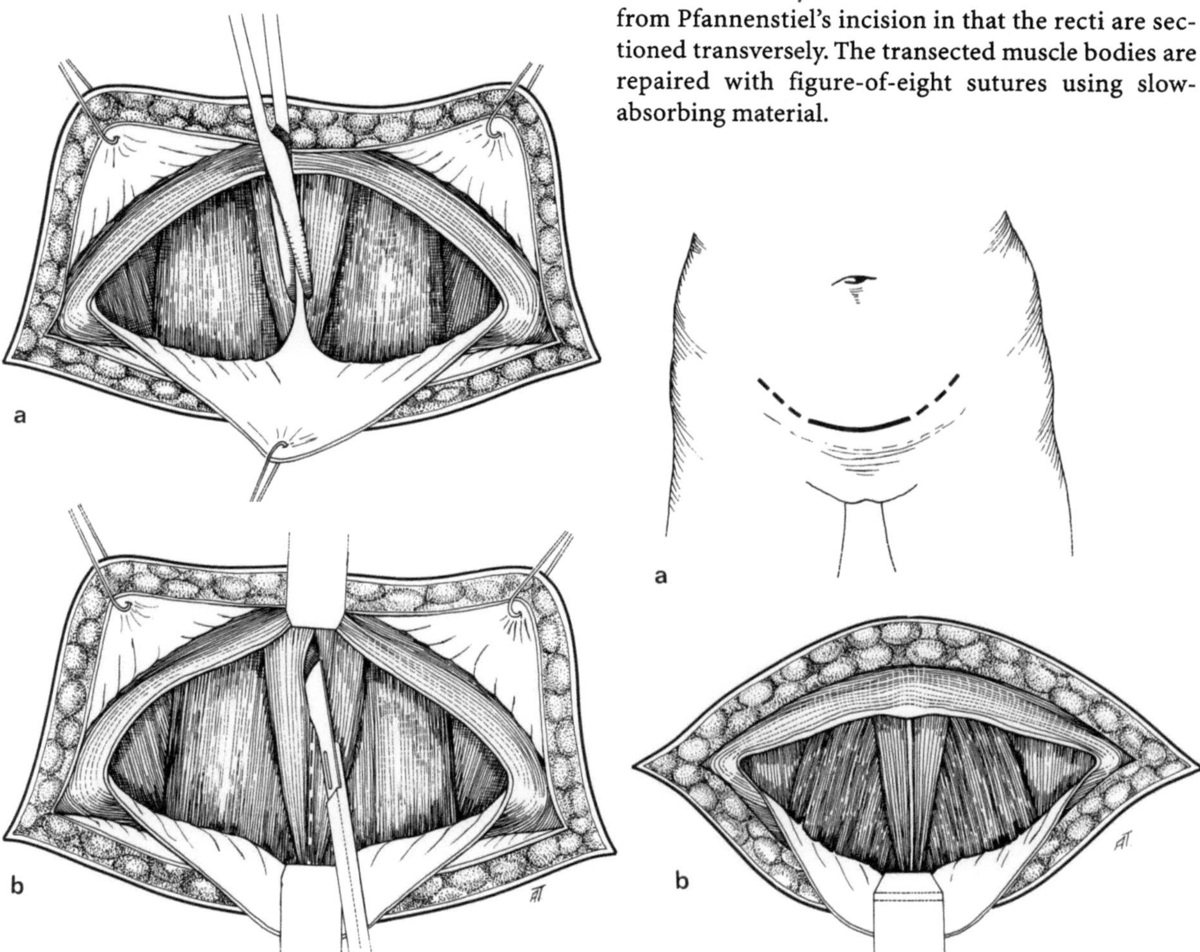

Fig. 4.3a, b. Pfannenstiel's incision. Transverse incision of the anterior lamina of the rectus sheath. **b** Sagittal incision of the muscle layer (recti abdomini and pyramidalis) allowing similar incision of the peritoneum

Fig. 4.4a–h. Cherney's incision. **a** The skin is incised one finger breadth above the pubis. The *dotted line* shows the enlargement in the extraepigastric variation of this incision. **b** Transverse incision of the rectus sheath

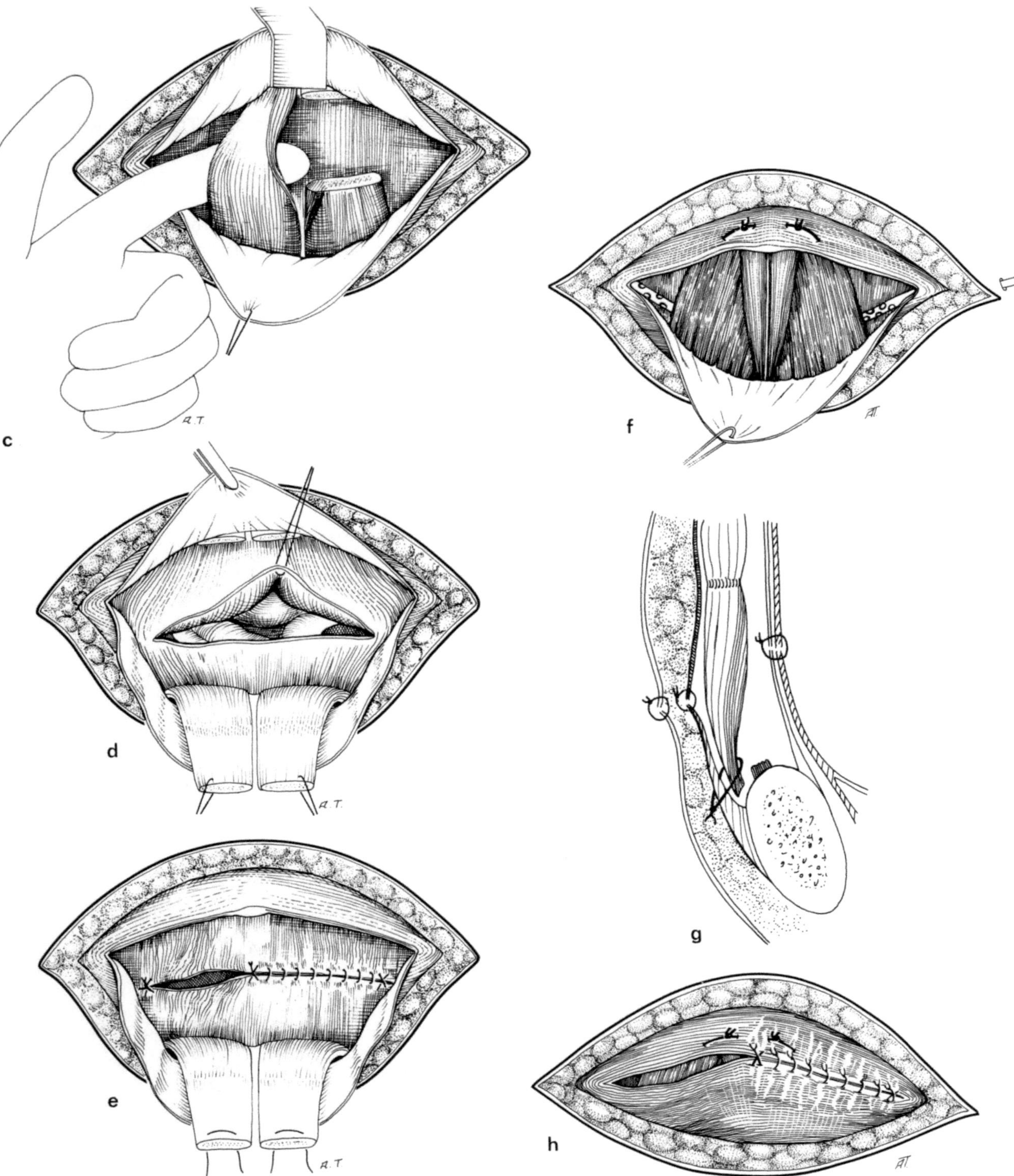

Fig. 4.4. c Disinsertion of the tendons of the recti abdomini and pyramidalis flush with the pubis. **d** Transverse incision of the peritoneum terminating at the epigastric vessels. **e** After closure of the peritoneum, two strands of suture are passed through the tendons of the recti abdomini to achieve their reinsertion. **f** The tendons are reinserted on the anterior lamina of the rectus sheath. **g** Sagittal section showing closure of the abdominal wall. **h** Parietal repair is completed by suturing of the anterior lamina of the rectus sheath

Cherney's incision (1946) consists of the stripping off of the recti flush with the pubis. Subsequent to blunt dissection of the posterior surface of the terminal tendons using the index finger, the insertions are cut with curved scissors to expose the insertion of the aponeurotic sheet on the posterior surface of the muscle bodies (Fig. 4.4a-c). The transverse fascia and peritoneum are then incised transversely at a point two to three finger breadths above the pubis to avoid injury to the bladder (Fig. 4.4d). On closure the insertions of the recti are repaired on the anterior lamina of their sheath using interrupted figure-of-eight sutures. Cherney incision allows more solid repair of the abdominal wall than does Bardenheuer's incision (Fig. 4.4e-h) and yields excellent exposure for all types of pelvic surgery [Chidichimo & Venuit de lo Scudo 1964; Bastien et al. 1965]. Furthermore, this approach can be extended laterally once the inferior epigastric vessels have been ligated.

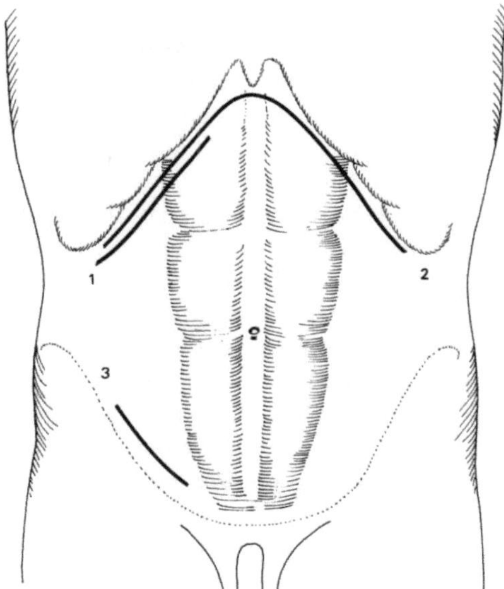

Fig. 4.5. Oblique incisions of the abdominal wall. *1* Subcostal; *2* bilateral subcostal (Leclerc's incision); *3* inguinal

C. Oblique

Subcostal incisions slanting obliquely downward and laterally are widely used in surgery of the supramesocolic viscera (Fig. 4.5).

1. Subcostal

The skin is incised two finger breadths below the costal margin. When used as an approach to the gallbladder, it is not necessary, in our opinion, to extend the incision to the midline. Accordingly, it can be stopped two finger breaths lateral to the midline so that it does not extend over the medial margin of the rectus. Conversely, in cases of more complex biliary surgery (for example, intrahepatic biliodigestive anastomosis) or difficult splenectomy, the surgeon should not hesitate to extend the incision beyond the midline. The subcostal incision can easily be enlarged laterally to the midaxillary line or even to the lateral boundary of the lumbosacral region. The size of the incision depends upon the surgical maneuvers to be performed. Cholecystectomy can be done through a small incision of 10 cm or less over the right rectus, whereas in other cases the incision can be extended laterally over the three flat abdominal muscles. *Exposure* is facilitated by the use of costal retractors (Cresson's or Olivier's retractor). The abdominal wall is *closed* in two layers in the region of the rectus and in three layers in the region of the flat abdominal muscles. Furthermore, we always use three figure-of-eight sutures of 00 Vicryl to reconstruct the two cut muscle surfaces to prevent hematoma formation within the rectus sheath and to avoid late postoperative formation of a small, unaesthetic depression. Subcostal incisions have been systematically used in our department for several years, on the right for surgery of the biliary apparatus and portal vein and on the left for surgery of the spleen, kidney, and adrenal gland.

2. Bilateral Subcostal

This approach, also referred to as Leclerc's incision, gives exceptional exposure of the supramesocolic viscera. The incision requires no special techniques. Scrupulous hemostasis is required and closure of the linea alba must be done meticulously. For this purpose we place two interrupted sutures on the linea alba, which are to be used as endpoints for the continuous sutures of the anterior and posterior laminae of the rectus sheath. This incision is used for gastric, hepatic, and pancreatic surgery.

3. McBurney's

This short, oblique incision, running downward and medially, begins two finger breadths in front of and below the anterior-superior iliac spine and is made parallel to the inguinal ligament for a distance of 4 to 5 cm. We prefer to use a low transverse approach rather than McBurney's incision.

4. Inguinal

These incisions are used for treating hernia of the groin. We use the approach described by Bassini in the nineteenth century [Bassini 1889; Chevrel 1983]. The incision, made 2 cm above the previously identified inguinal ligament, is begun at the level of the superficial inguinal ring and is then drawn upward and laterally parallel to the inguinal ligament. Its length varies according to the adiposity of the patient. The aponeurosis of the external oblique is incised with the plain knife from the upper end of the skin wound down to the superficial inguinal ring. The genital branches of the ilioinguinal and iliohypogastric nerves are then identified in order to avoid untoward injury to them. We have demonstrated, by postmortem and operative dissections, the frequent occurrence of a branch to the groin, which pierces the aponeurosis of the external oblique at the usual site of incision. This branch may be sectioned if care is not taken to systematically look for it. A similar suprapubic branch can also be found [Salama et al. 1983]. The aponeurosis of the external oblique is repaired using nonabsorbable interrupted sutures. The use of this procedure is based on our observation of recurrent hernia due to rupture of the suture of the external oblique at the level of the deep inguinal ring.

II. Lateral and Posterior Incisions

These incisions are used mainly for surgery of the kidney and for sympathectomy, but they are also useful for reintervention in cases where the anterior abdominal wall is in such a poor state that repeat laparotomy cannot be done. Before describing these approaches, it should be emphasized that a large subcostal incision extending more or less over the midline gives excellent exposure of the kidney. Indeed, this type of incision, on either the right or the left, allows the performance of extended nephrectomy for malignant tumor or adrenalectomy, under excellent conditions.

A. Lumbar Route

The patient is placed in the lateral decubitus position with an adjustable pad under the lower ribs. After identification of the 11th and 12th ribs, the incision is begun at a point lying at the level of the angle formed

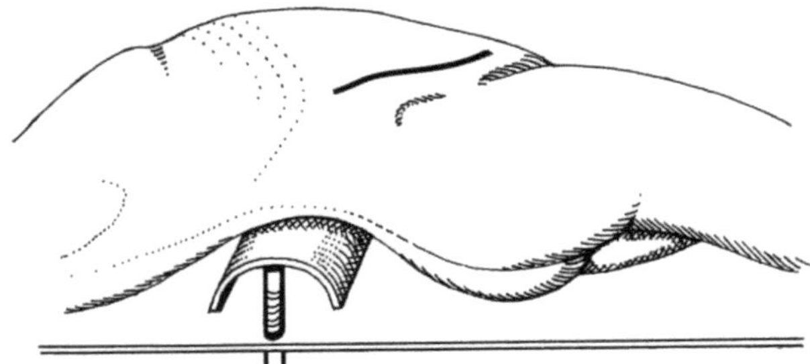

Fig. 4.6. Lumbar incision

by the inferior edge of the 12th rib and the lateral margin of the lumbosacral mass, i.e., practically at the anterior tip of the 12th rib when the latter is short (Fig. 4.6). The incision is then made downward to bisect this angle and terminates near the anterior-superior iliac spine, either above or medial to this easily identifiable landmark. The incision is usually about 15 cm long, but it can easily be enlarged downward by extending it parallel to the inguinal ligament or upward by partially resecting the 12th rib (at the level of its neck). Subsequent to the skin incision, the latissimus dorsi above and the external oblique below are successively transected, followed by a second layer comprising the internal oblique and posterior inferior serratus near the upper end of the operative wound. Finally, the aponeurosis of the transverse and Henle's ligament above it are sectioned. In cases where the 12th rib is short, it is best to stay a slight distance away from the rib owing to the proximity of the pleural cul-de-sac.

Closure is done in three layers using slow-absorbing continuous sutures. In some cases closure is hindered by anterior retraction of the internal oblique under the superficial layer. When this problem arises pick-up forceps should be used to pull the muscle back in place, thereby allowing proper closure of this second layer.

It should also be borne in mind that the iliohypogastric nerve skirts the posterior lip of the wound. Care should be taken not to compress this nerve when making a continuous suture, in order to avoid residual neuralgia.

B. Anterolateral Approaches

Among the numerous possible anterolateral incisions, those that we commonly use for surgery of the kidney, ureter, or colon (Fig. 4.7) are described below.

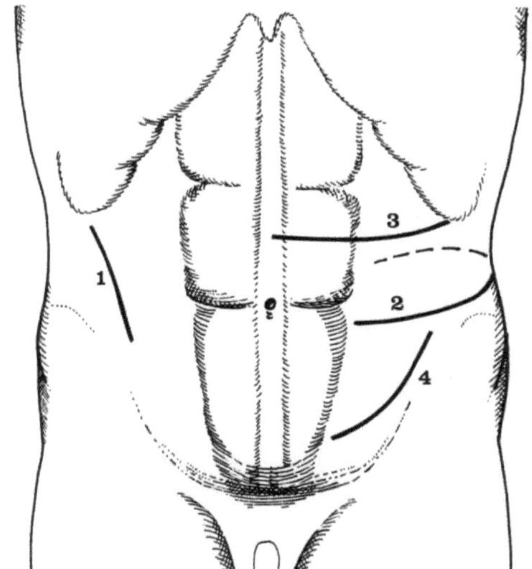

Fig. 4.7. Anterolateral incisions. *1* Oblique anterolateral (Chevassu's incision); *2* lateral transverse (Péan's incision); *3* horizontal (Bazy's incision); *4* iliac

1. Oblique Anterolateral Incision

This incision, also called Chevassu's incision, is begun at the inferior edge of the 10th rib just anterior to the tip of the 11th rib and continues obliquely downward and forward to terminate one finger breadth medial to the anterior-inferior iliac spine. This approach lies in a more anterior and vertical position than does the lumbar route. In the course of dissection the external oblique, internal oblique, and transverse are successively encountered. As in the lumbar route, parietal repair is a three-layered procedure using continuous slow-absorbing sutures. The incision can be enlarged inferiorly by terminating it like McBurney's incision. When made on the left side in the shape of a *J*, this approach allows good access to the descending colon and rectum.

2. Other Horizontal Incisions

Some of these incisions were proposed over 50 years ego by urologists. *Péan's large transverse incision* runs at the level of the umbilicus from the lateral margin of the lumbosacral region to the lateral edge of the rectus. This approach can easily be enlarged anteriorly and affords excellent exposure of the kidney and its pedicle. However, we prefer to use a large subcostal incision extending posteriorly to the lateral margin of the lumbosacral region when a wide approach to surgery of the kidney is required. Péan's incision can be used as an extra- or intraperitoneal route. The latissi-

mus dorsi and then the flat abdominal muscles are transected in this approach. Parietal closure is achieved layer by layer. A more anterior horizontal incision was described by Louis Bazy and corresponds to what is currently termed the "transverse subcostal incision" (see page 69). It is begun slightly below the tip of the 11th rib and is then drawn transversely forward to the midline at a level halfway between the umbilicus and xiphoid process. We use this incision, made about one finger breadth lower, in surgery of the right colon.

3. Iliac Incision

This incision, made parallel to the inguinal ligament, allows an approach to the iliopelvic segment of the ureter by the extraperitoneal route. It is begun one finger breadth medial to the anterior superior iliac spine and runs 2 cm above the inguinal ligament to terminate on the lateral margin of the rectus, one finger breadth above the pubis. Subsequent to successive incision of the external oblique, internal oblique, transverse, and transverse fascia, the peritoneum is bluntly dissected (with compresses or the fingers) and the ureter is identified near the bifurcation of the external iliac artery. This incision can easily be enlarged either upward or downward and medially.

III. Thoracoabdominal Incisions

These incisions can be used as emergency procedures or in surgery for tumors of the liver. They afford excellent exposure, and although specific complications arising from their use occur only occasionally, i.e., osteitis or septic chondritis, their severity should be kept in mind. Accordingly, we have abandoned these incisions as an approach to a portacaval shunt and use instead a large right subcostal incision which also gives excellent exposure. Likewise, in surgery for cancer of the esophagus, we prefer to combine the abdominal and thoracic approaches without transaction of the diaphragm.

A. Midline Abdominal Incision with Sternotomy

When it is desirable to enlarge a midline abdominal incision toward the thorax via midline sternotomy, the abdominal skin incision is carried upward to the superior margin of the sternal manubrium (Fig. 4.8). It is recommended that the xiphoid process be resec-

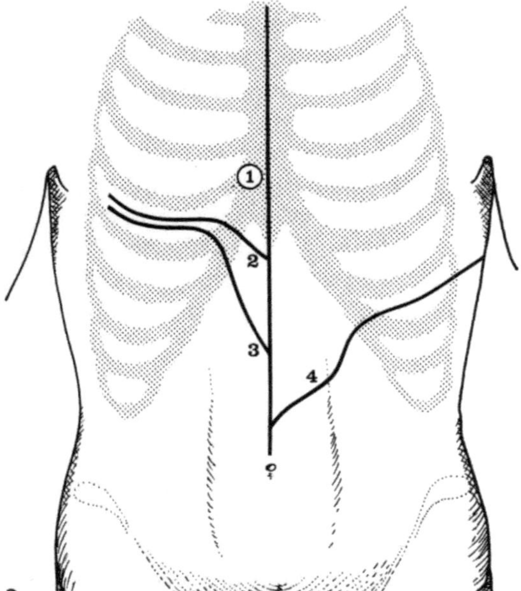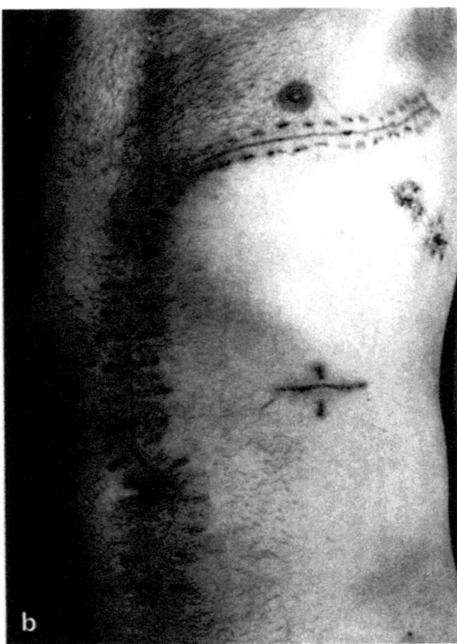

Fig. 4.8a, b. Thoracoabdominal incisions. **a** *1* Midline supraumbilical extended by full sternotomy; *2* midline supraumbilical extended by partial sternotomy to the right 5th intercostal space; *3* midline abdominal transformed into thoracophenolaparotomy (Bernard's incision); *4* thoracophrenolaparotomy via the left 8th intercostal space. **b** Midline laparotomy enlarged to left thoracotomy via the 5th intercostal space in a patient with a bullet wound of the heart (3rd postoperative week)

ted prior to sectioning of the sternum. A midline peritoneodiaphragmatic buttonhole opening is then made. Retrosternal dissection is started with scissors and followed by blunt dissection with a sponge stick or finger in contact with the sternum, according to the tunneling procedure described by Robertson and Sargent (1950) and introduced in France by Orsoni and Lemaire (1951). Dissection is then begun from above, posterior to the manubrium, to meet with the dissection already made below. The sternum can now be sectioned using either a costotome or cast-cutting saw, both of which can be used without risk of injury to the pericardium or left brachiocephalic vein. Partial sternotomy is also possible. In such cases the sternum is cut transversely where the thoracotomy was made, at the level of the forth or fifth intercostal space.

B. Midline Abdominal Incision
with Extension to Thoracophrenolaparotomy

As an emergency procedure, notably in cases of trauma to the liver, a midline incision of the abdomen can easily be transformed into a thoracolaparotomy with diaphragmatic incision (Fig. 4.8). Thoracotomy is made in the fifth intercostal space without rib resection, after which the sixth and seventh costal cartilages

are sectioned obliquely, allowing the thoracotomy to join the midline abdominal incision on the right edge of the base of the xiphoid process or slightly lateral to it. This approach, initially proposed by R. Bernard in 1958 for surgery of the esophagus, is not dangerous for the skin, regardless of whether the thoracic incision joins the upper end of the midline abdominal incision or connects almost perpendicular to it halfway between the xiphoid process and the umbilicus. We have often used this incision in cases of severe contusion of the liver. When the incision is made on the right side, the diaphragm is sectioned obliquely from its chondral insertions down to a point 1 or 2 cm above the inferior vena cava.

C. Oblique Abdominal Incision
with Extension to Thoracophrenolaparotomy

All types of laparotomy - horizontal, vertical, or oblique - which lie more or less obliquely along the costal margin, can be enlarged toward the thorax by section of the costal margin and diaphragm and opening of an intercostal space. This procedure for enlargement was described as early as 1919 by Anselme Schwartz and Jean Quenu. The initial oblique incision is made in the hypochondrium beginning on the linea alba, at the level of the umbilicus or slightly above it, to run upward and laterally and terminate roughly perpendicular to the thoracic ridge facing the sixth, seventh, or eight intercostal spaces, depending on the need. The incision is made through the skin and all layers, including the peritoneum. When enlargement toward the thorax is required, the incision need to be extended only a few centimeters onto the thoracic ridge, which is then easily cut with a bistoury, since at this level the site of incision lies over the costal cartilages. Subsequent to hemostasis of the corresponding intercostal vessels, the incision is extended above along the intercostal space and in depth through the diaphragm. A Finochietto retractor can now be installed to allow good exposure of the subphrenic fossa.

IV. Selection of an Incision

The selection of an incision is based on several factors. An appropriate approach should lead to clear exposure of the region or viscera to be operated on and allow for easy enlargement. Furthermore, it should not lead to weakness of the abdominal wall after closure, and the resulting scar should be as aesthetic as possible.

With these notions in mind the operator should run through a small checklist before commencing abdominal surgery. Such a checklist includes the following: the type of operation to be performed; the patient's morphology [Caix & Cubertafond 1978]; the risk factors for burst abdomen and incisional hernia (see page 118), including age, obesity, multiparity, and history of sepsis during a previous operation; the sites of incision of prior interventions; the probability of reintervention. In sum, the appropriate incision should give the best possible exposure with a minimum of inconvenience.

A. Operative Exposure

Operative exposure depends upon the site of the viscera to be operated on. Indeed, one need simply bear in mind the projection of certain viscera on the anterior abdominal wall to fully realize that it is more logical to incise the wall directly over the organ or structure requiring operation via a lateral, transverse, or oblique incision than to approach it from a distance via a midline incision, which may sometimes force the operator to work from an inappropriate position.

Surgery of the biliary apparatus and right colon is a good example of this point.

The morphology of the patient is another important factor guiding the type of operative exposure to be used. Over the past 40 years in Bordeaux and 30 years in Limoges [Caix & Cubertafond 1978], surgeons have emphasized the importance of topographical study of the thoracoabdominal viscera with respect to morphology. In short, stocky subjects the liver and biliary apparatus are largely covered by the chondrocostal ridge, these organs thus lying rather high in a large and deep thoracoabdominal region. Access to these structures is considerably facilitated by an oblique right subcostal incision, which can easily be enlarged over the midline to become a bilateral subcostal incision (Leclerc's incision). Accordingly, biliary and hepatic surgery and portacaval shunts can be achieved without special problems. In this same type of short stocky patient, wide exposure of the pancreas can be achieved with a large transverse subumbilical incision (e.g., Sprengel's incision), whereas radicular portacaval shunts can best be made via rather wide transverse incisions at an appropriately lower level of the abdominal wall.

From the practical standpoint, all types of abdominal surgery can be done via linear or arcuate oblique or transverse incisions [Hay et al. 1980]. A tentative quantification of their advantages compared with midline laparotomies is given below.

B. Disadvantages of Laparotomy

Laparotomy may lead to two types of complications, parietal and pulmonary.

1. Parietal Complications

The *aesthetic* appearance of an incision is often a minor detail because of the advanced age of many patients, although some young subjects will prefer an asymmetrical scar hidden in a skin fold rather than a perfectly symmetrical, but highly visible, midline scar. The *pain* arising from midline and transverse incisions was studied in a randomized trial by the Pollock team in Scarborough [Greenall et al. 1980]. However, the two testing techniques used in that study (pain scales filled in by the patient and amount of analgesics administered) were abandoned because of their lack of objectivity. The two major parietal complications of abdominal wall incision are burst abdomen and incisional hernia. These complications are studied in detail in Chap 8. The data given below are presented simply to help orient the choice of an approach to the abdominal wall.

Burst abdomen is a postoperative complication in 0.03%-3% of laparotomies and carries a mortality ranging from 0% to 85%, according to series. These statistics underline the severity of this complication. The numerical data given below point out the role of the site of abdominal incision with respect to the occurrence of burst abdomen.

In older retrospective studies on a total of 9,165 laparotomies, Grenier et al. (1971) and Maillet and Revelin (1974) reported 68 cases of burst abdomen (0.74%) resulting from 63 midline and five transverse incisions. However, these authors did not give the relative proportions of these two types of incision, and thus their data can be considered of only limited value.

We reported a retrospective study of 1,446 laparotomies performed in our hospital at Bobigny, France [Chevrel & Loury 1980]. Of the 1,055 incisions made between 1970 and 1973, a total of 19 cases of burst abdomen (1.8%) were recorded. Fifteen of these cases occurred after 948 midline incisions (1.5%), three were seen in a total of 20 oblique incisions (Barraya's incision), and no cases were observed subsequent to 37 transverse incisions and 50 thoracophrenolaparotomies (see page 120).

In the first half of 1979, transverse incisions accounted for 22.5% of the laparotomies performed at our hospital (88 of 391 laparotomies). Burst abdomen, observed in four of our patients (1%), arose in three of the 298 midline laparotomies and in one of the five thoracophrenolaparotomies, but in none of the 88 transverse or subcostal incisions. These findings suggest that the incidence of this complication is lower when a transverse approach to the abdominal wall is used.

Conclusions of greater validity can be drawn from the prospective randomized trial published in 1980 by Greenall et al. Of the 579 laparotomies performed, 557 allowed meaningful analysis, i.e., 276 midline and 281 transverse incisions. In this series two cases of burst abdomen (0.4%) occurred after midline laparotomy, whereas none were seen after transverse incision of the abdominal wall. These results confirm the retrospective data presented above and thus indicate that, in comparison with midline laparotomy, the risk of postoperative burst abdomen is lower when a transverse approach is used. However, the results of other published series suggest the absence of a significant relationship between the type of abdominal wall incision

and the occurrence of burst abdomen or incisional hernia [Richards et al. 1983].

It is quite difficult to quantify the incidence of *incisional hernia* according to the type of incision of the abdominal wall, its overall frequency varying between 4% (Chevrel: 120/3,000 procedures) and 8% (Pollock: 7%; Nyhus: 8%). Most cases occur after midline laparotomy, but it is also true that the latter is far more often performed than transverse incision of the abdominal wall [Chevrel 1983].

The reduced risk subsequent to transverse incision is also suggested on the basis of theoretical data. The forces of traction acting on the margins of a longitudinal incision are clearly greater than those acting on a horizontal incision. In a postmortem study by Greenall et al. (1980) it was shown that the force necessary to tear out a thread placed 5 mm from an incision of the rectus sheath was 0.93 kg in the case of a longitudinal incision and 1.78 kg in the case of a transverse incision. When the suture material was placed at a distance of 10 mm from the incision, the values were 2.65 and 5.75 kg respectively (Fig. 4.9). From the practical standpoint, the randomized study by Greenall et al. (1980) showed that the overall incidence of incisional hernia was 7% at 6 months' follow-up. There were 17 cases (7.3%) of incisional hernia in the 233 midline laparotomies, of which eight occurred subsequent to sepsis; 15 hernias (6.4%) were seen in the 234 transverse incisions, of which 13 were observed subsequent to sepsis. There findings clearly illustrate the widely

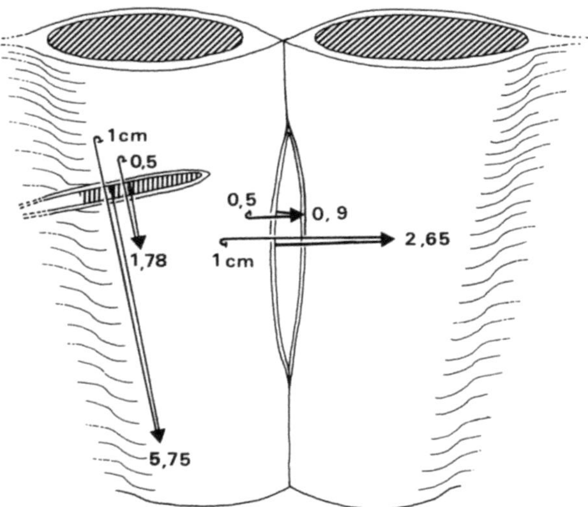

Fig. 4.9. Study of the forces required to tear a suture. Vertical incision: rupture occurs at a force of 0.9 kg or 2.6 kg when the suture is placed at a distance of 5 mm or 10 mm respectively. Horizontal incision: 1.7 kg at 5 mm, 5.7 kg at 10 mm

held notion that abscess of the abdominal wall is a major factor leading to incisional hernia. In this series the authors reported the occurrence of sepsis in 26% of the laparotomies, and its frequency was approximately the same in both types of incision. Conversely, in the absence of suppuration the transverse incision clearly offered greater protection against postoperative incisional hernia than did longitudinal laparotomy.

2. Pulmonary Complications

The second major complication of laparotomy involves respiratory function. There is widespread agreement that the site and length of the incision are major factors contributing to postoperative pulmonary complications.

Spirometric analysis performed in the Department of Anesthesiology of the Bicêtre Hospital in Paris [Edouard et al. 1979; Miraud 1976] showed that the decrease in vital capacity (VC) in the immediate postoperative period varies according to the type of incision used: there is a 25% reduction after minor laparotomy, a 45% reduction after lumbar surgery, a 60% reduction after midline subumbilical laparotomy, and a 70% reduction after midline supraumbilical laparotomy. Conversely, a major transverse incision led to a decrease in VC of only 50%.

The maximum expiratory flow rate (MEFR) per second and respiratory volume/minute (MRV) decreased similar to VC, whereas Tiffenau's coefficient ([MEFR $\times$ 100]/VC) was not modified, thus reflecting the purely restrictive syndrome caused by the incision. Such a decrease in VC obviously increases the risk of pulmonary complications in patients who already have a preoperative disturbance of ventilatory function. However, the randomized trial reported by Greenall et al. (1980) did not show a significant difference regarding postoperative pulmonary complications when the different types of incision of the abdominal wall were compared. Indeed, minor pulmonary complications occurred postoperatively with 29.4% of the midline laparotomies and 33.9% of the transverse incisions, while major complications were seen in 9.1% and 7.7% of cases respectively. Nevertheless, these data show a trend toward fewer major pulmonary complications subsequent to transverse incision of the abdominal wall.

In conclusion, the data presented above do not allow one to select between longitudinal and transverse incisions on the basis of their association with postoperative complications. Accordingly, the incision to be used must be adapted to each type of patient and operation. The possibility of a possible preoperative anomaly leading to an increased risk of parietal or pulmonary complications should also be taken into account, although it cannot be concluded that there is a significant correlation between the type of incision used and the occurrence of these complications, especially those of parietal nature.

The main advantage of the midline approach is the rapidity with which exposure and closure can be achieved [Lemercier 1981]. In our opinion, the strong point of the transverse incision is its apparently lower rate of pulmonary morbidity and the seemingly greater parietal solidity it affords in both the short and long term [Chevrel 1981].

Below is a list of the incisions we prefer according to the viscera to be operated on:

Biliary apparatus	- right subcostal
Portal vein	- enlarged right subcostal
Liver	- enlarged right subcostal
Spleen	- left subcostal
Adrenal gland	- subcostal
Stomach	- midline or bilateral subcostal, according to patient morphology
Pancreas	- bilateral transverse supraumbilical
Right colon	- right transverse paraumbilical
Left colon	- left transverse paraumbilical or oblique anterolateral
Rectum	- midline subumbilical or oblique anterolateral
Kidney (lithiasis)	- lumbar or oblique anterolateral
Kidney (malignancy)	- enlarged subcostal
Subrenal aorta	- bilateral transverse supraumbilical
Female genital apparatus	- transverse suprapubic

V. Procedures for Closure

In closing a laparotomy the operator must choose between several technical procedures regarding the number of layers to be closed, the type of suture material to be used and the types of sutures to be made. In certain special cases the use of prosthetic material or, conversely, the absence of closure may be discussed.

A. Layers to be Sutured

The number of layers to be closed varies according to the type of incision. The midline approach presents a maximum of four layers (peritoneum aponeurosis, subcutaneous layer, skin), while an additional layer (muscle) is added for the lateral approaches.

1. Peritoneal Layer

The main aim of closure of the peritoneal layer is to avoid the adhesion of the viscera to the deep surface of a poorly protected aponeurotic layer. Such closure requires careful work with continuous suturing using slow- absorbing material (00 Vicryl or Ercédex).

The simplest way to achieve proper apposition is to use an everting continuous suture (Fig. 4.10). The only site where this layer is difficult to close is the umbilical region, where the peritoneum adheres tightly to the deep surface of the abdominal wall. In this area the sutures should take up both the peritoneum and aponeurosis in order to avoid tearing of the peritoneum. When a transverse incision has been made, the peritoneum and deep aponeurosis are often closed as a single layer using stronger suture material (gauge 0). Although it is our opinion that proper closure of the peritoneum as a separate layer reduces the risk of subjacent visceral adhesion, some authors suggest that the opposite is true. Cases of postoperative occlusion apparently related to closure of the peritoneum as a separate layer have been published [Ellis 1971; Ellis & Heddle 1977]. Similarly it seems that closure of the peritoneum as a separate layer does not decrease the risk of burst abdomen or incisional hernia [MacFadden & Peacock 1983] and may even induce complications according to Keill et al. (1973). Accordingly, it has been suggested that suturing of the peritoneum is a futile procedure, which some authors feel should be abandoned in order to reduce the risk of postoperative occlusion without increasing the risk of wound dehiscence [MacFadden & Peacock 1983]. However, we firmly believe that an everting continuous suture of the peritoneum made with slow-absorbing material avoids adhesion of the bowel to the abdominal wall. This attitude is based on our own observations. Every time we have encountered visce-

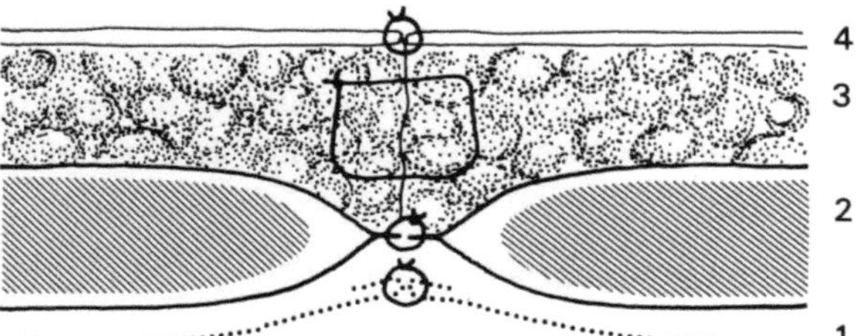

Fig. 4.10. Layer-by-layer closure of a midline incision. *1* Everting continuous suture of the peritoneum (gauge 00); *2* continuous or interrupted sutures of the linea alba (gauge 0 or 1); *3* continuous subcutaneous suture (gauge 000); *4* interrupted skin sutures

ral adhesions to the deep surface of the abdominal wall on reintervention it has been in a patient who did not undergo suturing of the peritoneal layer during the first operation. Of course, peritoneal suturing does not prevent the viscera from adhering to one another and it is this type of adhesion, in addition to a deperitonized surface, that is often responsible for cases of postoperative occlusion.

2. Fascial Layer

The aponeurotic structures can be closed as a single layer through a midline incision or as two layers, deep and superficial, when a paramedian, oblique, or transverse approach has been used. Careful suturing of this layer requires that it be clearly visible. Two questions arise regarding the closure of the fascial layer: Should interrupted or continuous sutures be used? Should nonabsorbable or slow-absorbing suture material be employed?

a) Interrupted Versus Continuous Sutures

A prospective randomized trial carried out by the *Association de Recherche en Chirurgie* (ARC) (Association for Research in Surgery) was designed to answer these questions [Konrat 1983].Midline laparotomy was performed in 3,135 patients. In 1,569 cases where absorbable interrupted sutures were used incisional hernia was seen in 32 (2%), while 26 cases of incisional hernia occurred (1.6%) among the 1,566 cases where closure was done with absorbable continuous sutures. Statistical analysis of these results demonstrated that closure by continuous suturing was at least as solid as that by interrupted sutures, if not more so. Furthermore, these patients were subdivided into three groups. In the group of high-risk patients (septic operation, general or local factors of severity) continuous sutures were statistically superior to interrupted sutures. Another randomized prospective trial by Richards et al. (1983), who studied 571 laparotomies, led to the same conclusion. In this work, the patients were also divided into three groups, and the judgment criteria were burst abdomen and wound dehiscence.

In practice we achieve fascial closure of midline incisions using two continuous sutures (one for each half of the wound) of gauge 0 Vicryl. Each suture is begun at one end of the wound and both are solidly anchored in the middle of the incision. When the transverse approach is used two-stage fascial closure is done, i.e. a posterior layer, where the sutures also take up the peritoneum, and an anterior layer. Each layer is closed using two continuous sutures as described above for midline incision.

b) Selection of Suture Material

Regarding the use of absorbable or nonabsorbable material, reference can be made to the study by Drouard et al. (1980) who analyzed 1,820 midline laparotomies. If one excludes the 204 patients in this series in whom single-layered mass closure was achieved, then in 572 cases fascial closure was done using nonabsorbable sutures (Dacron) and led to four cases (0.69%) of incisional hernia. Among the 1,044 patients in whom fascial closure was done using slow-absorbing sutures (polyglactine 910), five cases (0.47%) of incisional hernia were found. These results confirm the reliability of slow-absorbing sutures made of synthetic material, since the risk of incisional hernia was not higher with the absorbable than with the nonabsorbable sutures, regardless of the patient's condition or the type of lesion that was treated.

In routine practice we use sutures made of either polyglactine 910 (Vicryl) or braided polyglycolic acid (Ercédex, Ligadex). Gauge 0 is most often chosen, except for obese patients, for whom gauge 1 seems preferable.

Nevertheless, it is doubtful whether the incidence of incisional hernia is a sufficient criterion for evaluating the reliability of suture material. Recent studies seem to lead to conclusions opposite to those stated above and should temper the current vogue in favor of slow-absorbing suture material. A study by Bucknall and Ellis (1981) showed an 11.5% rate of incisional hernia when absorbable material (polyglycolic acid) was used compared with a rate of only 3.8% when nylon was used, whereas the rate of burst abdomen (respectively 0.9% and 0.94%) was the same regardless of the suture material employed. In a very recent study, Leese and Ellis (1984) reported on two groups of 53 patients who had undergone major laparotomy and were followed up for 1 year. The rate of incisional hernia was 8.5% after closure with nylon and 20% when polydioxanone suture was used. No cases of burst abdomen were found. According to the authors, nylon remains the best available material for closure of the abdominal wall.

3. Muscle Layer

The muscle is closed as a separate layer in incisions other than those made on the midline. When the muscle fibers have merely been dissociated, only a few stitches with fine, slow-absorbing material are needed to achieve approximation. Conversely, when the muscle fibers have been transected we prefer to use absorbable figure-of-eight sutures (gauge 00) for two reasons: The immediate purpose is to abolish the cavity between the two cut muscle surfaces and between the two aponeurotic layers, since such spaces may give rise to hematoma. In the long term, the purpose is to avoid the formation of a small depression which may be visible under an otherwise aesthetic scar.

4. Subcutaneous Layer

Separate closure of the subcutaneous layer seems to be of value only in patients with a very thick abdominal wall in order to avoid the formation of a tunnel under the skin which may lead to hematoma and subsequent suppuration. Two techniques may be used. First, one can simply close this layer by a few well-spaced interrupted sutures, taking up both the full thickness of the subcutaneous tissue and the skin. In this case the skin is only partially closed. Three of four stitches are usually sufficient to close a subcostal or midline incision and to avoid formation of hematoma or abscess. In the long term, the cicatrix resulting from this technique is identical to that obtained when full skin closure has been done (Fig. 4.11a). When hermetic skin closure is desired, the second technique consists of abolishing the tunnel using an absorbable continuous suture (gauge 2/0) to close off the fatty subcutaneous walls. In some cases a horsehair wick installed at both ends of the wound and left in place for 4 or 5 days is a simple measure to prevent the subcutaneous collection of serous or bloody fluid.

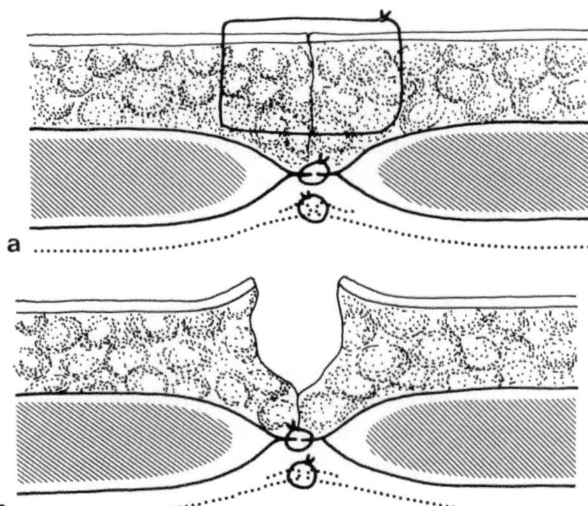

Fig. 4.11a, b. Closure of a thick subcutaneous layer of fat. **a** Superficial suturing of the skin and full thickness of the subcutaneous layer. **b** The skin and subcutaneous tissue are left largely open

5. Cutaneous Layer

Skin closure is performed according to the surgeon's personal preference. The use of wound clips gives a very aesthetic scar if the clips are loosened on the second postoperative day. In cases where the abdominal wall is rather thick we often prefer to alternate mattress sutures with plain interrupted sutures, using nylon with a straight needle (gauge 0 or 2/0). However, a more aesthetic scar is obtained with continuous intradermal suturing. In cases of a small incision devoid of traction, e.g., horizontal incision for appendectomy, adhesive dressings without skin sutures can be used to achieve an aesthetic scar. Regardless of the closure technique, it is essential to achieve good apposition of the wound margins without overly tight closure.

B. Special Cases

Parietal closure requires a special technique in cases of sepsis. When there is a risk of abscess of the wall in an obese patient with thick subcutaneous fat the skin should simply be approximated by 2 or 3 stitches leaving the subcutaneous layer largely open (Fig. 4.11b). Conversely, in certain cases of reintervention for peritonitis, only the skin is closed coupled with wide lateral cutaneofascial relief incisions [Nordlinger et al. 1980] (see Chap. 5, II).

In cases where the abdominal wall is weak many techniques of parietal reinforcement have been proposed to avoid immediate wound dehiscence leading to burst abdomen or late dehiscence causing incisional hernia. These techniques (Fig. 4.12) include mass-closure twin-loop suturing [Drouard et al. 1980], twin-loop extraperitoneal suturing [Burleson 1978], mass closure with far-and-near suturing [Samama et al. 1978], and atraumatic suturing [Chometowski 1975]. It should be borne in mind that reinforcement of a midline suture by full-thickness extraperitoneal suturing does not improve the solidity of the abdominal wall, as demonstrated in a randomized multicenter trial published by Maillard et al. (1980). Reinforcement of abdominal wall closure by pasting dressings around the wound decreases but does not entirely abolish the risk of postoperative burst abdomen [Guivarch & Mouchet 1969; Hay et al. 1980] (see Chap. 5, II B).

For several years now we have preferred full-thickness metal sutures (Ventrofil, Laboratories Bruneau), whose main advantage over traditional techniques of mass closure is that the forces of lateral traction are

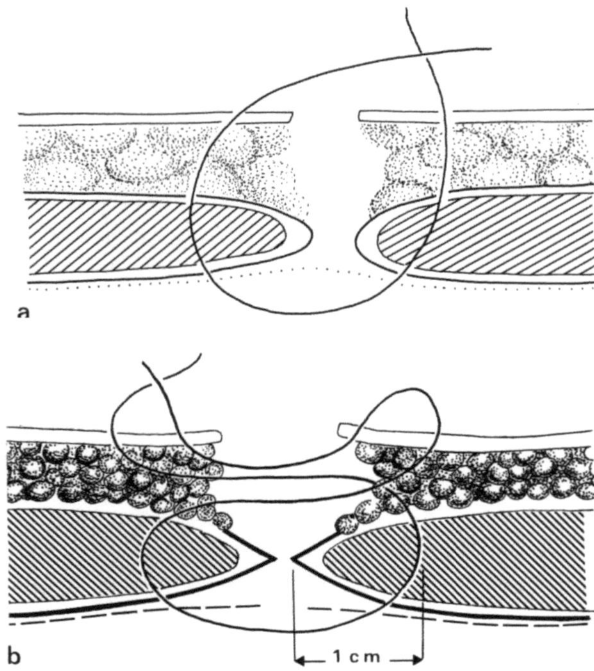

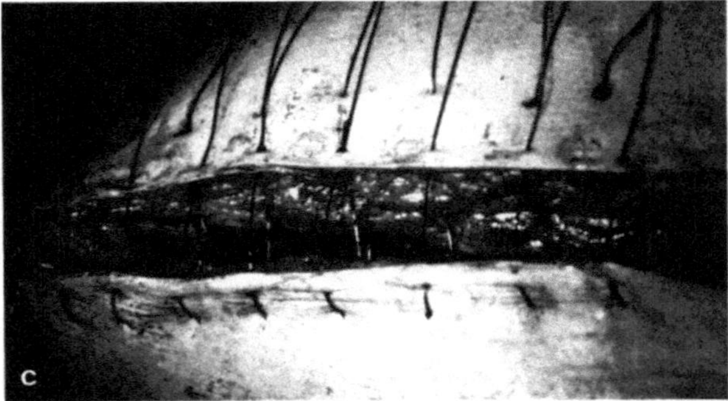

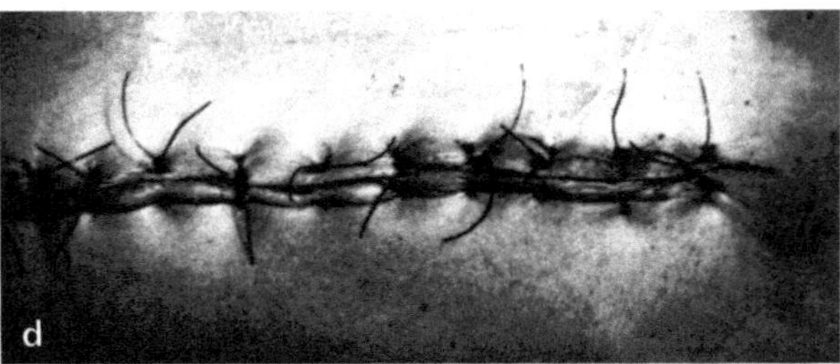

Fig. 4.12a-g. Procedures for reinforcement of parietal closure. **a** Simple full-thickness sutures. **b** Twin-loop mass closure (Drouard's technique). **c** Peroperative photograph of mass-closure sutures in place. **d** Mass closure after tying of sutures

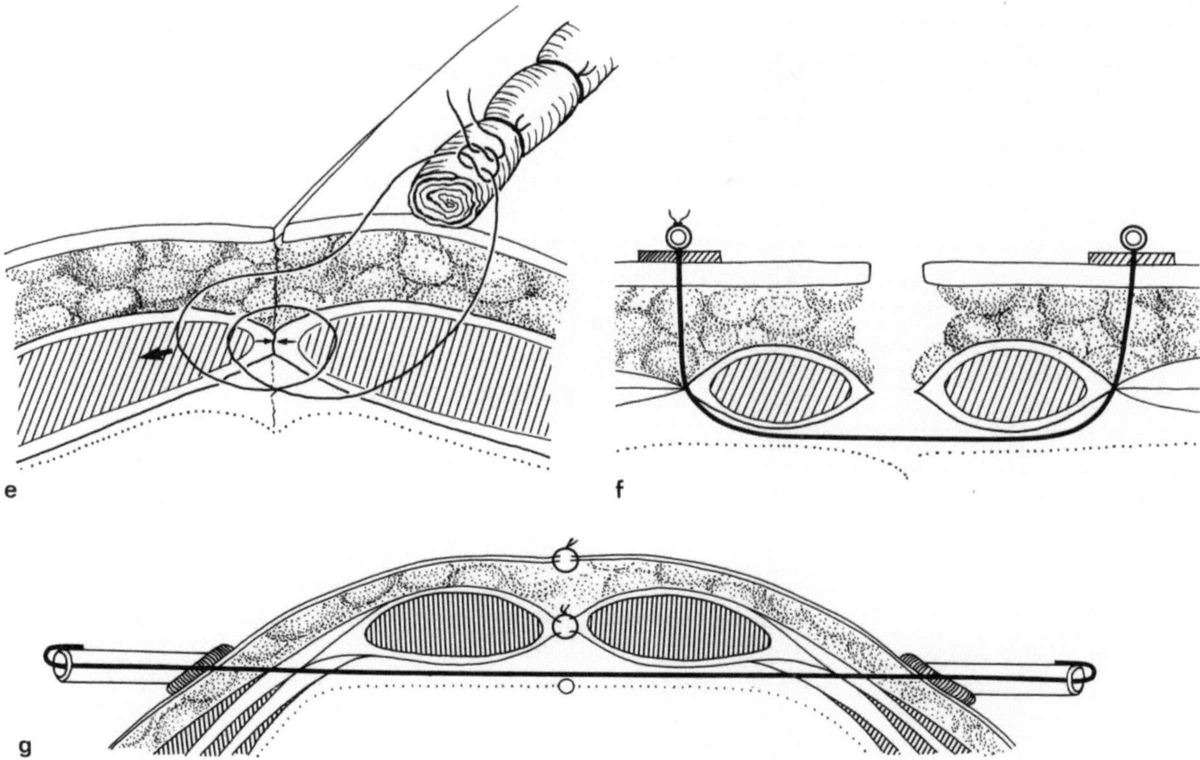

Fig. 4.12e Twin-loop mass closure (Burleson's technique): the inner loop closes the midline while the outer loop is tightened by contraction of the muscles of the abdominal wall. **f** Far-and-near suturing (Samama's technique). **g** Atraumatic suturing (Chometowsky's technique)

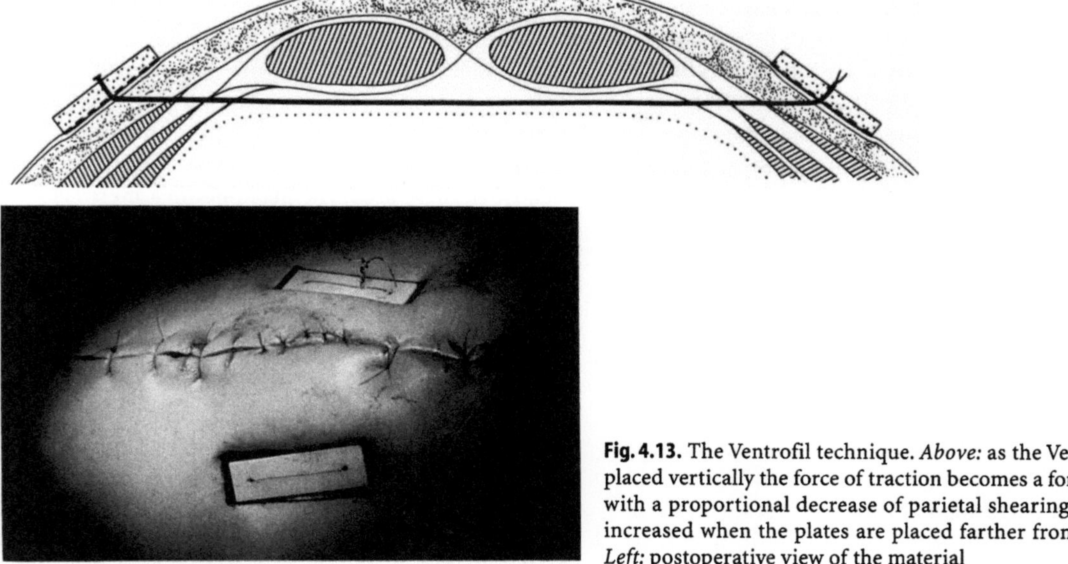

Fig. 4.13. The Ventrofil technique. *Above:* as the Ventrofil plate is placed vertically the force of traction becomes a force of pressure with a proportional decrease of parietal shearing. This effect is increased when the plates are placed farther from the midline. *Left:* postoperative view of the material

transmitted to rigid plastic plates resting on the skin, thereby avoiding any shearing effect. The traction acting on the plates can be broken down into two secondary forces: a shearing force which decreases as the plate is placed in a more vertical position (hence the need to position the plate in the region of the flank), and a pressure force which acts to press the plate against the skin (Fig. 4.13) [Saric et al. 1980]. When used in high-risk patients (see Chap. 5, II B) this technique prevents the occurrence of very early post-operative burst abdomen. However, left in place for 15 to 20 days, these plates do not fully protect against late burst abdomen.

The reader should consult the sections on incisional hernia (Chap. 5, II B) and burst abdomen (Chap. 5, II A) for a detailed discussion of closure using prosthetic material.

VI. Laparoscopic Surgery

G. Champault

Although the laparoscopic approach to the abdomen has been practiced for over three decades, notably in gynecological procedures and in the diagnosis of liver disease, it was not until the early 1990s that it became widely adopted, in an almost explosive fashion, following the first laparoscopic cholecystectomy carried out by Philippe Mouret in 1997.

Two factors were responsible for this sudden explosion of interest. First was the mini-invasive technique and important esthetic advantages in preserving the body image, particularly in a predominantly female population of patients suffering from symptomatic biliary disease. In the second place the images produced by the camera were easy to enlarge, reproduce and publicize, transferring the surgical act from the manual to the visual.

By 1997 virtually every abdominal surgical procedure, with the exception of transplantation, has been carried out via the laparoscope. Certain procedures were recognized early on as being much superior to conventional surgery and became 'gold standard' operations. These include cholecystectomy for symptomatic or complicated gallstone disease, appendicectomy in the obese, division of bands and adhesions, and suture of perforated hollow viscera, such as duodenal ulcers or following colonoscopic accidents. Additionally, treatment of gastro-oesophageal reflux, splenectomy for idiopathic thrombocytopaenic purpura, marsupialisation of hepatic cysts, Heller's ope-

ration for achalasia, the investigation of lower abdominal pain in young women and adrenalectomy, have been added to the list.

Others are still in the stage of development, including appendectomy, repair of inguinal hernia and other procedures on the abdominal wall, and colectomy for cancer, for which the results remain to be evaluated and compared with those of conventional surgery, in terms of feasibility, risk, cost and long-term results.

A. The Pneumoperitonium

The creation of a pneumoperitoneum with CO_2 is the common denominator in laparoscopic surgery. Its performance is modified by the general state of the patient, and the biological age (however these procedures have been carried out in centenarians) the cardiac and respiratory risk , closed angle glaucoma, blood dyscrasias, pregnancy and also by the local conditions including previous operations, the number and site of which may contraindicate both peritoneal puncture and the procedure to be carried out. In every case, the CO_2 insufflation must be controlled continuously and automatically in order to keep the intra-abdominal pressure between 7 and 15 mmHg, according to the patient's tolerance. Regular monitoring of CO_2 levels is mandatory.

1. Insufflation

a) Uncomplicated Situations

In the uncomplicated situation with a virgin abdomen, the pneumoperitoneum is induced by puncture with a Palmer or Veress type needle either at the level of the umbilicus or else in the left subcostal region, because in these areas the peritoneum adheres closely to the muscular layer. Having checked the function of the needle, the abdominal wall is pierced in two stages, the muscles and peritoneum. Safety checks are essential, including syringe aspiration to confirm that a vessel or hollow organ has not been punctured, and evacuation of the contents of the syringe while lifting up the abdominal wall. Insufflation is then started with a low flow of up to one litter of CO_2, the pressures being low to start with and progressively raised. The hepatic dullness disappears, whereupon flow can be speeded up until the desired pressure of 12 to 14 mmHg is obtained, according to the build of the patient, and the degree of obesity, up to a volume of 3.5 to 6 litters of CO_2. Total curarisation is essential.

b) Suspension of the Abdominal Wall
[Champault 1996]

In order to reduce the volume of the pneumoperitoneum, particularly in patients with poor respiratory function, it has been suggested to lift up the abdominal wall by vertical traction on the muscles, using a V shaped anchor placed within the abdominal cavity. This device creates a space identical to that of a CO_2 pneumoperitoneum. However, it has a number of disadvantages. Apart from a further limitation of the operative field which is already restricted by the introduction of a video apparatus and other devices, suspension of the abdominal wall may produce compression injuries on the muscular layers, particularly if the operation is prolonged. It also may produce a tendency to increased bleeding because of the lack of interabdominal pressure. On the other hand, it permits unrestricted use of the sucker.

2. The Trocars

These are composed of a sleeve of variable length and diameter containing a valve system which prevents escape of CO_2, with a pointed mandril of conical or bevilled shape. Some types are disposable, while others are made of metal and can be used again. They are introduced through the abdominal wall via a skin incision of the same or slightly larger diameter than that of the instrument, and directed towards the operative site (for instance the subhepatic region for cholecystectomy and the region of the hiatus for antireflux procedures). The introduction is made by progressively applied pressure and the correct position of the trocar is confirmed by a sharp escape of gas as the mandril is withdrawn. Introduction of the first trocar is blind, and hence potentially dangerous. It is usually carried out at the umbilicus, especially for cholecystectomy and apendicectomy where this is the usual site for introduction of the telescope.

B. General Principles of the Laparoscopic Approach

1. Orientation

The trocar should be passed towards the operative field, which frequently implies an oblique course through the abdominal wall. This partly explains the rarity of herniations though the trocar sight.

2. Disposition

The principle of "encirclement" is used. The trocars are inserted in a broad curve around the operative field. The optical sheath is usually placed at the center in order to provide direct vision. The paramedian ports are used for exposure of the operative field and the lateral ports, which are the furthest apart, are used for dissection, suture, etc. It is necessary to use a broad angle of more than 120» in order to carry out the different stages of the operation without tangling of the instruments.

3. Adaptation

The number, size and position of the trocars varies greatly according to the build of the patient, the usual custom of the operator, the extent of the pathology, and the need to have recourse to particular instruments such as clamps, mechanical forceps and so forth. For laparoscopic cholecystectomy one usually uses four trocars, but the operation can be carried out with three, five or six. The same applies to appendectomy, (three trocars) antireflux procedures (five trocars), splenectomy (five ports), colectomy (five ports or more). The addition of a supplementary trocar does not damage the abdominal wall, but may considerably improve the operative conditions, by widening the exposure or permitting the introduction of additional instruments such as a sucker.

4. Open Laparoscopy

Laparoscopy by mini incision or " open laparoscopy" is the best way of preventing the serious mishaps which are described below. This technique consists in carrying out a micro-laporotomy of 12 to 15 mm at the umbilicus, as far as the peritoneal level. A guide in the form of a metallic stalk with a blunt extremity is introduced into the abdomen. The sleeve of the trocar is slid along the stalk as far as the abdominal cavity and the stalk is then withdrawn. The trocar is then completed by replacing its valve and insufflation carried out through it. It is sometimes necessary to occlude the incision in the muscular layer by one or two stay sutures, in order to reduce leakage of gas. This orifice, which is slightly wider than a direct puncture, is useful for retrieving the operative specimen. Open laparoscopy is a very controlled technique which is often quicker to perform than a double puncture with the Veress needle and the first trocar. Many surgeons use it routinely for induction of the pneumoperitoneum, and it represents the basic technique for surgeons in training. It is essential in previously operated cases, but is of limited value in the obese.

5. "Laparo-assisted" Surgery

This combines a laparoscopic stage and a conventional open operation, reducing the size of the incision for the latter. The best examples are mobilization of the splenic flexure of the colon in sigmoid colon resections, where continuity may risk tension on the anastomosis, and right hemicolectomy and similar bowel resections. In these cases, following laparoscopic mobilization of the gut, the resection is carried out with the abdomen open and the anatomosis performed outside the peritoneal cavity, by the usual technique. Finally, mention should be made of the «dexterity glove» whereby the laparoscopic operator introduces a gloved hand through a short incision, which allows better mobilization of the specimen and assists hemostasis. It is particularly useful in the removal of a large spleen.

6. Advantages of Laparoscopy

Whatever the nature of the operation, the laparoscopic approach to the abdomen carries certain constant advantages over conventional surgery.

The postoperative course is less painful, as measured by verbal and visual scales and by the required dosage of analgesics [Benoit et al. 1994].

The hospital stay is reduced by 50% to 70% over that of conventional surgery, with less problems related to the abdominal wall [Champault 1996] as well as respiratory, septic and thromboembolic complications. Physical activity is resumed 50% earlier [Champault 1996].

C. Complications of Laparoscopic Surgery

1. Complications of the Pneumoperitoneum

Some of these are relatively unimportant, such as a «neumo-omentum» which is immediately apparent when the abdomen is explored, and puncture of the liver, colon or bladder. However others may be lethal, including:

• puncture of the great vessels, in particular the aorta, which lies only 3 cm to 4 cm from the umbilicus;
• massive gas embolus with immediate shock, cardiac arrest and abrupt lowering of the CO_2 pressure. This requires immediate cessation of the insufflation, administration of oxygen and prompt cardiac resuscitation. Gaseous microemboli have also been reported from injury to small vessels and may be responsible for transient neurological problems in the postoperative phase.

2. Complications Related to the Trocars

The most frequent is hemorrhage into the abdominal wall, which may require hemostasis and open invasion. This complication seems to be related to the type of mandril tip [Catheline et al. 1995] and is seen more frequently with the bevilled type rather than those with conical ends. The most serious are injuries to the vessels and viscera, following introduction of the first trocar. The aorto-caval axis and the iliac vessels are most often involved, depending on the direction of the trocar, but injuries to the mesenteric vessels, portal vein and epiploic vessels have also been reported. These injuries usually indicate immediate conversion to laparotomy so as to control hemorrhage and repair the vascular injury. This sort of injury may involve any of the abdominal organs, most particularly the digestive tract. Their incidence has been estimated at 67/100,000 [Champault 1996]. The stomach, small bowel and colon are most often involved but damage to the bladder, liver and spleen have all been reported. Once recognized, an intestinal injury requires immediate repair, usually by open laparotomy, but sometimes (particularly if the wound is small and the surgeon is experienced) it can be put right by laparoscopic suture. Overlooked wounds of this nature, sometimes quite small, run the risk of serious secondary sepsis (abscess or peritonitis) often serious and sometimes lethal. This type of trocar injury tends to occur in thin patients and those with abnormalities of the abdominal wall such as weak muscularity, poor relaxation or weakening by multiple pregnancies. Their incidence seems unrelated to the experience of the surgeon [Champault 1996]. Although the insertion of the first trocar is the one most dangerous from the point of view of vascular injury, subsequent trocars inserted under direct vision are not totally free of similar risks. The trocars should always been withdrawn under direct visual control. There is a risk of bleeding when the sleeve of the trocar is withdrawn, which can usually be corrected by mono or bipolar diathermy or by the insertion of hemostatic sutures. Major hemorrhage requires replacement of the trocar and introduction of a Foley balloon catheter which is placed under traction. These complications do not seem to be reduced by the use of the so-called "safety trocars"

3. Postoperative Complications

a) Early

The appearance of a portion of omentum through a 10 mm or 12 mm trocar site has been reported on several occasions [Champault 1995] so that all insertion sites greater than 10 mm should be closed by absorbable sutures in the aponeurotic layer. Infection is rare [Lauroy et al. 1994]. As with open surgery, laparoscopic procedures should be protected by routine prophylactic antibiotics in all clean or potentially contaminated procedures. Sepsis often occurs at the extraction site of a potentially contaminated specimen such as an appendix or gallbladder. It can be prevented by the routine use of plastic extraction bags and by the application of antiseptics to the trocar sites before the skin is closed. Infection is promoted by the presence of foreign bodies, particularly fragments of stone where there has been a difficult gallbladder extraction with a rupture of the wall.

b) Secondary

Unsightly scars may be avoided by using horizontal incisions along the skin tension lines, slightly broader than the diameter of the trocar. In fact, too small an incision is subject to tension forces when the trocars are manipulated. The length of the incision should equal the circumference of the trocar ($2\pi r$) and not its diameter (πr^2). Foreign bodies may be revealed later by inflammatory swelling or sepsis. They can be identified by ultrasound and removed by re-opening of the trocar site.

c) Late

Eventration is at less than 1% [Champault 1996] and is related to the size of the trocar (10 mm to 12 mm or more) and by failure to close the aponeurotic layer. It presents as an expanding swelling which is often tender, and is easily repaired, at the expense however of a good cosmetic result.

Port site metastases [Prasad et al. 1994] were first described by F. Drouard after cholecystectomy for a gallbladder which contained an unsuspected carcinoma [Drouard et al. 1991]. They were already known in gynecological surgery, particularly following ovarian cancers explored by laparoscopy. [Wexner & Cohen 1995]. Their incidence is not precisely known but varies according to the authors from 0.1% to 3% or more [Menducar 1994]. They appear between three and nine months postoperatively as an induration at the trocar site, the nature of which can be confirmed by ultrasound. It is necessary to carry out a wide excision of the area, but the prognosis is grave. They have been particularly prone to occur with Dukes Stage C or D tumors with carcinomatosis peritonei, but have on occasion followed a Dukes A tumor [Champault et al. 1994]. This situation has induced some units to abandon, at least for the time being, laparoscopic treatment of colorectal cancer, and others limit it to Dukes A or D cancers with synchronous hepatic metastases which are unresectable. Certain current studies [Barrat et al. 1983] suggest that this situation does not vary much from that which follows conventional surgery.

Peritoneal bands seem, in the absence of randomized studies, to be less frequent after laparoscopic than after conventional surgery, as is often noted at re-operation.

D. Conclusion

Laparoscopic abdominal surgery is now a routine and daily practice, even though not all of the operations have been completely validated. Its advantages as regards the abdominal wall are unquestioned, both from the esthetic and the functional point of view. Subject to restraints relating to the experience of the operator, this technique represents a way of preserving the integrity of the abdominal wall and preventing late complications such as eventration, the incidence of which may be expected to diminish rapidly.

References

Annibali R, Quinn T, Fitzgibbons RJ Jr (1994) Surgical anatomy of the inguinal region and lower abdominal wall: the laparoscopic perspective. In: Bendavid R (ed) Prosthesis and abdominal wall hernias. R G Landes, pp 82-103

ARC (1983) La fermeture des laparotomies médianes. Surjet contre points séparés. Essai contrôlé de l'ARC. Monographie CHU Créteil 10-12

Bassini E (1889) Nuovo metodo operativo dell'ernia limente. Prosperni

Bastien J, Hartglas L, Bastien B (1965) La désinsertion suspubienne des grands droits en chirurgie gynécologique. J Chir (Paris) 89: 181-188

Bernard R (1958) Un nouveau tracé de l'incision des grandes thoraco-phréno-laparotomies. Presse Med 66: 629-630

Bucknall TE, Ellis H (1981) Abdominal wound closure. A comparison of monofilament nylon and polyglycolic acid. Surgery 89: 672-677

Burleson RB (1978) Double-loop mass-closure technique for abdominal incision. Surg Gynecol Obstet 147: 414-416

Caix M, Cubertafond P (1978) Etude anatomique de la région thoracoabdominale considérée en fonction du type morphologique. Anat Clin 1: 185-188

Cherney LS (1974) A modified transverse incision for low abdominal operations. Surg Cynecol Obstet 72: 92-95

Chevrel JP (1981) Incisions verticales ou transversales en chirurgie abdominale. Les laparotomies transversales. 82ème Congrès Français de Chirurgie. Actual Chir Masson, Paris, pp 162-165

Chevrel JP, Loury JN (1980) Etiopathogénie des éviscérations et des éventrations. Monographie GREPA. Lab Bruneau, Paris, 9: 10-13

Chevrel JP, Duchêne P, Sarfati E (1983) L'opération de Bassini. Monographie GREPA. Bruneau, Paris, 5: 9-12

Chevrel JP (1983) Généralités sur les éventrations post-opératoires; table ronde (R Stoppa). 85ème Congrès Français de Chirurgie. Masson, Paris. Chirurgie 83: 1-2

Chidichimo G, Venuit de lo Scudo (1964) Indications, technique et avantages de la laparatomie transverse hypogastrique avec désinsertion des muscles droits au pubis. Ospedali d'Italia Chirurgia 10: 708-724

Chometowski S (1975) Fermeture abdominale par points totaux atraumatiques. Nouv Presse Med 4: 1645-1646

Detrie P (1982) Paroi abdominale, sutures digestives laparatomies. Nouveau traité de technique chirurgicale. Masson, Paris

Drouard F, Dufilho A, Bayle E, Moussalier K, Sequat M (1980) Etude comparative des risques d'éviscérations au décours des laparotomies médianes suturées au fil synthétique résorbable. Monographie GREPA 2. Lab Bruneau, Paris, pp 16-18

Edouard A, Miraud A, Place G, Noviant Y (1979) Evaluation spirographique du retentissement ventilatoire de la chirurgie générale. Cahiers Anesth 27: 25-36

Ellis H (1971) The cause and prevention of post-operative intraperitoneal adhesions. Surg Gynecol Obstet 133: 397-408

Ellis H, Heddle R (1977) Does the peritoneum need to be closed at laparotomy? Br J Surg 64: 733-736

Estour E (1995) Revue de 9221 cures laparoscopiques de hernie de l'aine réalisées chez 7340 patients. J Coelio Chir 16: 42-48

Greenall MY, Evans M, Pollock AV (1980) Midline or transverse laparotomy? A random controlled clinical trial. Br J Surg 67: 188-194

Grenier JF, Sava G, Kohler JJ, Gillet M (1971) Les éviscérations post-opératoires. Enseignement à propos de 40 cas. J Med Strasbourg 3: 201-206

Guivarch M, Mouchet A (1969) Sanglage abdominal par bas nylon dans l'éviscération post-opératoire. Presse Med 77: 101-102

Hay JM, Fagniez PL, Kaswin R, Mahoux P, Maillard JN (1980) Prophylaxie des éviscérations des laparotomies médianes par le bas collé. Etude contrôlée. Monographie GREPA 2. Lab Bruneau, Paris, p 22

Keill RH, Keitzer WF, Nichols WK, Henzel J, De Weese MS (1973) Abdominal wound dehiscence. Arch Surg 106: 573-577

Konrat A (1980) Comment fermer une laparotomie médiane: points séparés contre surjet de fils à résorption lente. Essai contrôlé de l'ARC. Monographie GREPA 2. Lab Bruneau, Paris, p 20

Leese T, Ellis H (1984) Abdominal wound closure. A comparison of monofilament nylon and polydioxanone. Surgery 95: 125-126

Lemercier M (1981) Incisions verticales ou transversales en chirurgie abdominale. Les incisions verticales. Face à face technique. 82ème Congrès Français de Chirurgie. Actual Chir Masson, Paris, pp 166-168

Luijendik RW, Jeekel J, Storm RK, Schutte P, Hop WEJ, Drogendijk AC, Huikeshoven FJM (1997) The low transverse Pfannenstiel incision and the prevalence of incisional hernia and nerve entrapment. Ann Surg 225: 365-369

MacFadden M, Peacock EE (1983) Preperitoneal abdominal wound repair: Incidence of dehiscence. Am J Surg 145: 213-214

Maillard JN, Hay JH, Fagniez PL, Prandi D (1980) Prophylaxie des éviscérations des laparotomies médianes par les points totaux. Etude controlée. Monographie GREPA 2. Lab Bruneau, Paris, p 21

Maillet P, Revelin P (1974) Les éviscérations post-opératoires. Journées Réa Med Chir Nancy, Spei, Paris

Miraud A (1976) Contribution à l'étude des conséquences ventilatoires de la chirurgie. Thèse médecine, Université Paris Sud

Nordlinger B, Levy E, Parc R, Bloch P, Cugnenc PH, Loygue J (1980) Traitement des éviscérations et prévention des récidives par la méthode des incisions cutanées de relaxation. Monographie GREPA 2. Lab Bruneau, Paris, p 23

Orsoni et Lemaire (1951) Oesophagoplastie rétro-sternale. J Chir Paris 67: 491

Quenu J, Perrotin J (1960) Traité de technique chirurgicale. Abdomen, vol VI. Masson, Paris

Richards PC, Balch CM, Aldrete JS (1983) Abdominal wound closure. A randomized prospective study of 571 patients comparing continuous versus interrupted suture techniques. Ann Surg 197: 238-243

Salama J, Sarfati E, Chevrel JP (1983) Les lésions nerveuses au cours des hernies de l'aine. Bases anatomiques. Anat Clin 5: 75-81

Samama G, Dupuis F, Bezard J (1978) Fermeture des laparotomies par points totaux en brandebourg. Nouv Presse Med 7: 2249-2250

Saric J, Charlopain G, Persissat J (1980) Intérêt du ventrofil dans la prévention des éviscérations postopératoires. Monographie GREPA. Bruneau, Paris, pp 26-29

Schwartz A, Quenu J (1919) Thoracolaparotomie. Paris Médical 9: 162

Tera H, Aberg C (1976) Tissue strength of structures involved in musculoaponeurotic layer sutures in laparotomy incisions. Acta Chir Scand 142: 349-355

5 Pre- and Postoperative Care

J. P. Chevrel

I. Preparation for Surgery of the Abdominal Wall

A. General

As does surgery of the abdominal viscera, surgery of the abdominal wall requires careful local and general preparation. It is not the purpose of this section to give a list of the routine investigative procedures that are done prior to surgery of the abdomen. However, emphasis should be given to the need for investigation of respiratory function and blood gas determinations prior to surgical repair of the abdominal wall in cases where the loss of tissue may lead to a modification of the infra-abdominal pressure and a subsequent disturbance of ventilatory capacity (see Chap. 8, II B on incisional hernia).

B. Skin

Preparation of the skin is begun on the afternoon before operation. The skin should be thoroughly but gently shaved and then cleansed with a lather of lauryl mercurothiolate (or an equivalent cleansing solution) with special emphasis given to the umbilical region. The skin is then painted with an aqueous solution of povidone iodine and finally protected by a sterile surgical towel.

Just before surgery is begun the skin should of course be disinfected once again with the iodinated solution. We do not place an adhesive plastic protector on the skin since removal of the latter prior to closure pulls off a fine superficial film containing the iodinated antiseptic.

Regardless of the type of surgery to be performed (repair of simple inguinal hernia or of complex incisional hernia), antisepsis is maintained throughout the operation with surgical towels soaked in povidone iodine.

C. Respiratory Apparatus

Ventilatory preparation is dependent upon many factors, including preexisting respiratory disease, such as asthma and chronic bronchitis, current respiratory status, and the type of operation to be done. A detailed discussion of respiratory function in major incisional hernia and of the consequences of visceral reintegration on respiratory function is given in Chap. 5, II B. Emphasis should be given to the importance of stopping smoking as soon as the operation is pro-

grammed and of performing respiratory exercises (physiotherapy), possibly coupled with the use of incentive spirometry [Celli et al. 1984]. Prior to surgery in cases of major obstructive herniation of the abdominal cavity, sessions of pneumoperitoneum according to the technique described by Goni-Moreno (1970; see page 143) allow evaluation of the patient's reaction to reintegration of the hernial mass and progressive adaptation of the diaphragm to functioning under normal conditions.

II. Postoperative Care

A. Drainage of the Abdominal Wall

At the end of surgery, drainage of the abdominal wall is required when the operation has been done under septic conditions in a patient with thick subcutaneous fat, or when there is a risk of secondary hemorrhagic effusion despite rigorous hemostasis subsequent to extensive dissection. Indeed, such effusion may give rise to a more or less voluminous hematoma. In cases where hemorrhagic effusion persists we use suction drainage with multiperforated Jost-Redon tubes. A single drain is sufficient in surgical repair of hernia via the inguinal route, whereas two drains positioned in Retzius' space are required when a preperitoneal prosthesis has been inserted via the midline subumbilical approach. Four drains are used after surgery for incisional hernia requiring "overcoat" repair and Mersilene prosthesis since surgical dissection is extensive in such cases. In order to avoid retrograde contamination we prefer to install the drains through a stab wound made about 10 cm from the operative field.

When closure is to be done on a thick abdominal wall with subcutaneous fat measuring 5 cm or more in depth it is advisable to drain the abdominal wall for a few days to prevent the collection of fluid. For this purpose a horsehair capillary drain brought out at both ends of the incision or a small flat rubber drain (3-4 cm wide) can be used.

In cases where extensive surgical dissection has been done our practice is to compress the dressed wound for 8-10 hours using one or two ice packs. The latter, when only partially filled, afford homogeneous compression and superficial vasoconstriction which reduce the risk of postoperative hemorrhage within the abdominal wall.

B. Transcutaneous Electrical Stimulation for Pain

This technique is based on the use of peripheral neurostimulation delivered by an external source during the early postoperative period. Use of electroanalgesia in surgery of the abdominal wall (as in visceral surgery) obviates the need for postoperative administration of analgesic drugs. Furthermore, postoperative depression of respiratory function does not occur and expectoration is not inhibited, thereby reducing the risk of bronchoalveolar obstruction.

Postoperative transcutaneous electrical stimulation is a recent step forward in the development of methods to control pain. The earliest descriptions of the effects of electric fish date back almost 2,000 years (torpedo fish, electric eels, etc.). Electrotherapy began in the nineteenth century (notably in the work of Duchenne de Boulogne) with the description of static electricity and the advent of the Volta battery. The modern era of electroanalgesia commenced in 1965 when Melzack and Wall (1965) introduced their theory, according to which pain transmission can be blocked by stimulation of the thick nerve fibers displaying rapid conduction (type-A beta fibers). Initially applied in the treatment of chronic pain, this theory is now the basis for relief or acute postoperative pain after a laparotomy for visceral surgery [Hymes et al. 1973; Van der Ark & McGrath 1975; Gestin 1979] or in cases of surgery of the abdominal wall only, e.g., treatment of inguinal hernia and incisional hernia.

We have recently begun to use transcutaneous electrical stimulation to treat postoperative pain resulting from abdominal surgery. Subsequent to skin closure, the disposable sterile electrodes (self-adhesive) are positioned on both sides of the wound margins at a distance of about one finger breadth (Fig. 5.1a). Stimulation is delivered by a miniature battery-powered external impulse generator (Neuromod 7718-220-Medtronic).

Stimulation is given at a fixed frequency, but the intensity is adjusted to each patient, the ideal stimulation being that at which the patient experiences a tingling sensation of the skin (tested before, and 6 h after operation). Electroanalgesia is given continuously or intermittently (1 h every 4 h), the intensity and duration of the stimulation being set by the patient beginning on the second postoperative day.

The excellent results obtained in nearly 75% of our patients are in agreement with those reported in two randomized double-blind trials [Hymes et al. 1973; Van der Ark & McGrath 1975]. The effects of transcutaneous electrical stimulation were judged on the following criteria: absence of subjective pain, suppression of analgesic drugs, decreased postoperative pulmonary complications, and decreased postoperative disturbance on pulmonary function tests.

In our opinion this technique of pain control is indicated mainly for patients at a high risk of postoperative respiratory complications, i.e., in cases of chronic bronchitis and asthma.

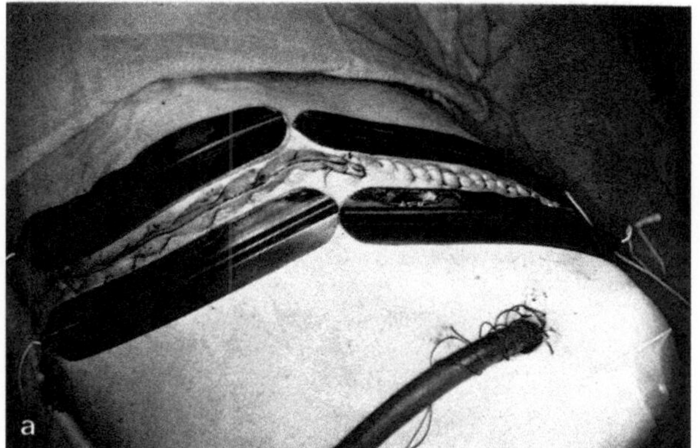

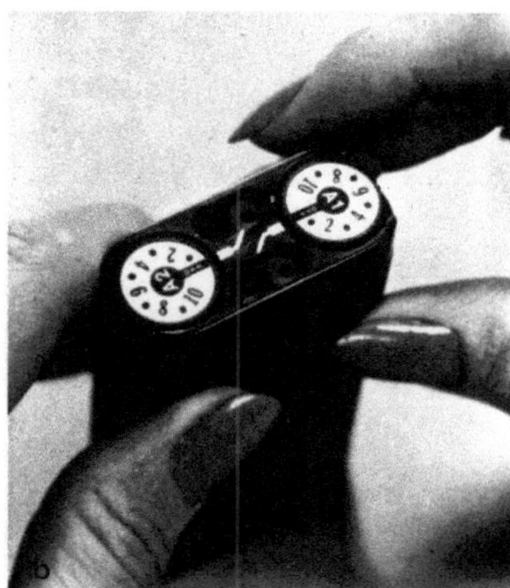

Fig. 5.1a Positioning of the self-adhesive surface electrodes on either side of the incisional wound. **b** The impulse generator used for postoperative transcutaneous electrical stimulation

References

Celli BR, Rodriguez KS, Snider GL (1984) A controlled trial of intermittent positive-pressure breathing, incentive spirometry, and deep breathing exercises in preventing pulmonary complications after abdominal surgery. Am Rev Respir Dis 130: 12-15

Chevrel JP, Pierrot M, Rathat C (1983) La radiographie des poumons dans la contention pariétale pharmacologique post-opératoire. Med Chir Dig 12 (2): 95

Gestin Y (1979) Electro-analgésie transcutanée post-ope-
    ratoire. Journées Franco-Marocaines d'Anesthésio-
    logie, Rabat, 21 (23): 1
Goni-Moreno I (1970) Les pneumopéritoines dans la pré-
    paration pré-operatoire des grandes éventrations.
    Chirurgie 9: 581-585
Hymes AC, Raab DE, Yonehiro EG, Nelson GD, Printy AL
    (1973) Electrical surface stimulation for control of
acute postoperative pain and prevention of ileus. Surg
    Forum 24: 447
Melzack R, Wall PD (1965) Pain mechanisms: a new
    theory. Science 150: 971
Van der Ark GD, McGrath KA (1975) Transcutaneous
    electrical stimulation in treatment of postoperative
    pain. Am J Surg 130: 338-340

The complications of laparotomy can be subdivided into early (hematoma, abscess, burst abdomen) and late complications (residual pain, incisional hernia, tumor growth in the scar tissue). Burst abdomen and incisional hernia are discussed in Chap. 5. Presented below are the classical complications, i.e., hematoma, abscess, and cicatricial tumors, in addition to the problem of residual pain, which is still poorly understood from both the clinical and therapeutic standpoints.

I. Early Complications Involving the Abdominal Wall

A. Hematoma

A small hematoma may be a benign complication of laparotomy without any further consequences. On the other hand, hematoma can lead to abscess or even burst abdomen. In exceptional cases where extensive dissection has been done hematoma can lead to severe blood loss, requiring transfusion and emergency reintervention.

Hematoma is usually clinically evidenced as a variable-sized bulging of the incisional wound. The patient sometimes complains of painful tension, while palpation gives the impression of thickening, resistance, or even true fluctuation of the abdominal wall. Full-blown hematoma presents as a pronounced ballooning of the abdominal wall, accompanied by bluish skin color and hypotension. Such a hematoma may contain more than a liter of bluish-black blood, often containing clots. The hematoma may extend throughout the rectus sheath when a presumably midline incision has not been made on the linea alba but rather has led to opening of the rectus sheath on one side.

The management of hematoma begins, of course, with its prevention, based on three points. First, thorough hemostasis of the vessels of the abdominal wall should be achieved during surgery. Second, at the end of surgery in patients with a thick abdominal wall one of the following two procedures should be used: evacuation via a small rubber drain, capillary horsehair drain, or suction drain, or partial skin closure with approximation sutures spaced 5-6 cm apart. In cases where extensive dissection has been done, i.e., cutaneomuscular (treatment of wound dehiscence) or peritoneomuscular dissection (treatment of hernia or incisional hernia), the spaces resulting from the surgical procedures must be evacuated by several suction drains (see preceding chapter). Third, local compression and cooling by partially filled ice packs produces homogeneous compression of the wound and any zones of subcutaneous dissection, as well as vasoconstriction of the abdominal wall vessels.

Once diagnosed, a hematoma should be evacuated immediately by removal of the skin sutures or clips, care being taken to ensure maximum asepsis to avoid secondary infection. In the exceptional cases where the volume of the hematoma increases hour by hour and the patient shows signs of hemorrhagic shock, emergency reintervention may be required to ligate a bleeding arteriole and remove the coagulated blood.

B. Abscess

The repercussions of abscess range from a simple prolongation of hospitalization to incisional hernia, burst abdomen, or contamination of prosthetic material. The incidence of abscess varies according to the type of surgery performed (septic or aseptic conditions), the circumstances of operation (emergency procedure or programmed in advance), and the type of hospital environment (public hospital or private clinic). Despite a maximum of risk factors in some cases, i.e., emergency surgery in septic conditions in a public hospital, certain precautions will yield a significant reduction of the incidence of abscess.

The well-known clinical signs of abscess are not discussed here. The main goal, in our opinion, is early diagnosis of abscess so that appropriate treatment can be given, minimizing the proteolysis which leads to weakness of the abdominal wall. Accordingly, the incisional wound should be examined and palpated daily, if possible, every morning and night. In this way, the early signs suggestive of abscess will not be overlooked: slight rigidity of the wound, a very slight feeling of thickening of the wound on palpation, a moderate reddening localized over part of the wound. In such cases, removal of a few skin sutures or clips allows the evacuation of a cloudy serous fluid before the next stage, which is that of the collected abscess. Unfortunately, diagnosis is often made only after the abscess has spontaneously opened through the skin. In such cases the wound must be completely opened to allow for appropriate treatment. It should be noted that the insidious development of an abscess beneath an apparently normal skin suture is a causal factor in one-third of cases of burst abdomen and as a antecedent factor in one-fourth of cases of incisional hernia.

Treatment of abscess is relatively simple. The wound must be opened over a sufficiently large area so that septic foci remain in contact with the fascial suture. During the next few days dressings soaked in Dakin's solution usually afford proper disinfection of the wound. We sometimes add continuous local infusion of lactic acid solution for 3-4 days. Bacteriological analysis is indicated, in our opinion, only in cases where septicemia is also present. Beginning on the 3rd or 4th day the use of absorbent dressings (dextran microspheres, Debrisan, Schering Laboratories) may accelerate wound cleansing (Fig. 6.1). Spontaneous closure subsequent to extensive opening of the wound is always a slow procedure and may take 4-6 weeks. However, in cases where there is a long, deep incisional wound through a thick subcutaneous fat pad, the skin can be closed again one week after saucerization. A flat rubber drain should be installed at both ends of the wound; this yields an acceptable cicatrix one week after closure.

The primary importance of *prevention* of abscess of the abdominal wall is obvious when one is aware of both its early and secondary complications. Accordingly, preoperative preparation of the skin must be scrupulous (see page 90). During surgery, towels soaked in iodinated solution (or circular wound protectors) are far more effective in preventing infection of the exposed abdominal wall than are dry towels, which afford no protection whatsoever, or adhesive plastic fields, which, when removed, strip off the antiseptic solution initially used to disinfect the skin. In cases of septic intervention, the systematic administration of prophylactic antibiotics significantly reduces the rate of abdominal suppuration and its subsequent complications. At the end of surgery hemostasis should be checked carefully in order to prevent hematoma formation. Postoperative dressings should be kept to a minimum; a compress containing iodinated solution is sufficient for this purpose. We now tend to leave wounds of the abdominal wall exposed, protection being afforded by a thin film of ethoxyethyl methacrylate sprayed over the site of skin closure. However, it must be borne in mind that the association of this film with iodinated polyvidone can lead to marked irritation of the skin.

C. Seroma

Certain techniques in the repair of inguinal hernias require extensive dissections and the placement of non absorbable prostheses which are apt to provoke a major inflammatory reaction which varies with the extent of the dissection and the prosthetic material used. Such is the case with the technique used by Rives in the treatment of midline abdominal hernias by the placement of a prosthesis behind the rectus muscles

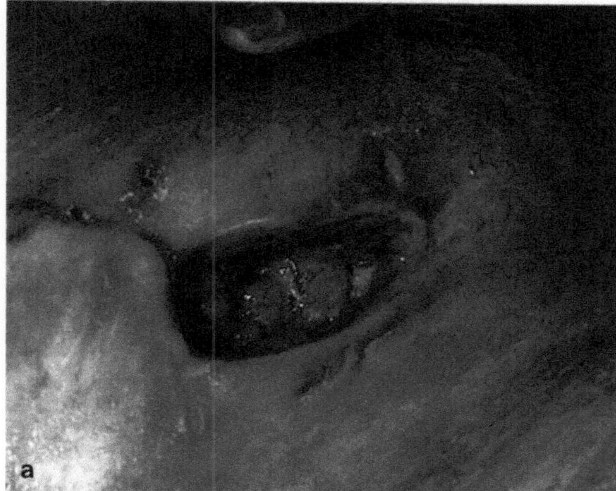
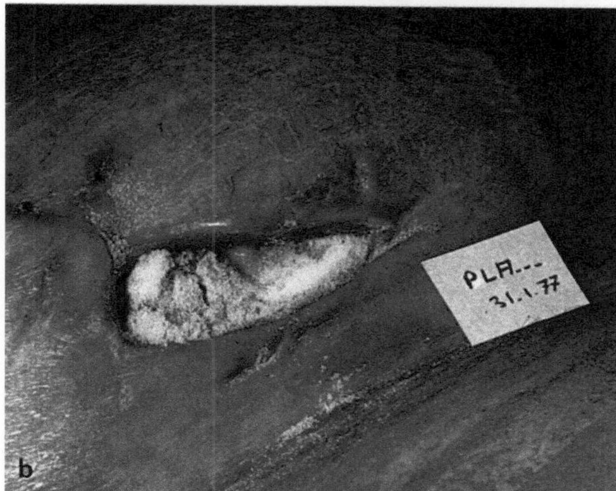

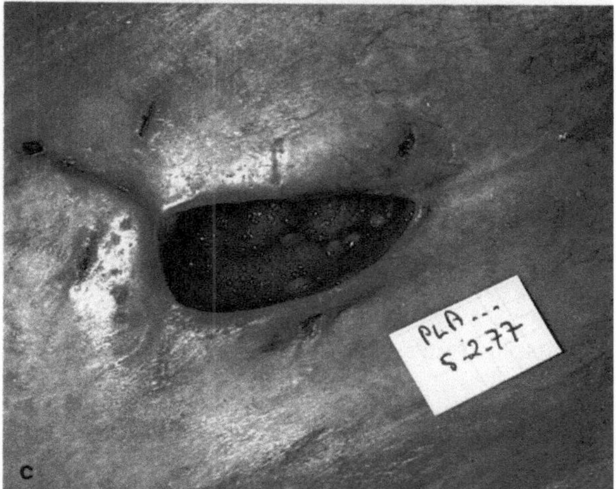

Fig. 6.1. a Midline laparotomy with subsequent abscess formation in the abdominal wall and partial wound dehiscence. **b** Wound dressing with dextran microspheres on the fourth postoperative day. **c** Picture taken 48 h later

and in front of the posterior rectus sheath, also of the technique used by Shiver in the treatment of such midline hernia by the placement of a prosthesis in front of the external oblique aponeurosis, and the Stoppa technique used in the treatment of certain inguinal hernias by the placement of a large prosthesis in the preperitoneal space. It also applies in the case of the lipectomies carried out by plastic surgeons, where there is often a major degree of tissue detachment. The inflammatory reaction, and the unavoidable division of small lymphatic vessels may lead to the formation of a seroma, the treatment of which is fairly straightforward. The role of the inflammatory reaction in contact with certain prostheses used in the cure of inguinal hernias is apparent from the reading of the publications on this subject whether the material involved is polypropylene [Kaufman & Weissberg 1985; Bendavid & Kux 1994; Capozzy et al. 1988; Usher 1962], Dacron [Casebolt 1975; Durden & Pemberton 1974; Lin & Vargas 1973], Teflon [Gibson & Stafford 1964], or PTFE [Debord et al. 1974; Law & Ellis 1990; Leblanc & Booth 1992].

In a personal series of 400 herniations, 240 received a reconstruction of the linea alba reinforced by a premuscular prosthesis, 107 of which were fixed by fibrin glue. We encountered six seromas in this series of 240 (2.5%) of which five occurred within a short series of patients operated on without drainage.

The diagnosis is clear on postoperative inspection. We have now returned to inserting 2 to 4 suction drains in every case where there has been extensive tissue dissection.

We also observed a serous discharge lasting for one month in a patient who had a combined operation including repair of an incisional hernia, dermolipectomy and liposuction. The leakage ceased spontaneously following simple elastic compression. The study of the literature concerning the frequency of seroma following surgery for inguinal hernia using a prosthesis reveals figures ranging from 0 to 20%. Seromas are also seen following the use of inert prostheses such as Tantalum, or fascia lata grafts [Lam et al. 1948; Lin & Vargas 1973; Peacock 1984].

1. Preventive Treatment

Two precautions help to reduce the risk of seroma formation.

• The suction drains should always be left in place when there has been extensive dissection involving different muscular layers. These drains, varying from two to four according to the extent of the dissection, should not be removed until serous discharge has ceased completely, which is usually around the fourth or fifth day. Persistence of any major leakage (20 to 30 ml per day or more) implies seroma formation, and drainage should be maintained until the area is completely dry, which may take several weeks.

• An elastic pressure bandage should be placed around the abdominal wall at the end of the operation, with the aid of a wide belt extending from the pubis to the xiphisternum. In order to prevent seroma, this belt should be worn continuously for 15 days, but as the repair does not attain a maximum degree of solidity until around the eighth week, it is advisable that patients whose abdominal wall has been weakened by multiple recurrent herniations, should wear the belt for two months.

2. Curative Treatment

There are various possibilities.

• Maintenance of elastic pressure may lead to absorption of the seroma after a period which may extend to three months [Bendavid 1986].

• Local injections of corticosteroids may induce rapid resorption of the collection. Graham has had success with a mixture of 10 ml Xylocaine plus 40 ml depomedrone in 500 ml normal saline (personal communication).

• Insertion of a suction drain together with abdominal compression may also hasten resolution of the problem.

• In case of failure, a further operation may be indicated, such as we have carried out in two of our patients and in two others referred to us because of persistent seroma. The operation consisted in resection of the seroma (which always presents as a pocket with a smooth, gliding avascular lining), insertion of a suction drain and a spray of cologne blue. Regardless of the technique chosen, cure is almost always obtained at between two and twelve weeks.

II. Residual Pain Subsequent to Laparotomy

Chronic pain persisting or occurring after the sixth postoperative month and lasting more or less for many years is rare after laparotomy. Treatment of such pain is difficult, and in most cases surgery is not indicated.

A. Pathophysiology

It is important to make a clear distinction between acute postoperative pain and chronic pain which is subsequent to laparotomy. To help make this distinction, the features of nociceptive stimuli and subjective pain, and the different reactions to these two types of pain are given below [Boureau et al. 1981; Gatt et al. 1982].

1. Painful Stimuli

Nociperception is not always related to the transmission of painful stimuli via a specific system similar to that transmitting visual or auditory information. The sensation of pain can be elicited via tactile stimulation acting through a mechanism of spatial or temporal summation [Boureau & Willer 1979; Zimmermann 1981].

Acute pain results from activation of a peripheral system, wherein the lesional site is the same as the painful focus. The stimuli causing such pain are of mechanical or chemical nature (inflammation with release of bradykinins and prostaglandins).

Chronic pain results from a defect in the inhibitory system controlling pain transmission in the spinal cord, as seen for example in cases of deafferentation (to be discussed further on in this chapter). In some cases chronic pain may be related to central mnesic retention of previous painful experience. Finally, this type of pain may also be related to hyperstimulation of nociceptors [Procacci 1969].

2. Subjective Pain

Regardless of the acute or chronic nature of pain, there is no correlation between the magnitude of the lesions and the intensity of the pain subjectively experienced by the patient. Pain is difficult to assess, and most investigational methods rely on verbal questioning or pain scales, wherein the intensity and not the qualitative features of the pain are given [Melzack & Torgeson 1971]. Emotion and distraction play an important role in exacerbating and attenuating chronic pain.

3. Muscular and Vegetative Reflex Response to Pain

Acute pain is often associated at the segmental spinal level with muscular (contraction) or vegetative manifestations, as well as with a generalized reaction of the sympathetic nervous system (the latter reaction is not specific to pain). In cases of chronic pain these manifestations may be totally absent, or present for only brief periods of time. Conversely, they may be more or less constant, thereby maintaining the painful state.

4. Emotional Reaction

In cases of acute pain, emotional reaction is not proportional to the causal stimulus but is dependent mainly on the patient's personality and prior pain experience. Depression and anxiety are often encountered in patients with chronic pain. Indeed, the analgesic effect of antidepressant drugs has been clearly established [Sternbach 1974].

5. Behavioral Reaction

The behavioral reaction to acute pain is often rather stereotyped, associating facial grimace with verbal and motor excitation. Such behavior is often exaggerated in cases of chronic pain owing to its effect on the patient's family, financial, and social life [Melzack & Wall 1965]. Accordingly, the acute pain symptom can be opposed to the chronic pain malady, although one should not confuse the former with organic pain and the latter with psychogenic pain. Acute pain can easily be treated with good results, whereas this is often not so in cases of chronic pain. The latter should be broken down into its constituent pathophysiological mechanisms in an attempt to find an appropriate and often more complex treatment regimen.

Two main mechanisms can be adduced to account for the occurrence of pain subsequent to laparotomy. However, both are often intricately related, thus rendering diagnosis difficult. One mechanism is the excessive stimulation of the system transmitting painful stimuli, while the other is the lesion of an inhibitory neural structure controlling somesthetic influx.

Reference to the general organization of nociception (Fig. 6.2) shows that the afferent fibers originating from the nociceptors (AS and C fibers) transmit painful stimuli to the spinal synapses (sites of sympathetic and motor reflex) and to certain ascending tracts (located in the anterolateral columns of the spinal cord). The painful stimuli then travel along these ascending paths to the regions of the brain that are the neurological basis of the perception of pain and related behavior. Spinal neurons can be inhibited by medullary interneurons or certain neurons of the brainstem.

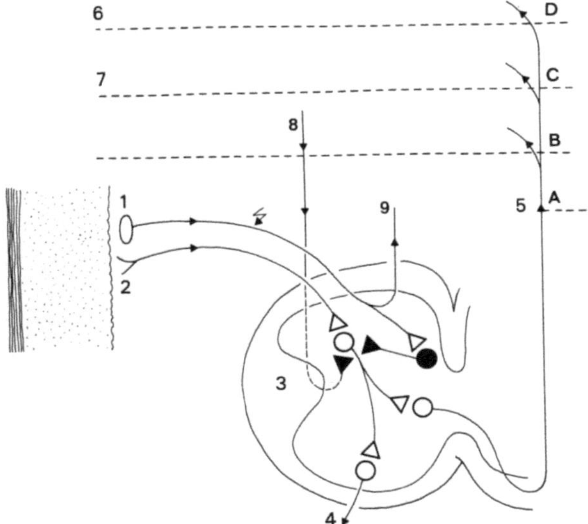

Fig. 6.2. Transmission of nociceptive stimuli in the spinal cord [Zimmermann 1981]. *1* Perception and experience of pain; *2* the morphinomimetic antinociceptive system; *3* mechanoreceptors; *4* nociceptors; *5* serotoninergic and morphinomimetic inhibition of painful information; *6* motor and sympathetic nociceptive reflexes; *7* transmission of pain input

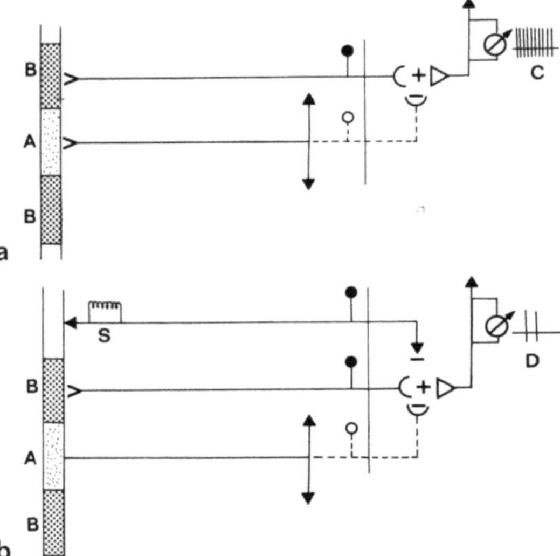

Fig. 6.3a, b. Deafferentation pain [Boureau & Willer 1979]. a Section of a nerve trunk *(arrows)* leads to a zone of cutaneous anesthesia *(A)* surrounded by a transient area of hyperalgesia *(B)*. Deinhibition is shown in the recording *(C)*. **b** The inhibitory effect shown in the recording *(D)* is elicited by stimulation *(S)* of the skin

B. Clinical Findings in Chronic Pain

Chronic pain can be subdivided schematically into two types: pain due to a peripheral nerve lesion and referred pain.

1. Peripheral Nerve Lesion

a) Pain of Neuroma

Pain of neuroma is well known to surgeons. These lesions result from the aberrant proliferation of nerve fibers beyond their neurolemma subsequent to partial or total section of the nerve without normal repair. The pain of neuroma is felt as permanent hyperesthesia or hyperpathia of variable intensity without paroxysm in the cutaneous territory corresponding to that of the involved nerve. Palpation over the neuroma triggers an exquisite pain resembling an electrical discharge [Head 1983; Wall & Guitnick 1974; Zimmermann 1981].

b) Deafferentation Pain

This type of pain occurs subsequent to partial or full interruption of a nerve, or to stricture induced by ligation. The pain is felt as a paroxysmal burning sensation in the corresponding sensory territory of the nerve accompanied by permanent background pain.

The deafferentation pain arises a few weeks after the initial lesion. On clinical examination one can initially note the existence of anesthesia in the corresponding area of cutaneous distribution with a surrounding ring of hypoesthesia due to the overlapping of the neighboring areas of cutaneous sensory innervation. This initial hypoesthesia gradually gives way to peripheral hyperpathia over a period of a few weeks. Palpation over the lesion site does not induce pain, although stroking of the skin in the spontaneously painful cutaneous zone will elicit a painful sensation [Boureau & Willer 1979; Lombard et al. 1977] (Fig. 6.3).

2. Projected Pain

In certain patients pain is reported at a site some distance from the causal lesion. Two terms are used to describe this topographical dissociation between the initial site of the lesion and that of the pain reported by the patient, i.e., reported pain and referred pain (Fig. 6.4).

a) Reported Pain Along an Intact Nerve

This type of pain results from the irritation of a fully intact nerve. e.g., compression of the nerve by a fibrous callus or a ligature. In such cases the pain originating along the nerve is reported by the patient in

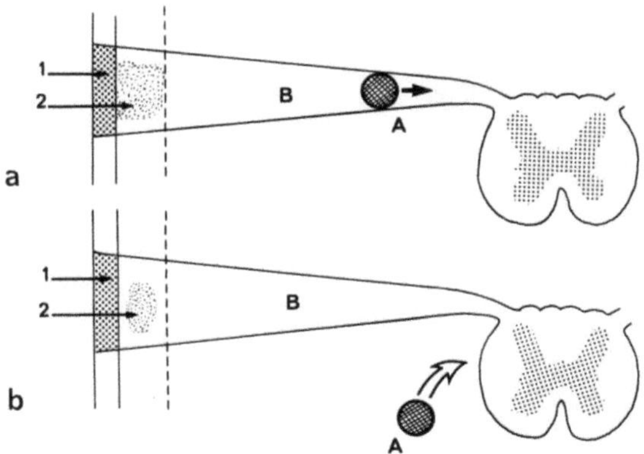

Fig. 6.4a, b. Pain projected at a distance from the lesional site [Boureau & Willer 1979]. **a** Reported pain. The lesion (*A*) is located on the peripheral tracts that transmit pain input (*B*). The latter is decoded as if it originated from a cutaneous or subcutaneous site. **b** Referred pain. The pain originates from a deep lesional site (muscle, joint, viscus) innervated by fibers which are different from those innervating a peripheral cutaneous or subcutaneous zone where the pain is erroneously localized

the cutaneous territory supplied by the nerve. The pain is felt as permanent, nonparoxysmal hyperalgesia and thus can be distinguished from the pain of deafferentation, which is paroxysmal. On clinical examination pain can be elicited by touch, and the absence of exquisite pain induced by palpation allows a distinction from the pain of neuroma [Head 1983; Ruth 1960].

b) Referred Pain at a Distance from the Lesion

This type of pain is due to a lesion located at some distance from the nerve, i.e., a lesion of a muscle (inflammatory granuloma in contact with suture material) or a visceral structure (intestinal loop fixed to the stump of the peritoneal envelope). The fact that the patient reports pain in the cutaneous territory of a nerve not in the region of the lesion can be accounted for by an error of integration of impulse transmission at the spinal level [Procacci 1969; Ruth 1960]. Two types of referred pain can be described.

Type-I referred pain is a permanent hyperalgesia without paroxysm in a limited neural territory. Certain nuances allow distinction to be made with respect to reported pain, i.e., touch triggers a disagreeable sensation rather than true pain, and muscle contracture is often noted in the area of the type-I referred pain. Analysis of cutaneous impedance will demonstrate the existence of a sympathetic reflex.

Type-II referred pain is also reported as permanent hyperalgesia, but in this case involves several metameric levels. Accompanying muscle contracture is not evidenced on clinical examination. Nociceptive stimuli (pinch, pin-prick) trigger intense pain lasting much longer than in type-I referred pain. No abnormalities are found on analysis of cutaneous impedance.

In clinical practice these different types of referred pain are obviously not always as stereotypic as described above. Precise diagnosis can be obtained in such cases by taking into account the features of the pain, surgical data, and the efficacy of any previous treatment. In certain cases, the latter may constitute a veritable diagnostic test.

C. Proposed Treatment

Regardless of the type of pain reported by the patient, two essential components, emotional and sensorial, must be considered with respect to treatment. General therapeutic strategy should begin with the simplest noninvasive procedures, with progression to more specific and invasive means when necessary. The simplest approach is the practically systematic use of nonsteroidal analgesics and eventually of narcotics with antidepressant drugs when other analgesics have failed.

1. Noninvasive Management

The initial treatment of *neuroma* consists of infiltration of local anesthetics with or without associated chemical sympathectomy in the area neighboring the lesion [Haberer 1977; Gatt et al. 1982].

Deafferentation pain can be treated by transcutaneous electrical stimulation, and it should be underlined that surgical intervention, which is always a failure in such cases, is contraindicated (Fig. 6.5) [Campbell & Long 1975; Hameroff et al. 1981; Legout et al. 1982]. When transcutaneous electrical stimulation fails, infiltration of local anesthetics and corticosteroids may be of help. Acupuncture may also relieve such pain in some cases. The beneficial effect of antiepileptic drugs remains to be substantiated.

Reported pain can be treated by neurolysis via local, truncal, or epidural infiltration of local anesthetics with corticosteroids.

Referred pain (types I and II) can be relieved by infiltration of the cutaneous territory with local anesthe-

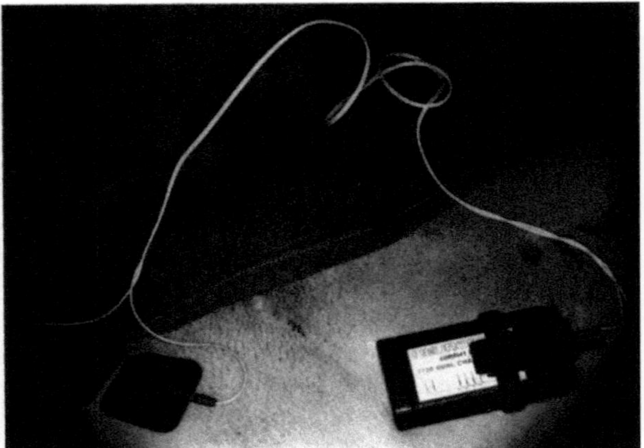

Fig. 6.5. Transcutaneous electrical stimulation in the territory of the genitofemoral nerve. The patient presented with intractable neuralgia subsequent to surgical treatment of left inguinal hernia

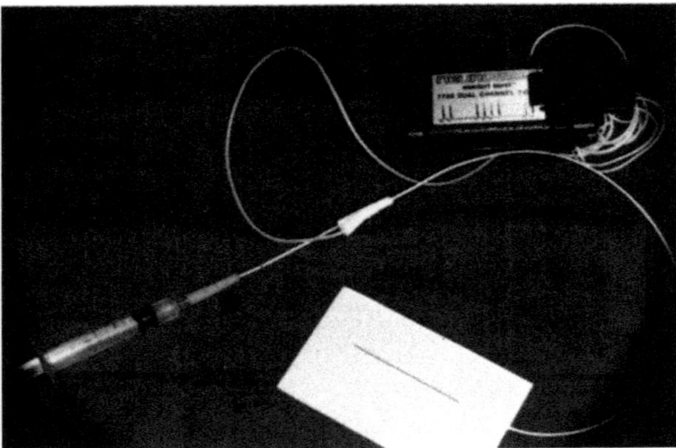

Fig. 6.6. Material used for truncal neurolysis. An electrical stimulus is delivered via the needle to confirm that the latter is correctly positioned in contact with the nerve, prior to injection of alcohol or phenol

tics or by transcutaneous electrical stimulation. Chemical sympathectomy allows improvement, but not full regression of the pain. Acupuncture is also indicated in cases of referred pain.

2. Invasive Methods

a) Neuroma

This easily diagnosed lesion is rather often an indication for reintervention with resection and bipolar electrocoagulation or burying of the proximal segment within a muscle. Neuroma is most often encountered as a sequela to surgical treatment of hernia of the groin [Chevrel et al. 1982]. In cases where it is not desirable to reoperate at the initial hernia site, the section can be made much higher up along the nerve, via the subperitoneal route, i.e., at its site of emergence from the lumbar plexus [Neidhardt 1982]. Certain orthopedists treat digital neuroma by burying the lesion in the bone marrow. This technique can be applied to neuroma of the ilioinguinal or iliohypogastric nerve, using the iliac crest as the site of burying. Finally, in certain cases transcutaneous phenolization of the neuroma can be done [Devaux et al. 1983].

b) Deafferentation Pain

When noninvasive methods of pain relief have failed, truncal neurolysis by injection of alcohol, or phenol or epidural neurolysis at the site of emergence of the involved nerves (using the same agents) may be beneficial (Fig. 6.6) [Sicard 1901; Smith 1964].

c) Projected Pain

Reported or referred pain can be relieved by truncal neurolysis with alcohol, phenol-induced sympathectomy (referred, but not reported pain), or differential truncal thermocoagulation. Intrathecal phenol has also been used [Nathan & Scott 1958; Wilkening 1977].

D. Results of Treatment

Since 1981 a series of 28 patients with intractable pain subsequent to surgery for hernia have been treated in our hospital departments. The results of the different modes of treatment used in these cases [Chevrel & Gatt 1983] are given below.

Full relief was obtained in ten of the *18 patients with deafferentation pain* by transcutaneous electrical stimulation. In seven other cases where this treatment failed, antidepressant drugs associated with local or paravertebral truncal infiltration afforded efficacious relief of pain. In the one remaining case all types of treatment failed.

Successful reintervention was done in *six cases of neuroma*.

Four patients presented with projected pain. In one of these cases reported pain was mistakenly diagnosed as neuroma and reoperation was performed. Relief was subsequently obtained in this case by infiltration of local anesthetic with corticosteroids. The pain in the remaining three cases (reported in one and referred in two) was successfully treated by a series of infiltrations.

As for all types of complications of laparotomy, prevention of pain should be borne in mind in the course of surgery. Such a preventive approach requires that the surgeon be familiar with the course of the nerves in the abdominal wall and their possible variations, and can identify the nerves during surgery of hernia of the groin [Moosman & Oelrich 1977; Salama et al. 1983].

In the presence of chronic neuralgia subsequent to laparotomy, careful analysis of the features of the pain should allow distinction to be made between the pain of neuroma, deafferentation pain, and that projected at a distance from the lesional site (referred and reported pain) in order to select the most appropriate form of medical or surgical treatment.

III. Tumors of the Scar Tissue

Four types of tumor may arise in the scar tissue of laparotomy, i.e., osteoma, endometriosis, inflammatory granuloma, and secondary malignancy.

A. Osteoma of the Abdominal Wall

Ossification of the abdominal wall is a rare complication of midline laparotomy, usually arising in cases where the incision has been extended to the xiphoid process or pubic symphysis.

The pathogenesis of these tumors is poorly understood. One suggested mechanism is the seeding of cartilage originating from the ribs or pubic symphysis along the incision. However, this theory would not account for osteoma arising in the scar tissue of an incision made at a distance from these cartilaginous zones. Indeed, we have seen a case of osteoma involving the scar of a McBurney's incision. It is often held that ossification results from the resection or longitudinal incision of the xiphoid process. Although no particular hypothesis has been confirmed, it may be reasonable to assume that some of these tumors are due to osseous metaplasia of calcified fibrous tissue [Guérin 1958]. These tumors are not preceded by any particular type of early postoperative complication, and investigative procedures do not demonstrate endocrine or biochemical disturbance.

From the *clinical standpoint*, osteoma presents as an induration running lengthwise along the abdominal scar, and in some cases may even constitute a veritable bony extension of the sternum down to the umbilicus. The lesion does not give rise to spontaneous pain but hinders movements of flexion. Lateral roentgenograms will confirm the diagnosis. *Treatment* is simple, consisting of full excision including the fibrous sheath around the osteoma, and leads to full cure without recurrence.

B. Endometriosis of Scar Tissue

Endometriosis of scar tissue usually occurs in cases of midline subumbilical laparotomy or Pfannenstiel's incision for hysterectomy, but it may also be seen in incisions made for other types of surgery.

From the *clinical standpoint*, endometriosis presents as a small, hard subcutaneous tumor which is tender to the touch. The main feature of these poorly limited tumors is their increased volume during menses. These lesions may lead to ulceration and bleeding. *Treatment* is also simple in these cases and consists of wide resection. In cases where no pathological cells persist, recurrence is not observed.

C. Inflammatory Granuloma

Inflammatory granuloma occurs as a small tumor which develops around a foreign body, e.g., silk, linen, or braided nylon suture material, talcum powder, micrograins of starch. The use of slow-absorbing sutures rather than nonabsorbable material and the removal of talcum powder from surgical gloves have led to a great reduction in the incidence of this complication.

Inflammatory granuloma is a small, generally painless tumor, often discovered by the patient. In some cases it is found on reoperation as a small roundish mass around the offending suture material. In such cases a small cavity containing puriform fluid that is most often free of microbes can be found near the causal foreign body. Full cure without subsequent recurrence is obtained by complete excision and closure using slow-absorbing sutures.

D. Secondary Malignancy of Scar Tissue

Secondary malignancy is a complication of surgery for abdominal cancer involving intraperitoneal (digestive tract, biliary apparatus, pancreas), retroperitoneal (urinary tract), or other structures (sarcoma of the abdominal wall). In some cases these tumors can be removed, but usually there are multiple lesions accompanied by tumors of the abdominal wall and/or metastases, rendering treatment futile. Tumors of the scar of a drainage wound usually result from exteriorization of a malignant infiltrate along the drainage tract.

In rare cases, resection of malignancy of the scar tissue can be achieved, although wide resection is most often unjustified, owing to the development of the cancer in this stage of disease. Minimum resection usually leads to recurrence within a few weeks of operation. Finally, in cases of radiosensitive lesions, radiotherapy may lead to stabilization over a variable period of time.

References

Bendavid R (1986) The "Fletching": a new implant for the treatment of inguinal hernias. Int Surg 71: 248-251

Bendavid R, Kux M (1994) Seromas and prostheses. In: Bendavid R (ed) Prosthesis and Abdominal Wall Hernias. R G Landes, Austin, pp 367-372

Boureau F, Willer JC (1979) La douleur: exploration, traitement par neurostimulation, électro-acupuncture. Masson, Paris

Boureau F, Gay C, Doubere JF (1981) Bases physiopathologiques des douleurs aiguës et chroniques. Similitudes, différences. RM 33: 2067-2073

Campbell JN, Long DM (1975) Peripheral nerve stimulation in the treatment of intractable pain. J Neurosurg 45: 692-699

Capozzi JA, Berkenfeld JA, Cherry JK (1988) Repair of inguinal hernia in the adult with Prolene mesh. Surg Gynecol Obstet 167: 124-128

Casebolt BT (1975) Use of fabric mesh in abdominal wall defects. Mo Med 72: 71-76

Chevrel JP, Gatt MT, Sarfati E (1982) Les névralgies résiduelles après cure de hernie inguinale. Monographie GREPA, Laboratoire Bruneau, Paris, pp 29-31

Chevrel JP, Gatt MT (1983) Que faire devant une névralgie après cure de hernie. Entretien de Bichat

Debord JR, Wyffels PL, Marshall JS, Miller G, Masrshall WH (1992) Repair of large ventral incisional hernias with ePTFE prosthetic patches. Postgrad Gen Surg 4: 156-160

Devaux C, Mangez JF, Attington K, Allibert F, Verdure L, Goldlewski G (1983) Diagnostic, techniques et moyens d'études de la douleur chronique bénigne. In: Andrien de Castro S, Balatoni E, Lecran L (eds) L'anesthésiologiste devant la douleur. Symposium International Ars Medici. Congress series no 3, vol II, 381-382

Durden JG, Pemberton LB (1974) Dacron mesh in ventral and inguinal hernias. Am Surg 40: 662-665

Gatt MT, Legout J, Boureau F, Pourriat JL, Cupa M (1982) Traitement des algies résiduelles après cure chirurgicale de hernies par les blocs nerveux. Monographie GREPA, Laboratoires Bruneau, Paris, pp 20-21

Gatt MT, Boureau F, Legout J, Pierrot M, Cupa M (1982) Mécanismes physiopathologiques des douleurs pariétales postlaparotomies. Monographie GREPA, Laboratoires Bruneau, Paris, pp 13-16

Gibson LD, Stafford D (1964) Synthetic mesh repair of abdominal defects follow-up and reappraisal. Am Surg 30: 481-486

Guérin P (1958) Tumeurs de la paroi abdominale. Encycl Med Chir 2011 B 10

Haberer D (1977) Importance de l'éclectisme dans le choix des anesthésiques locaux. Symposium International Tunis: Les anesthésiques locaux, 23-28 janvier

Hameroff SR, Carlson GC, Brown BR (1981) Ilioinguinal pain syndrome. Pain 10: 253-257

Head H (1983) On disturbance of sensation with special reference to the pain of visceral disease. Brain 16: 133

Kaufman M, Weissberg D (1985) Repair of recurrent inguinal hernia with Marlex mesh. Surg Gynecol Obstet 160: 505-506

Lam CR, Szilagyi DE, Puppendahl M (1948) Tantalum gauze in the repair of large postoperative ventral hernias. Arch Surg 57: 234-244

Law NW, Ellis H (1990) Preliminary results for the repair of difficult recurrent inguinal hernias using ePTFE patch. Acta Chir Scand 156: 609-612

Leblanc KA, Booth WV (1992) Repair of primary and secondary inguinal hernias using ePTFE. Comtemp Surg 41: 29-32

Legout J, Gatt MT, Boureau F, Cupa M (1982) Le traitement des douleurs chroniques après laparotomie. Technique d'électrostimulation. Monographie GREPA, Laboratoires Bruneau, Paris, pp 17-18

Lin BS, Vargas A (1973) Use of tempory prostheses to repair difficult hernias. South Med J 66: 925-928

Lombard MC, Sark C, Salman N, Nashold R (1977) Hyperesthésis chroniques provoquées chez le rat par la lésion des racines dorsales du plexus brachial. CE Acad Sci Paris 284: 2369-2372

Melzack R, Torgeson WS (1971) On the language of pain. Anesthesiology 34: 50-59

Melzack R, Wall PD (1965) Pain mechanisms: a new theory. Science 150: 971-979

Moosman DA, Oelrich RM (1977) Prevention of accidental trauma to the ilioinguinal nerve during inguinal herniorraphy. Am J Surg 133: 146-148

Nathan PW, Scott TC (1958) Intrathecal phenol for intractable pain. Lancet 76

Neidhardt JPH (1982) Traitement chirurgical des séquelles douloureuses des laparotomies. Monographie GREPA, Laboratoires Bruneau, Paris, pp 25-28

Peacock EE Jr (1984) Internal reconstruction of the pelvic floor for recurrent groin hernia. Ann Surg 200: 321-327

Procacci P (1969) A survey of modern concepts of pain. In: Vinken PJ, Bruyn GW (eds) Handbook of clinical neurology, vol. 1. Elsevier, Amsterdam, pp 114-146

Ruth TC (1960) Pathophysiology of pain. In: Ruth TC, Fulton HD (eds) Medical physiology and biophysics. Saunders, Philadelphia, pp 350-368

Salama J, Sarfati E, Chevrel JP (1983) The anatomical bases of nerve lesion arising during the reduction of inguinal hernia. Anat Clin 5: 75-81

Sicard A (1901) Les injections médicamenteuses extra durales par voie sacro-coccygienne. C R Soc Biol 53: 396-398

Smith MC (1964) Histological findings following intrathecal injections of phenol solution. Br J Arnes 36: 387

Sternbach RA (1974) Pain patients: traits and treatment. Academic, New York

Stoppa R (1989) The treatment of complicated groin and incisional hernias. World J Surg 13: 545-554

Usher FC (1962) Hernia repair with Marlex mesh: an analysis of 541 cases. Arch Surg 84: 325-328

Wall PD, Guitnik M (1974) Ongoing activity peripheral nerve: the physiology and pharmacology of impulses originating from a neuroma. Exp Neurol 93: 580-593

Wilkening M (1977) La neurolyse chimique dans le traitement des algies cancéreuses. Symposium International Tunis: Les anesthésiques locaux, 23-28 janvier

Zimmermann M (1981) Mécanismes physiologiques et traitement de la douleur. Triangle 21, No. 4

7 Closed Trauma of the Abdominal Wall

J. P. H. Neidhardt

Closed trauma results in more or less extensive subcutaneous rupture of the muscular part of the abdominal wall. The causes of such trauma vary greatly, from localized injury (abrupt impact, trauma from the handlebar of a two-wheeled vehicle) to major abdominal crush injury encountered in certain construction site accidents (compression by a mechanical shovel), farming mishaps (crush injury by a tractor), or explosions (blast injury). These different types of trauma lead to a wide variety of lesions of variable severity.

I. Hematoma

Simple hematoma of the muscle layers of the abdominal wall is diagnosed by elimination since loss of tissue per se is not observed. It is highly problematic whether surgery should be performed for such lesions. Such difficulty is related to the following factors: infiltration of the abdominal wall, which prohibits proper assessment of the possible muscle damage, and marked pain, which renders impossible the interpretation of the peritoneal irritation. In some cases severe blood loss and subsequent shock further complicate the clinical picture. *Hematoma in the sheath of the rectus abdomini* is usually easy to recognize, owing to its fusiform shape and paramedian position in the region of the sheath. *Hematoma of the flat abdominal muscles* spreads out within the muscles and posteriorly to the loin and is poorly circumscribed. In such cases secondary lumbar or inguinal ecchymosis confirms the presence of the hematoma. In cases of closed trauma of the abdomen it is very hazardous to conclude that the only lesion present is hematoma of the wall. Despite the current tendency to limit the indications for exploratory surgery, laparotomy should be done in any case where there is doubt as to the exact nature of the traumatic lesion. Indeed, peritoneal lavage alone may yield erroneous results. For example, the catheter used for lavage may enter the hematoma, thereby leading to the conclusion that the lesion is intraperitoneal (false-positive diagnosis). In other cases lavage may aggravate the lesion by causing progressive dilaceration. Finally, such hematoma is often accompanied by a bloody exudate within the peritoneal cavity, even though a genuine visceral lesion is absent. Under these conditions lavage may give inconclusive results. The best diagnostic procedure seems to be echotomography, which can identify the extraperitoneal site of the hematoma and the absence of intraperitoneal effusion. However, it should be emphasized that the presence of such a hematoma often hinders the interpretation of deep investigation by this technique.

II. Localized Rupture

Localized rupture leads to immediate or delayed herniation involving the anterior abdominal wall. Such hernias contain viscera displaying contusion or rupture. In most cases these lesions are accompanied by tearing of the parietal peritoneum, leading to hemoperitoneum. The purely parietal origin of the latter is always very difficult to confirm.

Localized ruptures can be divided into three types according to the level of the lesion: upper level - the abdominal wall is ruptured at or near its chondrocostal insertions or xiphoid process; middle level - rupture occurs in the center of the anterior abdominal wall; lower level - the recti muscles are disinserted from the pubis or there is traumatic laceration in the inguinal region (rupture of the aponeurosis of the external oblique and conjoint tendon).

From the clinical standpoint, localized rupture may manifest itself immediately after the traumatic event. In such cases there is a localized bulging of the abdominal wall, and on palpation the viscera can be felt beneath the skin and are more or less reducible. Diagnosis may sometimes be achieved only at a later stage when the hernia is fully formed, with a neck, and contains the visceral structures, which may be fixed in place. In the special case of traumatic inguinal hernia, it is often difficult to confirm that the hernia is the result of the traumatic event. The discovery of localized herniation in the course of surgery for abdominal contusion is a delicate situation from the medicolegal standpoint. Indeed, such a situation occurs when exploration of the deep aspect of the abdominal wall is insufficient. Accordingly, full investigation should be done in all cases of exploratory surgery of the abdomen.

Treatment of the above-described lesions is done either as an emergency or as a delayed procedure. *In an emergency setting*, the absence of indicative local or general signs may argue in favor of abstention from surgery. This attitude has been proposed by certain American authors who favor a general tendency to abstention in cases of open or closed abdominal trauma.

However, it should be emphasized that the presence of muscle rupture, even when it is localized, reflects the violent nature of the traumatic event. Pain in the abdominal wall and the resulting guard reaction, or the presence of blood in the peritoneal cavity are major arguments in favor of exploratory surgery. This should be done via a midline incision. At the end of exploration the wound (at least the deep layer) is closed. A special approach to repair the superficial myofascial layers may be required.

Cases of localized rupture in the upper or lower part of the abdominal wall near the bony or cartilaginous structures may require that the muscles be reinserted. Since marked retraction is absent at this stage, the use of mesh implants is indicated only in exceptional cases.

When these lesions are seen at a later stage (in some cases after unsuccessful primary repair, which is not always of best quality when tissue contusion was present) they often present as organized herniation. Treatment is usually achieved via edge-to-edge suturing of the hernial neck, whose surrounding fibrous ring allows solid anchoring of the sutures. Incision of the superficial layers must be done very cautiously, since the viscera may adhere to the cutaneous layer. A local approach is sufficient in most cases.

III. Extensive Subcutaneous Rupture of the Anterior Muscular Wall

This type of rupture is caused by major trauma where the impact to the abdominal wall is intense and widespread. One frequent type of accident is crush injury caused by a mechanical shovel or bulldozer. In such cases the lesions are rarely confined to the muscle wall but also involve the bony frame of the abdomen, i.e., fracture of the base of the thorax or pelvic bones. The resulting muscle tearing is so extensive that a systematized description cannot be given. The integument may show signs of necrosis and can be seen to "float" on a bed of bloody fluid. On palpation the viscera can be felt directly beneath the skin [Fredlund & Dahn 1967]. In the cases encountered in our department, lesions of the viscera (especially rupture of the small bowel and bladder) were consistently present. The clinical picture is commonly that of abdominal or thoracoabdominal contusion with severe shock. In such cases the need for surgery is rarely open to discussion since the lesions of the hollow viscera rapidly engender inoculation of the dilacerated muscles with fecal material, i.e., conditions leading to gangrenous cellulitis or myositis [Detrie 1982].

Surgery in such cases is aimed mainly at repair of the viscera. Indeed, surgical repair of lesions of the abdominal wall is not always possible, or, when possible, often leads to dangerous ischemia resulting from the muscle suturing in cases where the lesions are recognized late and are already infected. Thus, it is often better not to intervene on the abdominal wall, but to simply obtain cutaneous cover of the abdominal viscera. Owing to the precariousness of such closure, additional means of abdominal support are often required, e.g., adhesive elastic fishnet material. Respiratory assistance is frequently necessary due to the accompanying thoracic injury, as well as to the respiratory disturbances caused by any extensive lesion of the abdominal wall. The major muscle destruction in these cases necessitates the systematic use of antibiotics with a combination of β-lactamine, aminoglycoside, and imidazole drugs.

Extensive subcutaneous rupture naturally evolves towards the formation of massive, traumatic herniation of the abdominal wall [Dajee & Nicholson 1979; Dubois & Freeman 1981]. Treatment of marked muscle retraction may require the extensive use of prosthetic material. However, such secondary repair should be done only 6 months or more after the initial trauma to allow a sufficient period of peritoneal freedom and organization of the lesions involving the abdominal wall.

IV. Trauma of the Posterior Abdominal Wall

Such trauma may cause more or less extensive rupture involving the lumbar region. In most cases, however, trauma of the posterior abdominal wall leads to muscle disinsertion from the superior (lower ribs) or inferior (iliac crest) sites of attachment. The subsequent tissue loss is amplified by the contraction of the muscles resulting in the formation of pathological orifices, at least one boundary of which is formed by bone. These lesions are rarely identified at the initial stage, just after the traumatic event. At this early stage signs of lumbar trauma with marked hematoma are observed, and attention is naturally drawn to the possible existence of renal or spinal injury (fracture of the lumbar transverse processes). Accordingly, injury to the posterior abdominal wall is usually diagnosed at a later stage, when the lesions have become organized. As a general rule, treatment at this stage consists of suturing and reattachment of the affected muscles. Pronounced retraction or extensive tissue destruction requires complex reconstructive surgery. Inferior muscle disinsertion with suprailiac lumbar hernia can be managed by Koontz's operation [described in Detrie 1982]. This procedure involves cutting the upper part of the tensor fascia lata to form a large aponeurotic flap whose free edge lies roughly at the level of the tip of the greater trochanter. The flap is then turned upward and sutured to the upper edge of the destroyed muscle, the iliac crest acting as a hinge for this maneuver. This procedure can be used for repair up to the inferior part of the lumbar herniation but not higher. In cases where tissue destruction is more extensive or is located higher up, the above procedure can be supplemented or replaced using the lumbar fascia, which is incised along the spinous processes and turned forward along the lateral margin of the lumbosacral muscles (m. erector spinae) [Everett 1973].

V. Abdominointercostal Hernia

In these cases there is herniation through the lower intercostal spaces. Such herniation occurs when there is destruction of both the thoracic wall (rib fractures with tearing of the intercostal muscles) and the lateral chondrocostal insertions of the diaphragm. Intercostal herniation arises in cases of major destruction of the base of the thorax and is particularly frequent when thoracophrenolaparotomy has been done to explore lesions of the dome of the liver.

From the clinical standpoint, intercostal herniation is seen as an expansive bulging of the lower intercostal spaces, obviously containing abdominal structures. Treatment is not always achieved with ease, especially when costal resection has been done. In theory, surgery is performed via the intercostal approach. An incision is made along the axis of the intercostal space, followed by very cautious opening of the hernial sac, which may contain adherent viscera (especially the hepatic flexure of the colon which can ascend very high up when the right part of the liver has been resected).

Opening of the pleura cannot always be avoided, but this procedure does not lead to major complications. The key to a successful operation is obviously the repair of the diaphragm, which must be freed, clearly identified, and then sutured. Owing to the complexity and risk of the intercostal approach, it may be preferable to use an abdominal route. In such cases the diaphragm is sutured along its inferior surface. When marked destruction of the diaphragm is present a textile mesh can be used as a substitute. Abdominal pressure will force the material against the inferior surface of the diaphragm, thereby constituting an excellent mechanical obstacle to ascension of the abdominal viscera.

VI. Trauma Caused by Seat Belts

Accidents caused by seat belts are currently rare since the newer shoulder-lap designs cause little trauma to the abdominal wall. Most cases of injury related to the use of seat belts are reported in the work of Kokos (1978). The older lap belts similar to those used in commercial aviation have been found to be particularly dangerous.

In a study of 87 accident victims wearing transverse lap belts reported by Williams and Kirkpatrick (1971), 42 cases of infra-abdominal injury and eight cases of more or less extensive injury of the abdominal wall were observed. Conversely, in 24 accident victims who wore a simple over-the-shoulder belt, no cases of visceral lesions and only one case of abdominal wall contusion were recorded. Finally, in a group of 63 patients who used the modern three-point belt system, there were three cases of injury of the abdominal viscera and no cases of serious injury of the abdominal wall. In sum, most lesions of the abdominal wall directly attributable to the use of seat belts were seen when the now obsolete simple transverse type of lap belt was used.

Nevertheless, the currently used three-point seat belts do not protect against lateral shock, which gives rise to multiple pelvic lesions and may also cause disinsertion of the muscles of the flank.

A tentative systematization of the lesions of the anterior abdominal wall caused by seat belts leads to the following classification in order of increasing severity: band-like ecchymosis, also referred to as the "belt sign" - in itself, this lesion is perfectly benign, although assessment of any underlying lesion is more difficult in such cases; abdominal wall hematoma - the same remarks, but to a greater degree, apply to this type of lesion; cutaneous necrosis - this type of lesion is far less frequent in the abdominal than the thoracic region, where the skin is compressed between the narrow shoulder belt and the thoracic skeleton. In cases where the abdominal skin is involved, the lesion does not always present the same topography, owing to the occurrence of cutaneous detachment at a site some distance from the belted area, especially in adipose subjects. The precise limits of the lesion cannot be identified until a few hours or days after the traumatic event. Indeed, the lesion can present as mummification of the skin resembling a third-degree burn which rapidly becomes well limited, or may appear much later as necrosis whose full limits are difficult to identify. The final class is subcutaneous necrosis, which is true steatonecrosis without integumentary devitalization and may lead to more or less circumscribed effusion resembling classical Morel-Lavallée's effusion of the thigh.

Lesions of the Muscular Wall. These lesions correspond to more or less systematized traumatic dilaceration and hernia. For the reasons alluded to above, the published reports on these lesions are rather old [Hurrwitt 1965; Williams & Kirkpatrick 1971; Payne 1973]. The types of lesions that can be found are given below. The rectus muscles may show uni- or bilateral transverse ruptures (found in three of the eight cases of abdominal wall trauma reported by Williams and Kirkpatrick). Superior muscle rupture and disinsertion [Lemire et al. 1967] due to tearing of the part of the abdominal wall that is in contact with the longer edge of the thorax seem to occur when the belt is incorrectly positioned, i.e., inserted under the costal margin. This situation can lead to dilaceration of the anterior abdominal wall, which apparently induces rupture of the diaphragm in some cases [Dardik et al. 1973]. Inferior dilaceration involves the inguinal canal with tearing of the aponeurosis of the external oblique and disinsertion of the conjoint tendon or even the inguinal ligament. These injuries resemble the localized muscle lesions described above.

One very special case is the avulsion of the anterior-superior iliac spines. These normally act as points of support when the seat belt is properly positioned. However, when the subject is incorrectly seated, i.e., insufficiently upright, the transverse belt will ride up and over the iliac spines. Avulsion of the bone may then occur, similar to the disinsertion of the inguinal ligament or conjoint tendon described above.

In conclusion, the more recent shoulder-lap three-point seat belts offer little risk of abdominal wall injury. Furthermore, these belts support the abdominal wall during anterior projection of the visceral mass in head-on collision and thus probably protect against other lesions. In cases where there is injury to the abdominal wall caused by seat belts, the patient should be systematically examined for the presence of visceral lesions, and also for possible injury to the diaphragm in cases of upper abdominal trauma. When longer abdominal trauma is seen, one should systematically look for possible injury to the iliac or femoral vessels, bearing in mind that such lesions may appear with some delay.

References

Aubert M, Moaulle PY, Ravet D, Latreille K (1981) Ruptures sous-cutanées des muscles larges de l'abdomen et contusions de l'artère iliaque externe. Lyon Chir 77: 247-248

Dajee H, Nicholson DM (1979) Traumatic abdominal hernia. J Trauma 19: 710-711

Dardik H, Waren A, Dardik I (1973) Diaphragmatic visceral and somatic injuries following tear lap. Seat belt trauma. NY State J Med 73: 577-580

Detrie P (1982) Nouveau traité de techniques chirurgicales, vol. 9. Masson, Paris

Dubois BM, Freeman JB (1981) Traumatic abdominal hernia. J Trauma 21: 72-74

Everett WG (1973) Traumatic lumbar hernia. Injury 4: 354-356

Fredlund P, Dahn I (1967) Traumatic subcutaneous rupture of the abdominal wall with intestinal prolapse. Acta Chir Scand 133: 501-503

Hurrwit ES, Silver CE (1965) Seat belt hernia, ventral hernia following an automobile crash. JAMA 194: 829-831

Kokos A (1978) La ceinture de sécurité. Ses aspects médicaux, légaux, juridiques, psychologiques et techniques. Thèse, Lyon Grange Blanche

Lemire IR, Early DE, Hawley C (1967) Intra-abdominal injuries caused by automobile seat belts. JAMA 201: 735-737

Payne DD (1973) Seat belt abdominal wall muscular avulsion. J Trauma 12: 262-267

Williams JS, Kirkpatrick KJR (1971) The nature of seat belt injuries. J Trauma 2: 207-218

8 Defects of the Abdominal Wall

J. P. H. Neidhardt
J. P. Chevrel
J.B. Flament and J. Rives

I. Pathological Defects

J. P. H. Neidhardt

In this section, two main categories of pathological destruction of abdominal wall tissue will be discussed, i.e., open trauma (burns, shotgun wounds, dilaceration) and infection of traumatic, operative, or apparently spontaneous origin. These lesions raise difficult therapeutic problems regarding the extent of exeresis and the subsequent covering of the abdominal viscera.

A. Open Trauma

1. Burns

Burns of the abdominal wall are not, by themselves, specific lesions. The main problem encountered in such cases is a strategic one, concerning the possible need for laparotomy owing to the presence of accompanying traumatic lesions or burn-related pathology, e.g., stress ulcers, intestinal or biliary necrosis. When necessary, one should not hesitate to perform laparotomy. Indeed, midline celiotomy made through a fresh burn of the abdominal wall does not present any major difficulties, whereas incision through old or infected burn lesions is problematic. In the latter case the patient should be considered at a high risk for burst abdomen and appropriate precautions taken. Immediate closure may not be the best approach under these conditions and can thus be done as a deferred procedure, which we refer to as laparostomy.

2. Shotgun Wounds

Shotgun blasts made at a close distance result in multiple wounds of the anterior and posterior abdominal walls. Different factors of wound severity accompany the lesions. When the blast occurs at a short distance from the abdominal wall the projectiles cause high-speed trauma. Owing to their round form, the projectiles are suddenly arrested as they penetrate the integument and their kinetic energy is almost totally dissipated. These conditions lead to a complex shock wave from the multiple projectiles, causing widespread injury to the abdominal wall. This purely ballistic tissue destruction is complicated by the presence of foreign bodies in the abdominal wall, i.e., the projectiles, fragments of clothing, wadding from the gun cartridge. In some cases the projectiles traverse the abdominal cavity to become lodged in the posterior wall. In such cases the viscera are also damaged, especially the colon, thereby adding fecal contamination to the

mechanical injury. Under these conditions there is a high risk of gangrene of the abdominal wall. These extensive lesions cannot be managed by limited excision, and thus emergency treatment should include extensive debridement with drainage of the abdominal wall and the peritoneum.

3. Major Dilaceration

This type of lesion is rarely encountered outside a military setting. We have seen several cases due to farming accidents, i.e., mishaps with motorized cultivators where the victim has fallen to the ground and the abdominal wall and part of the viscera have been torn away by the teeth of the machinery.

Explosions cause complex lesions including more or less extensive avulsion of the abdominal wall, blast injury, and burns. This situation is sometimes encountered in civilian medicine, e.g., terrorist bombings. However, severe abdominal injury is found in only 2%-3% of such victims. Such injuries are obviously more frequent in a military setting, where approximately 10% of victims present with abdominal lesions, although they are not always of major severity.

Major therapeutic problems are encountered in cases of massive dilaceration of the abdominal wall. Indeed, attempts to achieve closure at any cost expose some patients to the risk of gangrene. Furthermore, artificial means of closure, such as cutaneous displacement with lateral counter-incision, are not always successful. Accordingly, closure can be deferred (laparostomy) in some cases.

B. Tissue Destruction Due to Infection

Three types of infection causing destruction of the tissues of the abdominal wall are discussed below: Fournier's disease, subcutaneous streptococcal cellulitis, and gangrene (gas gangrene and anaerobic cellulitis of the abdominal wall).

1. Fournier's Disease

Fournier's disease manifests as fulminating cutaneous necrosis of the genital integument (scrotum and penis) [Fournier 1884]. The deep structures of the region, perineal muscles and areolar tissue, testicles and erectile organs, are very rarely affected. Similar forms of the disease have been described in women. The existence of a specific causal organism is open to debate, although the frequent demonstration of hemolytic streptococci has led to this disease being considered a particular form of necrotizing erysipelas. The disease naturally progresses to a stage of toxic infection, with death occurring in about 50% of patients. Fournier's disease most often occurs in cases of severe systemic illness or immunosuppression. The major problem encountered with survivors concerns the difficulty of achieving cutaneous covering of the genital organs, whose deep structures remain intact.

This disease is discussed here because the lesions often extend to part of the anterior abdominal wall, forming a vast region of necrosis in the area covered by underpants. The lesion is initially seen as a bright red area sometimes accompanied by edematous swelling. In cases where death does not rapidly ensue, the lesion progresses to become a blackish eschar within 3-4 days. Fournier's disease is often mistaken for gangrenous cellulitis of the perineum, although in the latter case the cutaneous lesions are not of primary, but of secondary origin. Medical therapy, including antibiotics and intensive care, is the basis of management. Indeed, the use of relaxing incisions in the acute phase of disease has not proven worthwhile and thus, surgery should be considered only at the stage of sequelae, e.g., repair of tissue destruction that has led to denudation of the aponeurotic layer. Owing to the facts that islets of skin unaffected by necrosis persist and that epidermization is possible, skin grafting should be done only after the initial lesions have become stabilized.

2. Subcutaneous Streptococcal Cellulitis

This affection can be distinguished from Fournier's disease, since primary involvement of the integument is not observed. Subcutaneous streptococcal cellulitis is also different from anaerobic gangrene in that it is due mainly to hemolytic streptococci [Benmessaoud 1983], sometimes associated with other pyogenic organisms, especially Staphylococcus aureus.

Subcutaneous cellulitis tends to affect mainly the limbs, especially the lower limbs, but in some cases can extend to the anterolateral abdominal wall and flanks. The lesions are characterized by the presence of diffuse necrotizing cellulitis of the subcutaneous tissue, which is infiltrated by numerous abscesses. The infectious process leads to thrombosis of the veins and then the arteries, thereby giving rise to plaques of integumentary necrosis. However, the rather limited nature of the superficial necrosis belies the extensive subjacent tissue destruction. Affected patients consistently present with marked deterioration of their general condition, accompanied by septic shock and sometimes stress-related visceral lesions [Robin et al. 1976].

As opposed to Fournier's disease, surgical management is the basis of treatment in subcutaneous streptococcal cellulitis. Indeed, penicillin, which is theoretically active in almost all cases of streptococcal infection, does not produce a clinically obvious response in such cases unless all the lesions have first been widely exposed [Meneley 1929]. Accordingly, wide subcutaneous debridement is indicated, although this procedure may in itself induce necrosis of the integument. Owing to the risk of this formidable complication, surgery should be done without consideration being given to later covering of the abdomen, which can be achieved by skin grafting, if necessary.

Mortality is high for subcutaneous streptococcal cellulitis. Septic shock and intestinal necrosis were the cause of death in two of the six cases we have seen.

3. Gangrene of the Abdominal Wall

We use the term "gangrenous parietitis" to designate gangrenous disease of the abdominal wall where the major pathogens are anaerobic organisms. This definition thus includes anaerobic cellulitis and myositis (the latter refers to gas gangrene of the abdominal wall, according to the classical definition), which present many common clinical, bacteriological, therapeutic, and prognostic features.

a) Etiology

Gangrene of the abdominal wall is most often seen postoperatively, but may also arise after trauma or under apparently spontaneous conditions.

(1) Postoperative Gangrene

Postoperative gangrene accounted for the majority of cases seen in France that were reported at the International Symposium on Anaerobic Organisms (Paris, 1980). In our department in Lyon, specializing in emergency surgery, one quarter of all cases of gas gangrene occurred after surgery of the abdominal wall, i.e., in 52 of 210 cases seen over 13 years. As a general rule, these patients had undergone visceral surgery under septic conditions. Surgery of the small bowel was the most frequently involved procedure, and in all cases occlusion, perforation, or necrosis had occurred. Appendectomy was the second most frequent operative cause of gangrene. In about one-half of the latter cases only "moderate inflammation" of the appendix was seen initially. Thus, it is important to keep in mind that the appendix, even when it is apparently healthy, is part of the colon! Gangrene subsequent to colorectal surgery was less frequently observed, and this may have been due to the standard precautions taken in this type of operation. In such cases, gangrenous complications can arise seemingly unexpectedly, e.g., in simple colostomy opened prematurely. Surgery for gastroduodenal ulcer is almost always done in cases of hemorrhagic complications. This is also true in gynecological surgery for hysterectomy in cases of infected malignancy of the cervix or hemorrhagic fibroma. The presence of blood in the lumen of these organs contributes to the development of anaerobic organisms, which are especially common in the female genital tract.

In some cases, the point of origin of the anaerobic infection is at some distance from the site of operation. This may account for the retroperitoneal gangrenous cellulitis due to effraction of the lymphatic ducts seen after lumbar sympathectomy in patients with stage-IV ischemia accompanied by infected peripheral lesions.

When this redoubtable complication of surgery arises one should first try to identify its origin based on sound, common-sense evaluation, thereby often avoiding fruitless epidemiological investigations or analysis of the conditions of hygiene in the hospital.

(2) Trauma

Gangrene resulting from trauma is far less frequent than that seen postoperatively (12 of the 210 cases seen in our department). In rare cases, direct anaerobic inoculation of the abdominal wall may occur, or muscle attrition may be a causal factor, as discussed above in Sect. A, devoted to open trauma. Conversely, gas gangrene of the abdominal wall is more often encountered after traumatic injury when a visceral lesion has been overlooked. In such cases, the gangrene becomes exteriorized after the deep septic lesions have progressed. The prognosis is particularly grave under these conditions. The most frequent causes in these cases are wounds of the subperitoneal part of the rectum and retroperitoneal segments of the duodenum and colon.

(3) Apparently Spontaneous Gangrene

In the majority of such cases the gangrene of the abdominal wall results from extension of a gangrenous phlegmon originating from the perianal region, and sometimes the urethra [Boisbeunet 1941]. Subsequent to invasion and destruction of the scrotum, the gangrenous process diffuses to the abdominal wall via the inguinal regions, thereby infecting both the superficial and the deep structures. Such extension to the abdominal wall, although secondary to the initial perineal infection, merits special consideration. Indeed, the colostomies required in such cases of complicated perianal infection must be made at a distance from the initial lesion, e.g., at the level of the transverse colon, in order to avoid the risk of opening of the peritoneum in the midst of the gangrenous cellulitis. If this precaution is not taken anaerobic peritonitis may ensue.

b) Pathological Findings

Gangrenous infection develops in the areolar tissue and muscles. In about 50% of cases cellulitis is found in the deep areolar tissue (fascia propria). The infection then progresses along the incisional wounds in postoperative cases to invade the lumbar region, roots of the thigh, or inguinal regions, since these are zones of communication between the fascia propria and the superficial areolar layers of the abdominal wall. In the remaining 50% of cases both cellulitis and myositis are found. The myonecrosis may remain confined to the margins of the operative wound or, conversely, undergo propagation beyond the operative site. In the latter case, treatment requires wide excision, which prohibits parietal closure. Successive incisions of the abdominal wall compromise the vitality of a given sector and increase the risk of such gangrenous complications.

Gangrene consistently leads to burst abdomen in cases where midline laparotomy has been done. However, when McBurney's incision has been made burst abdomen is an infrequent sequela of gangrene, since the peritoneum shows much greater resistance in this region, even in cases where it is exposed subsequent to excision of the overlying muscle.

Gangrene leads to variable, secondary modifications of the superficial cutaneous layer of the abdominal wall. In some cases of fulminating gas gangrene the skin remains apparently intact. However, as in all types of gas gangrene, the skin most often presents phlyctenae containing a reddish-orange fluid and bluish-black plaques, while the integument appears taut and brownish-purple in color The resulting emphysema usually causes distension of the subcutaneous layer but in some cases may remain deep to this layer and rather limited for quite some time, especially when the causal organism is *Clostridium oedematiens* (*C. novyi*) or *Bacteroides fragilis*.

The status of the peritoneal cavity varies considerably between cases and may be perfectly healthy in some, with infection of only the abdominal wall.

Conversely, infection may spread from the abdominal wall to the peritoneum (peritonitis) or vice versa. In the latter case, the peritoneum is a permanent source of possible infection, especially when the peritonitis is due to visceral lesions that are either undiagnosed or secondary to surgical intervention. In cases where the infection has evolved over a certain period of time it is very difficult to identify the chronological sequence of the lesions.

The rapid extension of the gangrenous process allows identification of two forms of disease: relatively limited and highly invasive gangrene. The latter, which undergoes rapid extension over a period of 6-12 h, has a particularly poor prognosis.

c) Bacteriological Findings

The association of aerobic and anaerobic organisms is found in cases of abdominal wall gangrene. The aerobic organisms are the common gram-negative enterobacteria (*Escherichia coli*, Proteus, etc.) which may be accompanied by *Streptococcus fecalis* and sometimes by *Staphylococcus aureus*. The anaerobic organisms are opportunistic bacteria usually originating from the digestive or genital tract. Clostridium (*C. welchii* or *C. perfringens*) is the most common offending Gram-positive organism (about 80% of cases). In about half of such cases, Gram-negative anaerobes are also found, e.g., *B. fragilis*. The importance of the latter, known since the work of Veillon (1898), became apparent with the advent of newer methods of bacterial culture.

Clostridial infections are sensitive to β-lactamines, especially penicillin G. The Gram-negative and Gram-positive anaerobes are remarkably sensitive to the family of imidazole antibiotics.

d) Clinical Features

The clinical features are mainly those of the postoperative type of gangrene. The first signs usually appear 4-5 days after surgery, i.e., with a greater delay than in traumatic gangrene of the limbs. However, because of the postoperative context, this apparently longer latency period is often related to delayed diagnosis rather than to slower development of the infection. In fact, there seem to be three frequency peaks with respect to the onset of the gangrene: the first 24 h postoperatively - these cases are generally related to the prior existence of deep infection; 3-5 days after the operation - this so-called free period rarely exists. Earlier onset can usually be identified in these cases as shown by the patient's temperature chart and the nurse's notes, although it is true that the infection often undergoes sudden aggravation 3-5 days after surgery; 8-15 days after surgery - in these cases, late occurring gangrene of the abdominal wall is related to deep complications, or to undiagnosed visceral lesions which are often masked by prophylactic antibiotics.

It is often said that the patient's general condition is the best indicator of a possible postoperative complication. This worthy attitude may, however, give insufficient emphasis to careful local examination. Although pain is largely related to the patient's subjective interpretation, the existence of deep, dull pain of the constrictive type involving the abdominal wall may carry the same significance as similar pain felt in a limb. In any case, such pain should lead to removal of the dressing, systematic examination of the operative wound and removal of a few stitches. The identification of an ichorous and blood-stained discharge mixed with fatty globules and gas bubbles may allow diagnosis of gas gangrene at its very onset.

Subcutaneous emphysema can be identified by palpation, although the interpretation of this finding is often difficult. Indeed, noninfectious emphysema of mechanical origin is frequent, and if misinterpreted may lead to futile surgical procedures, while on the other hand the emphysema of certain highly invasive anaerobic infections may be rather inconspicuous. During local examination one should also carefully look for any abnormal discharge from the wound or the drains, since this may reflect the existence of an underlying peritoneal or subperitoneal infection. Unfortunately, diagnosis is too often achieved only, at a much later stage, when there is a change in the patient's vital signs. In such cases, pronounced fever is the rule and is almost always accompanied by a disturbed state of consciousness, dyspnea, and subicterus. These patients are sometimes admitted with a tentative diagnosis of delirium tremens or postoperative pneumopathy, while in other cases septic shock is the inaugural sign. The presence of acute renal failure indicates a very poor prognosis. This complication, occurring after a delay of a few days, is indicative of focal destruction of the kidney. Precious time is often lost by the administration of symptomatic treatment to these seriously ill patients.

The course of gas gangrene of the abdominal wall is highly variable. In nearly half of the patients death ensues within 48 h of diagnosis. In other cases the gangrene may remain more localized. Only moderate tissue necrosis is seen in such patients, and vital signs usually improve, although organic renal failure and clouding of the sensorium may persist for quite some time. A veritable "bacteriocycle" is established in the region of the wound with the successive appearance of different populations of bacteria and rapid disappearance of the initial anaerobic organisms. Massive colonization by *Pseudomonas aeruginosa*, despite the difficulties it causes, is often the sign that gangrenous development has terminated.

e) Prevention and Treatment

Prevention is the cornerstone of management, regardless of the etiology of the gangrene. In cases of traumatic origin, prevention requires identification of any deep visceral lesions, while in postoperative gangrene prophylaxie is based on avoiding bacterial contamination of the abdominal wall or on keeping such contamination to the strictly unavoidable minimum. Finally, in spontaneous cases of perineal origin, the abdominal wall should be protected against possible gangrenous extension by the performance of sufficient initial surgical procedures and via a colostomy at a distance from the lesional site.

Prevention can be specially efficacious regarding postoperative gangrene of the abdominal wall and should include full assessment of general risks, such as age, diabetes, and chronic renal insufficiency, as well as evaluation of the local risks related to the sepsis of the lesions.

During surgery full precautions should be taken to exclude the abdominal wall from the operative field. The traditional cloth toweling, which is a veritable source of bacterial diffusion, should be replaced by plastic protectors. In cases where septic inoculation cannot be avoided, e.g., surgery for peritonitis, it can be decreased in time and space by making an initially limited incision followed by thorough aspiration of septic fluid and adequate protection of the abdominal wall. In other cases, the traditional practice of full isolation of the abdominal wall during the stage of septic intervention should be kept in mind.

Attrition of the abdominal wall should also be avoided by gentle maneuvering of manual retractors and periodic relaxation of autostatic retractors. In cases of major contamination and lengthy intervention, the soiled wound margins can be resected prior to closure. Finally, parietal closure and drainage should be considered an integral step of the operation and constitute a second intervention with the use of new instruments and field protectors.

Drainage of the abdominal cavity requires the use of appropriate material, correctly installed and monitored. Three essential points must be respected when performing peritoneal drainage. First, the atraumatic drains should be silicon coated and nonadherent, and, if necessary, of the suction type. These drains must be correctly positioned in the lowermost part of the abdominal cavity and the patient must be kept supine. The drains should exit through stab wounds made at a distance from the operative wound in order to avoid contamination of the latter, and care should be taken to position the drains away from any sites of ileostomy. Second, closure of the abdominal wall should be modified in relation to the degree of sepsis. Indeed, there is a current tendency to overlook nonclosure as a therapeutic choice. Finally, subparietal evacuation via a flat, siliconcoated drain placed at one end of the operative wound avoids the stagnation of septic fluid and protects the viscera from direct contact with the suture material in cases where the omentum does not afford adequate protection. Thus, this system is drainage of the abdominal wall rather than drainage via the abdominal wall. Unfortunately, the latter is still done and regularly leads to septic contamination of the abdominal wall.

Once parietal gangrene has occurred medical therapy and surgical treatment are used to manage this condition.

(1) Medical Therapy

Medical therapy obviously includes general intensive care (volume and electrolyte re-equilibration, renal and respiratory assistance, if necessary) and administration of antibiotics. The usefulness of antibiotics as preventive therapy has not been demonstrated. Indeed, the systematic administration of "theoretically active" antibiotics does not protect against gangrene of the abdominal wall (the same is well known regarding gangrene of the limbs) in cases where insufficient or dangerous surgical procedures have been done or the basic precautions of sound surgical practice have not been taken. Of course, this does not mean that antibiotics are not useful in cases where gangrene of the abdominal wall has been diagnosed. The common finding of the association of different organisms in gangrene of the abdominal wall justifies a combination of three antibiotics: a β-lactamine, generally penicillin G at a dose of 40-50 million units per day; an aminoglycoside, such as gentamycin given at doses not inducing nephrotoxicity; and an imidazole, given via a nasogastric tube or intravenously (at a dose of 1,000-1,500 mg per os). In exceptional cases of intolerance to β-lactamines, erythromycin or chloramphenicol can be used, although these drugs are far less efficacious.

The therapeutic efficacy of hyperbaric oxygen is a controversial subject. To our knowledge, proof is lacking as to the efficacy of this approach, especially in cases of gas gangrene of the abdominal wall. Although this technique may be of limited use in gangrene of the limbs, we do not use it in cases where the abdominal wall is involved.

(2) Surgical Treatment

The problems of surgical treatment of gas gangrene of the abdominal wall are threefold and, as opposed to the limbs, "the ultimate therapy" of amputation is of course not applicable. The first problem encountered is that *treatment of the abdominal wall* requires wide exposure of the lesions and excision of all contaminated tissue (areolar tissue and muscle). Second, the peritonitis often accompanying the gangrene must also be treated. Finally, *any existing visceral lesions* require appropriate treatment as well. Given this context, suturing is absolutely out of the question and only the necessary surgical openings should be made.

Surgical procedures for treatment of gas gangrene of the abdominal wall very often lead to extensive parietal destruction. Even in cases where closure is physically possible, such a procedure should be likened to closure of a septic limb stump due to gas gangrene; such a procedure would of course not be done. Furthermore, the extent of the parietal destruction most often prohibits any attempt at closure, so that procedures referred to as laparostomy are needed in such cases. Parietal gangrene is probably the prime indication for these "open-abdomen" procedures, which are highly contested under other conditions.

It should be stressed once again that mobilization of the cutaneous layer must be avoided. As a general rule, any reconstructive surgery leading to the formation of a dead space will promote the recurrence of the gangrenous process. All contaminated tissue must be exposed, excised, and left open in accordance with the general principles of treatment of gangrenous affections.

Continuous surgical monitoring must be done, hence the usefulness of laparostomy. Additional procedures such as excision of sphacelous tissue and saucerization of new gangrenous foci may be required for several days until stabilization can be achieved. Thereafter, treatment consists of progressive assistance of the cicatrization which occurs as an invasive overgrowth of the wound, covering over and investing the abdominal viscera. At this stage, thin grafting can be done to ensure cutaneous cover, although incisional hernia is an inevitable sequela.

f) Sequelae

The sequelae of gangrene of the abdominal wall are complex and include major dehiscence and the frequent need to re-establish intestinal continuity. Accordingly, a standard therapeutic strategy cannot be defined, although some general rules will be outlined below.

Unless it is absolutely necessary, surgery should not be done again within at least the first three months following a severe peritoneal infection. If this rule is not respected, fresh, often inextricable adhesions will be encountered and any attempt at their removal may cause further damage to the viscera.

All types of plastic procedures, cutaneous displacement, and in general maneuvers which may cause hematoma, as well as inclusion of prosthetic material, should be avoided during at least the first six months following gangrene of the abdominal wall. Our current approach is to wait one year before these types of procedures are done.

At this stage of the recuperative process, the sequelae of gangrene can be included in the broader subject of treatment of major incisional hernia. The aim of this section was to discuss the acute aspects of major infections seen in an emergency setting. However, one should always bear in mind that a patient who has been salvaged under what are often very difficult conditions may be lost at a later stage owing to an overly ambitious and perfectionistic attitude with respect to reconstruction of the abdominal wall.

References

Boisbeunet T (1941) Contribution à l'étude de la gangrène spontanée foudroyante des organes génitaux externes. Thèse de Médecine, Montpellier

Benmessaoud F (1983) Cellulites gangréneuses à streptocoque bêta hémolytique (6 cas). Thèse, Lyon Nord

Fournier FA (1884) Etude clinique de la gangrène foudroyante de la verge et des diabétides génitales. France Médicale 1: 423

Meleney F (1929) Hemolytic streptococcus gangrene. Importance of early diagnosis and early operation. JAMA 92: 2009-2012

Neidhardt JPH, Morin A, Cuche P, Chadenson O, Latarjet J, Bouletrot P, Petit P (1974) Gangrène de paroi après chirurgie abdomino-pelvienne. In: Larcan A (ed) Problèmes de réanimation, vol 1. Spei, Paris

Neidhardt JPH, Morin A, Kraft F, Charroux B, Roubin C (1978) Remarques sur le drainage abdominal en chirurgie d'urgence. Urg Chir Commentaria I: 23-25

Neidhardt JPH, Kraft F, Rousson B, Morin A, Roubin C, Charroux B (1979) Actualité persistante de la gangrène gazeuse. Lyon Chir 75: 281-288

Robin M, Himmich H, Rapin M (1976) Cellulites streptococciques fulminantes. Importance du choc hypovolémique. Nouv Presse Med 5: 192-194

Sebald M, et al (1980) Symposium international sur les anaérobies. Les anaérobies. Masson, Paris

II. Iatrogenic Defects

A. *Postoperative Burst Abdomen*

J. P. Chevrel

Over the past 20 years progress in the techniques of surgery and intensive care has led to improved success of operation in patients of increasing age with evolving abdominal lesions requiring lengthy surgical intervention. Although major abdominal surgery can now be done in elderly patients often presenting with multiple visceral disturbances, the resulting rate of postoperative burst abdomen and subsequent mortality is significant. Indeed, the rate of burst abdomen has remained practically constant over the past 50 years, ranging from 0.03% to 3% of cases in 1932 and from 0.05% to 3.2% in recent years [Grenier et al. 1971; Estenne et al. 1971; Maillet & Revelin 1974; Mousseau et al. 1974; Rives et al. 1976; Chevrel 1979; Drouard et al. 1980; Flament et al. 1980]. In cases of surgical reintervention, the rate of burst abdomen reaches a level of 3%-18% of cases [Estenne et al. 1971].

We have treated 55 cases of burst abdomen in a series of 4,638 laparotomies performed between 1970 and 1982. The use of certain preventive measures has led to an almost 50% reduction in the frequency of this complication in our department, i.e., a rate of 1.8% of cases from 1970 to 1973 versus 1.04% from 1979 to 1982. These data emphasize the importance of adequate knowledge of the pathogenesis of this severe complication, in which mortality ranges from 0% to 85% of cases, according to the series [Grenier et al. 1971; Maillet & Rivelin 1974]. In our series the mortality was 52%, but it reached a level of 83% in cases of recurrent burst abdomen.

1. Clinical Features

Postoperative burst abdomen refers to the exteriorization of the abdominal viscera through a recent incision of the abdominal wall. In such cases the cutaneous sutures may not always display disunion. As a function of the delay before the burst abdomen occurs and the aspect of the lesion, three types of burst abdomen can be described.

a) *Free*

This type of burst abdomen arises in the early postoperative period, usually within 3 days of surgery. The inaugural event is often coughing or vomiting, subsequent to which a variable mass of abdominal viscera protrudes through a fairly large part of the incisional wound. In such cases all layers of closure show disunion. The protruding abdominal mass most often comprises small bowel, omentum, and transverse or sigmoid colon. The involved viscera may be totally free or partially adherent, according to the delay between surgery and the herniation. Major respiratory disturbances ensue and there is a risk of necrosis or fistulization of the herniated viscera. Treatment requires emergency reintegration and reinforcement of the abdominal wall.

b) *Fixed*

This type of burst abdomen occurs later, i.e., 8-10 days after surgery. In such cases the herniated viscera adhere to one another, as well as to the omentum and margin of the wound via false membranes and fibrinoid adhesions, which thus inhibit exteriorization of the viscera (Fig. 8.1a). The problem is less urgent, but the intestinal loops must be covered to prevent an exposed fistula from developing.

c) *Covered*

This variety of burst abdomen differs from the other two in that the cutaneous sutures remain intact. It can thus be considered a sort of precocious incisional hernia. In such cases there is a risk of strangulation of the viscera incarcerated in the wound of the abdominal wall.

2. Pathogenesis

Knowledge of the pathogenesis of burst abdomen is important if one is to decrease the incidence of this complication by appropriate prophylactic measures. Four factors contribute to the occurrence of burst abdomen: emergency surgery, site of abdominal wall incision, technique of closure, and quality of postoperative course.

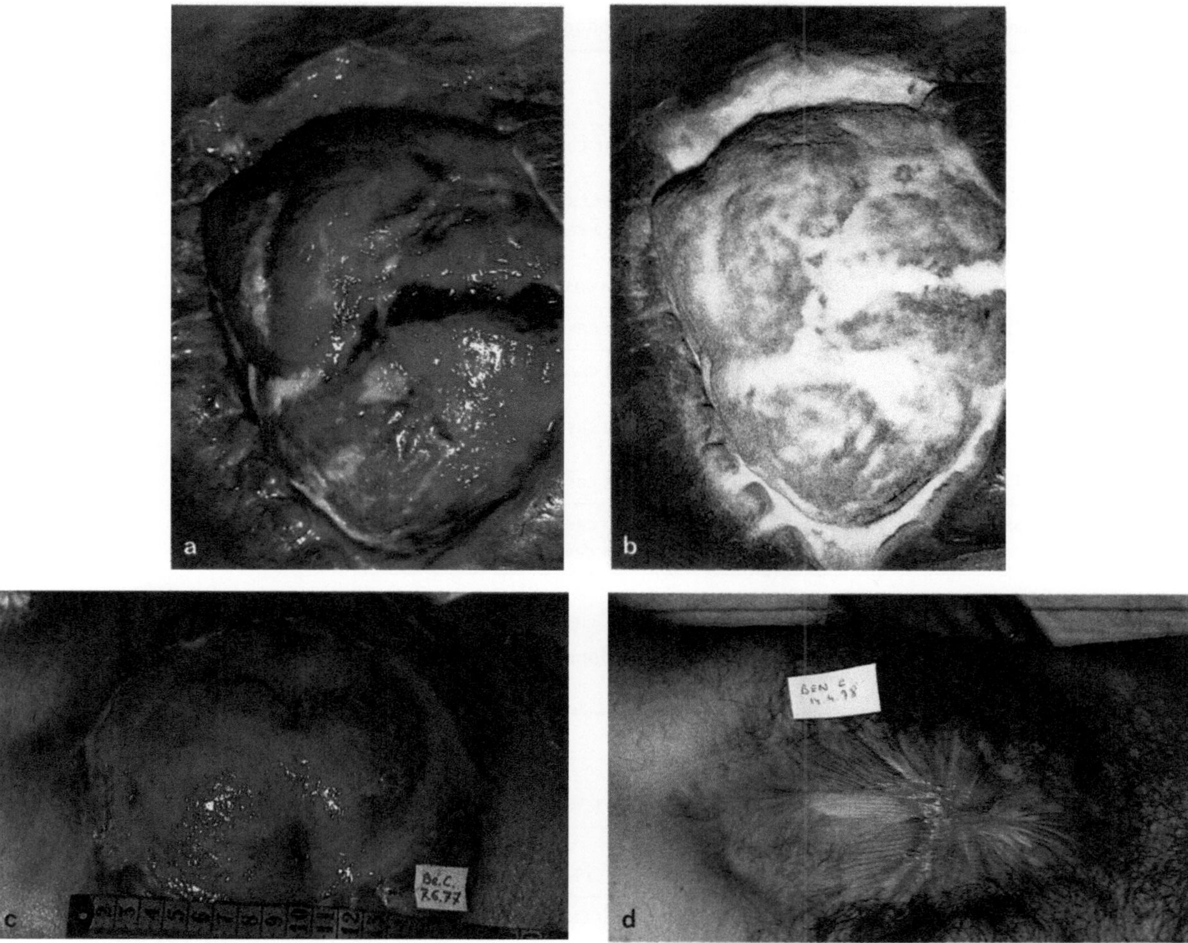

Fig. 8.1a-d. Treatment of fixed burst abdomen by simple dressings with right transverse colostomy. **a** Initial view of burst abdomen on the 12th postoperative day. **b** Dressings with dextran microspheres. **c** Abdomen 1 month later. **d** Definitive cicatrization accompanied by incisional hernia

a) Emergency Surgery

The risk of burst abdomen is highest in cases of emergency abdominal surgery, as shown by the following data: emergency surgery led to burst abdomen in 23 of 55 cases (41%) according to Chevrel and Fagniez (1979) and in 18 of 48 cases (48%) in a series published by Botella (1967). Furthermore, most patients who have burst abdomen subsequent to emergency surgery present with one or more additional risk factors which can lead to mechanical complications (increased abdominal pressure of various origins) or delayed cicatrization of the operative wound (Table 8.1). Alcoholism and malnutrition are often intimately related risk factors; i.e., about one-half of malnourished patients also present with signs of liver failure. To a lesser extent, successive surgical interventions also

Table 8.1. Organic disease in 55 cases of burst abdomen

Organic disease	No. of cases of burst abdomen
Chronic bronchitis	17 (31%)
Recent weight loss	11 (20%)
Plasma protein < 40 g/l	11 (20%)
Cirrhosis	12 (21%)
Cancer	9 (16%)

carry an increased risk of burst abdomen, evaluated at 3%-18% of cases [Estenne et al. 1971].

b) Site of Incision

Burst abdomen most often occurs after midline laparotomy. However, statistical data are difficult to inter-

Table 8.2. Occurrence of burst abdomen according to type of abdominal incision

			Present series (total = 55 cases)	Series from the literature
Vertical incisions (87.2%)	Midline incisions	Supraumbilical	18 cases	Botella (1967) 21/48
		Straddling umbilicus	13 cases	5/48
		Subumbilical	12 cases	21/48
		Xiphopubic	4 cases	
	Transrectus		1 case	Greniez 34/40
Transverse incisions (12.7%)	Subcostal		1 case	Botella (1967) 1/48
	Oblique (Barraya's incision)		3 cases	
	Thoracophrenolaparotomy		3 cases	
Repeat laparotomy	Short interval (21 days)		7 cases	
	Long interval (21 days)		4 cases	

Table 8.3. Frequency of burst abdomen according to type of abdominal incision (author's personal series)

	1970-1973	1979	1982
Total no. of laparotomies	1055	391	468
Total no. of burst abdomens	19 (1.8%)	4 (1%)	4 (0.8%)
Vertical incisions	948	298	283
Burst abdomens	15 (1.5%)	3 (1%)	4 (1.4%)
Transverse incisions	37 (3.5%)	88 (22.5%)	185 (39.5%)
Burst abdomens	0	0	0
Oblique incisions	20	0	0
Burst abdomens	3	–	–
Thoracophrenolaparotomies	50	5	0
Burst abdomens	0	1	–

pret in this respect since vertical incisions are used far more frequently than horizontal ones, especially in cases of emergency surgery. Almost 85% of the burst abdomens seen in our department have occurred subsequent to vertical incision of the abdominal wall. Furthermore, since oblique incisions and thoracophrenolaparotomy were abandoned in our department in 1979, all subsequent cases of burst abdomen were seen in patients who had undergone midline laparotomy (Table 8.2).

The transrectus incision, used systematically by certain surgeons, does not avoid burst abdomen [Grenier et al. 1971] and may even carry twice the risk of this complication compared with midline laparotomy [Maillet & Revelin 1974]. Transrectus incisions have not been used in our department. Furthermore, our tendency over the past few years has been to replace vertical incisions by transverse ones. This approach, coupled with other preventive measures, seems to have led to a decreased incidence of burst abdomen, as shown in Table 8.3.

c) Technique of Closure

The technique of closure may be a factor in burst abdomen, although it is quite difficult to evaluate precisely the role of this parameter with respect to the incidence of this complication. A recent prospective study by the *Association de Recherche en Chirurgie*

[ARC 1983] evaluated the incidence of burst abdomen in a series of 3,135 patients who had undergone midline laparotomy. The patients were divided into two groups according to the type of closure used (continuous or interrupted suturing) and each group was stratified as a function of the degree of risk of burst abdomen (three strata per group). No difference was seen between the two groups, except in the subgroups at high risk where the incidence of burst abdomen was significantly lower in the cases of closure by continuous suturing (96 cases of burst abdomen in 1,566 patients: 1.6%) than in those of closure by interrupted sutures (32 burst abdomens in 1,569 patients: 2%).

The possible role of the number of layers of closure as a factor of burst abdomen is also difficult to evaluate. In a prospective study of 1,129 laparotomies, Bucknall et al. (1982) reported a decreased incidence of burst abdomen when closure (excluding the cutaneous layer) was done as a single-layered rather than a two-layered procedure, i.e., 0.95% versus 3% incidence of burst abdomen. In a retrospective study of 1,820 patients, Drouard et al. (1980) confirmed the efficacy of *mass closure* in the prevention of burst abdomen and reported no difference in the incidence of this complication when the use of nonabsorbable suture material was compared with that of slowly absorbable material. Conversely, in a prospective multicenter trial of 211 high-risk patients, Maillard et al. (1980) compared three-layered closure and mass closure and found no difference between the two techniques. Furthermore, mass closure can lead to certain other complications (cutaneous necrosis, fistula of hollow organs in contact with the suture material), and in the study by these authors mortality was significantly higher in the mass closure group.

We prefer to use layer-by-layer closure (see Chap. 4) under conditions of rigorous asepsis and hemostasis, possibly coupled with abdominal wall reinforcement, as described further on.

d) Postoperative Course

The quality of the postoperative course plays a major role in the occurrence of burst abdomen [Hollender et al. 1972]. Two factors, increased abdominal pressure and infection, contribute to weakening of the sutures of the abdominal wall.

Increased abdominal pressure is amplified in the postoperative period, if recovery from anesthesia is difficult, and in patients with respiratory obstruction (frequent in cases of chronic bronchitis) or postope-

Table 8.4. Postoperative septic complications in 55 cases of burst abdomen

Abdominal wall abscess	20 cases	(36%)
Postoperative peritonitis	13 cases	(23%)
Prolonged fever	9 cases	(16%)
Positive blood cultures	6 cases	(10.9%)

rative ileus accompanied by meteorism, which may be highly pronounced. Furthermore, efforts of coughing or vomiting can induce peak values of abdominal pressure of 100 mmHg.

Infection has been emphasized by many authors as a factor contributing to weakness of the abdominal wall [Vilain et al. 1967; Grenier et al. 1971; Mousseau et al. 1974; Rives et al. 1976; Flament et al. 1980]. Such infection is often due to septic intervention, hence the frequency of intestinal tract organisms found on bacteriological examination. Infection of the abdominal wall is a frequent cause of dehiscence. However, burst abdomen is often only one of the signs of a septic postoperative complication (other signs include anastomotic fistula, for example) that must be taken into account in the decision to reoperate (Table 8.4).

Analysis of the mechanisms of burst abdomen thus allows identification of certain risk factors, which, when present, should lead the surgeon to take maximum precautions. The main risk factors are as follows: septic operation (frequently seen in emergency surgery); early surgical reintervention; malnutrition and alcoholism; major respiratory insufficiency. A special patient sheet on abdominal wall closure was introduced a few years ago in the Saint Quentin Hospital (France). This record displays a list of the main risk factors of burst abdomen, thereby guiding the surgeon to select the most appropriate type of closure to minimize the incidence of this complication [Drouard et al. 1980].

3. Treatment

The treatment of burst abdomen involves different stages of surgery. Prophylaxis is of utmost importance before, during, and after operation. Curative therapy varies according to the type of burst abdomen and its cause. Discussed below are these two aspects of treatment.

a) Prevention

Preventive measures must be taken pre-, per-, and postoperatively.

(1) Preoperative

The prophylaxis of burst abdomen is based on the quality of both general and local preparation.

General Preparation. When emergency surgery is not necessary the surgeon should be prepared to delay operation in patients presenting with advanced age, malnutrition, anergy, systemic disease, or respiratory insufficiency - i.e., high-risk candidates for burst abdomen. General preparation may require enteral or parenteral nutrition to obtain positive nitrogen balance and positive skin tests, in addition to respiratory physiotherapy, treatment of bronchopulmonary infection, and of diabetes. A period of 3 weeks is sometimes required to achieve adequate general health of the patient.

Local Preparation. On the day before operation the skin should be shaved and thoroughly cleansed with a foam disinfectant (lauryl mercurothiolate or equivalent solution) and then protected by a dressing containing a solution of povidone iodine.

(2) Peroperative

Although no technique offers full protection against the occurrence of burst abdomen, several precautions should be taken to minimize the risk of this complication. Whenever it is feasible to do so, an oblique or transverse incision should be used, especially in surgery of the biliary apparatus, portal hypertension, right colon, stomach, duodenopancreas, kidney, or subrenal segment of the aorta. In the course of incision it is imperative to achieve full hemostasis and excellent protection of the abdominal wall (wound protectors) using towels soaked in povidone iodine and an appropriate selection of atraumatic retractors.

At the end of the operation it is important to achieve correct relaxation of the abdominal wall, thereby allowing closure to be accomplished under good conditions. It is obviously impossible to propose an ideal procedure for closure (if such were the case, the numerous available techniques would not exist). However, it is possible to weigh the merits of the different techniques. As discussed above, the preferred number of layers of closure varies according to the author; each is able to expound the advantages of his technique and the disadvantages of the other procedures. The following have been proposed: mass closure including the skin [Grenier et al. 1971; Drouard et al. 1980], mass closure excluding the skin [Bucknall et al. 1982], extraperitoneal mass closure, and layer-by-layer closure. In

our opinion, it is very difficult to identify any difference between these techniques with respect to the risk of burst abdomen. However, there is certainly no difference when interrupted and continuous suturing [ARC 1983] and absorbable and nonabsorbable suture materials are compared [Drouard et al. 1980; ARC 1983]. In our department, closure of vertical and transverse incisions is currently done layer by layer (peritoneum, aponeurosis, subcutaneous layer, skin) using slow-absorbing continuous suture (see page 80). We have abandoned the use of extraperitoneal mass-closure reinforcement since this technique has led to small bowel fistula in our experience. On the other hand, we have had no experience with the multiple types of reinforced closure that have been proposed, e.g., mass closure using pledgets [Berutti & de Saint Julien 1978]; mass closure with over-and-under suturing [Samama et al. 1978]; twin-loop extraperitoneal closure [Burleson 1978]; atraumatic mass suturing [Chometowski 1975]; peg reinforcement [Ewald et al. 1978]. However, subsequent to a report by Saric et al. (1980), we now reinforce closure of the abdominal wall in patients at a high risk for burst abdomen using mass-closure wire suturing (Ventrofil technique). This material consists of two rigid plastic plates placed parallel to and at some distance from the incision. The plates are connected by a braided steel wire passing through the abdominal wall in a strictly extraperitoneal position. The wire is placed through the abdominal wall using two large curved needles with a triangular tip (see Chap. 4 V B). Two or three of these 7-cm-long plates can be positioned along a midline incision. In a series of 90 operated patients at a high risk for wound dehiscence no cases of free burst abdomen were observed when this closure technique was used [Perissat in Saric et al. 1980]. In our experience, based on a smaller series of patients in whom closure was achieved with this technique, only one case of burst abdomen occurred, i.e., on the day when the Ventrofil was removed too early. These sutures must be left in place for 20 days. This technique protects against the occurrence of free, but not covered burst abdomen. Prevention of burst abdomen should also include, when necessary, the use of efficacious abdominal drainage at the end of surgery and suction of the digestive tract until intestinal transit is re-established in order to minimize abdominal distension.

(3) Postoperative

The use of adhesive nylon strips initially designed to achieve external reinforcement in cases of burst abdomen [Guivarch & Mouchet 1969] can be applied as preventive treatment [Mousseau et al. 1974]. We systematically use this technique at the end of operation and maintain the material in place until the skin sutures are removed. However, burst abdomen is not always prevented despite the use of this technique (three cases of burst abdomen in our series of 55 patients).

Prevention of bronchopulmonary obstruction and infection will reduce coughing, especially with daily respiratory physiotherapy for smokers or patients with chronic bronchitis. Adequate nutrition must also be given as soon as possible. Early parenteral nutrition can be given for this purpose in patients with protein deficiency.

b) Curative

The treatment of burst abdomen is dependent upon the anatomical type of lesion and the state of the peritoneal cavity.

(1) Free Burst Abdomen

Treatment of early free burst abdomen requires emergency surgical reintervention. Three different situations can be encountered in this respect.

In cases of *purely mechanical burst abdomen* without suppuration of the peritoneum or the abdominal wall, closure can usually be achieved by interrupted extracutaneous suturing, leaving the skin open. In cases where the closure is free of traction we achieve reinforcement using one or two Ventrofil plates. When the closure is under tension we prefer to make two large cutaneoaponeurotic relaxing incisions in the flanks, according to the technique proposed by Levy et al. (1981). This technique allows simple cutaneous cover of the abdomen under traction-free conditions. The relaxing incisions are made slightly outside the lateral margin of each of the recti and from the inferior thoracic ridge to the inguinal ligament. The incisions should be slightly concave medially and should involve the skin, subcutaneous layer, and anterior lamina of the rectus sheath (1 cm from its lateral margin and over its entire length). This technique allows midline aponeurotic suturing without traction.

In cases of *suppuration of the abdominal wall* we prefer to simply close the skin in order to cover the small bowel. The relaxing incisions are covered with vaseline dressings. Cicatrization occurs without difficulty a few weeks later.

In patients presenting with *progressive peritonitis* or acute necrotizing pancreatitis we do not try to close the abdominal wall; scrupulous prolonged peritoneal lavage is performed, after which the bowel is reintegrated into the abdomen and protected by a sheet of polyurethane foam. Pasted nylon strips are then used to reinforce the abdominal wall. This technique, which we refer to as "laparostomy", allows repetitive peritoneal lavage to be done [Fagniez et al. 1979; Guivarch et al. 1979; Neidhardt et al. 1979; Champault et al. 1979], while closure of the abdominal wall or the skin is deferred until the peritonitis has regressed. Once repetitive peritoneal lavage is no longer required, synthetic mesh (polyglactine 910) can be installed intraperitoneally to maintain the bowel in place. Oily dressings placed on the mesh promote the development of granulation tissue, which progressively occludes the defect [Levasseur et al. 1979]. Details of this technique are given elsewhere in this book (see page 166).

(2) Delayed Burst Abdomen

The problems encountered in delayed burst abdomen are different from those of the free type. *In cases where the viscera are not exposed* there is a risk of strangulation of the bowel incarcerated in the parietal defect. The condition requires emergency surgery with reintegration and reinforcement using an adhesive elastic dressing that can be applied at bedside with the patient under analgesia. *Impending burst abdomen* should also be managed with this technique. Although prevention can be achieved, incisional hernia may ensue in certain cases. In the absence of subjacent peritoneal suppuration, *fixed burst abdomen* raises the problem of protection of the exposed visceral structures, which are highly prone to erosion and fistulization, especially in cases where the protective omentum has been removed during a prior operation. Two techniques are used to achieve atraumatic covering of the viscera. One method is simple cutaneous cover, which can be facilitated by large lateral relaxing incisions, similar to those used in the treatment of free burst abdomen. A second technique is to initially protect the exposed viscera by sheets of humidified polyurethane foam (Lyomousse, Peters Laboratories) followed 6 days later by dextran microspheres (Debrisan, Schering Laboratories). The foam sheets must be changed every 48 h due to saturation. Dressings of dextran microspheres (now commercially available in the form of paste) should be renewed once or twice daily since they are highly absorbent (Fig. 8.1). When these techniques are used granulation tissue progressively grows to cover the bowel. As a general rule, full cutaneous cover is attained after 3 months. Of course, this thin layer of newly grown tissue is of poor quality,

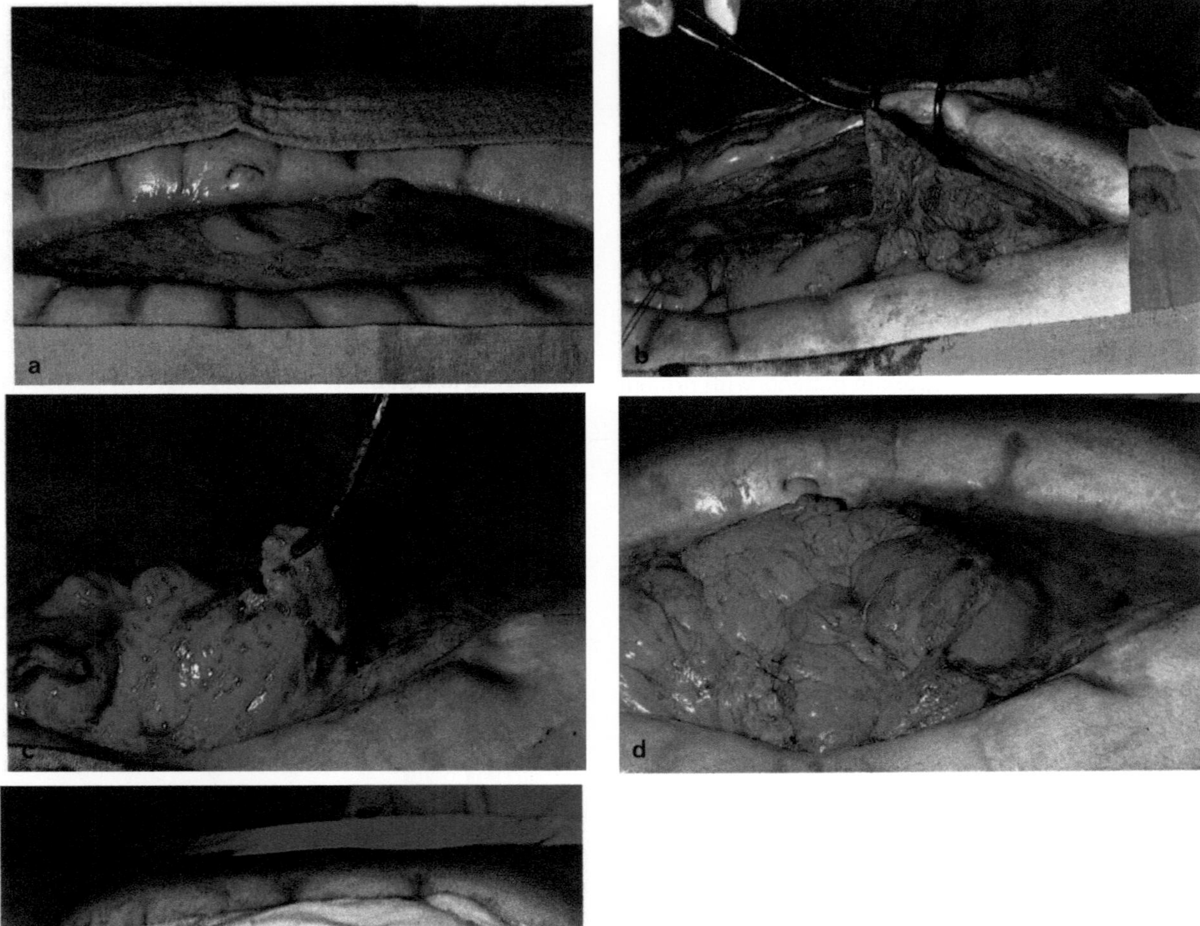

Fig. 8.2a-e. Treatment of fixed burst abdomen with external small bowel fistula. **a** Exposed fistula of the small bowel. **b** Initial dissection near the periphery of the overlying tissue. **c** Dissection of the overlying tissue. **d** Appearance of the wound after dissection and segmental resection of the small bowel. **e** At end of operation the defect is covered by vaseline compresses

and the loops of small bowel adherent to the deep surface and their peristalsis are visible.

At this stage further therapeutic management varies greatly. In some patients, poor general health contraindicates reoperation; in other cases, the extent of the parietal damage is such that repair would be a hazardous procedure. Under these conditions appropriate management consists of prescribing an abdominal truss. In other cases the special incisional hernia resulting from the cicatrization of the fixed burst abdomen can be repaired when no surgical contrain-

dications are present. The first step of this phase of treatment is dissection, which is less difficult than often believed. The abdominal wall is incised one finger breadth away from the granulation tissue covering the defect (Fig. 8.2); the peritoneal cavity can now be opened easily. After dissection around the residual incisional hernia, the overlying plaque can be easily freed from the adhering bowel loops using Metzenbaum's scissors.

The operative conditions are now similar to those for any abdominal wall defect of variable size. The

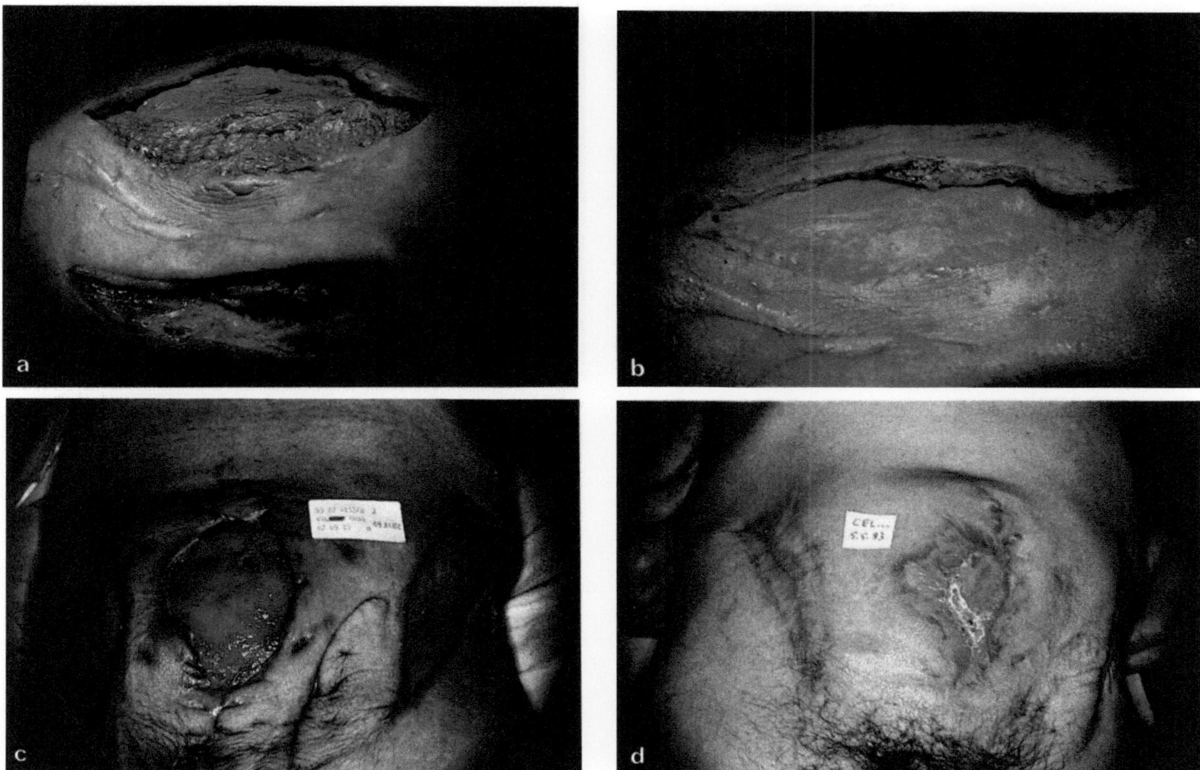

Fig. 8.3a-d. Repair of fixed burst abdomen by reconstructive surgery and polyglactine mesh (midline herniation with abscess of Douglas' pouch). **a** Single-layered midline closure with two relaxing incisions through the skin, muscle, and aponeurosis. **b** Reinforcement of the suture with polyglactine mesh. **c** Appearance of the wound 1 month later. **d** Appearance of the wound six months later; note solid abdominal wall

margins of the defect are generally limited by the recti abdomini, since burst abdomen occurs in the midline in most cases.

We generally use one of the following two techniques to achieve parietal repair: edge-to-edge interrupted suturing of the defect subsequent to longitudinal incision of the anterior lamina of the rectus sheath, which flattens out the muscle and allows tension-free closure; turndown of the anterior lamina of the rectus sheath using Welti's procedure. Both of these techniques require extensive subcutaneous dissection beyond the lateral margin of the rectus abdominis. In certain cases closure of the abdominal wall can be reinforced by a mesh of polyglactine 910 (Fig. 8.3).

(3) Free Burst Abdomen and Fistula

The association of precocious burst abdomen and bowel fistula is a grave complication arising under three special conditions.

Rupture of the sutures of an anastomosis leads to peritonitis, which in turn generally causes early, i.e., free burst abdomen. *Initial burst abdomen,* either of the free type (treated by dressings and external reinforcement) or of the fixed type, may undergo secondary complication with fistulization of one or more poorly protected bowel loops in cases of incomplete cutaneous cover, or when irritative dressings are used. This complication is referred to as external fistula of the small bowel.

Therapeutic evisceration, i.e., the open-abdomen technique used to treat a special case of very severe peritonitis, may be secondarily complicated by fistulization, as described above.

The association of burst abdomen and fistula, the latter involving the small bowel in 80% of cases, raises two major problems with respect to treatment, i.e., the problem of intestinal repair and that of the fistula. Burst abdomen secondary to peritonitis due to suture rupture is a surgical emergency requiring segmental bowel resection on each side of the rupture, followed

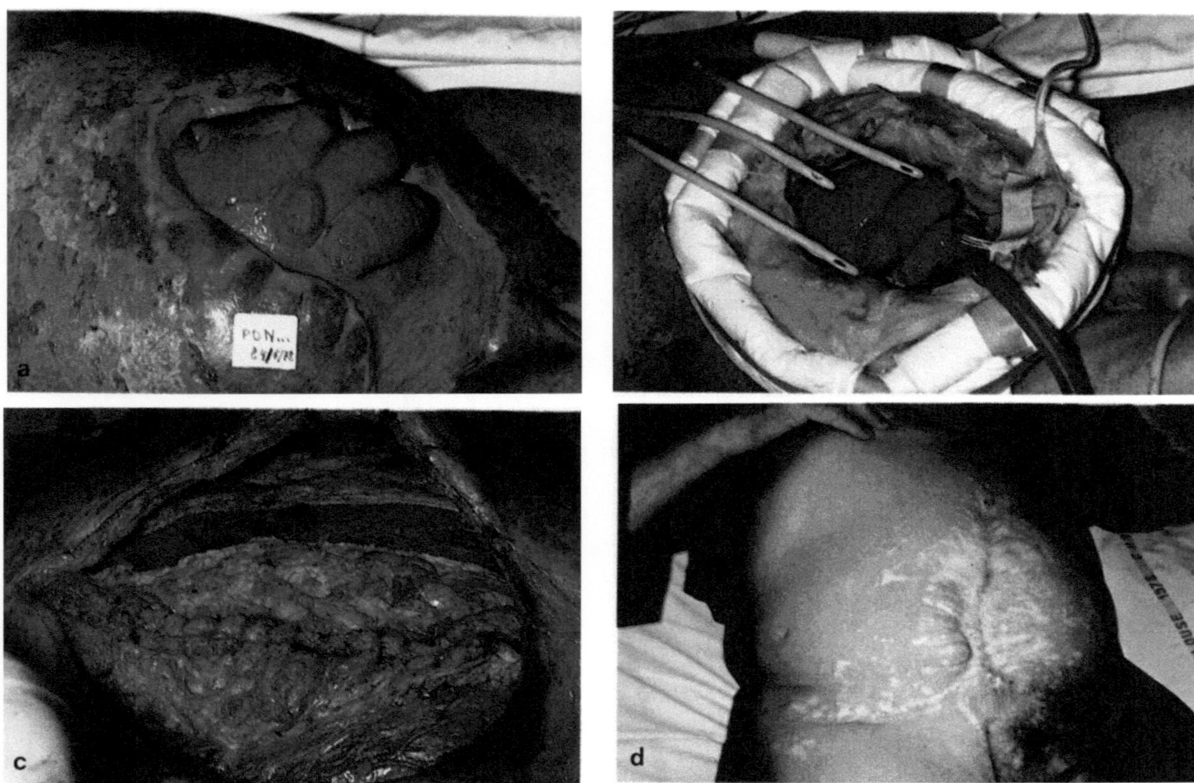

Fig. 8.4a-d. Repair of external small bowel fistulas in a case of burst abdomen. **a** Six fistular orifices (secondary to mass closure) in the region of the burst abdomen. **b** Enteral and parenteral nutrition are given for 10 days. **c** Subsequent to segmental resection of the small bowel and immediate anastomosis, abdominal wall repair is done by single-layered closure with relaxing incisions of the aponeurosis. **d** Appearance of the wound 6 months later; note solid abdominal wall

by double ileostomy. Once the fistula has been treated in this way, management corresponds to that of free burst abdomen. Thorough peritoneal lavage over a sufficient period of time is done using isotonic saline and, when necessary, appropriate drainage. The next step is parietal repair according to the condition of the abdominal wall. In cases where the margins of the wound are in a very poor condition it is best to achieve simple reinforcement of the wall using adhesive nylon mesh, with protection of the small bowel by a polyurethane plate or synthetic mesh (polyglactine 910) covered by simple cutaneous suturing. Conversely, when the abdominal wall shows less damage the defect can be repaired by extracutaneous mass closure with large lateral relaxing incisions of the myoaponeurotic layer.

(4) Fixed Burst Abdomen and External Fistula

Although these cases are not an indication for emergency surgery, they are just as difficult to treat as those discussed above. It should be noted that, contrary to deep fistula, these cases of external fistula never show spontaneous healing. Furthermore, any attempt to close the orifice of the fistula by suturing, with adhesive material, or by grafting consistently fails. When preparation of the fistula and general preparation (enteral nutrition whenever possible, if not parenteral nutrition) have been done correctly the fistula(s) can be repaired at the same time as the abdominal wall. Indeed, in such cases the peritoneal cavity is usually free at the periphery of the herniated viscera, and thus it can be approached at this level to achieve segmental resection of the fistulized bowel with immediate re-establishment of intestinal continuity (Figs. 8.2b & 8.5b). The abdominal wall is then repaired by suturing with relaxing incisions of the aponeurosis (Fig. 8.4) or by reconstructive surgery, using the anterior lamina of the rectus sheath (Fig. 8.5), similar to the secondary treatment of fixed burst abdomen uncomplicated by fistula. In cases where the abdominal wall is severely damaged, simple skin closure or synthetic mesh can be used, but it is absolu-

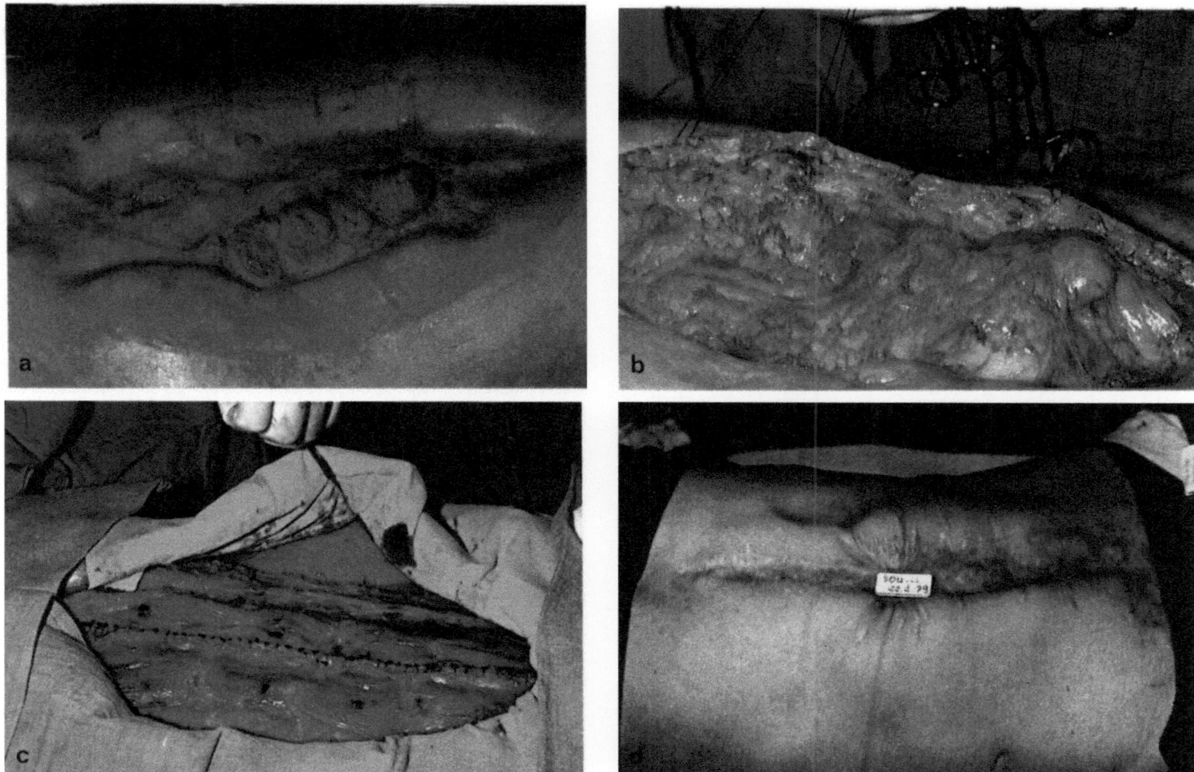

Fig. 8.5a-d. Repair of external small bowel fistulas in a case of burst abdomen. **a** Multiple external fistulas. **b** Appearance of the wound after resection of the overlying tissue by the peripheral approach. **c** After segmental resection of the small bowel and immediate anastomosis, abdominal wall repair is done by reconstructive surgery using the anterior lamina of the rectus sheath. **d** Definitive cicatrization with solid abdominal wall

tely mandatory to cover the intestinal suture, regardless of the technique employed.

c) Postoperative Care

Decubitus complications are a major cause of mortality in burst abdomen, where the mean death rate is about 40%-50% of cases. The incidence of such complications highlights the necessity of physiotherapy of the respiratory apparatus and lower limbs, coupled with systematic heparin prophylaxis.

References

Alexander H, Prudden JF (1966) The causes of abdominal wound disruption. Surg Gynecol Obstet 122: 1223-1229

ARC (1983) La fermeture des laparotomies médianes: surjet contre points séparés. Monographie ARC

Berutti A, de Saint Julien J (1978) Procédé de prévention des éviscérations. Nouv Presse Med 7: 465-466

Botella R (1967) Les désunions pariétales après laparotomies. Thèse de Médecine, Paris

Bucknall TE, Cox PJ, Ellis H (1982) Burst abdomen and incisional hernia: a prospective study of 1,129 major laparotomies. Br Med J 284: 931-933

Burleson RL (1978) Double-loop mass-closure technique for abdominal incisions. Surg Gynecol Obstet 147: 414-416

Champault G, Magnier M, Psalmon F, Roche JY, Patel JC (1979) L'éviscération: élément thérapeutique dans les péritonites. Nouv Presse Med 8: 1349

Chevrel JP (1979) Sur les fistules exposées du grêle. Chirurgie 105: 366-367

Chevrel JP, Fagniez PL (1979) Les éviscérations. Chirurgie 105: 149-154, Masson, Paris

Chevrel JP, Duchene P, Pfughaupt M, Rathat C, Legout J (1980) Problèmes pariétaux des fistules exposées du grêle. Med Chir Dig 9: 323-324

Chevrel JP, Loury JN, Fagniez PL (1980) Les éviscérations post-opératoires. 81ème Congrès Français de Chirurgie Actual. Chir 11: 77, Masson, Paris

Chevrel JP (1994) Loss of substance of the abdominal wall. In: Bendavid R (ed) Prosthesis and Abdominal Wall Hernias. R G Landes, Austin, pp 311-320

Chometowski S (1975) Fermeture abdominale par points totaux atraumatiques. Nouv Presse Med 4: 1645-1646

Drouard F, Dufilho A, Bayle E, Moussalier K, Seqat M (1980) Etude comparative des risques d'éviscération au décours des laparotomies médianes suturées au fil synthétique résorbable. Monographie GREPA, Lab Bruneau, Paris 2: 16-18

Estenne B, Botella R, Charles JF, Hirschmann F, Houdard C (1971) Les éviscérations aiguës post-opératoires. Ann Chir 25: 1241-1246

Ewald N, Langlois-Zantain O, Cacolyris T, Koseleff B (1978) Traitement des éviscérations par la technique des broches. Nouv Presse Med 7: 1553-1554

Fagniez PL, Hay JM, Regnier B, Renaud J (1979) La laparostomie: une technique d'exception dans le traitement des péritonites dépassées. Concours Méd 28: 4569-4573

Flament JB, Palot JP, Rives J (1980) Etiopathogénie des éviscérations. Rôle du facteur infectieux. A propos de 40 observations. Monographie GREPA, Lab Bruneau, Paris 2: 19

Germain A, Julien M, Fagniez PL (1980) A propos des fistules intestinales exposées au sein d'une éviscération. Chirurgie 106: 377-381

Grenier JF, Sava G, Kohler JJ, Gillet M (1971) Les éviscérations post-opératoires. A propos de 40 cas. J Med Strasbourg 3: 201-206

Guivarch M, Mouchet A (1969) Sanglage abdominal par bas nylon dans l'éviscération post-operatoire. Press Med 77: 101-102

Guivarch M, Roullet-Audy JC, Chapmann A (1979) La non fermeture pariétale dans la chirurgie itérative des péritonites. Chirurgie 105: 287-290

Hollender LF, Sava G, Guillet M (1972) Les éviscérations aiguës post-opératoires. MEd Chir Dig 1: 189

Levasseur JC, Lehn E, Rignier P (1979) Etude expérimentale et utilisation clinique d'un nouveau matériel dans les éviscérations graves post-operatoires. Chirurgie 105: 577-581

Levy E, Parc R, Cugnenc PH, Bloch P, Hannoun L, Nordlinger B, Huguet C, Loygue J (1981) La couverture cutanée abdominale sans traction. Ann Chir 35: 99-101

Maillard JN, Hay JH, Fagniez PL, Prandi D (1980) Prophylaxie des éviscérations des laparotomies médianes par les points totaux. Etude contrôlée. Monographie GREPA 21. Laboratoires Bruneau, Paris

Maillet P, Revelin P (1974) Les éviscérations post-operatoires. Journées Réa Méd Chir Nancy. Spei, Paris

Mousseau M, Le Neel JC, Pannier M (1974) Problèmes pratiques posés par la prévention des éviscérations. Journées Réa Méd Chir Nancy. Spei, Paris

Neidhart JH, Kraft F, Morin A, Rousson B, Charroux B, Roubin M (1979) Le traitement "à ventre ouvert" de certaines péritonites et infections pariétales abdominales graves: note technique sur le procédé personnel de la jupe plastique. Lyon Chir 75: 272-274

Rives J, Convers G, Croix JC, Hibon J (1976) Le rôle de l'infection dans les éviscérations. Lyon Chir 72: 117-122

Samama G, Dupuis F, Bezard J (1978) Fermeture des laparotomies par points totaux en brandebourg. Nouv Presse Med 7: 2249-2250

Saric J, Charlopain G, Perissat J (1980) Intérêt du ventrofil dans la prévention des éviscérations post-opératoires. Monographie GREPA, Lab Bruneau, Paris 2: 26-29

Vilain R, Elbaz JS, Singier P, Gueriot JC, Le Lirzin R (1967) Etude critique des complications des laparotomies, l'élimination des fils de suture, l'éviscération, l'éventration, les désunions cutanées suppurées. Ann Chir 21: 262-288

B. Major Incisional Hernia

J.B. Flament and J. Rives
with the collaboration of
J. P. Palot, A. Burde and C. Avisse

Eventration is defined as the postoperative protrusion, beneath the skin, of viscera normally contained within the abdominal cavity. The protruding viscera are always enveloped in a serous sac in continuity with the peritoneum via an abnormal orifice in the abdominal wall. The term incisional hernia, found in the English language literature, is more appropriate in our opinion and will therefore be used throughout this section.

Progress in surgical techniques, even with laparoscopic surgery, has unfortunately not led to the disappearance of incisional hernia. On the contrary, the frequency of this complication seems to be on the increase, as increasingly major and lengthy operations are performed, especially in elderly patients with concomitant organic disease. Indeed, incisional hernia is rarely the result of errors in surgical technique, but in most cases is rather related to various disturbances resulting from marked deterioration of the patient's condition.

These seemingly benign lesions in fact display a formidable tendency to undergo aggravation and recurrence and thus are almost always an indication for surgical intervention. This may be a simple procedure in cases where the hernial orifice is narrow and the sac of limited volume. On the other hand, surgical repair is difficult in cases of a large abdominal defect and when the herniated viscera have "lost their right to reside" in the abdominal cavity. Finally, in exceptional cases incisional herniation is beyond the scope of surgical repair, owing to severe deterioration of the patient's condition, notably due to old age, disabling obesity, and disturbances of respiratory function.

Closure of an incisional hernia has nothing in common with closure of a laparotomy. Surgical repair must take into account the irremediable weakening of the abdominal wall and the possible consequences of decreased abdominal pressure on diaphragmatic mobility and respiratory function, even in cases where such pressure decrements are intermittent and of low amplitude. The surgical repair of incisional hernia must be considered as a difficult procedure whose results can be assessed only in terms of the widely differing lesions to be treated. This part of the book is devoted to the most difficult cases of incisional hernia. Treatment of a major incisional hernia begins with careful evaluation of the patient's general health coupled with a general preparation which may last several weeks prior to operation. Surgical techniques of repair should be based largely on the use of prosthetic substitutes; therefore, the precautions that must be taken when artificial material is introduced into the human body should be kept in mind.

1. Definition

It is important to give a clear definition of these lesions in order to avoid any misinterpretation of the results of surgical treatment. Major incisional hernia, as discussed below, refers to cases where the hernial orifice is greater than 10 cm in diameter; often it reaches or exceeds a diameter of 20 cm. Protrusion of the hernial sac may be moderate in some cases of recent major subumbilical incisional hernia. However, in most cases, the swelling is of considerable size. The hernial mass is often mushroomshaped in appearance. In such cases, its cutaneous envelope displays trophic changes or even ulceration near the apex of the mass. In practically all cases pruriginous intertrigo is seen at the periphery of the swelling. Patients with major incisional hernia are often obese and in poor general health. These lesions must always be regarded as severe, and the surgical treatment they require may sometimes be a truly "formidable procedure" [Cokkinis 1958]. Accordingly, all patients must be clearly informed of the risks entailed in surgical repair. As a general rule, most of them accept these risks due to their disabling condition. However, it is the surgeon's role firmly to refuse certain candidates for surgery where deterioration in general condition, due especially to respiratory and cardio-vascular disease, renders the risks prohibitive.

2. Introduction

Over a long period of time, surgical progress was confined to the development of new techniques of excision or visceral repair, with little attention being paid to the consequences of surgical intervention on the abdominal wall. Incisional hernias were all the more frequent at the time when anesthesia and techniques of closure were largely imperfect. In the past, incisional hernias were treated by turndown or overlapping surgery using neighboring aponeurotic structures. Statistical series and long-term follow-up have been introduced only recently. These procedures gave manifestly unsatisfactory results, as can be judged by the frequency of very large recurrent herniation, considered to be beyond the scope of surgical repair. Affected patients would sometimes hide their lesions with a sense of guilt, under the misconception that the failed operation was somehow due to some special weakness of their abdominal wall. Some of these older techniques should not be forgotten, however, and will be mentioned later on since they may still be of value. Judd's technique (1912) is one such case: we still use this approach as first-line therapy in minor forms of incisional hernia or when sepsis is present.

Nevertheless, large hernial orifices and recurrent herniation require treatment using replacement material. Following the failure of fascial autografts, the skin seemed to be the material of choice in this respect, either as free sutured grafts, buried grafts, or band grafts. The technique of skin band grafting was introduced in France by Gosset (1949) and modernized by Banzet et al. (1979). This technique is very occasionally indicated to achieve closure of diastasis. Though, we have serious doubts regarding its efficacy in cases of wide diastasis or defects of the abdominal wall.

The failure of autografts naturally led surgeons to investigate the possible usefulness of prosthetic material. Early prostheses were constructed of metal or nylon. The former material was well tolerated, but its rigidity was a major drawback. Early nylon prostheses were also too rigid and led to infection. The advent of Marlex mesh, used in the United States, and later of Dacron-Mersilene, widely used in France, has clearly brought great progress. We investigated this type of prosthetic material as soon as it was introduced in France in 1966 and at that time used large sheets sutured in place to reinforce the abdominal wall.

In the early 1970s better knowledge was also acquired regarding the serious consequences of respiratory insufficiency, thanks to the important contribution to this field of the work by Goni-Moreno (1970), later publications by us on paradoxical abdominal respiration [Rives et al. 1973], and studies by Italian authors on disturbances of pulmonary compliance [Trivellini et al. 1978]. The commercial introduction of absorbable prosthetic mesh (Dexon, Davis and Geck; Vicryl, Ethnor Laboratories) has opened up new therapeutic possibilities in cases of infected lesions [Loury & Chevrel 1983]. However, the recurrence rate of incisional hernia is high when this material is used, and thus it cannot be applied routinely.

Surgery has progressed considerably in this field, although current results are still unsatisfactory. Continued progress requires that we strive for stricter definition of indications and improvement in technical details, in order to reduce the rate of infection and to eliminate recurrence of incisional hernia.

3. Natural History

Surgical responsibility for the occurrence of incisional hernia may be obvious in cases where laparotomy has been done with no regard to anatomical conditions. In such cases herniation results from the transection of neurovascular structures with resulting atrophy of the abdominal wall. The quality of suturing can also be considered when incisional hernia occurs rapidly in the absence of infection. In such cases, an obvious cause is a poor closure, where the spacing and bite of the sutures have been incorrectly evaluated. However, these technical errors are rare.

Incisional hernia is almost always *initiated by infection* along the suture of the operative wound. Such cases can be avoided by withdrawing one or more of the sequestered sutures which promote infection. The affected zone is a weak point giving rise to a small orifice due to the outward push of abdominal pressure. The orifice continues to enlarge until a state of equilibrium, i.e., major incisional hernia, is reached.

However, the force of abdominal pressure (or abdominal traction) should not be likened to that of an expanding balloon, where herniation would correspond to the bursting of the balloon. Indeed, measurements made within the abdomen demonstrate that intra-abdominal pressure is rather low (2-12 mmHg); thus, it can play only a minor role at the onset when the orifice is still narrow. The force most frequently involved in incisional hernia is *lateral traction*, measured in kilograms, dependent mainly upon the contraction of the flat abdominal muscles, i.e. external oblique, internal oblique and transversus. These lateral forces act particularly in cases of midline laparotomy because of the transverse arrangement of the fibers of these muscles. It should be kept in mind that all midline laparotomies are in fact *the equivalent of tendinous detachment of these muscles from the linea alba*. The effects of such contraction are obvious when one observes the contours of a laparotomy in a poorly relaxed patient; in the midst of the rigid abdomen the laparotomy wound takes on the circular appearance of the orifice of incisional hernia. Traction forces act in a similar way on bedridden obese patients who have undergone abdominal surgery, owing to the sheer weight of the fat-laden skin folds. Finally, the weight of the viscera themselves should also be taken into account in cases of major subumbilical herniation. Added to this effect are the force of the diaphragm, and especially the contraction of the lateral muscles. Indeed in cases of major incisional hernia, the walls of the abdomen open like sliding doors, allowing passage of the viscera. The flat abdominal muscles have become "sagittalized", and their contraction no longer offers resistance to the protrusion, but tends instead to push the viscera out of the abdominal cavity (Fig. 8.6).

These conditions easily account for the fact that incisional hernia has a natural tendency to progress. However, in some cases the herniation may remain limited, when the scar tissue consolidates the rim of the narrow orifice, thereby preventing its enlargement and affording solid insertion for the lateral abdominal muscles. These lesions can be likened to epigastric hernia. In most other cases, muscular traction and the weight of the viscera lead to progressive enlargement of the orifice, which may reach a diameter of 10-20 cm. At this stage the shortening of the muscle fibers reduces their ability to contract. Fatty degeneration of these fibers is often seen, accompanied by retraction of the involved aponeurosis. These lesions are irreversible. The abdominal defect undergoes organization, at which stage its margins present a sharp, resistant sclerotic edge, even in cases where the orifice is apparently subdivided by fibrous bands. It is of interest to note that the circumference of the defect may be partially formed by a bony (pubic symphysis) or cartilaginous structure (chondrocostal margin). The hernial sac resembles a thick, vascularized serous envelope, while the cavity within it often presents adhesions which may hinder the return of the herniated viscera. In such cases the swelling may be as large as the head of an adult. The skin over the apex of the protrusion is thin and poorly vascularized and may be the site of circular trophic ulceration (see Fig. 8.14a). This ulceration, always presenting as a single lesion, should not be mistaken for erosion due to friction against the skin. There is an increased risk of infection when ulceration is present, leading to burst

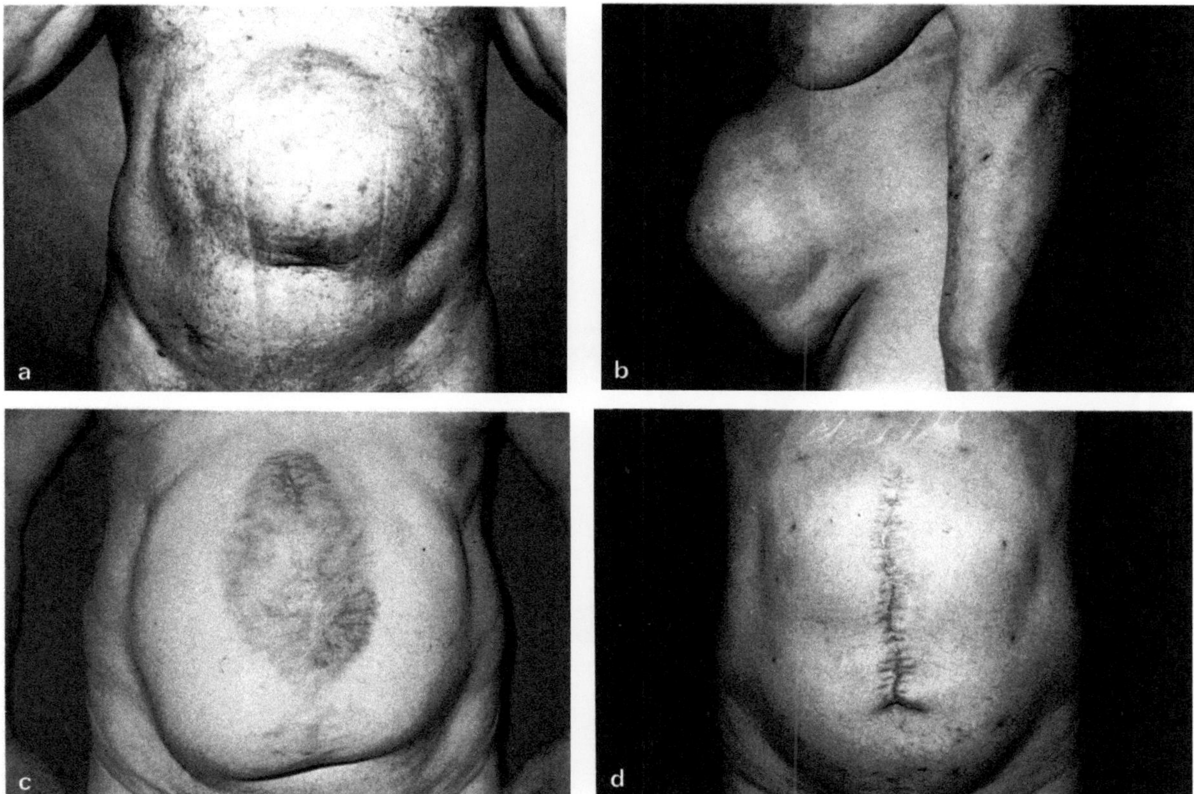

Fig. 8.6a-d. The abdominal muscles in major midline incisional hernia. The recti abdomini come to lie in the sagittal plane (**a** and **b**). The lateral muscles retract, but surgery allows their reattachement and apposition of the wound margins (**c** and **d** are from the same patient)

abdomen and fistulization. These voluminous disabling lesions accompany and aggravate obesity, and the deep skin folds constitute a reservoir for pathogenic organisms. Such sources of infection obviously complicate the management of incisional hernia.

4. Physiopathology

The loss of abdominal wall integrity leads to disturbances in general health which in the past were overlooked by many surgeons. We have referred to these disturbances in our earlier publications as incisional hernia disease or "eventration disease" [Rives et al. 1973; Rives et al. 1977; Flament & Palot 1994]. The disturbances are due to a decrease of intra-abdominal pressure resulting from the creation of the orifice and the extra-abdominal protrusion of the viscera contained in the hernial sac. However, the resulting pressure drop is not pronounced since normal abdominal pressure is never very high. Normal resting abdominal pressure measured beneath the diaphragm does not exceed 6-8 mmHg and is only slightly higher in the

pelvic region when the subject is standing (approximately 12 mmHg). This increase on standing is due to the hydrostatic pressure of the viscera, to which is added to the force of contraction of the abdominal wall muscles [Caix et al. 1982].

a) Respiratory Disturbances

(1) Disturbed Respiratory Function

These disturbances are related to the normal contributions of the abdominal muscles, abdominal pressure, and diaphragm to respiratory function. In some cases of reducible major epigastric incisional hernia the disturbed functioning of the diaphragm can be observed. Our illustrations of these anomalies have been widely reproduced in the medical literature. An analogy can be made with the changes seen in thoracic trauma. Such illustrations show the constituent movements of the "abdominal flap" and identify the four phases of paradoxical abdominal respiration, which replace the two phases of normal respiration (Fig. 8.7). These disorders illustrate the inefficacy of

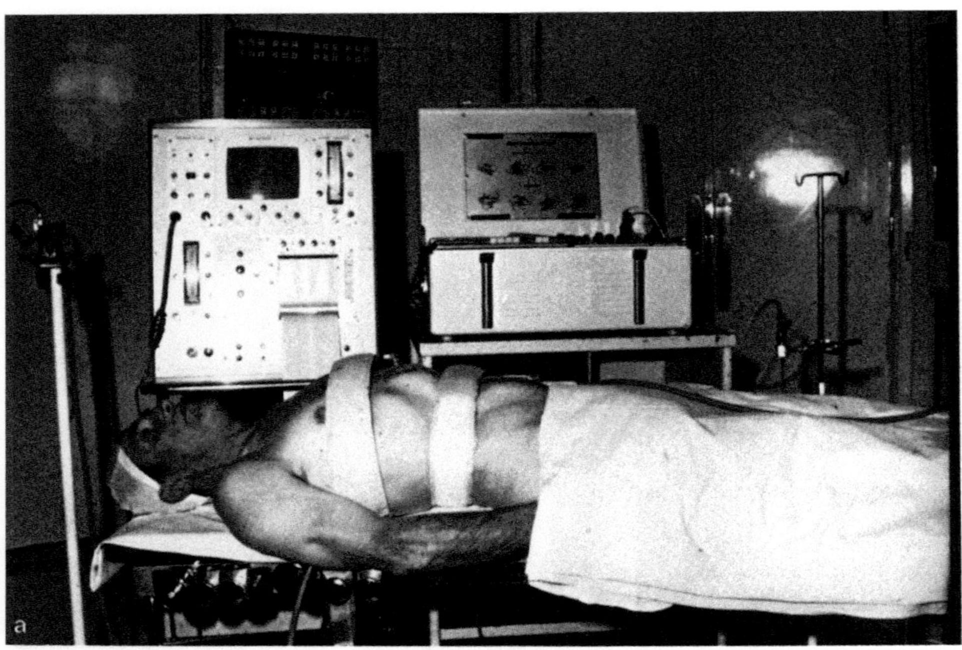

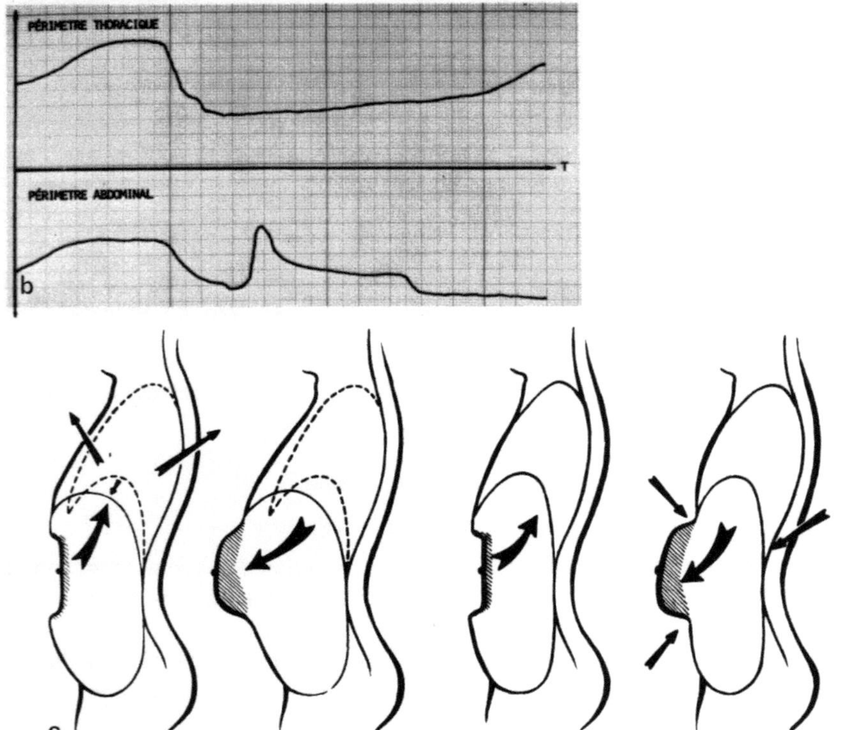

Fig. 8.7a-c. Paradoxical abdominal respiration. Recordings of thoracic and abdominal movements (**a**) show a fourphase curve of respiration (**b**). The drawings (**c**) illustrate this phenomenon; *left:* inspiration, *right:* expiration

the diaphragm and abdominal muscles when they contract in an open-abdominal cavity, and the diaphragm fails to contract against the viscera since these are no longer retained by the muscular wall. In most cases the respiratory dysfunction is not manifest and must be evaluated by appropriate respiratory function tests, in order to avoid a catastrophic postoperative course. Where these functional tests give satisfactory results, attention should be paid to the arterial (O_2, CO_2).

(2) Effects of Repair on Respiratory Function

In some patients, bulky hernias can be easily kept reduced by wearing a corset. In our experience, this is the case in active males of average corpulence with midline supraumbilical hernia. Reduction of this type of herniation is well tolerated. In other cases, however, the contents of the sac are fixed in place by adhesions and thus cannot be reduced: the herniated organs have lost their "right to reside" in the abdomen. Two abdominal cavities can be considered to exist in this situation (Fig. 8.8). If specific precautions are not taken, the consequences of hernial reduction are disastrous, i.e., increased abdominal pressure and diaphragmatic immobilization. This problem can be evaluated in a different light. In a previous study (Table 8.5) we have shown that in obese patients (many cases of incisional hernia are seen in the obese) the associated respiratory disturbances of obesity could be compensated or masked by the presence of a major incisional hernia. In such cases, vital capacity is increased (P = 0.001) as is the ratio of residual volume to total capacity (RV/TC). In other words, the obese patient with an incisional hernia is better able to ventilate the lungs (when pulmonary, and not abdominal, ventilation occurs) than is the obese person with an intact abdominal wall. Reduction of the hernia abolishes the beneficial effect of this compensation and exposes the patient to serious postoperative complications which may not be predicted by the results of preoperative

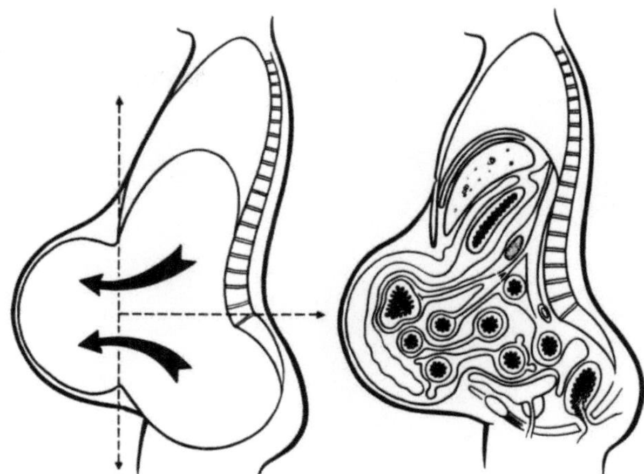

Fig. 8.8. The abdominal cavity in incisional hernia [after Stoppa, Rives et al. 1977]

pulmonary function tests.

Finally, coughing efforts, which normally increase abdominal pressure considerably (up to 80 mmHg), offers assistance when these patients have bronchial obstruction, since such a pressure increase cannot occur when there is a defect in the abdominal wall.

b) Visceral Disturbances

Less study has been devoted to this subject, although such disturbances certainly exist. The pressure within a hollow viscus results from a state of equilibrium. The latter is disrupted when abdominal pressure decreases. We observed a twofold increase in intravesical pressure (measured with a balloon) in cases of subumbilical incisional hernia. It can be deduced that similar modifications occur in the hollow digestive viscera, especially the colon, as evidenced on peroperative examination. Distension of these organs obviously has a negative effect on their vascularization and function, e.g., disturbed intestinal transit and disturbed micturition. Trouble with defecation, which is directly related to the incompetence of the abdominal

Table 8.5. Incisional hernia and obesity. The incisional hernia compensates the respiratory dysfunction induced by obesity (values shown are the mean of measurements made in 90 cases of incisional hernia)

	Obesity w/o herniation	Obesity plus herniation	Significance
VC	90.8% ± 16.4%	116.1% ± 19.3%	P ≤ 0.0000001
TC	97.4% ± 30.2%	110.7% ± 17.3%	NS
RV/TC	38.1% ± 5.8%	30.2% ± 7.9%	P ≤ 0.00001
MIFR/VC	82.4% ± 10.9%	78.6% ± 12.6%	NS
MEFR/VC	71.6% ± 13.1%	68.9% ± 11.8%	NS

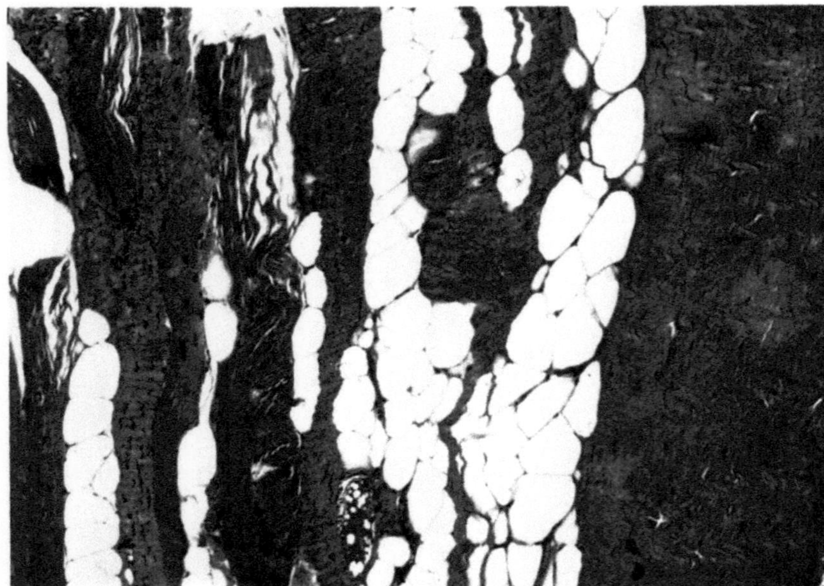

Fig. 8.9. Lesions of the lateral abdominal muscles in incisional hernia. Note the fibroadipose modifications of the muscle; this is more pronounced when the hernial orifice is large (cf. Table 8.6). (Courtesy M. Pluot) x 150

Table 8.6. Influence of diameter of hernial orifice on histological changes in muscles of the abdominal wall (90 biopsies)

	Normal muscle	Modest alterations	Pronounced alterations
Reference group ($n = 13$)	12	1	0
Diameter < 10 cm ($n = 33$)	19	8	6
Diameter > 10 cm ($n = 44$)	10	9	25

wall musculature, is another unpleasant consequence of incisional hernia.

c) Vascular Disturbances

Although we lack precise data on vascular disturbances, it is conceivable that major incisional hernia hinders caval and portal venous return, assuming, as suggested by physiologists, that maintenance of correct abdominal pressure plays a role in normal venous circulation.

d) Muscular Disturbances

Incisional hernia has too often been considered as a simple defect requiring closure, with little thought being given to the function of the abdominal wall muscles. In order to act correctly, these muscles must have solid insertions. Incisional hernia always involves detachment of these muscles and shortening of their fibers. These disturbances lead to histological changes in the muscles, which must be taken into account during surgical repair. The degree of muscle impairment is a function of the length of the involved fibers and of the size of the hernial orifice (Fig. 8.9, Table 8.6).

e) Static Disturbances

Some anatomists [Kapandji 1977] have proposed that the abdominal muscles act as anterior braces for the spine when the subject is standing (Fig. 8.10). Accordingly, weakness of these muscles, especially of the recti abdominis, will lead to exaggeration of lumbar lordosis. During flexion of the spine contraction of the rectus muscles relieves the strain on the spine by "the compression of an inflatable structure" created by the closure of the glottis and contraction of the abdominal muscles. This static function is compromised in cases of major incisional hernia, and many of these patients thus suffer from spinal pain.

f) Surgical Lesions

Little comment will be made on these well-known lesions which include the following: irregularity of the hernial sac, omental or visceral adhesions (in the hernial sac or abdominal cavity), trophic disturbances, and sometimes ulceration of the skin.

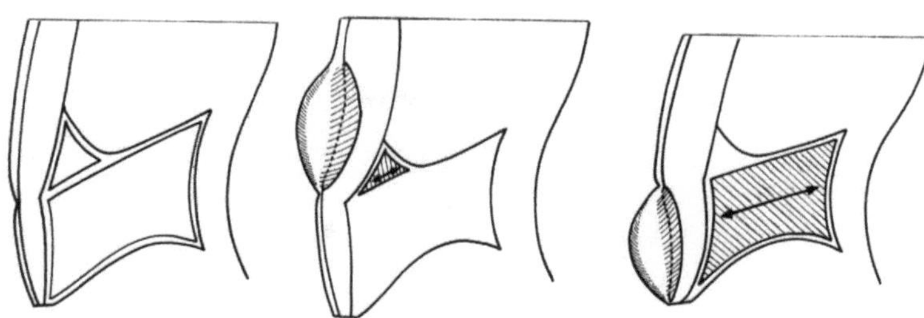

Fig. 8.10. Retraction of the abdominal muscles. The effects of retraction are different above and below the umbilicus

g) Medicolegal Considerations

Incisional hernia leads to a certain degree of invalidity which has to be evaluated by an expert. According to French legislation, permanent partial incapacity is assessed differently according to the legal category to which the patient belongs: in civil law the incapacity can range from 5% to 20%; in workmen's compensation, from 15% to 50%; in military law, from 30% to 60% [Myon 1981]. These percentages of incapacity are used by the medical experts and by specialists in occupational medicine. Any court decision must be based on the patient's professional situation. Conversely, residual incapacity after surgical repair is difficult to evaluate from the legal standpoint, since there are no reference scales on this aspect of the problem.

5. Anatomicoclinical Subtypes

In 1990, we were, with J. P. Chevrel, the editors of the annual report of the French Association of Surgery (AFC). We had the opportunity of collecting cases from many surgical teams in France. These data form the basis of this anatomoclinical classification.

a) Midline

This is the most frequent type of incisional hernia (Figs. 8.11 and 8.12) representing 77.5% of the figures of the French Association of Surgery.

(1) Supraumbilical Incisional Hernia

This type of incisional hernia is equally frequent in both sexes and represents 51.4% of AFC experience. Supraumbilical herniation is seen as a complication of surgery of the stomach and biliary apparatus, and sometimes of the lower part of a sternotomy. The hernial orifice undergoes rapid enlargement owing to the contraction of the powerful muscles in this region. The muscle fibers retract in front of and behind the costochondral margin, and the latter thus often forms the upper margin of the hernial orifice. The recti abdominis undergo atrophy in the affected part of the abdominal wall. However, the protrusion is moderate since the underlying viscera deep in to the incision are adherent. Surgical repair of this type of incisional hernia should be done without delay, as the defect eventually renders surgical apposition impossible, and a prosthesis is always required.

(2) Subumbilical Incisional Hernia

This type of incisional hernia is more frequently seen in women (28% of our cases), following one or more gynecological operations. The defect may be very large and the protrusion voluminous. The herniated viscera rest on the pubis like an apron. The hernial sac sometimes contains part of the colon or urinary bladder and almost always omentum and small bowel. Apposition of the wound margins is easier to obtain in these cases, since instrumental traction involves the longest abdominal muscle fibers. However, the rectus sheath is weakened in this area owing to the displacement of the deep lamina under Douglas' line, and the rectus sheath is prone to scarring and infection, which may lead to atrophy of the inferior fibers of the rectus abdominis near its pubic insertion. Such atrophy may expose much of the bone, especially in cases where operative repair has been unsuccessful. As in the preceding case, this complication may constitute a veritable mass defect of the lower abdominal wall.

(3) Massive Supra- and Subumbilical Midline Incisional Hernia

This type of hernia arises subsequent to single or successive operations involving the supra- and subumbilical regions (70 of 250 cases: 28%). We have seen a few cases of such massive hernia after operation on the abdominal aorta. However, most cases are seen in women (45 of our 70 cases) who have undergone multiple operations. These hernias may reach monstrous proportions and contain almost all of the abdominal viscera. Complications, such as cutaneous erosion and intertrigo, are frequent. Some cases may be beyond the scope of surgical repair.

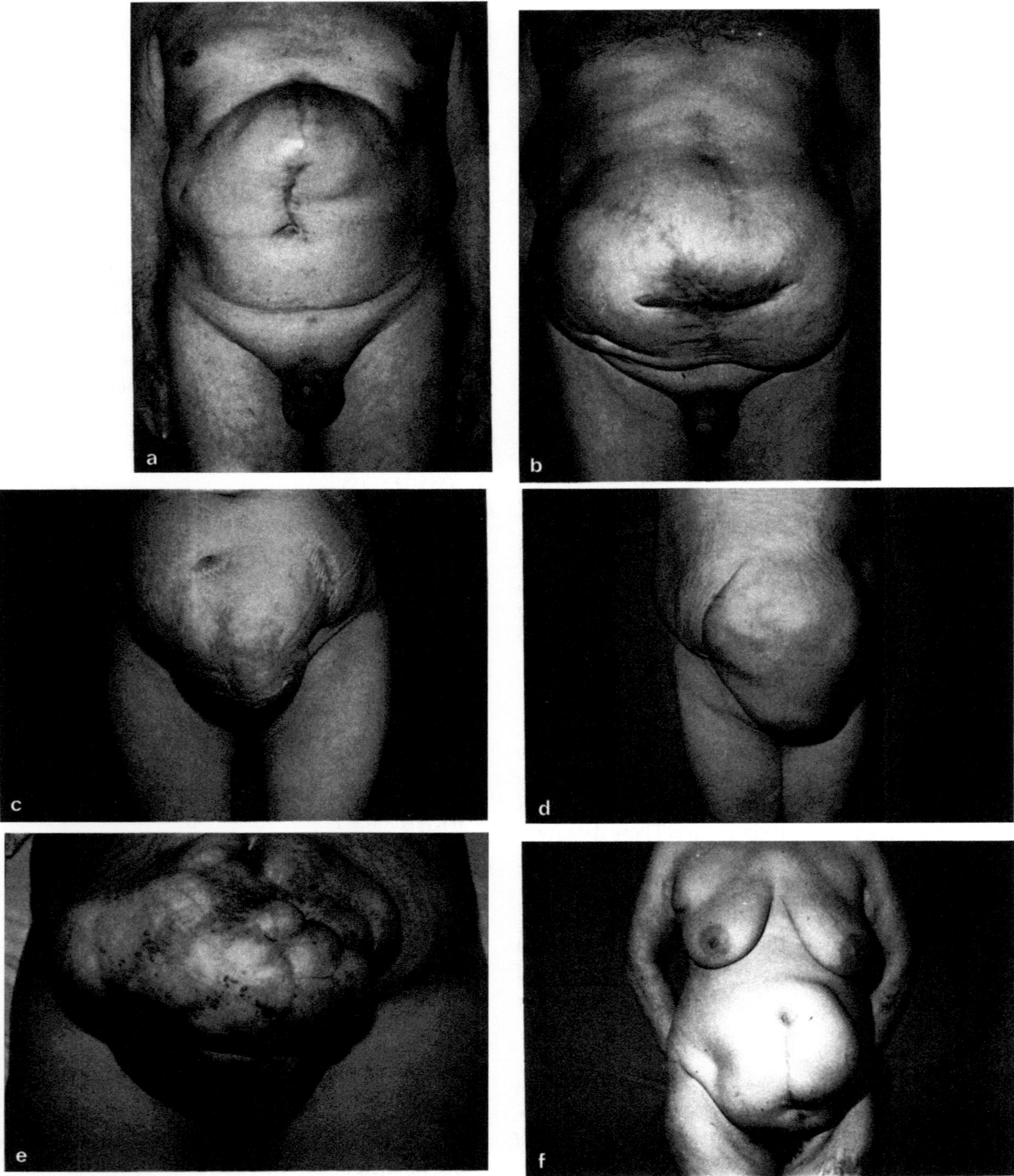

Fig. 8.11a-f. Examples of supra- and subumbilical midline incisional hernia

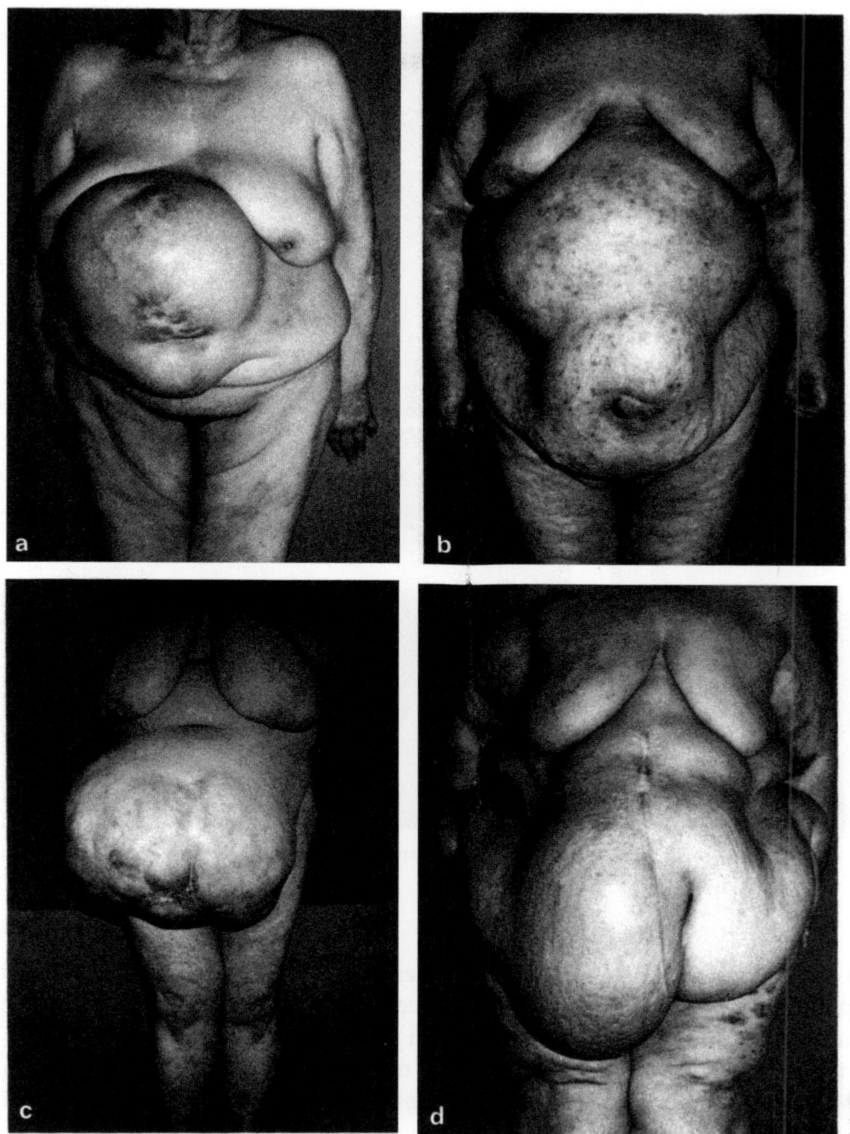

Fig. 8.12a-d. Examples of massive midline incisional hernia

b) Lateral

This type of hernia (Fig. 8.13) is less frequent (17%) than that which occurs in the midline, but often raises difficult problems with respect to treatment.

(1) Subchondral Incisional Hernia

These hernias (6.2%) usually lie under the right costal margin (80% of cases) and a rise following biliary surgery. Although it is conceivable that subchondral laparotomy carries a lower risk of incisional hernia than does the midline approach (we have little experience with subchondral incision), when incisional hernia does occur in this lateral position it is often pronoun-

ced and sometimes difficult to repair. The upper muscle flap of the defect undergoes atrophy and retraction, and the upper margin of the hernial orifice is formed by the costal margin. In some cases the linea alba is pulled over to the left by the traction of the muscles that remain intact.

(2) Inguinal Incisional Hernia

Incisional hernia of the inguinal region (7.6%) was seen more often on the right (20 cases) than on the left (one case) in our experience, and occurs in patients who have undergone successive major operations for appendicular peritonitis, inguinal hernia, or gyneco-

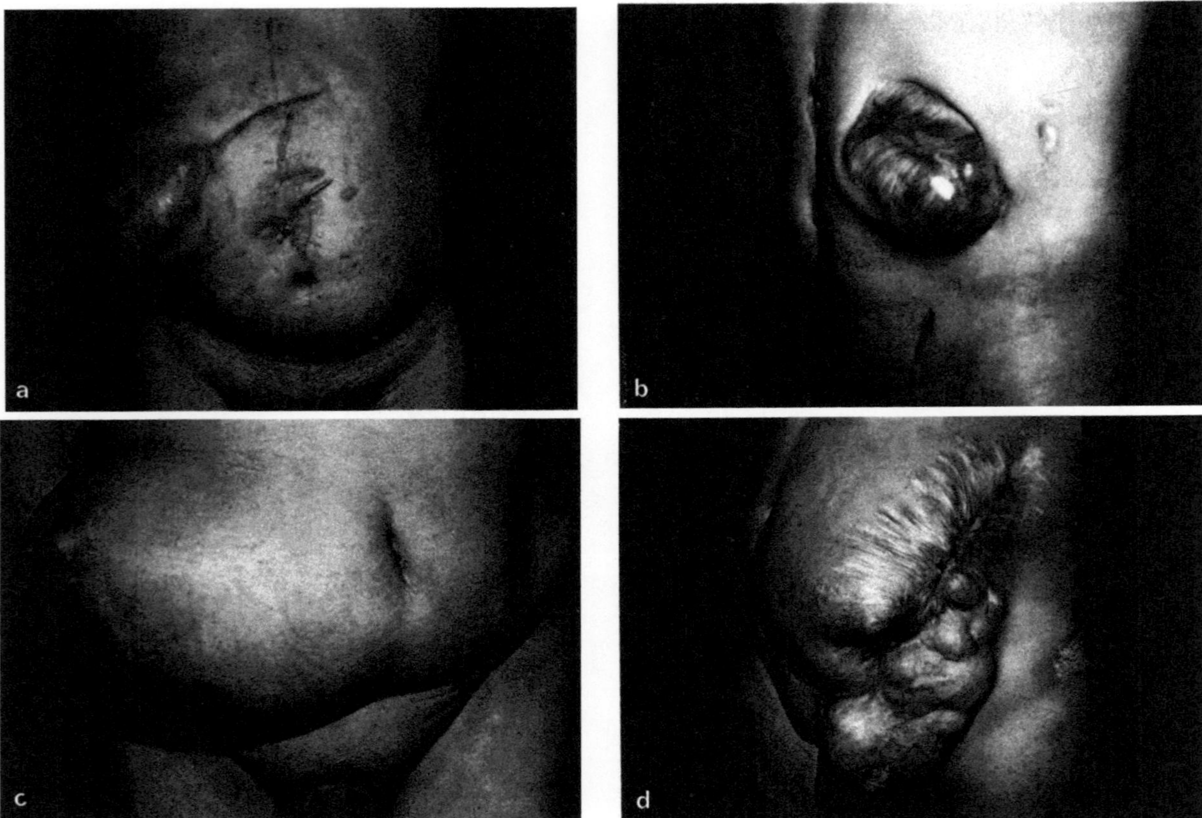

Fig. 8.13a-d. Lateral incisional hernia. These lesions are difficult to repair when they are located at the outer limits of the abdominal cavity, as shown in these examples

logical disorders; an associated midline subumbilical incisional hernia may also be present. In such cases, the inguinal ligament disappears and the abdominal muscles become detached. The inferior margin of the hernial orifice is formed by the psoas major, the vascular pedicle, and the horizontal ramus of the pubis. Repair can be achieved only by using prosthetic material.

(3) Incisional Hernia of the Flank

Incisional hernia of the rectus sheath (1.4%; the sheath is always much wider than imagined) is accompanied by pronounced disruption of the abdominal wall. Retraction and degeneration of the muscle fibers, which are usually free within the sheath, and loss of abdominal wall tissue are seen. This type of incisional hernia resembles that of a midline laparotomy, and often both types occur in the same patient.

Another type of lateral hernia occurs between the thorax and the iliac crest, in a narrow zone corresponding to the course of the 11th and 12th intercostal

nerves. Such herniation is often of modest size. Repair is easily achieved by apposition of the myoaponeurotic flaps, which remain large and supple.

A final type of lateral incisional hernia, seen in the posterior region near the costal ridge, occurs subsequent to urological surgery. Such herniation may be voluminous. The hernial orifice often shows a bony margin (10th and 11th ribs).

6. Complications

In the preceding section, the anatomicoclinical forms of incisional hernia are described, on the assumption that the hernia has reached the stage where it is a stable, organized lesion. Under such conditions the surgeon and intensive care specialist are able to evaluate the lesions and select an appropriate therapeutic procedure. However, other situations can be found (Fig. 8.14). Regardless of the type of hernia, the emergency context must be taken into account, since intensive care is difficult in such cases. Furthermore, septic lesions, or surgical maneuvers in septic conditions,

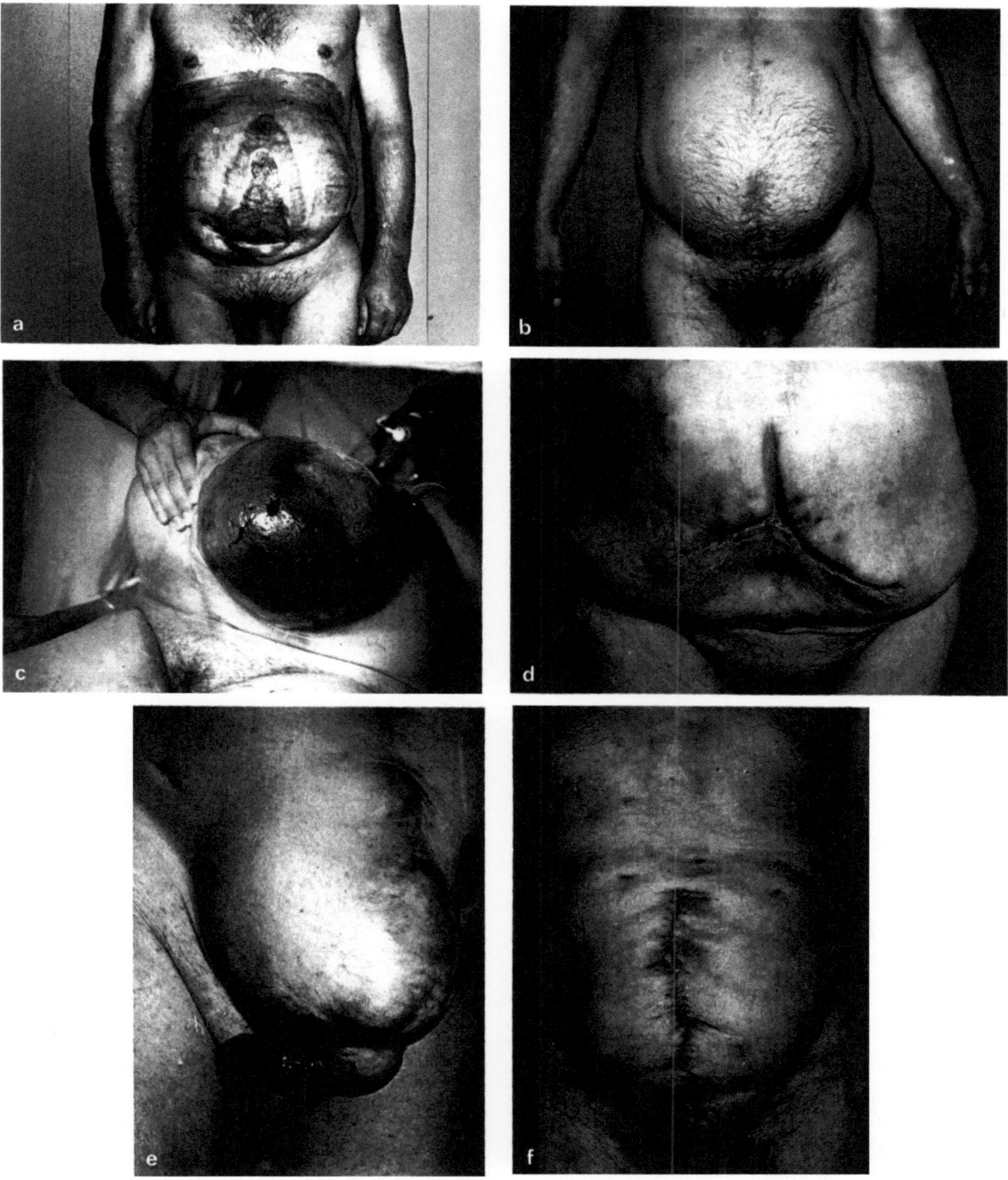

Fig. 8.14a-f. Complicated forms of incisional hernia and the results of surgery. **a** and **b** Large trophic ulceration. **c** and **d** Strangulated hernia with cutaneous necrosis: the skin has been left open. **e** and **f** Burst abdomen with incisional hernia

contraindicate the use of prosthetic material, thereby preventing a repair under the most favorable conditions.

a) Strangulation

Strangulated incisional hernia is a very serious complication. especially in elderly bedridden patients or in cases of bulky herniation with intestinal necrosis (Fig. 8.14c, d). We do not insert a nonabsorbable prosthesis in these cases, because of the lack of skin preparation and the presence of septic fluid within the hernial sac. The use of an absorbable prosthesis may offer an adequate alternative.

b) Trophic Ulceration

The skin often becomes ulcerated with large protrusions through the abdominal wall. The ulceration is seen over the middle and at the apex of the protrusion, and results from weakening of the subcutaneous cellular tissue and occlusion of blood vessels due to the pressure of the viscera. Our histologic data confirm the thrombosis of small vessels. The ulceration itself may be uninfected, but culture of the skin always reveals the presence of potentially dangerous pathogenic organisms (Fig. 8.14a, b).

Treatment requires wide skin resection around the ulcerative lesion. A change of drapes and instruments may tempt one to run the risk of installing a prosthesis at this stage, but we prefer to carry out repair at a later date.

c) Secondary Burst Abdomen

Neglected trophic ulceration will lead to burst abdomen (Fig. 8.14e, f). We have encountered one such case, where luckily the omentum acted as a barrier. In a less fortunate case referred to us a jejunal fistula was found. Treatment requires at least two separate operations.

d) Incisional Hernia with Colostomy

An incisional hernia that develops around an artificial anus can be of gigantic proportions. The hernia must be surgically approached at a distance from the colostomy and in the midline. Provided that scrupulous preparation has been carried out and the colostomy has been fully isolated under plastic protectors, a perforated intra-abdominal prosthesis can be installed with success.

An incisional hernia that occurs in the midline in proximity to colostomy causes more difficult problems. In these cases, where there is only a small dis-

tance between the colostomy and the operative site, we prefer not to use prosthetic material.

e) Associated Forms

Associated Abdominal Emergency. The presence of a lesion requiring emergency surgery in a patient with major incisional hernia is not rare. Treatment of the hernia may have been previously refused by the patient or the surgeon. Most of these patients present with peritonitis of various forms. Local and general preparation are obviously not possible under these emergency conditions. As in the case of strangulated herniation, the surgeon can do only what is in his power; nonabsorbable prostheses are contraindicated because of the risk of septic complications.

Elective Abdominal Surgery, with a Risk of Sepsis. The associated disease involves either the biliary apparatus, the stomach, small bowel or the colon. Prudence is mandatory and it is preferable to use classical procedures and absorbable prosthetic material.

7. Principles of Surgical Management

a) Chronic Incisional Hernia without Sepsis

(1) Nonprosthetic Repair

In cases where the hernial orifice is very small and undergoes only slow enlargement, management is simple. These patients have a large, supple abdominal wall with little muscle. It is of the utmost importance that they follow a regimen of strict body hygiene and that the skin be prepared and disinfected over a long period of time. Good results can be achieved by a classical technique of repair (e.g., a Welti-Eudel procedure). Successful repair requires that the abdominal wall be fully intact postoperatively and that the sutured flaps be apposed without tension.

(2) Difficult Management

Management is difficult in cases of bulky hernia with a large orifice. Prosthetic material is obviously necessary in these cases. Precautions must be taken similar to those used with orthopedic prostheses.

Some patients present *a loss of abdominal wall tissue* (Fig. 8.15a), which is almost always related to atrophy or retraction of the recti abdominis. Preparation and traction do not suffice to close the defect, and a large prosthesis is required to replace the missing tissue. We prefer to insert the prosthesis using transfixing sutures, under tension, which decreases its area of exposure to the overlying skin. This type of fixation can assist partial recovery of lateral muscle function, since the tension lost because of the midline detach-

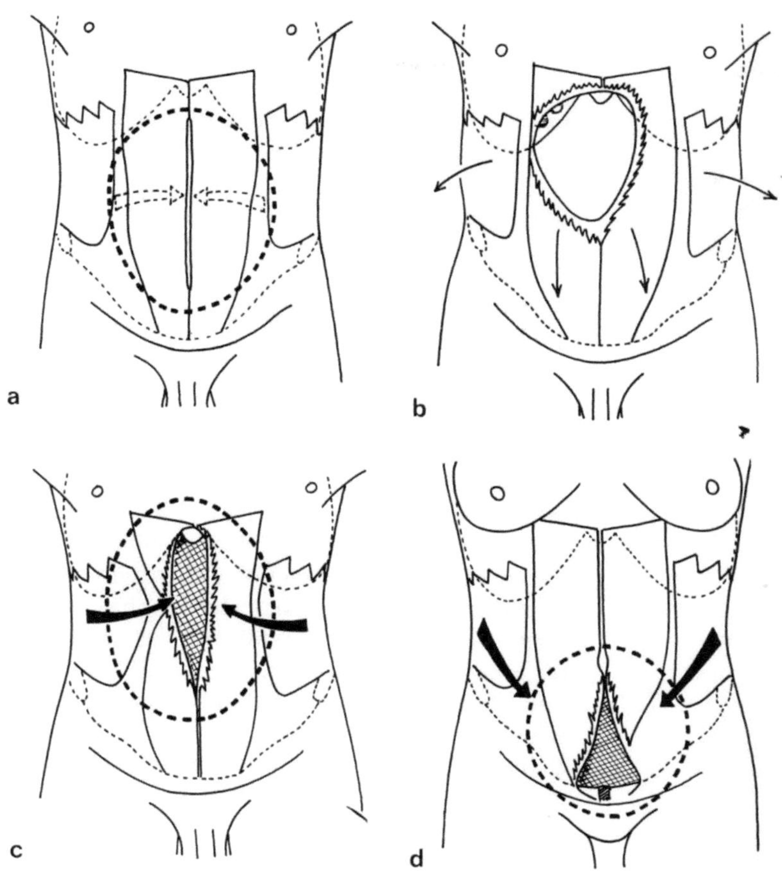

Fig. 8.15a-d. Abdominal wall defect in incisional hernia. Loss of tissue may be only apparent (a), in which case closure is possible. Other cases show a true defect due to muscle destruction (b-d) and the orifice can only be made somewhat narrower

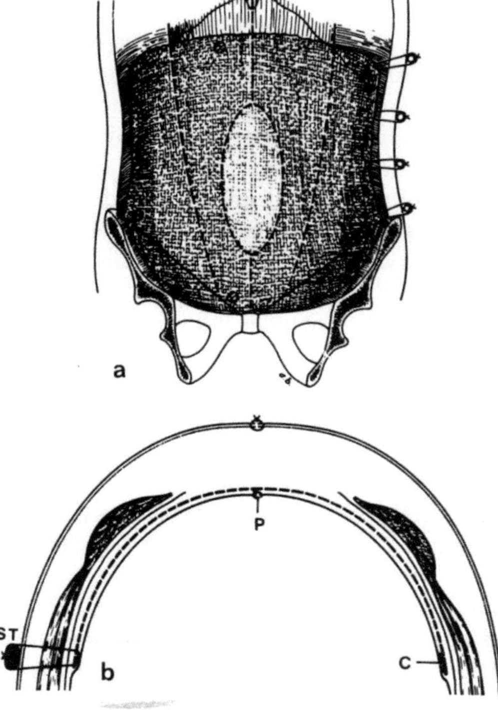

ment of the muscles is re-established. We therefore prefer to use a large prosthesis extending 8-10 cm beyond the margins of the defect. Abdominal pressure assists the integration of the prosthetic material. However, the prosthesis should not be so large that it "freezes" the lateral muscles into a fibrous reaction. The problem of abdominal wall reinforcement can be examined from a different point of view, as proposed by Stoppa et al. (1980). They consider the prosthesis a reinforcement of the peritoneal envelope and thus use larger prostheses allowing greater envelopment. These prostheses are not attached as solidly as with our technique. Transfixing sutures or biological glue can be used for this purpose (Fig. 8.16).

In some cases there is only *an apparent loss of abdominal wall tissue* (Figs. 8.15a, 8.17). Such patients

◀

Fig. 8.16a, b. Stoppa's procedure. A large, enveloping prosthesis is placed in the subperitoneal space and fixed in place by transfixing sutures or biological adhesive. [Stoppa et al. 1980; courtesy of Nouvelle Presse Médicale]

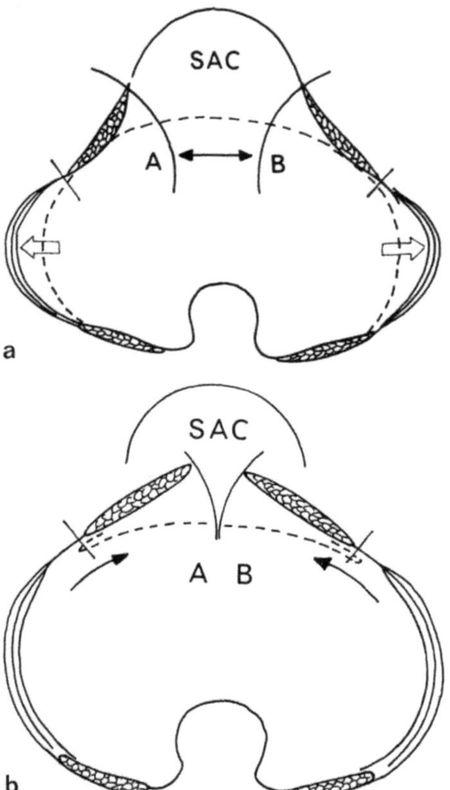

Fig. 8.17a, b. Principles of surgical treatment of midline incisional hernia. Our technique recreates tension on the retracted lateral abdominal muscles and allows us to appose the "sagittalized" recti abdomini. The prosthesis is solidly anchored to the semilunar line (Spigelius line) and extends widely beneath the deep surface of the recti

usually present with major midline incisional hernias, which can be likened to pronounced diastasis. There is no true loss of tissue, although the wall is scarred. Subsequent to appropriate preparation using the technique of pneumoperitoneum and adequate curarization during anesthesia, it is possible to achieve apposition of the margins of the hernial orifice, although the degree of traction required carries the risk of recurrence. Use of a prosthesis allows the forces of traction to be transferred to the edge of the implant. The abdominal wall can then be sutured over the prosthesis without tension. This procedure can be termed *prosthetic reinforcement*, since the prosthesis protects the midline suture.

b) Septic Incisional Hernia

Nonabsorbable prostheses should not be used for infected incisional hernias, at least in the primary stage of repair. The risk of recurrent herniation is preferable to the much more serious risk of infection. We prefer classical repair procedures under these conditions, coupled with the use of absorbable prosthetic material after an appropriate interval.

8. Treatment

a) Preparation

(1) Role of the Anesthesiologist-Intensive Care Specialist

On initial contact with the patient the specialist evaluates respiratory function and notes the existence of cough, expectoration, history of smoking, etc. Respiratory status is then assessed by appropriate tests. Clinical examination, chest X-rays, and radioscopy will evaluate diaphragmatic mobility. However, testing of respiratory function yields a more precise assessment. We place particular emphasis on the minute respiratory volume (MRV) and the ratio of forced expiratory volume to vital capacity (FEV/VC). The results obtained are compared with theoretical normal values using standard tables developed by Baldwin et al. (1948). Blood gas determinations are also of prime importance. Measurements should include partial oxygen pressure (normal value = 100 Torr), CO_2 partial pressure (normal value = 40 Torr), pH (7.4), and O_2 saturation (> 75%). The results of blood gas measurement are used to evaluate ventilatory efficacy and to identify latent respiratory insufficiency (Table 8.7).

Preparation of the patient is begun on the first day of hospitalization. The results of respiratory exploration on admission are compared with those obtained at regular intervals thereafter. In this way the respiratory status and the efficacy of preparation can be assessed. Electronic spirometry (Sandoz M-4-03) allows daily evaluation of residual volume (RV), forced expiratory volume (FEV), and minute volume (MV).

Preparation also includes withdrawal of tobacco; respiratory physiotherapy, i.e., costal exercise, diaphragmatic exercise (deep inspiration in different decubital positions), assistance of coughing and expectoration by clapping exercises, in some cases postural drainage; instrumental physiotherapy using a pressure-relaxation breathing apparatus (Bird Mark 8 or Bennet PR1, PR2) to facilitate coughing and decrease secretion by increasing alveolar ventilation (the breathing apparatus is driven by pressurized gas and can be used at home); prescriptions of a mucolytic agent (we use cyclohexyl methylammonium chlo-

Table 8.7. Acceptable values

Spirometry		Blood gas measurements		
VC	80%	PaO2	95 Torr	40 years
RV	40%		80 Torr	50 years
RV/TC	30%		85 Torr	60 years
FEV/VC	75%	SaO2	70%	
		PaCO2	40 ± 5 Torr	
		pH	7.40 ± 0.05	

Table 8.8. A 40-year-old woman, 161 cm, 75 kg presenting with major incisional hernia of right hypochondrium and right iliac fossa; postoperative course uneventful; discharge 1 month later

Respiratory function: theoretical values		Sept. 14, 1982	Dec. 12, 1982
VC	2,800 ml	2,700 ml	3,375 ml
FEV	2,160 ml	1,500 ml	2,850 ml
FEV/VC	77%	55.5%	84.5%
RV		1,950 ml	4,475 ml
TC	3,766 ml	4,650 ml	4,775 ml
RV/TC		42%	29.3%

Table 8.9. A 71-year-old woman, 158 cm, 94 kg; presenting with major supraumbilical incisional hernia complicated by diabetes, congestive heart failure, and ischemic heart disease. Preparation was carried out for 30 days. 48 hours after surgery the following were noted: polypnea, normocapnic hypoxia followed by hypercapnia, and heart failure requiring prolonged artificial ventilation and intensive care. The patient was discharged 1 month later

Respiratory function: theoretical values		Dec. 9, 1982	Jan. 3, 1983
VC	2,360 ml	2,250 ml	2,200 ml
FEV	1,620 ml	1,750 ml	1,550 ml
FEV/VC	68.5%	77.8%	70.5%
RV		1,700 ml	1,500 ml
TC	3,520 ml	3,950 ml	3,700 ml
RV/TC		43%	40%
PaO2/SaO2		83 Torr/96%	76 Torr/95%
PaCO2		41 Torr	37 Torr

Table 8.10. A 70-year-old woman, 155 cm, 90 kg, alcoholic, was refused operation due to disturbed alveolocapillary diffusion of O2 and CO2, confirmed by the CO2 compliance test

Respiratory function: theoretical values		April 17, 1982	April 26, 1982
VC	2,340 ml	1,200 ml	1,180 ml
FEV	1,600 ml	800 ml	780 ml
FEV/VC	68.5%	66.7%	67%
RV		1,600 ml	—
TC	3,460 ml	2,800 ml	—
RV/TC		57%	—
PaO2/SaO2		56 Torr/96%	50 Torr/84%
PaCO2		55 Torr	52 Torr

ride given as an oral solution); and antibiotics (in cases of infection). Where initial results are satisfactory the operation need not be further delayed. In other cases, improvement is seen only after several weeks of preparation, in which case the operation should be postponed until then. Such a case is illustrated by the results of respiratory function tests shown in Table 8.8.

In patients presenting with poor health who show no improvement after respiratory preparation, the decision to operate must be made with great care, since the postoperative course may have severe complications, as in the case outlined in Table 8.9. In other cases the results of respiratory function tests lead to a refusal to operate, despite the patient's insistence, as in the case outlined in Table 8.10.

(2) Role of the Nursing Staff

The nursing staff play a major role in preparation of the patient by ensuring proper hygiene and treatment of skin lesions and by encouraging the patient to ambulate, to use the stairs, etc.

(3) Role of the Surgeon

In cases where the hernia has "lost the right to reside in the abdominal cavity", the technique of pneumoperitoneum described by Goni-Moreno (1970) is useful. The premedicated patient is placed in the supine position. A blunt trocar (Palmer's needle) is introduced into the abdominal cavity on the line joining the umbilicus to the left anterior-superior iliac spine. The point of penetration should be closer to the umbilicus than to the iliac spine. Penetration into the peritoneal cavity can be easily achieved by requesting the patient to tense the abdominal muscles during the puncture (subsequent punctures are facilitated by the presence of residual pneumoperitoneum). A syringe is then used to inject sterilized air (taken over an open flame) into the peritoneal cavity until the patient feels discomfort, which is usually signaled by difficult respiration and sometimes the occurrence of scapular pain. The amount of air that can be injected during each session varies greatly according to the patient (from a few hundred milliliters to more than a liter). The pneumoperitoneum is reinduced every 2-3 days and the patient is monitored with X-rays (subdiaphragmatic air shadows). We prefer to use air rather than CO2, which is more rapidly resorbed, thereby allowing a greater time interval between injections.

With this technique we can assess the patient's tolerance to reduction of the hernial mass. The diaphragm can be readapted to work in physiological conditions and, according to the author of the technique, dissection of the hernial sac is facilitated.

b) Surgical Intervention

(1) Anesthesia

General anesthesia and artificial respiration are used. Operative analgesia is obtained by administration of a morphinomimetic drug (phenoperidine). Muscular relaxation is achieved with a curarimimetic (pancuronium bromide, 0.07-0.10 mg/kg). The advantages of this technique include its safety, reversibility and controllability, rapid awakening, and early return of intestinal transit.

(2) Exposure and Exploration

Skin Incision. The direction of the incision is of little importance and is chosen as a function either of the previous incision or of the major axis of the swelling. Our practice is to make the incision in the direction of the previous one, and to resect (at least in cases of major incisional hernia) a fairly large diamond-shaped area of skin, since the hernial sac always adheres to the skin. There is no point in trying to cut these adhesions to free the overlying skin, which will not be needed once the hernia is reduced. The skin over the sac is stretched thin and poorly vascularized and has lost its subcutaneous supportive tissue. In cases of cutaneous ulceration, the resected area should be as large as possible, extending well beyond the area of lymphatic drainage.

Dissection of the Hernial Sac. As described above, the sac is sometimes bulky and is always irregular. One should expect to find adherent and intertwined bowel loops within it, and in some cases sterile or infected fluid. This danger must be kept in mind when one proceeds to isolate the sac. It is preferable to approach the sac from without, beginning the dissection at a solid part of the abdominal wall. Work then progresses from the periphery to the center and the sac is approached via its neck. However, in the course of these maneuvers, the peritoneum often presents in such a way that it can be opened without apparent danger; the surgeon should seize such an opportunity when it arises.

Exploration of Contents of Hernial Sac. Once the limits of the sac have been defined and opened, the exploration of its contents can begin. Different situations can be encountered, which are discussed below.

In some cases, no adhesions are found within the sac. In this case the surgeon should simply identify the limits of the hernial orifice and explore it from within. For this purpose the hand is slipped inside the abdominal cavity to test the solidity of the abdominal wall from its posterior to its anterior part.

Sometimes a few loose, isolated adhesions are found, and these can easily be broken or divided. In some cases, however, major fleshy adhesions are encountered. After appropriate dissection, these can often be broken down, although this carries a risk of postoperative peritonitis. In the course of these procedures, care should be taken to protect the omentum, which may be needed later on.

In some cases the adhesions are numerous and involve major segments of intestine. Such patients run a high risk of visceral rupture, and it is better to resect the omentum and involved bowel. When the resections are done at the proper sites under good conditions, including adequate protection of the abdominal wall, there is less risk of operative failure than when there is unexpected opening of a hollow viscus, or an area of necrotic omentum. Although omental necrosis may be aseptic, one should assume the opposite. Indeed, highly pathogenic organisms can be found, e.g., *Pseudomonas aeruginosa* (pyocyanic bacillus) in one of our patients.

Exploration of the Abdominal Cavity. In cases of major incisional hernia the defect is large enough to allow thorough examination of the abdominal cavity, which may reveal other lesions that must be taken into account. Should repair of the incisional hernia be coupled with treatment of an ovarian cyst or gallstones? The answer depends on the condition of the patient, the surgical approach, the nature of the lesion and its severity, as well as on the risks of septic contamination, especially where nonabsorbable prosthetic material is to be used.

Exposure of the Margins of Hernial Orifice. The margins of the orifice must be carefully identified. Secondary orifices, when present, should be opened, since the aponeurotic bands extending from one side to the other are of no structural significance and cannot be used for repair. The contours of the defect thus identified must be solid, i.e., able to be grasped by strong forceps.

(3) Nonprosthetic Repair

Classical methods of repair are based on aponeurotic or muscular reconstructive surgery using the anato-

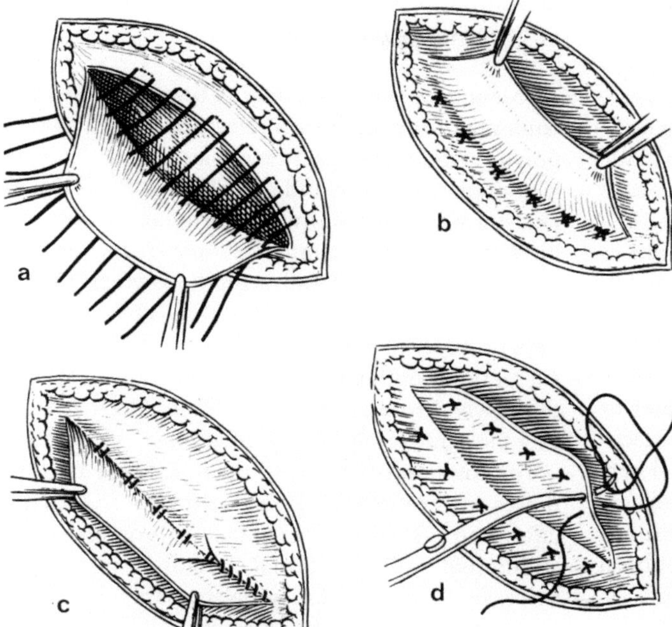

Fig. 8.18 a-d. Judd's procedure. Repair is achieved by overlapping of the existing aponeuroses. [Rives et al. 1977; courtesy of Encyclopédie Médico-Chirurgicale]

mical structures of the abdominal wall. These procedures may still be indicated in certain cases. Simple suturing of the aponeurotic margins after reduction of the herniated viscera and treatment of the hernial sac may be useful when the orifice is narrow, e.g., incisional hernia at a drainage site. In such cases, relaxing incisions in the anterior aspect of the rectus sheath [Gibson 1920; Welti & Eudel 1941; Clotteau & Prémont 1979] may be of help.

Suturing by Judd's technique also requires that the aponeuroses be solid. Furthermore, it is necessary that these fascial structures be stretched (as is almost always the case around the hernial sac) and that the margins of the orifice be brought into apposition without difficulty (Fig. 8.18). This technique is mainly applicable to the treatment of lateral incisional hernia, although it can be used in cases of midline hernia.

Reference is often made by French authors to the technique of Welti and Eudel (1941), and some reports on this technique have been published [Eudel 1979; Hureau et al. 1975]. The procedure is used for midline repair and consists of making two lateral incisions (parallel to the midline) through the anterior surface of the rectus sheath. The two resulting aponeurotic flaps are then sutured together over the midline defect. Finally, the medial margins of the rectus sheath are sutured together over the aponeurotic repair.

Gosset's technique (1949) of suturing full-thickness autografted skin bands is mainly indicated for the repair of midline incisional hernias. Results published by Banzet et al. (1979) demonstrate that the strips of skin are not rejected. This procedure of reinforced suturing can be very useful (Fig. 8.19).

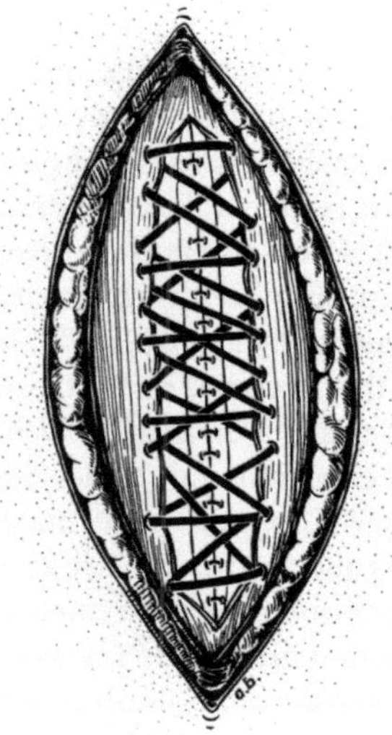

Fig. 8.19. Gosset's procedure. Suturing is done with bands of autografted skin, inserted like laces into the wound margins. [Banzet et al. 1979; courtesy of Nouvelle Presse Médicale]

For patients prepared by preoperative pneumoperitoneum, the various procedures described above can be used to treat relatively simple incisional hernia when there is neither a loss of abdominal wall tissue nor sclerotic retraction of the muscles. These techniques do not have the inconvenience of prosthetic repair and do not require the same precautions. In comparable groups of patients, infection is less frequent and less severe, but these classical procedures carry a high recurrence rate, and much attention has been given to prosthetic surgery. Nonprosthetic repair is still indicated where there is an obvious risk of sepsis. Under such conditions we prefer to use Welti Eudel's procedure with reinforcement of the anterior rectus sheath with an absorbable prosthesis. This technique can be applied to most types of incisional hernia. Furthermore, in cases of recurrent incisional hernia a prosthesis can be placed under good conditions since the retromuscular prefascial space has not been breached.

(4) Prosthetic Repair

Prostheses can be used to treat lesions which are often considered beyond the scope of surgery. The use of prosthetic material has been the subject of much controversy, but it is now widely accepted.

The choice of an appropriate prosthesis is based on the physical and biological properties of the material to be used. The ideal material should be as light and solid as possible, with a certain degree of elasticity and suppleness. Elasticity allows the prosthesis to conform freely to the curvatures of the visceral sac and to "accompany" the movements of the muscles into which it is incorporated, thereby avoiding undue friction leading to inflammation. It is also important that the material be of a fairly open mesh structure so as to induce a rapid fibroblastic response. For these reasons, we have chosen to use Dacron (Mersuture) over the past decades, since in our opinion it is the least inappropriate material commercially available. The results of our experience with this material in the treatment of hernia of the groin and major incisional hernia have been confirmed by experimental studies done by workers in Amiens (see Chap. 9, page 200) and Strasbourg [Adloff & Arnaud 1976; Petit et al. 1974]. They demonstrated that fibroblastic investment of the prosthesis is best when mersilene mesh is used, i.e., the index of fibroblastic reaction is high and much greater than the index of inflammatory reaction, which remains low (Fig. 8.20). Furthermore, we have never observed intolerance to this type of prosthetic

mesh, and the cases of rejection that have been seen were due to operative sepsis.

A recent experimental study [Chevrel & Rath 1997] compares four different materials, namely Dacron, polypropylene, polyglactine 910 and composite materials, namely Dacron and polyglactine 910. The comparison was based on two criteria: on the one hand biomechanical tests aiming to compare the resistance of normal abdominal walls with those which had been reinforced with different prostheses at 30, 60 and 90 days postoperatively, and on the other hand histological sections aiming to assess resistance by measuring the newly formed collagen and tolerance by estimating the acute foreign body inflammatory reaction.

The comparative study of the nonabsorbable prostheses with resorbable polyglactine showed that the latter can restore the resistance to pressure on the abdominal wall to normal, but does not actually increase it, as do the nonabsorbable prostheses. Furthermore, resistance to traction is less than that obtained by nonabsorbable meshes, particularly polypropylene. Its tolerance increases parallel to the rate of dissolution, but remains less than that of Dacron after the first month.

The comparative study of the two nonabsorbable prostheses which were tested shows that whereas Dacron is distinctly better tolerated, abdominal walls reinforced by polypropylene are three times more resistant to traction and the increase in resistance to pressure is extremely high. Polypropylene achieves a maximal degree of fibrosis earlier than does Dacron, but at the same time is more easily deformed. Thus Dacron seems to be the prosthesis of choice when maximum resistance is required, for example in those cases where the abdominal wall is so weak that a small increase in its resistance would be sufficient. In fact, Dacron only offers an increase of 55% in resistance to pressure, while maintaining resistance to traction at a physiological level.

Combination of an absorbed material (polyglactine) with nonabsorbable Dacron seems to confirm no advantage, whether on resistance or tolerance. The authors have not found any reliable criterion to indicate a preference for composite Dacron over simple Dacron.

All the prosthetically reinforced abdominal walls which were studied achieved their maximum resistance at the end of the first postoperative month, both to pressure and to traction. They all maintained a physiological level of elasticity comparable to that of a normal abdominal wall. The prostheses were equally

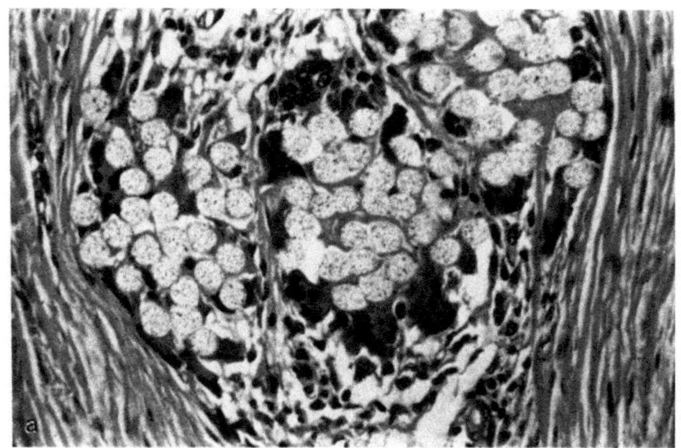

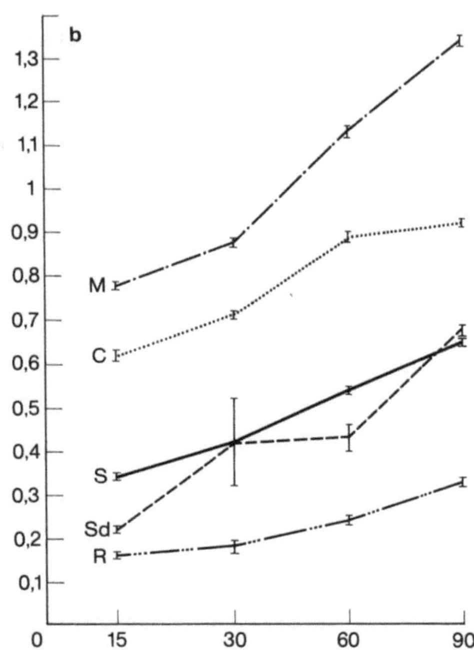

Fig. 8.20a, b. Tolerance for dacron-mersilène prostheses. Comparative histological study (**a** courtesy of T. Caulet) shows that dacron offers the best relationship of fibroblastic to inflammatory reaction. **b** Experimental study by Adloff and Arnaud (1976) of the resistance to and tolerance for prosthetic materials used in repairing defects of the abdominal wall. *R* Siliconized velvet-dacron plate; *Sd* silastic-dacron plate; *S* siliconized plate; *M* dacron mesh; *C* nylon mesh

well tolerated at the end of the third month. The choice must therefore rest on the resistance/tolerance ratio during the two first postoperative months.

The polyglactine prosthesis is only indicated in the presence of sepsis. The Dacron prosthesis confers good resistance to the wall, nonetheless limited, and its use in extremely obese or muscular subjects does not give complete protection against recurrent herniation due to tearing of the prosthesis. The polypropylene prosthesis, which is three time stronger, is clinically equally well tolerated and at present appears to be the nearest approach to the ideal. The composite Dacron polyglactine prosthesis seems to have no particular advantages over either of the simple types.

The site of Prosthetic Implantation. A prosthesis can be positioned intraperitoneally by attaching it to the deep surface of the abdominal wall, or under the skin by fixing it to the superficial aspect of the abdominal wall. However, insertion of the prosthesis within the wall itself obviously requires that the existing anatomical conditions be taken into account. The best planes of cleavage within the abdominal wall are found in the rectus sheath, between the lateral abdominal muscles and in the subumbilical part of the preperitoneal space.

Intraperitoneal Positioning. This has been recommended by Bourgeon et al. (1972). In a study published in

1997, Arnaud reported on this procedure in 220 patients. Good results (two deaths, infection in five cases, recurrence in eight cases) were obtained in that study, considering the magnitude of the lesions that were seen. We do not believe that intraperitoneal implantation has any advantages. Although the peritoneum rapidly envelops the prosthesis and offers a good defense against infection without hematoma formation, it is also true that this process is accompanied by adhesion of the bowel loops, thereby hindering intestinal transit and complicating further surgery. We have seen cases of intraluminal migration of such a prosthesis. Interpositioning of the omentum between the viscera and the prosthesis protect against these complications.

Premuscular Positioning of the Prosthesis. This has been defended by J.P. Chevrel (1979), who advances the following arguments:
• Placing the prosthesis in this position requires wide mobilization, which abolishes the lateral traction on the rectus muscles exerted by the oblique and transverse muscles. This dissection increases the effect of the counter-incisions, whether they be of the large Gibson type or the multiple incisions described by Clotteau-Prémont.
• The anterior rectus sheath should be considered as the principle tendon of insertion of the flat muscles into the linea alba.

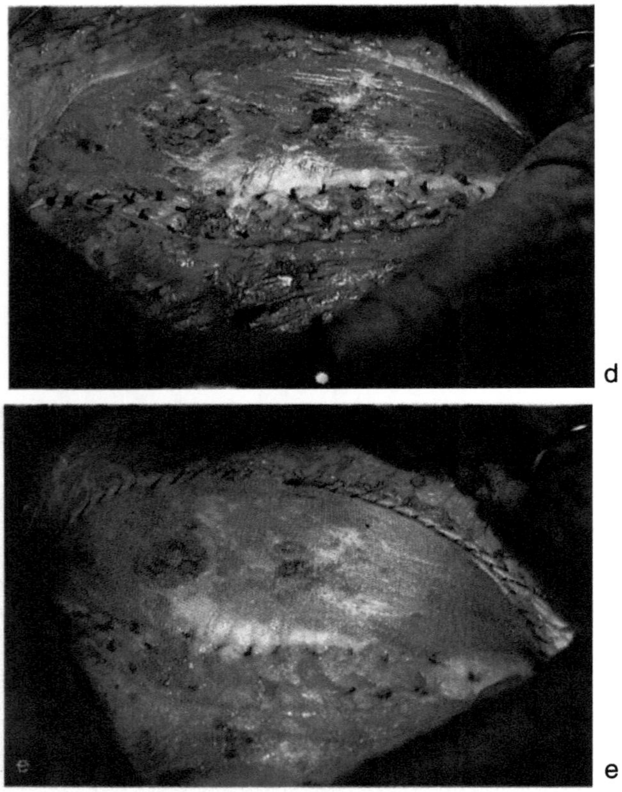

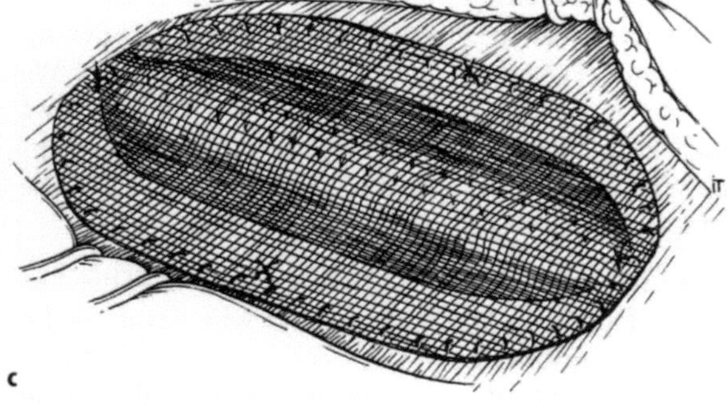

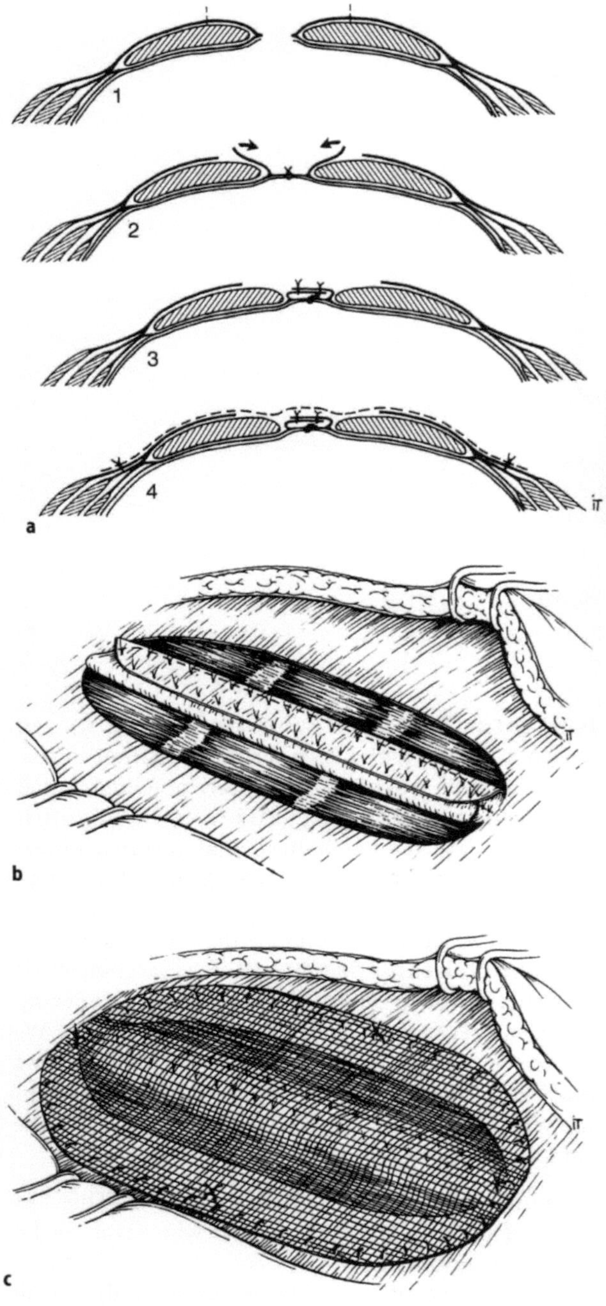

Fig. 8.21a-e. Chevrel's procedure: mantle reconstructive surgery and prosthesis. **a** _1_ Incision on the anterior rectus sheath. _2_ Approximation of fascial edges and turndown of the anterior rectus sheath. _3_ Mantle suturing of rectus sheath. _4_ Reinforcement with a nonabsorbable prosthesis, in the premusculoaponeurotic position, sutured and glued. **b** Appearance of the abdominal wall following suture of the fascial edges and mantle repair. **c** Appearance of the abdominal wall, following placement of a premusculoaponeurotic prosthesis (Mersilene, Prolene or Marlex). **d** Operative view. Subcutaneous dissection is widely extended laterally; note two rows of sutures in middle of operative field [courtesy of J. P. Chevrel]. **e** Fixation of ligalene-tulle mesh using four slow-absorbing sutures

• The superficial position of the prosthesis allows tension to be adjusted correctly when it is fixed in place.
• The use of a fibrin glue sprayed on to the prosthesis immediately consolidates the fixation.
• When a superficially placed prosthesis becomes infected it is simply managed by local measures, and does not require to be removed.

• In contrast, a deeply placed prosthesis may, if there is any defect in the peritoneum, come into contact with the viscera and favor formation of a fistula.

The operation includes a first stage of dissection during which it is necessary to resect the peritoneal sac, freshen the margins of the defect and free up the underlying viscera as widely as possible so that the abdominal wall can be reconstructed with no risk of visceral injury. This stage of the dissection is completed by carrying out a wide detachment of the plane in front of the muscles and aponeurosis upwards as far as the costal margin, downwards to the iliac crests and laterally to the mid-axillary line. Rigorous asepsis is mandatory, achieved by the use of Povidone-iodine soaked swabs and meticulous hemostasis so as to avoid postoperative hematomas.

The actual repair comprises reconstruction of the linea alba, which has almost always been possible in our series. Only four patients had a loss of substance which in three cases required the use of a patch and in one the construction of a flap from the rectus sheath. This reconstruction of the linea alba is carried out either in one layer by the Gibson or Clotteau-Prémont technique, using interrupted nonabsorbable sutures, or in two layers as described by Welti and Eudel, or as a "wrapover plasty" (Fig. 8.21).

J. P. Chevrel emphasizes this wrapover plasty which is carried out in four layers. The first layer, following large counter incisions in the anterior rectus sheath strengthens the margins of the defect, then a double aponeurotic layer constructing the wrapover with nonabsorbable 2/0 interrupted sutures, finally a fourth layer which is represented by the prosthesis itself in front of the muscles and aponeurosis.

The linea alba having been reconstructed, the abdominal wall is reinforced by a large Dacron or polypropylene prosthesis, which is fixed by four sutures of 2/0 absorbable suture material, reinforced by paramedian stitches which apply the patch firmly to the muscular layer and linea alba. The patch is also fixed by spraying with 2 ml of fibrin glue. Two to four suction drains are inserted. The subcutaneous tissues are approximated firmly with absorbable material, and the skin is closed with metal staples. Before recovery from anesthesia, a supporting abdominal girdle is put in place, and sepsis is prevented by an injection of 1 g of Vancomycin at the beginning of the operation in the case of recurrence and of cephamandol for primary operations. The dressing is not removed until the 6th postoperative day.

J.P. Chevrel has reported a series of 389 incisional hernias operated upon between 1980 and 1993, 236 of whom were managed with a prosthesis. Among these last, a series of 110 patients operated upon since 1989 received a collagen glue spray to fix the prosthesis in position. The series includes 328 midline hernias (84.31%), 68 lateral hernias (17.48%) and five parastomal hernias (1.28%). Twelve patients had multiple her-

niations. Various complicating factors rendered the surgery more difficult, in particular the inclusion of 23 infected cases and 143 which had recurred one or more times (36.76%). In the series of patients receiving prosthetic reinforcement, various techniques of suture or plastic repair were carried out, the choice depending upon the site of the hernia, its size and whether or not it was recurrent. Simple herniorrhaphy was employed 44 times, large Gibson type counter-incision 24 times, small multiple Clotteau-Prémont type incisions 31 times, a Gersuni-Welti-Eudel plasty 39 times, a Chevrel wrapover plasty 77 times, and other techniques including the Judd, Quénu patch and sandwich prosthesis 21 times.

Results (Fig. 8.22). The total follow up was 93.89% of the patients, and 98.18% of a recent series of 110 patients treated with prosthetic replacement and fibrin glue. The analysis of the series of patients treated by suture or hernioplasty plus prosthetic reinforcement shows that:
• The overall morbidity included twelve cases out of 236 of superficial sepsis (5%), three of which occurred in the 110 patients treated with the fibrin glue. There were ten hematomas (0.84%), one skin necrosis (0.42%), and seven seromas (2.96%). Six of these occurred in the fibrin glue group, at the beginning of the series when external drainage was not used.
• There was an overall benefit when the prosthesis was fixed with fibrin glue, as regards recurrences. Chevrel reports 28 recurrences in 153 repairs without prosthesis (18.3%), a figure which fell to 5.5% when a premuscular prosthesis was inserted. In this latter group there were twelve recurrences out of 133 operations where fibrin glue was not used (9.2%), and only one definitive recurrence in 110 patients where the glue technique was included (0.97%).

Preperitoneal implantation has been widely used by Stoppa et al. (1979, 1980). In his view the aim of the operation is to reinforce the peritoneum. Accordingly, the abdominal wall is closed over a large prosthesis placed between the abdominal muscles and the peritoneum, so that the prosthetic material envelops and reinforces the peritoneum. A biological adhesive is sometimes used to fix the material in place, although this procedure is not mandatory since the prosthesis is firmly held in place by the intra-abdominal pressure and later by fibrous ingrowth. Very good results have been obtained by Stoppa: among a total of 287 cases published, two deaths occurred postoperatively, six cases of suppuration were seen (leading to recurrence

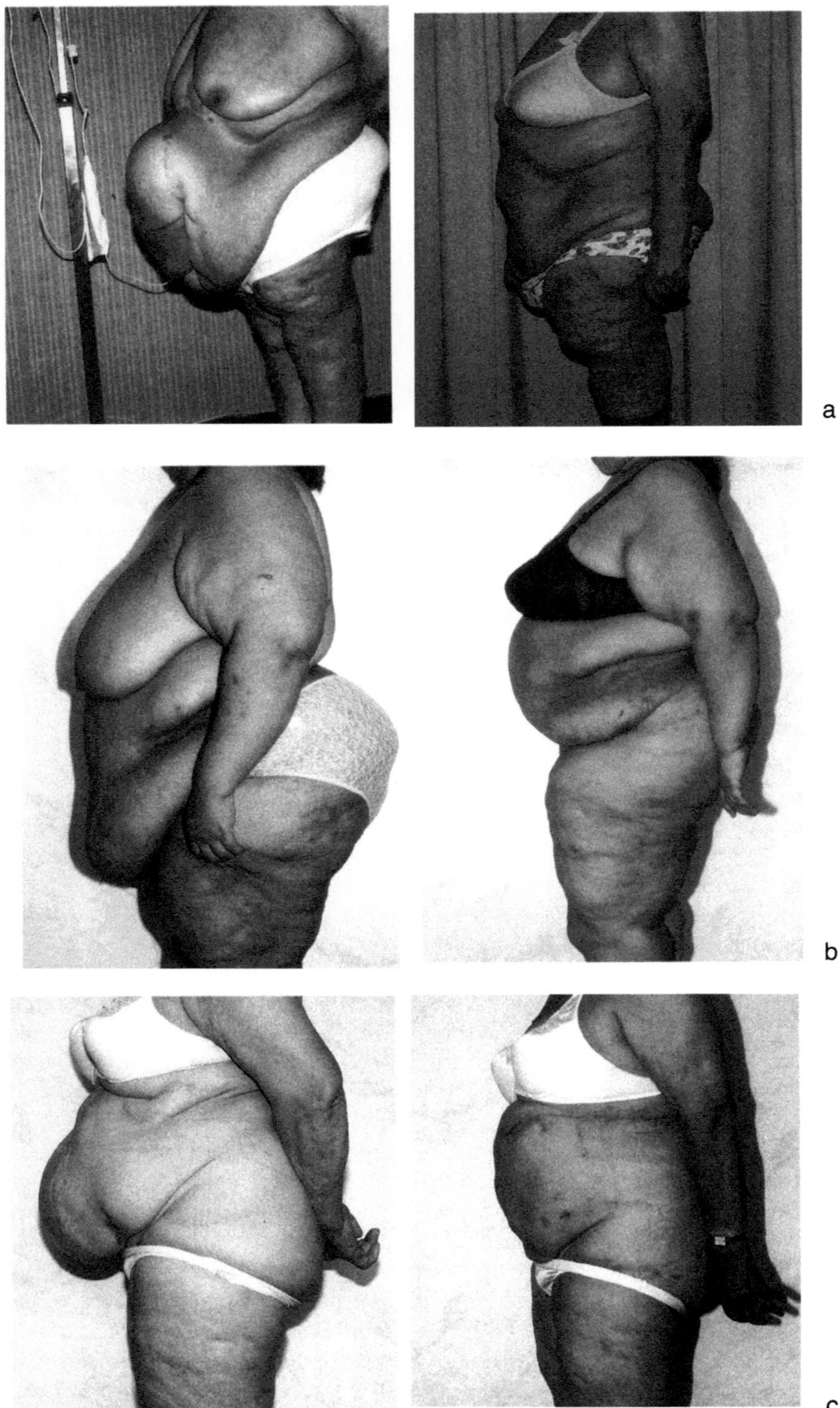

Fig. 8.22 a-c. Results obtained in three cases using Chevrel's procedure

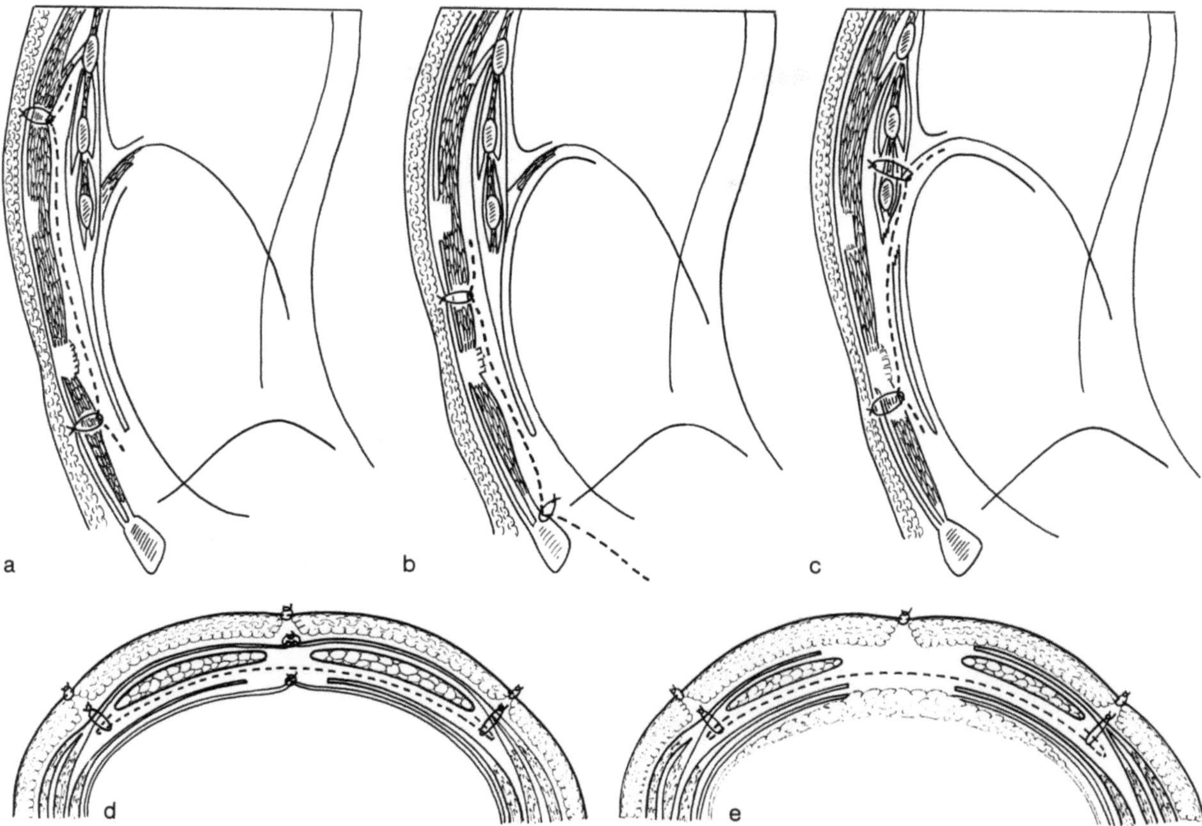

Fig. 8.23a–e. Author's procedure. **a** Paramedian sagittal section showing position of prosthesis (*dotted line*) in subumbilical midline eventration. **b** Paramedian sagittal section showing position of prosthesis in subumbilical eventration. **c** Paramedian sagittal section showing position of prosthesis in subchondral eventration. **d** Horizontal section showing position of prosthesis in case where abdominal wall can be closed over it. **e** Position of prosthesis is case where abdominal wall cannot be closed over it

in two patients), and five cases of aseptic recurrence were noted.

Retromuscular prefascial prosthesis. In the cases reported below the prosthesis was implanted deep to the muscles of the abdomen, i.e., in the rectus sheath or the preperitoneal space whenever possible, and if not, in the peritoneal cavity, in cases where peritoneal dissection was not possible (this was sometimes the case in the periumbilical region and always so in the subdiaphragmatic region). The space for implantation may differ for the upper and lower parts of the prosthesis.

In cases of midline incisional hernia (Figs. 8.23 & 8.24) we position the prosthesis in contact with the muscle fibers, i.e., in the interval between the rectus abdominis and the plane of contact between the peritoneum and the posterior lamina of the rectus sheath. This requires opening of the rectus sheath near the linea alba to gain entry to the retromuscular space and exposure of the posterior belly of the rectus muscle.

Closure anterior and posterior to the prosthesis. The peritoneal cavity must be closed prior to implantation of the prosthesis. In most cases, apposition of the peritoneal margins can be achieved when the peritoneum has been correctly and widely freed. In the midline, the peritoneal layer is much thicker since it is here covered by the posterior lamina of the rectus sheath. When peritoneal apposition cannot be achieved, we close the defect with an absorbable prosthesis. Omentum, when present, can be used to separate the viscera from the prosthesis. The posterior surface of the omentum allows good peritonization, while its anterior surface offers a source of granulation tissue which invests the prosthesis. Every attempt should be made to achieve an intervening surface of cover between the prosthesis and the skin, though this is not always possible.

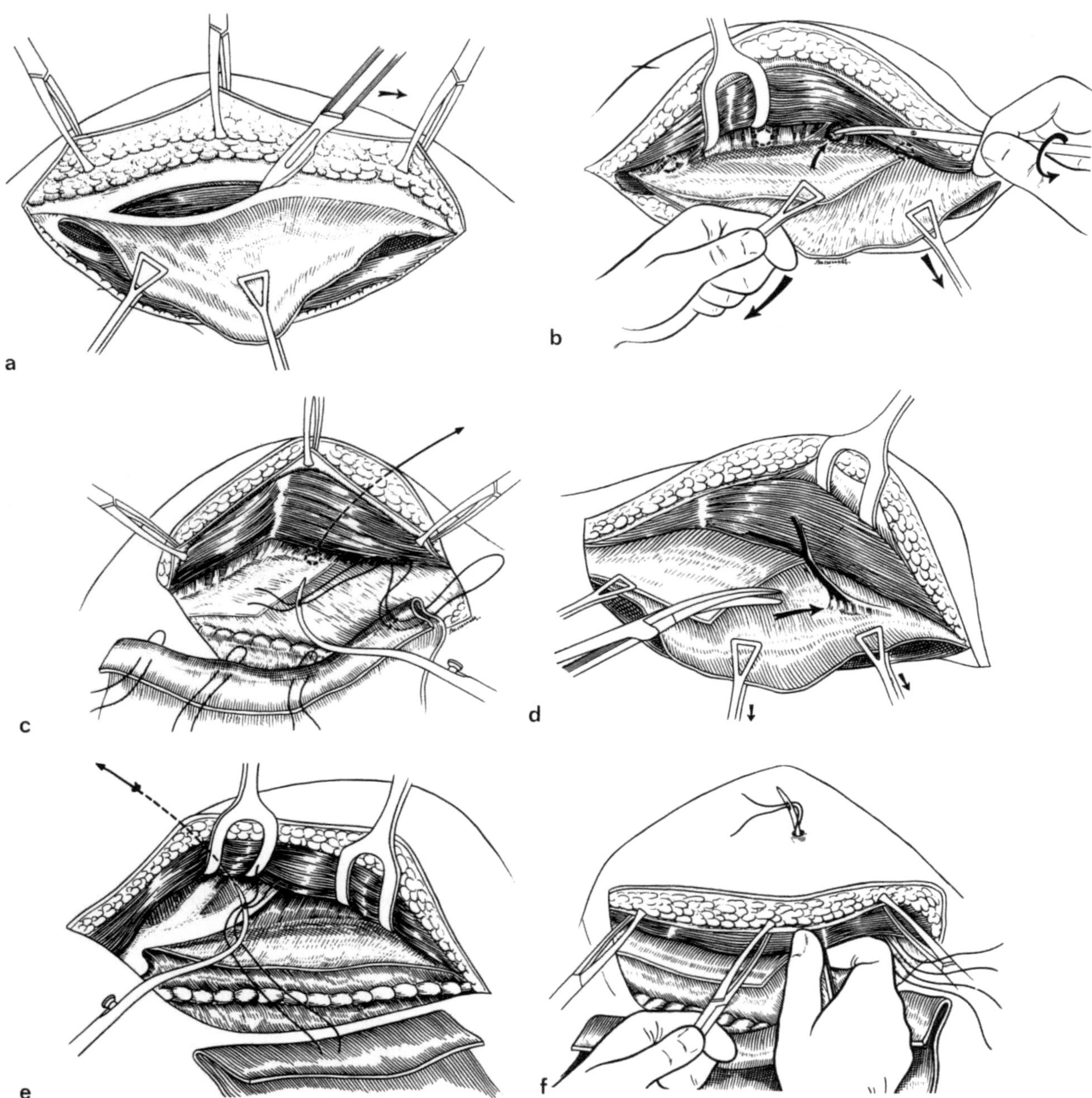

Fig. 8.24a–f. Implantation of prosthesis in the midline using the technique described by the authors; the stages are shown. [Rives et al. 1977; courtesy of Encyclopédie Médico-Chirurgicale]

Placement of the prosthesis. The upper part of the prosthesis is placed between the rectus abdominis anteriorly and the thorax and internal oblique posteriorly. The lower part of the prosthesis is fixed to Cooper's ligament and extends into the pelvic region in order to prevent its detachment; i.e., the prosthesis is implanted in the rectus sheath above the arcuate line and in the preperitoneal space below it.

In cases of lateral incisional hernia, the abdominal muscles may provide only one part of the circumference of the hernial orifice. With a subchondral hernia, it is often necessary to position the upper part of the prosthesis beneath the diaphragm and attach it to the rib cage using transfixing costodiaphragmatic sutures. The lower part of the prosthesis then lies anterior to the peritoneum, while the upper part is in the peritoneal cavity. In cases of inguinal incisional hernia it is necessary to position the prosthesis so that it envelops the peritoneum and extends into the iliac fossa and pelvis. The prosthesis is sutured above to the deep surface of the muscles and below to Cooper's ligament or the iliac crest. The patch of mesh should extend well beyond the area of the defect (in all directions) in the preperitoneal space.

The area of insertion of the prosthesis must be as large as possible. Our experience has shown that suturing of the material to the margins of the defect offers no guarantee of solidity and usually results in a recurrence due to lateral detachment. Accordingly, the mesh should extend well beyond the myoaponeurotic hernial orifice, with intra-abdominal pressure being used to ensure its insertion. The force of abdominal pressure holds the prosthesis against the deep surface of the muscles, thereby achieving a sort of "suture by apposition". However, this pressure-induced apposition is not sufficient to maintain the prosthesis in correct position during the first few postoperative weeks, and thus it is necessary to ensure that the prosthetic material is firmly stitched in around the edges. For many years we used pledgets to attach the prosthesis, which allowed removal of the sutures on the 20th postoperative day. However, we later discovered that these pledgets could give rise to complications and that they were not absolutely necessary. We changed our practice and now tighten each transfixing suture of the abdominal wall through a cutaneous buttonhole which is then closed by a single stitch. In cases of midline incisional hernia the semilunar line (Spiegel's line) is used as the site for peripheral attachment of the prosthesis.

The conditions for these surgical procedures should obey the rules of prosthetic implantation. The problems encountered are identical to those seen in orthopedic surgery. The risks of infection can be minimized by operating under conditions of scrupulous asepsis. Prosthetic surgery thus requires: perfect hemostasis, absence of direct manipulation of the prosthesis and overnight formalin vaporization of the operating room. Overhead light should not be manipulated during operation. A sucker should not be used during surgery so as to avoid the displacement of dust or other contaminated airborne particles.

c) Postoperative Care

Monitoring of body temperature. There may be an initial moderate rise due to inflammatory reaction.

However, persistence of fever beyond the 4th postoperative day usually indicates infection.

Aspiration drains should also be monitored. These drains, placed in contact with the prosthesis and/or beneath the skin, are used to evacuate fluid and blood in the areas of dissection, which may be very large. We remove the drains around the 6th postoperative day.

The skin and abdominal incision must be examined, and should be exposed as soon as possible so as to identify any slight early sign of infection.

Respiratory physiotherapy should resume as soon as the patient leaves the operating room.

Early ambulation is recommended in most cases, but precautions should be taken initially. It may be wise to replace early ambulation by mobilization in bed, with guidance by the physiotherapist whenever possible.

Finally, all sports activity and physical stress are contraindicated during the period of connective tissue cicatrization, i.e., for 3-6 months after the operation.

d) Treatment of Complications

Early postoperative infection. We obtained full cure in some cases of early postoperative infection (the last been observed in 1987) by wide saucerization and irrigation, thereby allowing the developing granulation tissue to invest the mersilene prosthesis. It is our impression that long-lasting wound suppuration results from overly conservative postoperative treatment (limited disunion, removal of a few stitches, etc.).

9. Results

Our experience with modern procedures for repair of incisional hernia dates back to 1964. During the 1970-1995 period, we observed 1,018 cases of major abdominal incisional hernia, although this figure is manifestly low since it represents those cases where a specific procedure was done to treat only the incisional hernia, and does not take into account the numerous small incisional hernias that were identified and treated during operation for some other reason.

Discussed below are the results of 478 major incisional hernias treated between 1971 and 1995. These cases have been selected for presentation as they constitute a homogeneous series with respect both to the type of surgical procedure performed and the surgical team who performed the operation (five senior surgeons implanted 93.3% of the 332 prostheses in this series). Critical analysis of previous failures permitted more selective indications and resulted in improvement of our results.

447 of our patients were elective cases, and 31 were emergencies. 347 (72.6%) were primary repair. 131 (27.4%) were recurrent incisional hernias. Recurrence occurred after nonprosthetic repair in 79 patients (60%), and after prosthetic repair in 52 patients (40%). The repair was nonprosthetic in 98 patients (20.5%). We used an absorbable mesh in 45 patients (9.4%). All the other patients (332) were treated with a nonabsorbable mesh (Mersuture Ethicon).

a) Using Prosthetic Material (332 cases)

(1) Early Postoperative Course

With stricter indications, we observed a dramatic improvement in our results: 325 (97.6%) of the patients had an uneventful postoperative course.

The mortality in our series was 0.9% (3 of 332 cases). Only one death is directly related to a complication of the procedure (female, 71 years, deep wound infection, septicemia with staphylococcus aureus). Two other deaths were not related to the operative repair:
• male, 73 years, necrotizing enteritis, necropsic confirmation;
• female, 69 years, cardiac arrest in recovery room.

Death from respiratory failure was not observed in this series of 332 patients.

Local Complications. Superficial infection occurred in 2 cases (1.2%). Deep infection is a serious complication since it affects the prosthesis. We observed, during the last 5 years, only 2 cases of deep infection, one being fatal. Special emphasis should be given to one case, in which wound suppuration occurred at a later date, (2 years after operative repair). This late complication demonstrate the need for prolonged follow-up of patients having undergone prosthetic surgery.

Recurrence of aseptic herniation was seen in 5.2% of our patients (16 of 304 cases available for follow up). In 13 of these patients, definitive repair was achieved by reoperation. In 3 other cases, reoperation was not done because of the minor degree of the recurrent hernia.

(2) Long-term Results

Excellent long-term results (Fig. 8.25) were seen in 98.6% of the patients. Evaluation was made possible by a careful follow-up of our patient with only 25 (7.5%) lost to follow-up.

These favorable results were often obtained from the onset of treatment. In a few cases (4.2%), the definitive result was not achieved for some time, owing to the need for local procedures (cure of superficial infection) or reoperation for small uninfected recurrences (13 cases). The discomfort of these complementary procedures and of the sensory disturbances reported in some cases is balanced by the satisfaction of having corrected a major lesion (sometimes of monstrous dimensions), which up to that time had often been considered untreatable (one to six recurrences had been noted in 30 patients).

b) Using Nonprosthetic Technique (143 cases)

Prosthetic surgery was contraindicated in some patients, so that sutures, plasties or absorbable mesh procedures were used. The 143 cases in this series were among the most difficult we have seen: 57 emergency cases (39%), and 43 cases of associated septic procedures (44.9%). Some of these patients presented with an enormous strangulated hernia and were bedridden, while others presented as emergencies, with an incidental large incisional hernia. The poor results in this series were seen in unprepared patients, which underlines the importance of adequate local and general preparation and of the precautions that should be taken in infected cases.

The mortality was 6.2% (nine cases) in this series. In seven of these cases death occurred after surgery to treat an accompanying lesion of the small bowel or colon.

Infections were seen in 11 cases, including seven emergencies, infected recurrence with impending rupture on two occasions, and accompanying septic procedures on five occasions. The overall infection rate was thus 7.6% (11 of 143 cases).

Recurrence of hernia was seen in 33 cases (23% of all 143 patients or 24.6% of the 134 who lived. Nonabsorbable prosthetic surgery was contraindicated because of the emergency situation and the associated septic procedures that were required.

c) Emergency Operation

Emergency surgery on a patient with a major incisional hernia is a grave situation. Local and general preparation is not possible and the procedure often involves intestinal obstruction or peritonitis. In our series of 478 patients, 6.5% (31 cases) underwent emergency surgery. Most of these patients presented with strangulation of the hernia (75%), though in some a visceral emergency (20%), occlusion due to band adhesions (2.5%) or abscess (1 of 14 cases: 2.5%) was the indication for the operation.

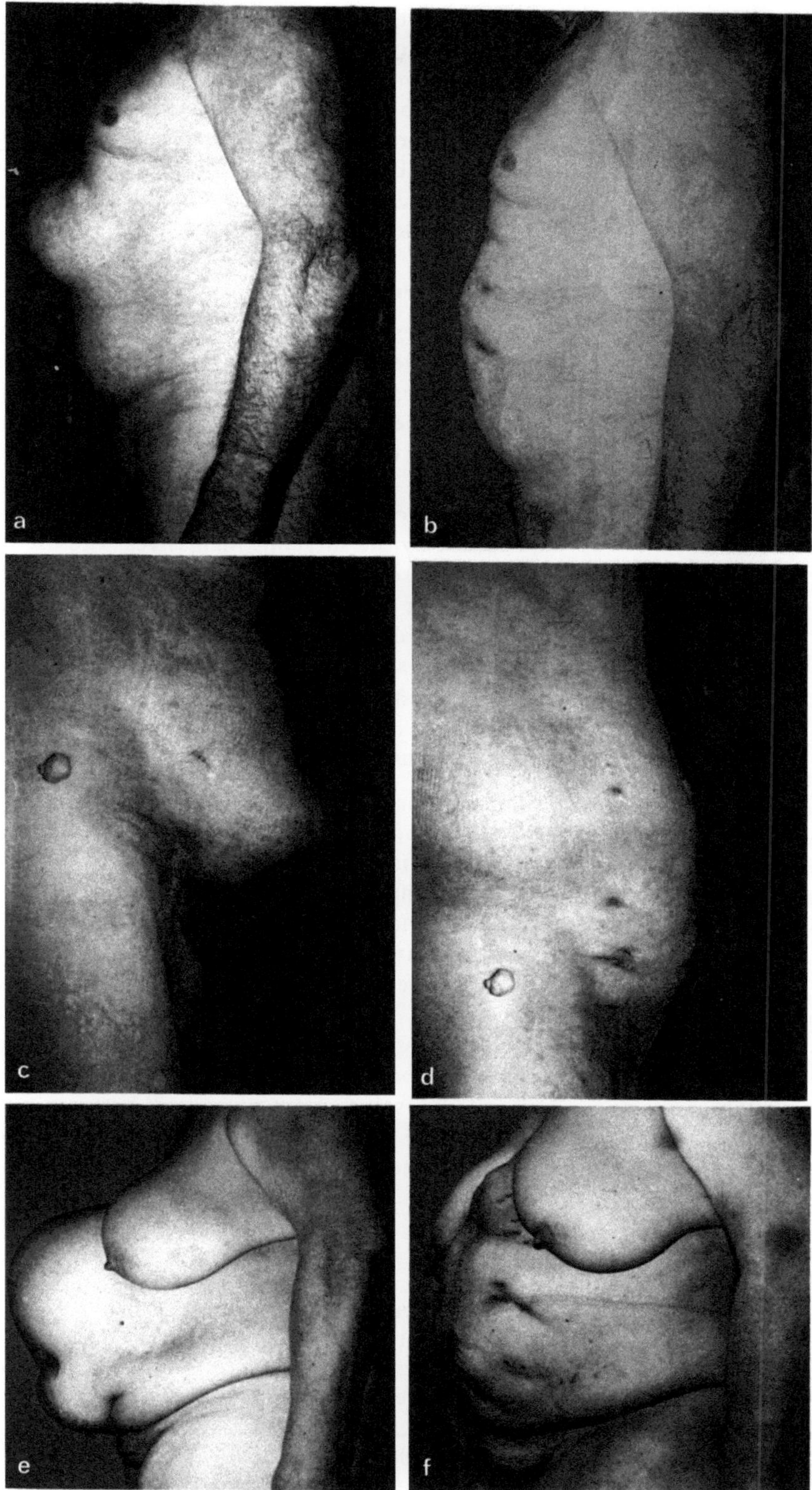

Fig. 8.25a-f. Results obtained in three cases using the technique described by the authors

Over the 5 past years, we never used a mersilene prosthesis. Mortality, in this group, was high (25.8%) and the recurrence rate, among the survivors was 23%.

10. Comments

a) Analysis of Results

Prostheses

The results described above were obtained using a personal procedure the principles of which have been explained and whose technical features have been codified. This technique, which we have used for over 25 years, has given satisfactory results. Minor details have been modified over the years, such as abandonment of pledgets, and the use of suction drainage. However, critical analysis of these results, especially of the failures, has led us to reconsider the indications for this procedure. Indeed, the attendant risks of such repair can be decreased by informed narrowing of the indications.

A reduction in mortality was achieved by taking into account the fact that many of the patients were elderly and obese and suffered from cardiopulmonary insufficiency. A careful preparation, if necessary with pneumoperitoneum is therefore mandatory. Aseptic recurrence of incisional hernia (mechanical) was rare (13 of 332 cases: 5.2%). These cases seem to be difficult to avoid, at least when the recurrence is due to rupture of the prosthesis or abdominal wall. Such rupture always occurs at the points of fixation of the prosthetic material. However, prevention of this complication may be possible by placing larger prostheses fixed to the ribs or the pubic bone.

The rate of infection was dramatically improved, however. In ten of our patients the prosthesis was implanted with associated septic procedures. We observed no infections, thanks to vigorous precautions.

b) Better Selection of Indications

We have modified our operative indications over the years: prosthetic surgery was indicated in 100% of cases in 1971 as against 56.5% in 1981 and 69.5% in 1995.

In our department, prostheses are reserved for cases that cannot be treated by other means. The main indication is the multiple, recurrent incisional hernia, where special attention must be paid to the identification of latent sources of infection and to disturbances of general health (especially diabetes). We have thus abandoned the use of prosthetic repair in emergency surgery and when operation is indicated primarily for reasons other than the incisional hernia. However, in some of these cases closure cannot be achieved using classical procedures for repair [Judd 1912; Welti & Eudel 1941]. For such cases we have recently adopted the use of resorbable prosthetic material. Repair using autograft skin bands may also offer a solution to these difficult cases, although we have had no experience with this method.

c) Technical Precautions

The need for extreme vigilance in prosthetic surgery cannot be overemphasized. Standard precautions include thorough disinfection of the operating room, prohibiting the use of vacuum aspiration of air and movements of the overhead lights, proper training of all personnel in sound hygienic practice, and "no touch" rules. So called "unexplained" accidents are in fact caused by the surgeons themselves. The use of laminar flow seems to reduce the incidence of such events; in our experience, the rate of unexplained infection has fallen from 11.2% (14 of 127 cases) to 5.5% (2 of 36 cases) since its introduction, although this difference is not statistically significant ($X^2 = 1.48$).

11. Conclusions

Major incisional hernia is a significant lesion affecting general health; in some cases it is a disabling lesion, previously considered to be beyond the scope of surgical repair. Improved understanding of the physiological disturbances induced by these lesions (especially respiratory insufficiency) and the judicious use of prostheses, offer a reasonable therapeutic solution for these patients. The results obtained reflect the considerable progress that has been made in this area, since some 90% of patients can now be cured. Critical analysis of failures demonstrates that still better results are obtainable by stricter definition of the operative indications and more precise codifying of surgical techniques.

References

Adloff M, Arnaud JP (1976) Etude expérimentale de la résistance et de la tolérance biologique de matériaux prothétiques utilisés dans la réparation des pertes de substance de la paroi abdominale. Chirurgie 102: 390-396

Amid PK (1997) Classification of biomaterials and their related complications in abdominal wall hernia surgery. Hernia 1: 15-21

Arnaud JP, Cervi C, Tuech JJ, Cattan F (1997) Surgical treatment of post-operative incisional hernias by intra-peritoneal insertion of a Dacron mesh. A report of 220 cases.. Hernia 1: 97-99

Arnaud JP, Patsopoulof J, Adloff M (1983) Traitement des volumineuses éventrations de la paroi abdominale: treillis de Mersilène en position intra-péritonéale associé à une plastie aponévrotique (à propos de 96 observations). Ann Chir 5: 337-340

Baldwin E, Cournand A, Richards DW (1948) Pulmonary insufficiency. I. Physiologic classification, clinical methods of analysis, standard values in normal subjects. Medicine 27: 243

Banzet P, Flageul G, Lelouarn C, Le Quang C, Dufourrnentel C (1979) Traitement chirurgical des éventrations par laçage avec de la peau totale autogène (36 observations). Nouv Presse Med 8: 3227-3229

Becouarn G, Szmil E, Leroux C, Arnaud JP (1996) Cure chirurgicale des éventrations post-opératoires par implantation intra-péritonéale d'un treillis de Dacron. J Chir (Paris) 133: 229-232

Bendavid R (1997) Composite mesh (polypropylene - ePTFE) in the intraperitoneal position. A report of 30 cases. Hernia 1: 5-8

Bendavid R (1994) Prostheses and abdominal wall hernias. R G Landes, Austin, p 591

Bendavid R (1990) Incisional parapubic hernias. Surgery; 108: 898-901

Body C (1976) Problèmes posés à l'anesthésiste par la chirurgie des grandes éventrations. Thèse inaugurale. Faculté de Médecine de Reims, France

Bourgeon R, Borelli JP, Lanfranchi JP (1972) Utilisation des prothèses de Mersilène dans le traitement des éventrations post-opératoires. Ann Chir 26: 541-545

Caix M, Outrequin G, Descottes B (1982) Anatomie fonctionnelle de la paroi abdominale: analyse électro-myographique et histoenzymologique, relations entre la tonicité pariétale et la pression intra-cavitaire abdominale. Report, 65th Congrès de l'Association des Anatomistes, Limoges, May 23-27

Champetier J, Laborde Y, Letoublon Ch, Durand A (1978) Traitement des éventrations abdominales post-opératoires: bases biomécaniques élémentaires. A propos de 51 cas traités par treillis de Mersilène. J Chir 11: 585-590

Chevrel JP (1994) The treatment of midline incisional hernia by a mantle herniorraphy and premusculoaponeurotic prosthetic implant. In: Bendavid R (ed) Prostheses and abdominal wall hernias. R G Landes, Austin, pp 479-483

Chevrel JP, Flament JB (1990) Les éventrations de la paroi abdominale. Rapport au 92ème Congrès Français de Chirurgie, A.F.C., Masson, Paris

Chevrel JP, Flament JB (1995) Traitement des éventrations de la paroi abdominale. Editions Techniques, Encycl. Med. Chir. Techniques Chirurgicales - Appareil digestif, 40-165, 14p

Chevrel JP (1979) Traitement des grandes éventrations médianes par plastie en paletot et prothèse. Nouv Presse Med 8: 695-696

Chevrel JP, Rath AM (1997) The use of fibrin glues in the surgical treatment of incisional hernias. Hernia 1: 9-14

Clotteau JE, Prémont M (1979) Cure des grandes éventrations cicatricielles médianes par un procédé de plastie aponévrotique. Chirurgie 105: 344-346

Cokkinis AJ (1958) Surgical technique of closure for extremely large abdominal hernias. J Int Coll Surg 30: 638-643

Dufilho A (1981) Les complications des prothèses en tulle de Dacron. A propos de 414 observations. Thèse inaugurale, Paris, Fac de Méd Pitié Salpétrière

Estour E (1995) Revue de 9221 cures laparoscopiques de hernies de l'aine réalisées chez 7340 patients. J Coelio Chir 16: 42-48

Eudel F (1979) A propos de la communication de R Stoppa et coll sur le traitement des éventrations post-opératoires. Chirurgie 105: 369-370

Flament JB, Palot JP, Burde A, Delattre JF, Avisse C (1995) Treatment of major incisional hernias. Problems in General Surgery 12: 151-8

Flament JB, Palot JP (1994) Prostheses and major incisional hernias. In: Bendavid R, Prostheses and major incisional hernias, Austin Landes Biomedical publisher

Godquin B (1979) Une technique sûre de réparation des éventrations abdominales post-opératoires: plastie aponévrotique associée à une prothèse. A propos de 38 observations. Chirurgie 105: 721-724

Goni-Moreno I (1970) Le pneumopéritoine dans la réparation pré-opératoire des grandes éventrations. Chirurgie 96: 581-585

Gosset J (1949) Bandes de peau totale comme matériel de suture autoplastique en chirurgie. Chirurgie 75: 277-279

Guyon P, Giraud O, Cariou JL (1997) Intérêt du lambeau en îlot fascio-cutané de tensor de fasciae latae dans le traitement des grandes éventrations abdominales. J Chir (Paris) 134: 27-30

Hornant P, Le Du J, Chaperon J, Lavenac G, Mambrini A (1996) Traitement des éventrations abdominales post-opératoires par prothèse non résorbable. A propos de 160 observations. J Chir (Paris) 133: 311-316

Hureau J, Vayre P, Muller JM (1975) L'utilisation du feuillet antérieur de la gaine du muscle grand droit dans les réparations pariétales abdominales. A propos de 865 interventions pour hernies et éventrations. Ann Chir 29: 1113-1119

Judd ES (1912) The prevention and treatment of ventral hernia. Surg Gynecol Obstet 15: 175-182

Kapandji JA (1977) Physiologie articulaire du membre inférieur. Le rachis, 4th edn; Maloine, Paris

Le Bouëdec, Kauffmann P, Mill P, Scherrer C, Raiga J, Dauplat J (1995) Les hernies incisionnelles post-cœlioscopiques. A propos d'un cas. J Chir (Paris) 132: 259-263

Loury JN, Chevrel JP (1983) Traitement des éventrations. Utilisation simultanée du treillis de polyglactine 910 et de Dacron. Nouv Presse Med 12: 2116

McLanahan D, King LT, Weems C, Novotney M, Gibson K (1997) Retrorectus prosthetic mesh repair of midline abdominal hernia. Am J Surg 173: 445-449

Myon Y (1981) Les éventrations abdominales post-opératoires et le préjudice corporel. Mémoire pour le diplôme d'études médicales relatives à la préparation juridique du dommage corporel. Lille

Palot JP, Flament JB, Avisse C, Greffier D, Burde A (1996) Utilisation des prothèses dans les conditions de la chirurgie d'urgence. Etude rétrospective de 204 hernies de l'aine étranglées. Chirurgie 121: 48-50

Petit J, Petit J, Stoppa R, Baillet J (1974) Evaluation expérimentale des réactions tissulaires autour des prothèses de la paroi abdominale en tulle de Dacron en fonction de la durée d'implantation et du siège en profondeur. J Chir 107: 667-672

Pire JC, Body C, Flament JB (1977) La capacité vitale, un piège dans le bilan des grandes éventrations. Nouv Presse Med 6: 3641

Porrero JL (1997) Cirurgia de la pared abdominal. Masson, Barcelone, p 313

Rath AM, Zhang J, Amouroux J, Chevrel JP (1996) Les prothèses pariétales abdominales. Etudes biomécanique et histologique. Chirurgie 121: 253-265

Read RC (1994) Prosthesis in abdominal wall surgery. In: Bendavid R (ed) Prosthesis and abdominal wall hernias. R G Landes, Austin, pp 2-32

Reith HB, Dittrich H, Kozuschek W (1995) Morphologie et intégration biologique des autodermoplasties dans les grandes éventrations. J Chir (Paris) 132: 229-236

Rives J, Pire JC, Flament JB, Palot, JP, Body C (1985) Le traitement des grandes éventrations. Nouvelles indications thérapeutiques à propos de 322 cas. Chirurgie 111: 215-225.

Rives J, Lardennois B, Pire JC, Hibon J (1973) Les grandes éventrations. Importance du "volet abdominal" et des troubles respiratoires qui lui sont secondaires. Chirurgie 99: 547-563

Rives J, Pire JC, Flament JB, Convers G (1977) Traitement des éventrations. Encycl Med Chir, Paris, 4.0.07, 40165

Rives J, Pire JC, Palot JP, Flament JB (1987) Surgery of the abdominal wall. Major incisional hernias. Ed. by JP Chevrel, Springer-Verlag, Heidelberg

Ronat R, Fingerhut A, Pourcher J (1978) Cure des grandes éventrations abdominales par plaque de mersilène haubannée. Nouv Presse Med 7: 2165-2167

Stoppa R, Henry X, Canarelli JP, Laguerche S, Verhaeghe P, Abet D, Ratsivalaka R (1979) Les indications de méthodes opératoires sélectionnées dans le traitement des éventrations post-opératoires de la paroi abdominale antéro-latérale. Propositions fondées sur une série de 326 Observations. Chirurgie 105: 276-286

Stoppa R, Henry X, Odimba E, Verhaeghe P, Laguerche S, Myon Y (1980) Traitement chirurgical des éventrations post-opératoires. Utilisation des prothèses en tulle de Dacron et de la colle biologique. Nouv Presse Med 9: 3541-3545

Stoppa R, Moungar F, Verhaeghe P (1992) Traitement chirurgical des éventrations médianes sus ombilicales. J Chir 129: 335-43

Sturniolo G, Versace GA, Gagliano E, Tonante A, Cacciola R, Fragomeni A, Sulvestro A, Biviano A (1994-1995) Actualité de la plastie en paletôt dans le traitement des hernies de la ligne blanche et des laparocèles. Chirurchie 120: 320-324

Trivellini G, Cantono GM, Zanella G, Arienti E (1978) Importanza della pressione endoaddominale e della compliance toraco-pulmonare nella terapia delle ernie post-operatorie. Chirurgia Arch Trim 3: 273-284

Vilain R, Soyer R (1964) Traitement chirurgical des éventrations. Ann Chir 18: 277-288

Wantz GE (1994) Prosthetics: their complications and management. In: Bendavid R (ed) Prosthesis and abdominal wall hernias. R G Landes, Austin, 326-329

Wantz GE (1991) Incisional hernioplasty with mersilene. Surgery 172: 129-37

Welti H, Eudel F (1941) Un procédé de cure radicale des éventrations post-opératoires par auto-étalement des muscles grand-droits après incision du feuillet antérieur de leurs gaines. Chirurgie 28: 791-798

III. Therapeutic Defects of the Abdominal Wall

J. P. Chevrel

Resection of tumors of the abdominal wall has been included in this chapter since the procedures of tumor removal create a veritable defect. The rather uncommon arrangement of this chapter is justified by the major therapeutic problems regarding repair that arise subsequent to wide excision of a tumor of the abdominal wall. Conversely, anatomical diagnosis of the tumor, whether it be a benign or malignant lesion, is generally not problematic.

The discussion is divided into three parts. The first part is a review of the different types of tumors that can be found in the abdominal wall. The second part covers the procedures commonly used to achieve repair. The last part of this section presents the technical features and indications for the therapeutic open-abdomen procedure referred to as laparostomy.

A. Tumors

Tumor of the abdominal wall is a rare finding. These lesions are quite diverse from the histological standpoint. Benign tumors are the most frequent, whereas malignant lesions raise more difficult therapeutic problems.

All possible types of benign tumor can be found in the abdominal wall including naevus, sebaceous cysts or neuroma developed in the cutaneous tissue, lipoma, fibrolipoma, myoma, neurofibroma, and deep lesions such as angioma of the muscle. These tumors display no special features related to their position in the abdominal wall as compared with other sites, and treatment can usually be done without difficulty.

1. Hydatid Cyst

The abdominal wall is a rare site for hydatid cyst. The lesion presents as a hard cystic tumor deep in the skin and may attain considerable size. The only appropriate treatment is cystectomy with the usual precautions of surgery for hydatid cyst, i.e., protection of the operative field by towels soaked in hypertonic saline.

2. Desmoid Tumors

Desmoids are proliferative nonencapsulated tumors of mesenchymal origin. These lesions are usually found in the abdominal wall, especially in the sheath of the rectus abdominis The lesion may be an isolated finding or one of the components of familial polyposis (3.5% of cases, according to Smith 1954) or Gardner's syndrome (17.3% of cases, according to Jones & Cornell 1966 & Chevrel et al. 1983; see Fig. 8.30).

Desmoid tumor is far more frequent in women, especially during pregnancy or postpartum, and in some cases it arises in the abdominal scar of a cesarean section [Loygue & Adloff 1977; Guérin 1958; Amouroux & Kemeny 1981]. Cases have been reported in men and in children of both sexes. Other possible sites include the deltoid, latissimus dorsi, and muscles of the lower limbs.

Despite the absence of histological signs of malignancy and metastatic potential, these tumors display very special features which render the prognosis rather poor; local recurrence is seen in about 30% of cases [Germain 1978]. Furthermore, when desmoid tumor is seen in Gardner's syndrome there is a tendency for tumor development within the peritoneal cavity, with invasion of the abdominal viscera and mesentery or retroperitoneal space, leading to external compression of the vascular axes [Delamarre et al. 1980].

In some cases the development of these tumors is so great that resection is impossible, especially in the recurrent type of tumor. Intestinal occlusion or necrosis results in these cases and is beyond the scope of therapeutic management.

The local invasive potential of desmoid tumors has led to their being referred to as "fibrosarcomatous" lesions, although their histological features and the absence of metastatic potential classify them as benign tumors.

From the clinical standpoint, the patient is often the first person to notice the lesion of the abdominal wall. The tumor is a firm round mass that is apparently well limited and does not invade the skin. A single tumor or multiple lesions may be found. These tumors develop slowly, and it is precisely this feature that renders them dangerous since the only successful treatment is wide resection performed at an early date. However, many patients consult a physician only when the tumor has become voluminous. At this stage repair is problematic.

Appropriate treatment is wide excision extending well beyond the limits of the tumor, which are not always easy to identify. Insufficient excision probably accounts for certain cases of apparent local recurrence due to the subsequent growth of residual tumor tissue [Loygue & Adloff 1977]. Unfortunately, excision is impossible in some cases, e.g., intra-abdominal and retroperitoneal tumors and mesenteric fibromatosis. Radiotherapy has been proposed to treat inoperable lesions, especially in women, where it has been suggested that it may act via a decrease in ovarian hormonal output. In fact, radiotherapy seems to be totally inefficacious Hormone therapy has also been proposed but proof of efficacy is lacking [McAdam & Goligher 1970]. Testolactone seems to have given good results in one female patient treated by Waddel (1975). This author also reported successful results with a combination of theophylline and chlorthiazide, but such treatment was a failure in one patient we treated [Chevrel et al. 1983]. In some cases chemotherapy may yield good results [Rignault 1982, personal communication].

3. Dermatofibroma of Darier and Ferrand

This is a rare tumor (0.1% of malignant skin tumors) [Pétoin et al. 1985], which develops in the dermal connective tissue. The lesion is slow-growing, progressively invading the superficial dermis and the underlying structures [Brabant et al. 1993]. The dermatofibroma occurs most frequently on the trunk and at the roots of the limbs [MacPeak et al. 1967]. Its principle characteristic is the high recurrence rate which varies from 10% to 80% in the various series. In fact these recurrences are usually due to inadequate initial excision.

As regards treatment, radiotherapy has not proved effective and may be regarded as an adjuvant to surgery in the case of a second recurrence [Rowsell et al. 1986]. The treatment is essentially surgical and involves a very extensive resection. It should be understood that the microscopic extent of the Darier tumor always exceeds the macroscopic lesion [Pétoin et al. 1985]. The risk of recurrence diminishes with the extent of the excision. Thus, MacPeak, who uses a clearance margin of 3 cm from the outer limits of the lesion, reports a recurrence rate of 10%, whereas Banzet and Servant [Brabant et al. 1993] who use an excision margin of 5 cm and also remove underlying healthy tissue such as aponeurosis and fascia, obtain a recurrence rate of 1.75%.

Repair of the large area of tissue loss following a resection of a Darier tumor requires a full thickness graft when the receptor area permits it, or a musculo-aponeurotic flap of rectus femoris or tensor fascia lata when the defect is of full thickness. This flap will require prosthetic repair if its aponeurotic component is not sufficiently strong (Latissimus dorsi, rectus abdominis). When the reconstruction involves almost the entire anterior abdominal wall the use of free flaps provides a solution to the various problems created. These include a free flap of tensor fascia lata [Caffee 1983], or of latissimus dorsi connected with a micro-anastomosis [Pannier 1996, personal communication] which as it contains no aponeurotic component needs to be reinforced by a nonabsorbable prosthesis. When the loss of substance is full thickness, many authors carry out the excision and reconstruction at a single stage, repair being effected by one or more pedicled flaps [Freedman et al. 1990; Gottlieb et al. 1990] or more rarely by a free flap [Neven et al. 1993; Piza et al. 1993]. Others prefer a two stage operation because of possible failure of a microsurgical flap [Revol et al. 1993; Pannir 1996], the first stage consisting in the preparation of as delayed flap near to the area of future loss of substance, in the shape of a slipper as described by Servant. At a second stage the lesion is excised and the defect repaired, provided that the vitality of the flap is assured.

4. Primary Malignancy

Cutaneous carcinoma and fibrosarcoma are the most common types of primary malignant tumors of the abdominal wall. *Spindle cell carcinoma* is the most

serious type of skin cancer since it spreads to the lymphatic system and at a late stage gives rise to distant metastases. These tumors often arise in the area of a pre-existing lesion, e.g., laparotomy scars, burns, radiodermatitis, psoriasis, dyskeratosis. Treatment requires wide excision of the lesion. Conversely, basal cell carcinoma seen in elderly patients carries a better prognosis, since successful treatment can be achieved by radiotherapy and minor excision.

The clinical features and development of *sarcoma* of the abdominal wall resemble those of desmoid tumor. As does the latter, sarcoma tends to recur locally in cases where surgical excision is insufficiently wide. These lesions are also complicated by distant metastasis or invasion of regional lymphatics. As does carcinoma, sarcoma can develop on pre-existing lesions. Diagnosis is usually achieved at a late stage since sarcoma develops in the deep structures of the abdominal wall and thus is not apparent for quite some time. From the histological standpoint, the following types of sarcoma of the abdominal wall can be seen: fibrosarcoma, neurosarcoma (sometimes associated with Recklinghausen's disease), nevocarcinoma, or even synovial sarcoma [Berkheiser 1952]. Clinical examination reveals a hard, irregular tumor with poorly defined limits. The mass adheres to the skin and deep layers and may undergo ulceration. As in all cases of malignant tumor, treatment is wide excision, sometimes coupled with radiotherapy or chemotherapy, according to the histological findings [Germain 1978].

5. Secondary Malignancy

Similar to malignant invasion of scar tracts (see page 91), secondary malignancy of the abdominal wall is a complication of primary abdominal cancer of various origins. Prognosis is very poor in cases of multiple tumors of the abdominal wall, which are often associated with pulmonary or hepatic metastases.

Conversely, certain types of abdominal wall invasion by malignancy of a subjacent abdominal organ (transverse or sigmoid colon, small intestine) can be treated by excision en bloc of the primary tumor and the abdominal wall lesion. We have performed this procedure in several cases, using techniques of repair to be described further on (Figs. 8.26, 8.28 & 8.29).

B. Abdominal Wall Repair
After Resection

Regardless of the histological type of tumor, the immediate therapeutic problem involves repair in

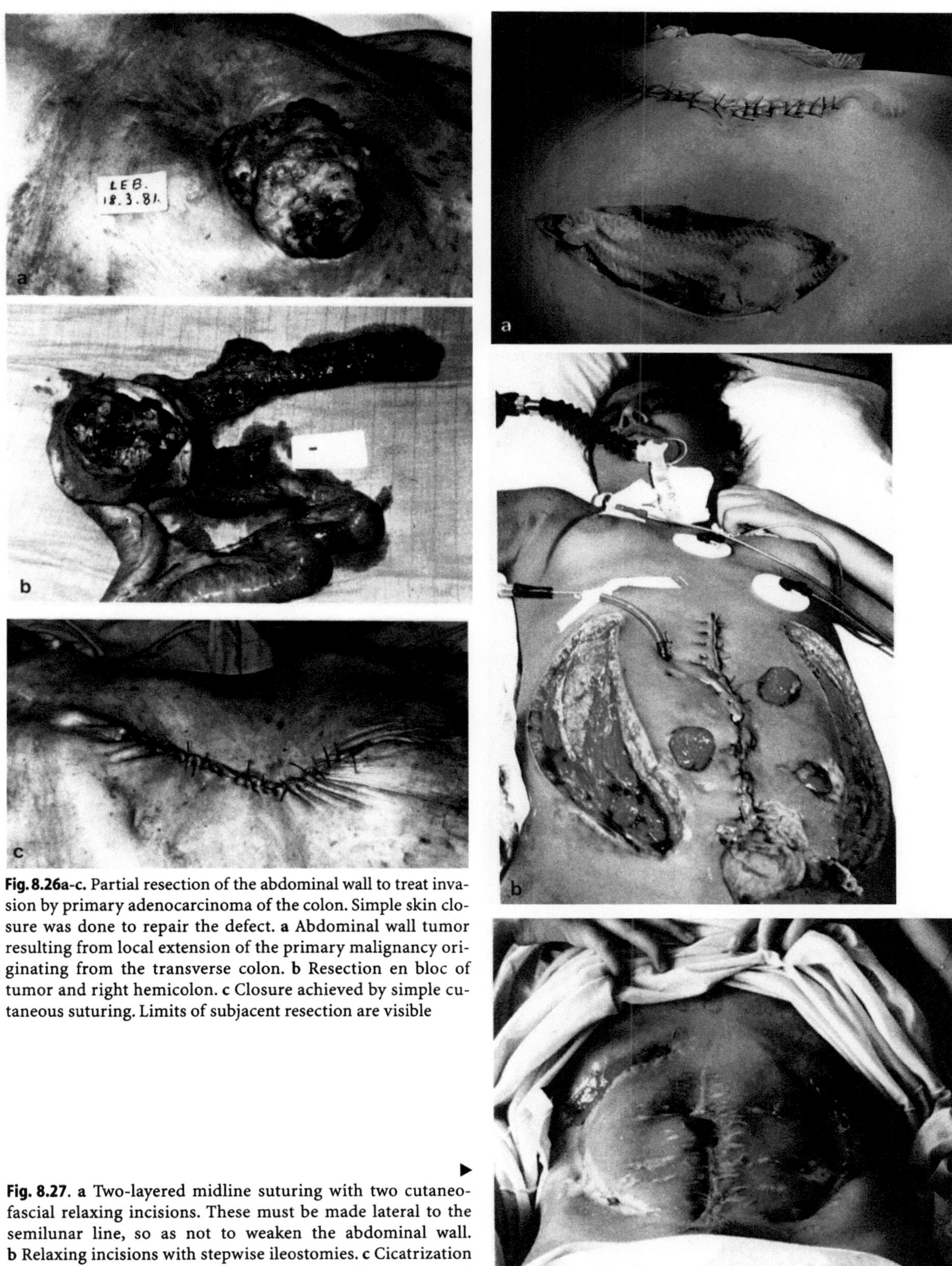

Fig. 8.26a-c. Partial resection of the abdominal wall to treat invasion by primary adenocarcinoma of the colon. Simple skin closure was done to repair the defect. **a** Abdominal wall tumor resulting from local extension of the primary malignancy originating from the transverse colon. **b** Resection en bloc of tumor and right hemicolon. **c** Closure achieved by simple cutaneous suturing. Limits of subjacent resection are visible

Fig. 8.27. a Two-layered midline suturing with two cutaneofascial relaxing incisions. These must be made lateral to the semilunar line, so as not to weaken the abdominal wall. **b** Relaxing incisions with stepwise ileostomies. **c** Cicatrization of the relaxing incisions (same patient as in **b**) [Hannoun et al. 1984; Anatomia Clinica]

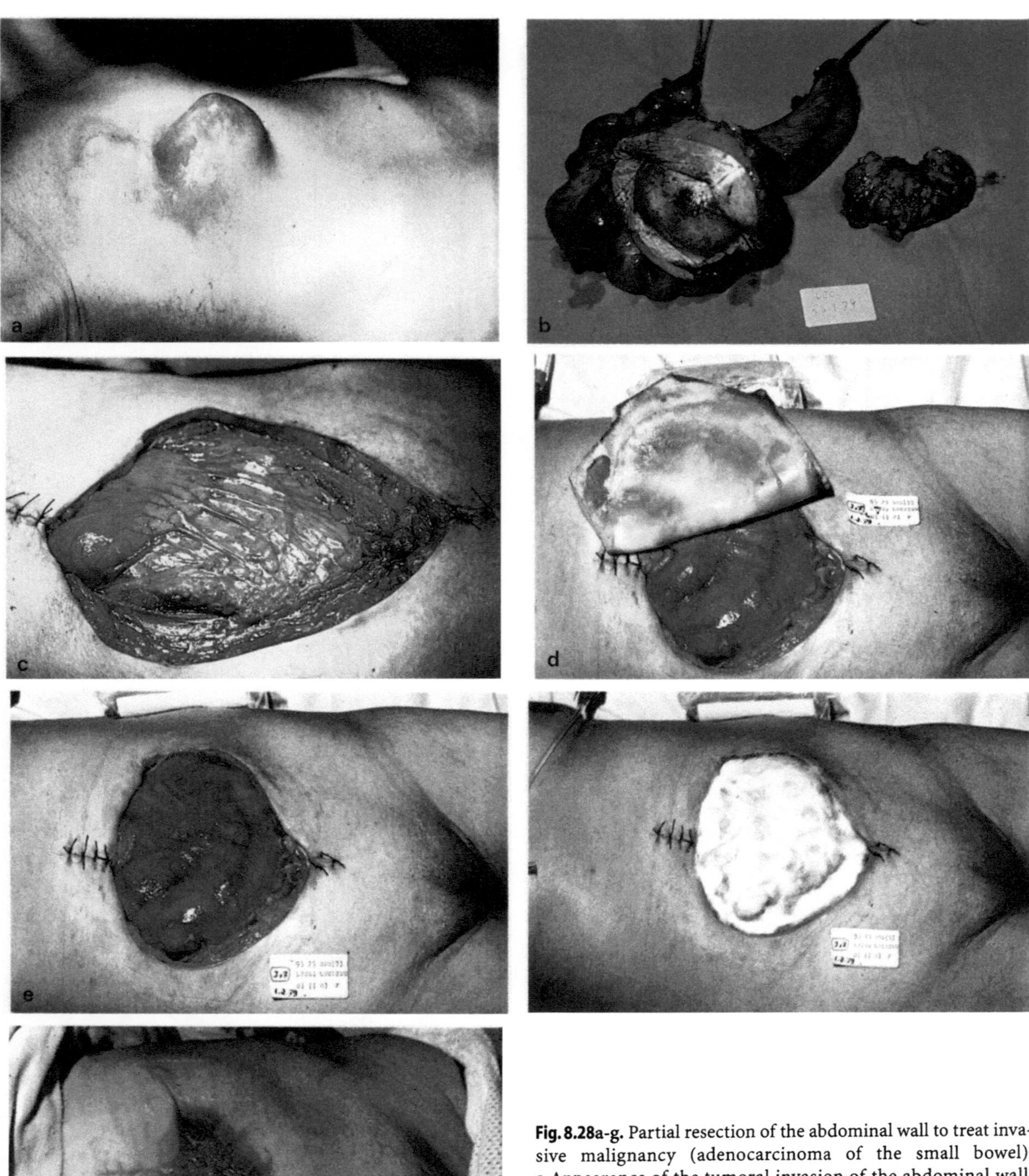

Fig. 8.28a-g. Partial resection of the abdominal wall to treat invasive malignancy (adenocarcinoma of the small bowel). **a** Appearance of the tumoral invasion of the abdominal wall. **b** Resection en bloc of the tumor and primary malignancy. **c** The resulting defect; note that the greater curvature of the stomach and greater omentum are exposed. **d** Appearance of the defect after 7 days of external cutaneous reinforcement and protection by polyurethane foam. **e** The same day as in d. **f** Dressing with dextran microspheres (Débrisan Shering). **g** Appearance of the cicatrix 3 months after operation

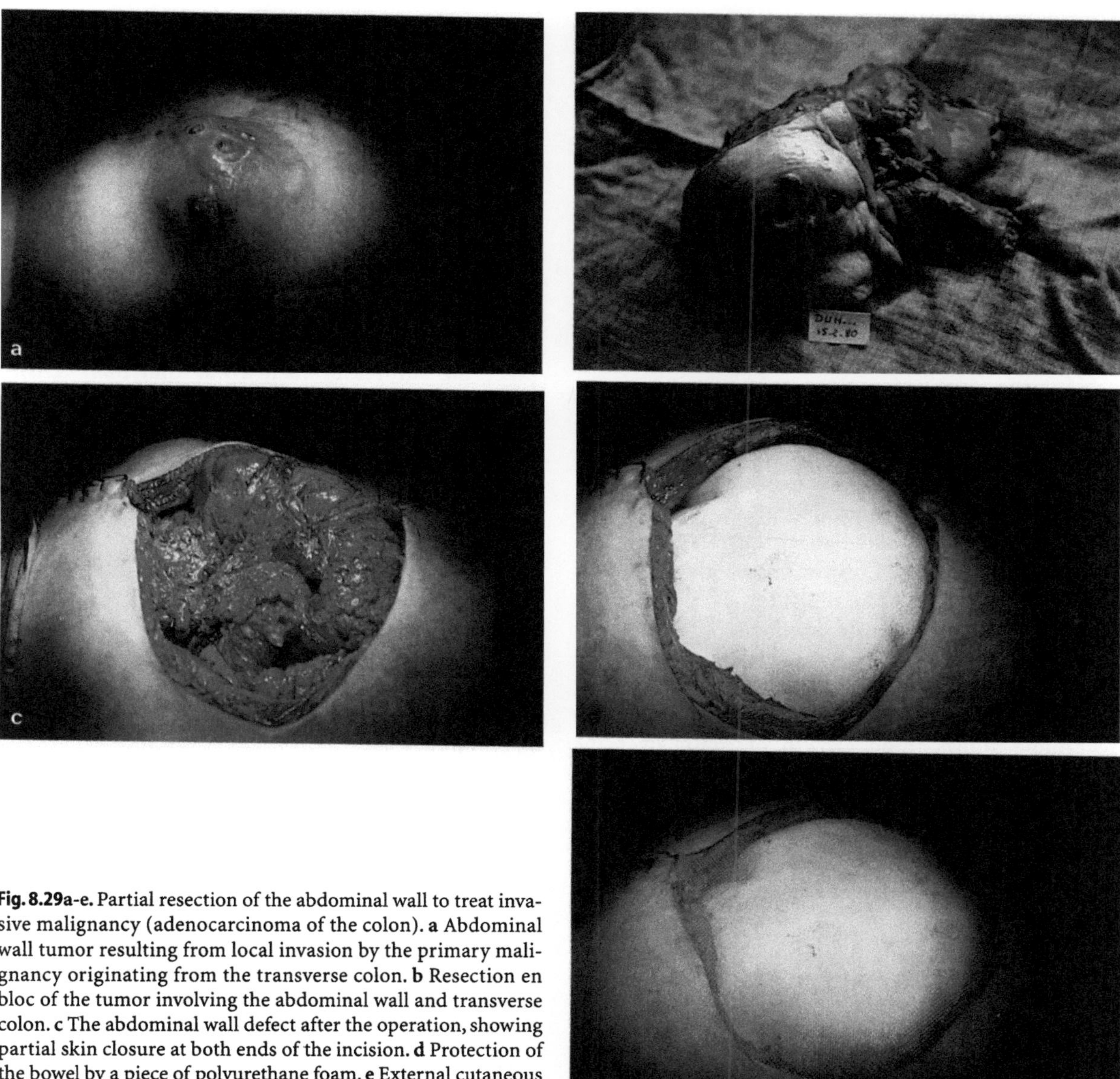

Fig. 8.29a-e. Partial resection of the abdominal wall to treat invasive malignancy (adenocarcinoma of the colon). **a** Abdominal wall tumor resulting from local invasion by the primary malignancy originating from the transverse colon. **b** Resection en bloc of the tumor involving the abdominal wall and transverse colon. **c** The abdominal wall defect after the operation, showing partial skin closure at both ends of the incision. **d** Protection of the bowel by a piece of polyurethane foam. **e** External cutaneous reinforcement using adhesive jersey-knit material

cases where wide resection has been done. This situation can be likened to that of pathological destruction of the abdominal wall and is especially analogous to the defects caused by gas gangrene. Several types of surgical repair are possible, depending on the size of the defect and the sepsis of the abdominal wall. The surgical repair of septic and aseptic defects is discussed separately below.

1. Under Septic Conditions

Plastic procedures or nonabsorbable prostheses such as mersilene or ligalene mesh cannot be used. In cases where the defect is large we use one of the procedures described below.

a) Simple Skin Closure

Ideal cover of the bowel loops requires traction-free closure (Fig. 8.26). Large lateral relaxing incisions can be made through the skin and the aponeurosis to relieve the tension on the abdominal wall. These incisions are made from the inferior thoracic ridge to the iliac crest and run at a distance of about 10 cm from midline. Vaseline dressings are placed over the incisions for about 2 weeks (Fig. 8.27). The persistent incisional hernia resulting from this type of repair can be treated by a second operation 10-12 months later.

b) External Cutaneous Reinforcement

In cases where the defect is very large and major sepsis is present, it may be wise to simply protect the bowel by the omentum and a plate of polyurethane foam. The edges of the foam piece should extend for some distance beneath the margins of the defect. External reinforcement is achieved by sticking polyamide mesh over the abdominal wall [Guivarch et al. 1979]. The dressing is changed daily for about 10 days. The defect will progressively take on the aspect of a fixed burst abdomen (Figs. 8.28 & 8.29). Once the viscera have become covered by granulation tissue (at the end of the first week) we dress the wound with a powder or paste of highly absorbent dextran microspheres, as in cases of fixed burst abdomen. The dextran paste (Débrisan, Shering) forms a gel which is clearly less traumatic than moist towels, although the protection it affords is incomplete. Therefore, it is necessary to place dry or vaseline compresses between the dextran dressing and the external reinforcement band. The latter is kept in place for 3 or 4 weeks. This technique allows rapid growth of tissue over the bowel, thereby forming the support for definitive epidermization. Cicatrization can be accelerated by a split-thickness skin graft (or skin net). Incisional hernia also persists when this technique is used. Full cicatrization is attained after 2-3 months.

c) Internal Cutaneous Reinforcement with Polyglactine Mesh

In cases of a very large defect, external reinforcement with mechanical protection of the intestines may prove insufficient to inhibit protrusion of the viscera. The viscera may become irritated by the dressings; this can lead to formation of an external fistula. In other cases, subsequent to successive operations or maintenance of laparostomy for several days, the defect resembles more or less pronounced fixed burst abdomen. When these different situations arise we achieve repair by internal reinforcement, using an absorbable prosthetic mesh (polyglactine 910). This procedure, developed by Levasseur et al. (1979) provides protection of the viscera and temporary parietal reinforcement. As described by its author, this technique consists first of full trimming of the margins of the defect. The mesh (whose edge is folded over so that the suturing needle passes through a double thickness of the material) is then anchored to the deep

surface of the parietal peritoneum and should extend as far laterally as possible. U sutures through pledgets are used for this purpose (the sutures are tied over the pledgets). It is also possible to tie off the sutures over the aponeurosis of the external oblique. In this case, small incisions of the skin and subcutaneous tissue (2-3 cm long) are made over the site of each aponeurotic suture. We use gauge 0-1 polyglactine 910 for the sutures. It is preferable to position all of the sutures on one side and then to tie them off. Once the mesh has been securely fixed on one side, the procedure is repeated on the opposite side, care being taken to place the sutures in such a way that their tension achieves perfect maintenance of the abdominal viscera, as evidenced by a flat abdominal wall. The prosthetic mesh is then covered by an oily dressing, which is changed once or twice daily. The sutures used to anchor the prosthesis are removed on the 8th postoperative day. Abdominal pressure maintains the prosthesis solidly in place by pressing it against the peritoneum. The latter will progressively adhere to the prosthesis after a short period of time. Fibrinoid tissue invests the prosthesis, rendering it fully hermetic in about one week's time. At this stage we replace the vaseline dressings with a gel of dextran microspheres, as in the procedure for external reinforcement (see page 159). Full closure of the defect takes about 2-3 months and is due to partial apposition of the muscle and growth of granulation tissue.

2. Aseptic Defects

In cases where peritoneal and abdominal wall infection is absent, the defect can be closed using reconstructive surgery and a nonabsorbable prosthesis. One of the procedures described below is used, according to the size of the defect.

a) Simple Suturing with Relaxing Incisions

In cases where the defect does not exceed 10 cm in diameter and its margins are sufficiently solid to be sutured, i.e., composed of aponeurosis, tension-free suturing can be done. Lateral cutaneofascial or purely fascial relaxing incisions, coupled with subcutaneous dissection, allow the suturing to be done under traction-free conditions. We prefer mass-closure (extracutaneous) interrupted suturing with slow-absorbing material for this purpose.

b) Turndown of Anterior Lamina of Rectus Sheath

This procedure can be used in cases of larger defects lying on the midline. The incisions are made 1 cm

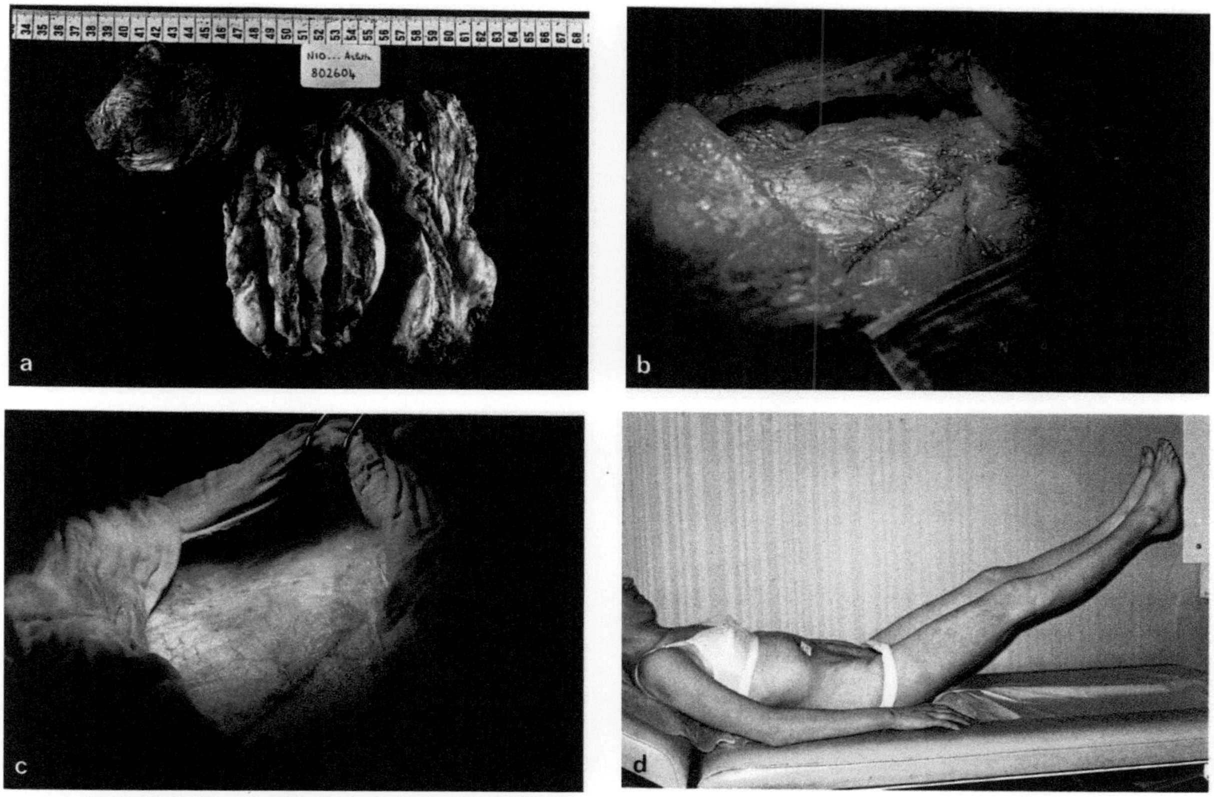

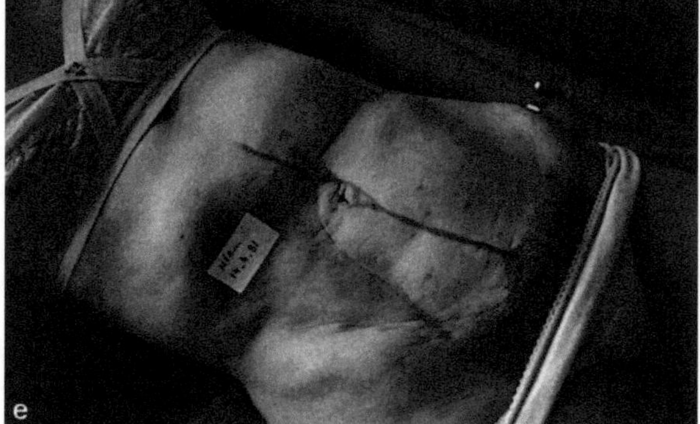

Fig. 8.30a-e. Resection of the abdominal wall from the inguinal ligaments to the inferior thoracic ridge in a case of desmoid tumor. **a** The two resected tumors. **b** The abdominal wall defect; note that the peritoneum has been preserved (except in a small area closed by edge-to-edge suturing). **c** Repair of the defect using a large mersilene mesh. **d** Functional result 1 year after operation. **e** Reoperation via the midline for total colectomy. The vertical incision of the prosthesis was closed with nonabsorbable sutures

from the lateral margins of the recti abdomini. The anterior lamina of the rectus sheath can then be turned down easily, except at the level of its fibrous intersections, where very careful hemostasis is required. The medial margins of the incision are joined together on the midline using interrupted sutures of polyglactine 910 (gauge 0). This procedure allows repair of a defect measuring up to 15 cm wide. In cases where there is traction on the sutures, two relaxing incisions are made as far lateral as possible (beyond Spigelius' line so as not to weaken it). Indeed, in the region of the semilunar line, there is a risk of opening all three fascial layers in a single step, thereby exposing the peritoneum. This complication will obviously give rise to lateral incisional hernia.

We have used this procedure in a few cases of resection en bloc of a colonic malignancy with invasion of the abdominal wall.

c) Prostheses or Autograft

In cases where the defect involves half or more of the abdominal wall, plastic surgery alone is insufficient.

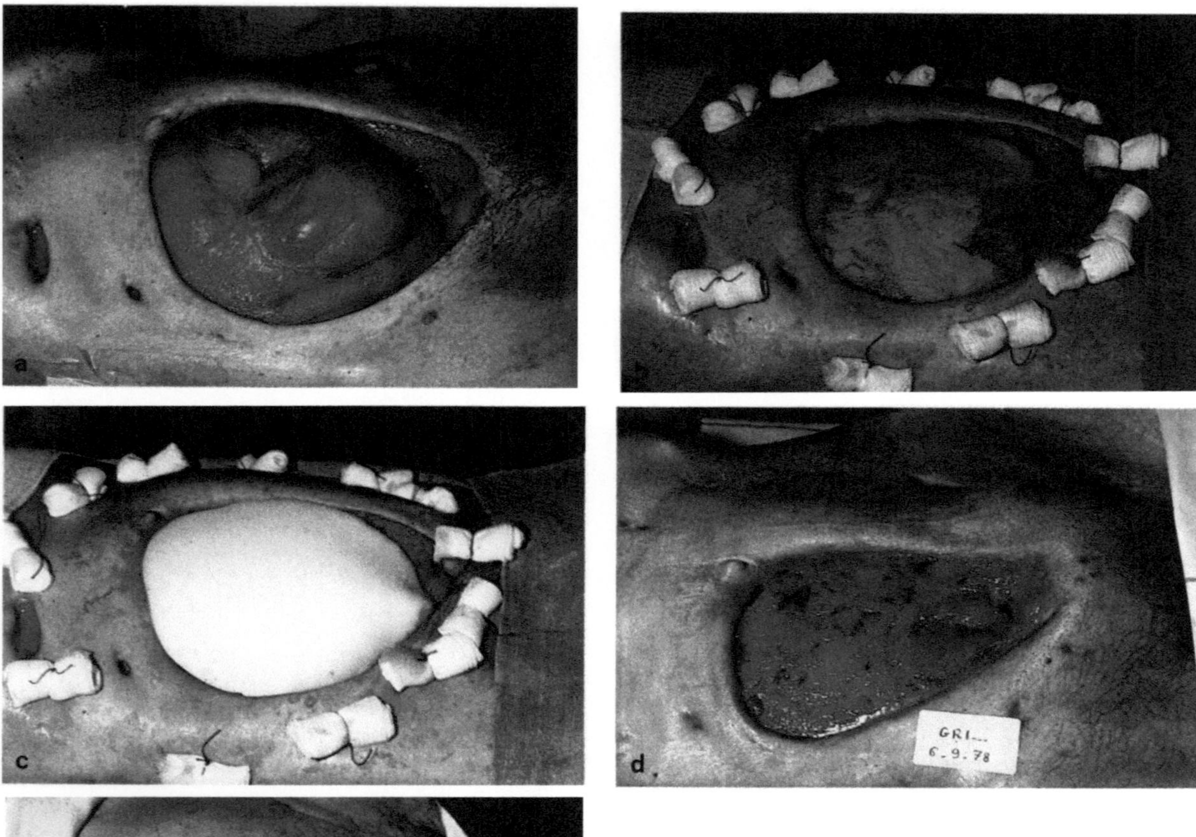

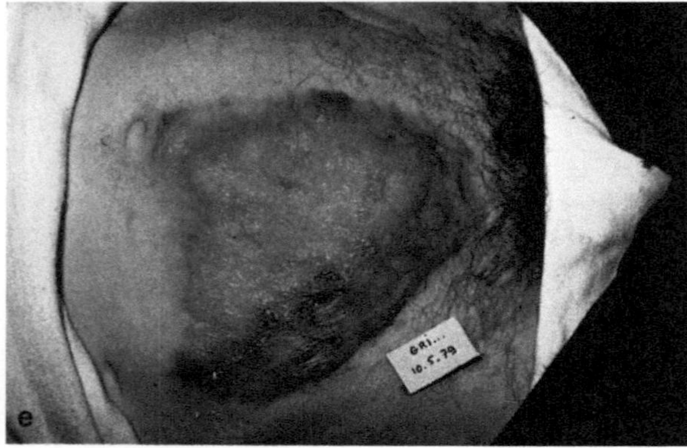

Fig. 8.31a-e. Resection of half of the anterior abdominal wall in a case of gas gangrene. **a** The abdominal wall defect 30 days after resection. External reinforcement using adhesive material; bowel protected by vaseline compresses. **b** Internal reinforcement with mersilene mesh. **c** Dressing with polyurethane foam, replaced on the 8th postoperative day by dextral microspheres. **d** Appearance of the defect 6 weeks later; note the full overgrowth investing the prosthesis. At this stage, cicatrization can be accelerated by thin-layer skin grafting. **e** Final result

Repair in these cases can be done with a prosthesis or by autografting. The choice of the procedure depends on whether the omentum and peritoneum have been preserved. Resection of the abdominal wall in cases of desmoid tumor (which usually does not affect the peritoneum) can be repaired by a large mersilene or ligalene mesh. We have performed such repair in a patient presenting with Gardner's syndrome (Fig. 8.30).

A similar procedure can be done to repair the defect of wide abdominal wall resection done in cases of gas gangrene where the omentum is intact. The defect is closed by implanting mersilene or ligalene mesh along the deep surface of the peritoneum (Fig. 8.31). As described above, the wound is initially dressed with vaseline compresses, followed by dextran gel from the 8th postoperative day onward. About 3 weeks later, i.e., when the prosthesis is completely invested by new tissue, cicatrization can be accelerated by thin skin grafts.

d) Myoplasty

In addition to turndown of the anterior lamina of the rectus sheath, myoplasty can be used to repair certain atypical defects of the abdominal wall.

Gracilis Myoplasty. Midline subumbilical defects can be repaired by myoplasty of the gracili muscles. This old procedure, described by Comolli in 1931 [in Quenu & Perrotin 1955], consists of sectioning the distal end of the two muscles at their myoaponeurotic junction, then turning the muscle bodies upwards. A subcutaneous tunnel is made to pass the lower end of the muscles (now the superior part of the myoplasty) over the defect. The muscle is then sutured to the margins of the defect.

Tensor Fascia Lata. Defects in the lumbar region of the abdominal wall can be repaired by tensor fascia lata pedicle flaps [Koonts 1955]. A U-shaped skin incision is made; the anterior and posterior parts of the U-shaped incision descend from the anterior-superior iliac spine and the middle of the iliac crest respectively, and are joined together (horizontal part of the U) over the greater trochanter. The superior part of the fascia lata is dissected free, but its insertion on the iliac crest is preserved. The fascia lata is then sectioned at a more or less inferior site and then turned upwards. The fascial sheet can be brought up as far as the inferior costal ridge. In cases where the fascia lata is not wide enough to cover the defect, the repair can be completed by using the aponeurosis of the lumbar muscles.

Tensor Fascia Lata Myocutaneous Pedicle Flaps. Some authors have successfully used tensor fascia lata myocutaneous flaps pedicled to a branch of the circumflex artery [Nahai et al. 1978; Caffee & Asokan 1981; Luce et al. 1983]. The neurovascular bundle approaches the fascia lata near the medial margin of its upper quadrant. The tensor fascia lata must be detached from the iliac crest and sectioned below at a point about 10 cm from its inferior end. Rotation 180° brings the flap to the abdominal wall to cover a massive defect. This procedure is indicated in exceptional cases, i.e., young patients in whom no other technique is possible. If necessary both of the tensor fascia lata muscles can be used to achieve total abdominal wall reconstruction [Luce et al. 1983].

C. Therapeutic Evisceration (Laparostomy)

1. History of Treatment of Burst Abdomen

This subject can be divided into three main periods. During the first period, lasting up to 1960, emergency reoperation was done to achieve closure at all costs. The mortality was 50% under these conditions. The second period was one of systematic refusal to reoperate. During this phase, techniques of abdominal belting and external cutaneous reinforcement were introduced [Guivarch & Mouchet 1969]. In the third period, abdominal wounds were made to treat underlying peritonitis. Many reports have been published recently on this subject [Fagniez 1978; Guivarch et al. 1979; Neidhardt et al. 1979; Champault et al. 1979].

Two therapeutic situations requiring an open-abdomen procedure can arise. In cases where burst abdomen complicates peritonitis, the abdominal opening can be maintained for a certain time to allow daily treatment of the peritonitis. In other cases (which are the most frequent) the laparotomy made to treat severe peritonitis is deliberately left open for several days, also to allow appropriate treatment. We refer to these open-abdomen procedures by the term "laparostomy".

The basic idea behind this technique was a result of the high mortality seen when closely spaced successive operations were done to treat grave peritonitis. Nonclosure allows visceral exploration and cleansing of the peritoneum to be done on a daily basis. This technique, which can be done at the bedside, is pursued until total cleansing of the peritoneum is obtained. The open-abdomen is then treated like free or fixed burst abdomen with adhesive external reinforcement bands until cicatrization occurs. At this stage the patient has an incisional hernia that may be treated a few months later.

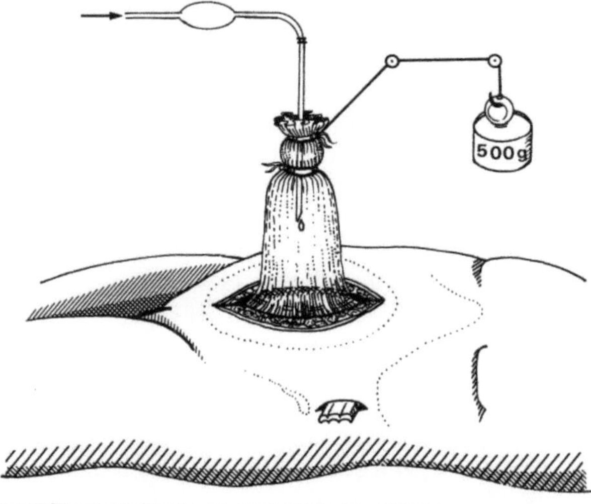

Fig. 8.32. The "plastic skirt" technique (according to Neidhardt). The open wound is covered by the plastic wound protector, through which irrigation fluid is delivered

2. Technique

This simple technique is done at the end of the operation for peritonitis. During surgery all septic foci are removed, intestinal sections are brought out to skin, and efficacious drainage of the peritoneal cavity is done subsequent to lengthy and thorough peritoneal lavage.

The viscera are then protected by polyurethane sponge, as proposed by Fagniez (1978). This material is apparently less traumatic than the traditional towels soaked in povidone iodine [Champault et al. 1979]. Reinforcement of the wall is achieved using adhesive jersey cloth (Contensor). We have performed laparostomy in 18 patients with a mean exposure time of one week (range: 4-18 days). Six of these patients died from peritonitis. However, we firmly believe that the mortality would have been much higher if repetitive laparotomy (not allowing daily peritoneal cleansing) had been done.

The "plastic skirt", a procedure developed by Neidhardt, was used in two of our patients. This technique has given satisfactory results, if one takes into consideration the dramatic situations in which it has been used [Neidhardt et al. 1979; Champault et al. 1979]. At the end of the operation, the semi-rigid ring of a plastic field protector (Wound Protector) is slipped under the margins of the defect (or incisional wound). The plastic sheet is then raised up and tied to a tube through which irrigation fluid is delivered. The upper end of the plastic skirt is also suspended by vertical traction to ensure a hermetic seal between the ring of the wound protector and the deep surface of the abdominal wall. The margins of the wound become everted, thereby facilitating local cleansing (Fig. 8.32). The irrigation fluid introduced via the tube is evacuated by drains placed in the lowermost part of the abdominal cavity. The plastic skirt is left in place for about a week. Irrigation fluid is usually isotonic saline (500 ml/24 h) [Neidhardt et al. 1979] or greater amounts of diluted (10%) povidone iodine (18-30 liters/day) [Champault et al. 1979].

References

Berkheiser SW (1952) Tumeur analogue à un synovialiome de la paroi abdominale. Ann Surg 135: 114-117

Bradant B, Revol M, Vergote T, Servant T, Banzet P (1993) Dermofibrosarcoma protuberans of the chest and the shoulder: wide and deep excisions with immediate reconstructions. Plast Reconstr Surg 71: 348-351

Caffee HH, Asokan R (1981) Tensor fascia lata myocutaneous free flaps. Plast Reconstr Surg 68: 195-200

Caffee HH (1983) Reconstruction of the abdominal wall by variations of the tensor fasciae latae flap. Plast Reconstr Surg 71: 348-351

Champault G, Magnier M, Psalmon F. Roche JY, Patel JC (1979) L'éviscération: élément thérapeutique des péritonites. Nouv Presse Med 8: 1349

Chevrel JP (1994) Loss of substance of abdominal wall. In: Bendavid R (ed) Prostheses and Abdominal Wall Hernias. R G Landes, Austin, pp 311-320

Chevrel JP, Sarfati E, Saglier J, Kemeny JL (1983) Tumeur desmoide et syndrome de Gardner. A propos d'une observation. J Chir 3: 159-164

Delamarre J, Dupas JL, Capron JP, Remond A, Lorriaux A (1980) Fibromatose mésentérique et syndrome de Gardner. Revue de la littérature à propos d'un cas d'évolution mortelle. Gastroenterol Clin Biol 4: 45-51

Fagniez PL (1978) La prévention des lésions intestinales lors des éviscérations. Nouv Presse Med 7: 1117

Freedman AM, Gayle LB, Vaughan ED, Hoffman LA (1990) One stage repair of the anterior abdominal wall using bilateral rectus femoris myocutaneous flaps. Ann Plast Surg 23: 299-302

Germain M (1978) Les tumeurs de la paroi abdominale. Enc Med Chir Estomac-Intestin 9049, A 10

Gottlieb JR, Engrav LH, Walkinshaw MD, Eddy AC, Herman CM (1990) Upper abdominal wall defects: immediate or staged reconstruction? Plast Reconstr Surg 86: 281-286

Guenn P (1958) Tumeurs de la paroi abdominale. Enc Med Chir 2011, B 10

Guivarch M, Mouchet A (1969) Sanglage abdominal par bas nylon dans l'éviscération post-operatoire. Press Med 77: 101-102

Guivarch M, Roullet-Audy JC, Chapmann A (1979) La non fermeture pariétale dans la chirurgie itérative des péritonites. Chirurgie 105: 287-290

Jones EL, Cornell WP (1966) Gardner's syndrome. Arch Surg 72: 287-300

Koonts AR (1955) Une opération pour grosse hernie lombaire sur cicatrice d'incision. Surg Gynecol Obstet 101: 119-121

Levasseur JC, Lehn E, Rignier P (1979) Etude expérimentale et utilisation clinique d'un nouveau matériel dans les éviscérations graves post-operatoires. Chirurgie 105: 577-581

Levasseur JC, Lehn E, Rignier P (1979) La contention interne par prothèse resorbable dans le traitement des grandes éviscérations. J Chir 12: 737-740

Loygue J, Adloff M (1977) Polypose intestinale. Masson, Paris

Luce EA, Hyde G, Gottlieb SE, Romm S (1983) Total abdominal wall reconstruction. Arch Surg 118: 1446-1448

MacPeak CJ, Cruz T, Nicastria AD (1967) Dermato-fibroma protuberans. An analysis of 86 cases - 5 with metastasis. Ann Surg 166: 803

NlcAdam AF, Goligher JC (1970) The occurrence of desmoid in patient with familial polyposis coli. Br J Surg 57: 618-630

Nahai F, Silverton JS, Vasconez LO (1978) The tensor fascia lata musculocutaneous flaps. Am Plast Surg 1: 372-379

Neidhart JH, Kraft F, Morin A, Rousson B, Charroux B, Roubin M (1979) Le traitement à ventre ouvert de certaines péritonites et infections pariétales abdominales graves. Lyon Chir 75: 272-774

Neven P, Shepherd JH, Tham KF, Fisher C, Breach N (1993) Reconstruction of the abdominal wall with a latissimus dorsi musculocutaneous flap: a case of a massive abdominal wall metastasis from a cervical cancer requiring palliative resection. Gynecol Oncol 49: 403-406

Pétoin DS, Verola O, Banzet P, Dufourmentel C, Servant JM (1985) Dermatofibrosarcome de Darier et Ferrand: étude de 96 cas sur 15 ans. Chirurgie 111: 132

Piza H, Rath T, Hausmaniger C, Walzer RL (1993) Wound closure at the trunk by microvascular free flap transfer. Microsurgery 14: 230-235

Revol M, Vergote T, Servant JM, Banzet P (1992) Transferts tissulaires libres en chirurgie plastique (urgences exclues). A propos d'une expérience de dix ans. Ann Chir Plast Esthet 33: 119-126

Rowsell AR, Poole MD, Geoffrey AM (1986) Dermatofibroma protuberans: the problem of surgical management. Br J Plast Surg 39: 262

Smith WG (1954) Desmoid tumors in familial multiple polyposis. Proc Staff Meet Mayo Clin 34-31

Waddel WR (1975) Treatment of infra-abdominal and abdominal wall desmoid tumors with drugs that affect the metabolism of cyclic 3-5 adenosine monophosphate. Ann Surg 3: 299-302

9 Hernia of the Abdominal Wall

R. Stoppa

With the collaboration of
P. Amid, R. Bendavid, G. Champault, J. P. Chevrel,
J. B. Flament, A. Gilbert, C. Meyer, J. P. Palot, G. E. Wantz

I. Groin Hernias in the Adult

Since the work of Henri Fruchaud (1956), we have used the term inguinal hernias to include all hernias of the inguino-femoral region, the region that Fruchaud called "inguino-crural". This concept arose from the fact that all of these hernias, which classically are divided into direct, indirect and femoral hernias, are caused by damage to the tranversalis fascia layer in the area of the myopectineal orifice. This region is known to be weak anatomically. The debate continues, and has recently became more active. Controversies concern the classification of hernias, over which there is no universal agreement, the indications for classical surgical procedures, the value of different laparoscopic procedures which still await proper evaluation, and the decisions regarding the general directions of hernia surgery. This is the most commonly performed surgery nowadays, and is thus of great social and economic importance.

Hernias have been known since the beginning of the medical history. In ancient civilizations, the need for urgent measures to deal with the catastrophe of strangulation, was well recognized. The modern surgical era, which was facilitated by the advent of anesthesia, began with Bassini in Padua in 1887. His procedure was well founded anatomically. Progress continued through the work of Halsted in Baltimore (1889), Lucas Champonnière in Paris (1892) and Marcy in Boston (1892) who described different types of reconstruction of the inguinal canal after excision of the peritoneal sac. Lotheissen (1898) was the first to use the pectineal ligament "Cooper's ligament" in surgical repair. Cheatle (1920) and Henry (1936) proposed the posterior abdominal approach. This technique was extensively used by Nyhus (1959) and developed in France by Stoppa (1969). Up until the Second World War, there followed a period during which each surgeon made up his technique based on personal criteria, with little regard to results.

Thereafter, the surgical community became more concerned about recurrence. Surgeons such as McVay and Anson (1949) in the USA, Fruchaud (1956) in France and others carried out anatomical researches which led to a revolution in hernia surgery.

Among the most important technical innovations was the use of synthetic material to repair difficult cases [Usher 1958; Koontz & Kinberley 1960]. Don Acquaviva (1949) introduced Nulon mesh into France, then Rives et al. (1965) brought in the modern polymeric mesh. Stoppa (1969) further applied these techniques and spread their use. Most recently, Lichtenstein developed multiform patches and plugs for hernia repair in the USA. His procedure generated great enthusiasm which is spreading throughout Europe progressively. Since 1990, mini-invasive and video-assisted surgical procedures have developed rapidly. Their effectiveness is still to be determined, but they need to be taken into account.

One might ask: "Should there be a subspecialty in hernia surgery based on rich historical background?" One might recall, in this connection, the view of Shuh (1804-1865), a Viennese surgeon, quoted by Halsted (1883) and Ravitch (1968): "If no other field was offered to the surgeon for his activity other than herniotomy it would be worthwhile to become a surgeon and devote an entire life to this service".

A. Principles of Treatment

1. Some Aspects of Surgical Anatomy of the Inguinal Region

Details regarding the surgical anatomy can be found in Part 1 of this book. Here are some considerations concerning inguinal hernia in particular.

Fruchaud (1956) considered the groin as a transitional region between the abdomen and the thigh. The importance of the groin is related to the resistance of its structures to abdominal pressure. Anatomical studies of the inguinal region have already demonstrated that voluntary striated muscle is absent and that it is an area of support where two dissimilar structures are superimposed, namely the external oblique muscle aponeurosis and the deep myofascial layer. The latter is far more important in surgical repair. The transversalis fascia is, in some respects, the only layer to resist abdominal pressure. The inguinal region is also the passageway for the spermatic cord and femoral vessels, which adds to its inherent weakness. The funnel-shaped "abdominofemoral fascia of Fruchaud", occupying the myopectineal orifice, is an anatomical passage between the abdomen and the thigh. All inguinal hernias occur within this passage.

Some anatomical variations contribute further to the constitutional and structural weakness of this region, such as the patency of the processus vaginalis (20% of young adults, Cloquet 1819), and/or the increased size of Hesselbach-Ferguson triangle, which lacks voluntary striated muscles. Retroparietal planes of cleavage [Bogros 1923; Odimba et al. 1980; Hureau 1991; Mertl 1996] are the logical deep prolongation of the normal anatomy of the inguinal region. They are important from the surgical point of view, as they delineate the posterior surgical approach for repair and are the ideal site for preperitoneal prostheses.

There are two anatomical approaches to the groin region.

- The earlier anterior approach was widely used and depended for its good results on the possibility of identifying the structures of the inguinal canal so as to effect a sound repair, preserve important organs (nerves, spermatic cord, etc.) and not to miss other hernias.

- The posterior or abdominal approach leads to the preperitoneal spaces and was developed more recently. It has the advantage of allowing direct access to the defect. The different surgical procedures are discussed later on. This approach is particularly useful when problems with the anterior approach are foreseen.

Each of these approaches has its own features. Griffith (1964) expressed this by saying: "Equal familiarity with these two approaches allows one to suit the operation to the patient rather than the patient to the operation".

2. Hernial Lesions

The multiple nature of groin hernias is well recognized. This should encourage surgeons to be meticulous in the description of hernias in their reports. It is necessary to look for all hernia lesions systematically. These are the size of the deep inguinal ring, the solidity of the posterior layer, the dimensions of the "myopectineal orifice of Fruchaud" and the femoral canal (Fig. 9.1).

Bulky hernias cause the two inguinal rings to become superimposed. Sliding hernias may be associated with sliding of intraperitoneal as well as retroperitoneal organs into the scrotum. A very large scrotum may require reduction by resection to prevent recurrent hematomas.

Surgery for recurrent hernias endangers regional nerves and spermatic cord components which are usually difficult to dissect because of scar tissue and fibrosis. This is particularly true of the anterior approach. Reoperations by the posterior approach, especially after the rare failure of a previous prosthetic repair, may be difficult due to loss of the preperitoneal plane of cleavage. These difficulties are resolved by the exclusion of the adherent area [Trivellini 1991], or by dissecting behind the pubis or even beneath the periosteum [Stoppa 1995].

Systemic and local microanatomical abnormalities should be mentioned, such as abnormalities of collagen synthesis and the "metastatic emphysema of

Read". These hypotheses are interesting but do not have a direct bearing on surgery, except to support the more radical use of prosthetic mesh. Postoperative scarring is another interesting feature which has an important surgical significance.

3. Classification of Hernias

The classical division of inguinal hernias into direct, indirect and femoral hernias does not adequately reflect the multiplicity of these lesions, and it is important to devise a universally accepted classification for inguinal hernias. An agreed nomenclature would make possible a comparative evaluation of different surgical procedures.

Many classifications have been already proposed in the medical literature but none has been universally accepted. Here is the result of many years of discussions accomplished by the GREPA. The advantage of a

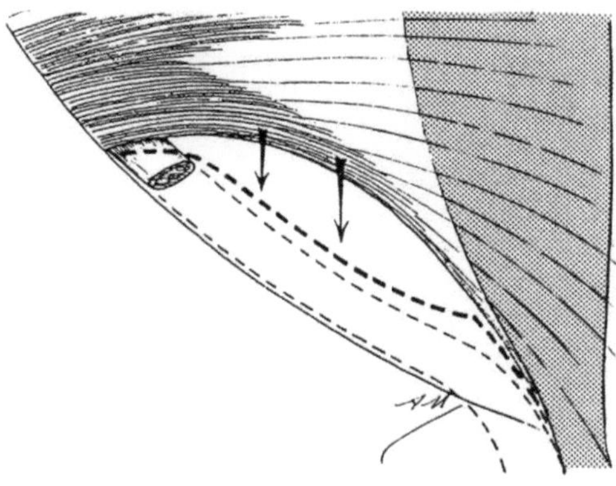

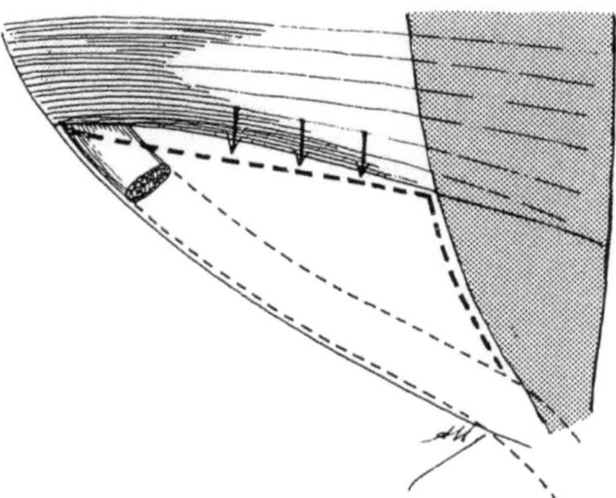

Fig. 9.1. Variations in the position of the inferior margin of the internal oblique (according to Fruchaud, Doin, Paris 1956). *Above*: The internal oblique lies in a rather low position and the inguinal triangle is rather narrow: efficiency protection mechanism of the inguinal canal; *below*: the internal oblique lies in a rather high position and the inguinal triangle is large: inefficient protection

universal classification would be the evaluation of different surgical procedures by comparing their results in homogeneous groups of patients. On the other hand, hernias are very common and are usually treated by many surgeons of unequal surgical experience. Such comparative studies might help to indicate the operation of choice. This effort is even more important when we consider that treatment of inguinal hernias seems to be on the increase, while other operations have recently became less often practiced. Moreover, the hernia surgeon is individually and personally involved in all aspects of the patient's management, while therapeutic decisions in many other fields are now often discussed and managed by multidisciplinary teams. Finally, laparoscopic hernia surgery has recently developed and could, in the absence of a classification, become as hard to evaluate as is open surgery.

Among the many proposed classifications, those of Fruchaud, Berger, McVay and Chapp, Harkins, Casten, Gilbert (Table 9.1), Cristinzio and Bendavid should be mentioned. The Nyhus scheme (1991) deserves close attention (Table 9.2), as it is fairly complete and well balanced concerning the indications for hernia repair with or without prosthetic mesh respectively. In this classification, groin hernias are divided into four types according to the state of the posterior wall of the inguinal canal. We agree with Nyhus, except on two points: (1) the choice between anterior or posterior approach is based on an accurate clinical distinction

Table 9.1. An anatomical and functional classification (Gilbert's) for the diagnosis and treatment of inguinal hernia

Type	I	II	III	IV	V
Internal ring	< IFB	IFB	> IFB	Norm	Norm
Peritoneal sac	Y	Y	N	N	N
Canal floor	I	I	DES	DES	DES (IFB)

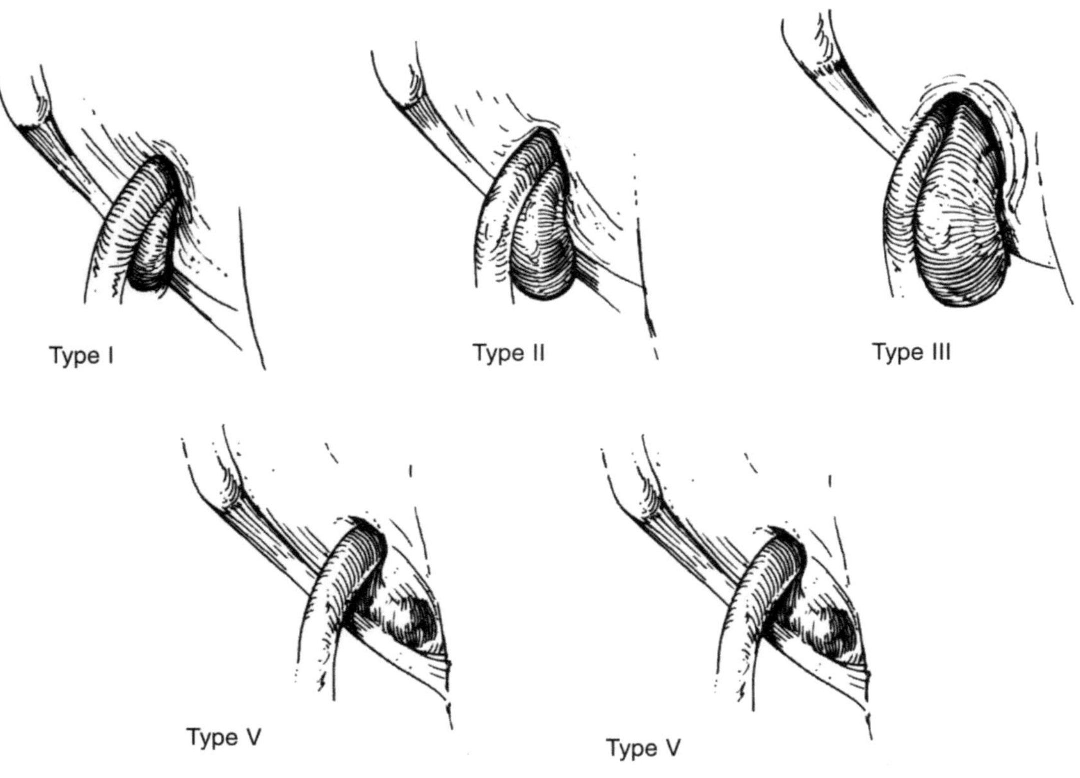

Table 9.2. Nyhus' classification of groin hernias (1991)

Type of hernia	Type of repair
I. Indirect	
Normal deep inguinal ring	High ligation of the sac without parietal repair
II. Indirect	
Widened deep inguinal ring	High ligation of the sac, closing of the inguinal ring
III. Lesions of the posterior wall	
A) Direct	Anterior approach: herniorrhaphy using ilio-pubic bandelette, or Shouldice or McVay procedures
B) Large indirect	Posterior approach: herniorrhaphy + prosthesis, or Stoppa procedure
C) Femoral	Posterior approach: herniorrhaphy
IV. Recurrent	Posterior approach: herniorrhaphy + prosthesis

between direct and indirect hernias in type III, which is unfortunately unreliable. (2) Femoral hernias and recurrent hernias are underestimated.

Our personal proposition for the classification of groin hernias (Table 9.3) is derived from the Nyhus classification, with special attention to the aggravating factors. These factors include some complex injuries related to the hernia (its size, degree of sliding, multiplicity, etc.), patient characteristics (age, activity, respiratory diseases, dysuria, obesity, constipation), special surgical circumstances (supposed technical difficulties, infection risks) or any other unfavorable factor which could modify the choice of treatment. Finally, it seems logical to include in the group IV "the group of recurrent hernias", the subgroups proposed by Campanelli (1996).

The fact that every hernia should be considered and treated individually must be emphasized. However, the general indications that we believe suitable for our four types of hernia, are as follows:

- Type I: indirect hernia with normal deep inguinal ring (admitting one finger at the most) in young patients. They are treated by excision and closure of the peritoneal sac.

- Type II: indirect hernia with widening of the deep inguinal ring (admitting more than one finger) and a solid canal floor. They are treated by repair of the deep inguinal ring, or a Bassini-Shouldice type procedure.

Table 9.3. Stoppa's classification of groin hernias

Type	Site	Anatomic characteristics		Treatment
		Deep inguinal ring	Inguinal floor	
I	Indirect	admitting one finger	solid	ligature resection of the sac
II	Indirect	admitting more than one finger	solid	closing of deep inguinal ring
	Type I hernia + aggravating factor*			
III	Indirect	large	± weak	Bassini/Shouldice
	Direct	± large	weak	
	Femoral	± normal	± weak	} Prosthesis to be discussed
	Type II hernia + aggravating factor*			
IV	Indirect	large	± weak	
	Direct	± large	weak	} Prosthesis
	Femoral	± normal	± faible	
	Type III hernia + aggravating factor*			

* Local aggravating factors: voluminous, multiple, complex hernias
  General aggravating factors: massive obesity, abdominal distention, collagenosis

- Type III: all direct or indirect inguinal hernias and femoral hernias associated with an impaired canal floor, or type II hernias associated with an aggravating factor. They are treated by a retroparietal prosthetic mesh placed by the inguinal or preperitoneal approach, and for femoral hernias, by a Lytle or plug procedure.

- Type IV: all recurrent hernias and type III hernias associated with an aggravating factor. According to Campanelli (1996), this type should be further divided into three subgroups: R1: first recurrence of an external oblique hernia of a small size in a non obese patient. It is treated by an anterior approach with the patch/plug procedure. R2: first recurrence of a suprapubic direct hernia of small size in a nonobese patient. It is treated via an inguinal approach with a plug or a prosthetic mesh (Rives or Wantz). R3: all other cases, including recurrent femoral hernias, hernial orifices of large size, groin eventrations, hernias with multiple recurrences, strangulated hernias, bilateral hernias and finally, all those associated with an aggravating factor (obesity, etc.). They are treated by a prosthetic mesh placed between the muscle and the peritoneum (Wantz or Stoppa operation).

4. Mechanisms of Inguinal Hernias

The congenital origin or predisposition is true of indirect inguinal hernias, generally because of a patent processus vaginalis which occurs in 20% of adults, according to Cloquet. Russel's theory (1906), according to which the peritoneal sac is the sole or principal factor responsible of the development of inguinal hernias, is not true in adults. Weakness of fascia transversalis around the deep inguinal ring [Keith 1924] is an important factor.

Direct inguinal hernias are acquired lesions. They are caused by failure of the "shutter mechanism" induced by contraction of the transverse myoaponeurotic arcade (Keith, Lytle). This failure exposes the central area of the transversalis fascia in the inguinal region to periodic rises in abdominal pressure. A low insertion of this myoaponeurotic arch strengthens this defense mechanism and explains the lower rate of inguinal hernias in women. More recently, acquired modifications of the fibrous structures of the groin have been studied. Peacock described changes in collagen metabolism as causing weakness of the fascia tranversalis "metabolic defect" (1974). Read (1970) noted an increased elastolytic activity in the lungs due to a disturbed ratio between circulating proteases and antiproteases, in smoking patients with direct hernias. These disorders resulted in a "metastatic emphysema" which was responsible for the impairment of fibrous tissue throughout the body, especially in the groin. Barbin discussed the "myoaponeurotic and tendinous dystrophy" found in patients with direct hernias. His works are cited in a thesis by Panou de Faymoreau (1976). Finally, the fact that inadequate operations in the inguinal region can cause damage resulting in recurrent or multiply recurrent hernias, should be emphasized.

With femoral hernias, the protrusion usually begins at the level of the femoral canal (of Anson and McVay). A prehernia lipoma is thought to take part in the genesis of such hernias by exerting traction on the peritoneal sac. Psoas muscle atrophy explains the increased rate of femoral hernias in old women, as it broadens the femoral canal which lies medial to the vascular sheath, under the inguinal ligament.

Finally, general factors, such as increased intra-abdominal pressure, dysuria, intestinal obstruction, chronic systemic disease, peritoneal dialysis, obesity, cachexia, old age, connective tissue inflammations, etc., are common to all types of hernias.

Thus, acquired hernias are of multiple origin, and the greater the number of adverse factors, the higher the risk of recurrence.

5. Epidemiology

Inguinal hernia repair is the commonest operation to be carried out on adult males. It is the third most common surgical procedure in Europe and the USA. Precise figures of the prevalence are lacking. A frequency of 3-4% of hernia in men of 65 years age or more has been reported. The frequency is at least three times greater in Africans than in Europeans.

The incidence and prevalence of hernias may be reflected by the annual number of operations carried out every year. For example, in 1987, 80,000 hernia repairs were done in the UK, 25,000 in Belgium, 120,000 in France, 150,000 in Germany and 550,000 in the USA. Estimated costs are US$ 28 billion, about 3% of the total health budget. The rates of operation varies from 100 per 100,000 persons in England, 200 in Norway and Australia to 300 in the USA. Studies from the United Kingdom [Kingsnorth 1995] reveal that the greatest frequency is between 55 and 85 years old. Strangulation rate is about 13% in 80 year old patients. 90% of operated patients are males, 65% of hernias are indirect and 55% are located on the right. Bilateral hernias are often direct. Femoral hernias are three times more common in females than in males. These numbers are almost the same in all developed countries.

The mortality of strangulated hernia is still high, more than 20,000 patients every year (1964-1967) in the USA [Heydorn 1990]. In the United-Kingdom, postoperative mortality is as high as 10-15% in 1990-1994 [Campling 1994]. Of femoral hernias, more than 40% are admitted because of strangulation [Royal College of Surgeons of England 1993], while only 3% of direct hernias arrive for the same reason. The risk of strangulation seems to vary according to the duration of hernia and is greatest during the first three months of its appearance [Allen 1987].

The Royal College of Surgeons of England recommended priority in waiting lists for hernia patients who had had a previous repair during childhood, the elderly, smokers, patients with aortic aneurysms and patients with recent hernias.

6. Length of Hospital Stay

The first report of an inguinal herniorrhaphy performed on an outpatient basis came from England. In 1909, Nicoll published a series of 9,000 young patients, many with hernias. He reported similar results as for hospitalized patients. In 1955, Faquharson showed that early return to normal activity did not lead to recurrence. This was confirmed earlier by E. Shouldice. Nowadays, most hernia surgery in the USA is performed on an ambulatory basis, because of the pressure from the insurance companies and the development of hernia centers.

Ambulatory herniorrhaphy has not been so popular in Europe, in spite of the economical advantages and the fact that this type of surgery is ideal for day case care. The reasons for this include lack of political and of appropriate units. Traditions in medical practice are difficult to alter and hospital managements are notoriously resistant to change. Patient's attitudes to ambulatory surgery vary widely. The Shouldice Hospital has not favored ambulatory herniorrhaphy, where the length of hospital stay is three days for unilateral and five days for bilateral repair. In 1993, the Royal College of Surgeons of England estimated that 30% of hernia patients could be treated on an ambulatory basis. This rate is almost similar to that of Germany, but it is higher in Belgium. In France, there are only 6,000 beds for all ambulatory surgery, an average of seven places for each unit. So that the possible rate of ambulatory herniorrhaphy is far lower than in other countries, and the mean hospital stay is about 2-3 days for unilateral repair. Reports on this important subject are scanty.

It should be emphasized that the surgeon's responsibility remains the same in all circumstances, whether or not the operation is performed on an ambulatory basis. Careful follow-up is mandatory.

7. Verification of Results and Quality

Bassini's written observations in the Clinica Chirurgica di Padova in 1889 and his other publications testify to his concern about recurrence after hernia repair (3.8% of recurrence at 4 years). For many years, his ideas were not pursued. It was only after the Second World War, and especially at Shouldice Hospital, that surgeons began to be concerned about recurrence, perhaps, because of more innovative and exciting techniques. It is now acknowledged that postal questionnaires reveal at best half of recurrences. Visits by general physicians are not the best solution. We know, however, that results of self-audit are better if some medical staff other than surgeons participates in follow-up.

In retrospective studies, a surgeon should have examined 90% of the patients, with at least 5 years follow-up. Publications from the Shouldice Hospital, whose objective methods are hard to reproduce, accumulated 130,000 operated patients since 1945. The long-term follow-up was 98% of patients at one year, 70% at 5 years, 70% at 10 years and 50% at 20 years.

Degeneration of the inguinal anatomical structures due to ageing could account for recurrences, ten years after the first herniorrhaphy. This factor was absent during the first repair. These are new hernias and not late recurrences. From their own retrospective results, Halverson and McVay developed a coefficient system in order to predict recurrence rates for up to 25 years. The recurrence rate at 1 year should be multiplied by 5, then by 2.5 at 10 years and by 1.2 at 10 years. However, this system applies only to the authors' own herniorrhaphy. In our experience, results of the prosthetic repair remain unchanged after the first postoperative year.

8. Informing the Patient

Patients undergoing surgical hernia repair should be given precise information. This is a medico-legal obligation and patients are eager to take part in medical decisions.

However, surgeons and patients do not always share the same opinion concerning medical problems. Therefore, all aspects of the surgery including the anesthetic technique, the surgical options, the type of approach, the necessity of a prosthetic repair, the advantages of a short hospital stay and the return to normal activity, should be addressed. The preopera-

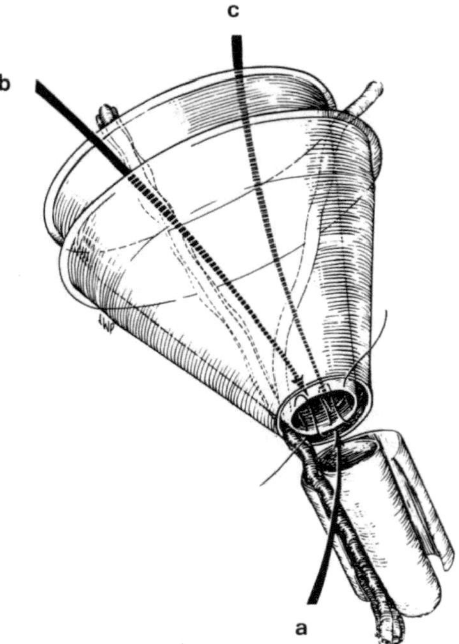

Fig. 9.2. The main surgical approaches to groin hernia: (*a*) inguinal approach; (*b*) preperitoneal abdominal approach; (*c*) transperitoneal approach [Griffith 1964]

tive consultation is the best occasion at which to give the hernia patients, who used to be considered as having a very standard disease, full consideration and explanation about their condition and its treatment. This helps the surgeon to achieve a perfect herniorrhaphy.

B. General Principles of Herniorrhaphy

1. The Choice of Approach

It depends on the surgeon's experience, the type of hernia and the procedure to be performed (Fig. 9.2).

a) The Anterior Inguinal Approach

This approach has been used for many years. It allows the performance of herniorrhaphies, autografts, myoplasties and classical prosthetic repairs. It can be carried out under local anesthesias.

The incision should be long enough, but not excessive. It needs to be appropriate for the technique (some plug techniques could be performed with a 2 to 3 cm incision). Surgeons and patients are more and more concerned about the length of the incision. Shouldice et al. incise low in the inguinal region in order to be within the pubic hair. For bilateral hernias, the incision can run horizontally over the midline. The nerves and the spermatic cord elements must be preserved. The sac is dissected and divided. The posterior myofascial layer is carefully palpated. The transversalis fascia is opened in Hesselbach triangle. All associated hernial defects and orifices are then thoroughly explored. Palpation around the tranversalis fascia is very important. A relaxing incision on the deep layer of the anterior rectus sheath is sometimes useful. Some authors believe that it should be always done (Chevrel).

In the anterior approach, the dissection goes through intact anatomical structures whose integrity could be compromised. In recurrent hernias, it is sometimes difficult to visualize the spermatic cord and other important structures because of scarring brought about by repeated dissection and suturing. Technical difficulties are even greater in cases of multiple recurrences, and if the surgeon is unaware of the previous technique used.

b) The Transabdominal Approach

It was reported in detail by Nyhus (1964) and Read (1989). Marcy (1891) and Laroque (1919) suggested high ligation of the hernial sac and closure of the deep inguinal ring by this approach.

c) The Preperitoneal Approach

This approach is better for groin hernia repair. It was first described by Annandale (1876). Then Tait (1891), Cheatle (1920) and Henry (1936) spelled out its advantages. For a long time, little interest was shown apart from Mahoner and Goss from England in 1962, and Huguier from France in 1963, until the work of Nyhus (1964, 1978, 1989 and 1995) achieved a world-wide acceptance of this approach. Since 1965, we have followed Rives in promoting the development and application of this approach (Fig. 9.3).

There are many advantages to the preperitoneal approach, especially if it is done by a midline or a Pfannenstiel incisions. The retroperitoneal spaces are easily entered and the preperitoneal cleavage is facilitated, especially in cases of complex recurrent hernias previously operated on by the anterior approach. This wide dissection gives an excellent exposure of all relevant structures and orifices without further damage to the inguinal structures (nerves, cord and vessels) nor to the already weak inguinal floor. All the hernial defects in the myopectineal hole are then easily visualized, and any associated hernias can be detected and treated. Simultaneous bilateral hernia repair is also possible by this approach.

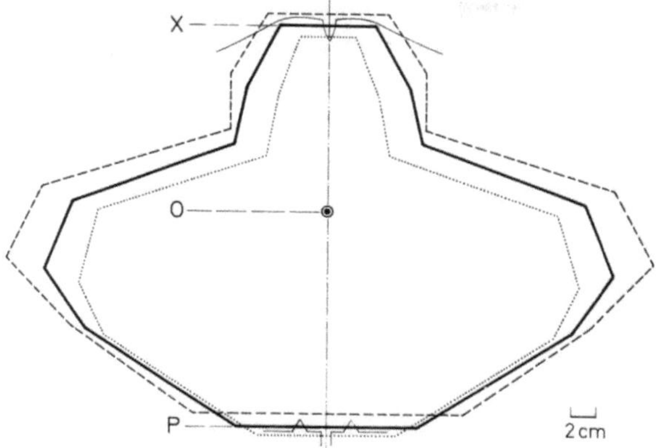

Fig. 9.3. The spatial plane of the preperitoneal and prevesical retrofascial space obtained by measurement in 20 dissections [Odimba et al. 1980]. The *heavy line* represents the mean dimensions of this space, the *dashed line* refers to the maximum dimensions, and the *dotted line* to the minimum dimensions. *X* xiphoid process; *O* umbilicus; *P* pubis

Midline incisions under local anesthesia are laborious, risky and uncomfortable for both surgeon and patient. General anesthesia is preferred but spinal anesthesia can be adequate. This approach is often proposed to patients who have a complex hernia with multiple recurrences. The risks of anesthesia are thus balanced against the need to perform a more radical operation with a lower recurrence rate.

Incisional hernias are one of the possible complications of the midline abdominal incisions. The use of a giant preperitoneal prosthetic mesh, nonabsorbable and biologically well tolerated prevents such complications. This prosthesis will treat all hernial defects and at the same time protect the midline incision.

Neater skin closure is achieved by an intracuticular running suture which helps patients to forget the unpleasant moments of the operation. However, it should be noted that some sero-sanguinous oozing occurs during the first postoperative day. Patients should be warned that this is not "bleeding".

d) Advantages of the Laparoscopic Approaches

These approaches, discussed below, are posterior and thus, have certain advantages. They are divided as follows.

(1) The Transabdominal Approach

It is a true "laparoscopic" approach as the operative field is the insufflated peritoneal cavity. All inguinal hernias can be detected and repaired by this method. Furthermore, associated abdominopelvic lesions are

visualized and if necessary treated. The possible risk of peritoneal or abdominal organ injury, however, rules it out as an ideal method of hernia repair.

(2) The Totally Extraperitoneal Approach

This one seems to be more difficult to perform. Insufflation is done in the preperitoneal space which is relatively small. The peritoneum must not be breached because this makes it turn difficult to induce a pneumoextraperitoneum.

The possibility of performing laparoscopic herniorrhaphy without an abdominal incision is one of the potential advantage of this method. However, although trocar site hernias are rare, the cosmetic result in young women is probably worse than that of a low suprapubic approach. It should be emphasized that laparoscopic herniorrhaphy is more difficult to learn, to teach and to perform than conventional herniorrhaphy. Individual surgeons, with different degrees of laparoscopic experience, do not have the same results.

Conversion from a laparoscopic to a more conventional surgical repair should not be considered as a complication, but as a deliberate decision. All patients should be informed of this possibility before the operation.

2. Dissection of the Spermatic Cord

Most of the ancient strolling operators used to divide the spermatic cord, and eliminate the testis, in spite of condemnations by Paracelus, the government and the church. This practice had progressively declined since the Renaissance. For more than twenty years, Heifetz (1971) divided the spermatic cord in elderly patients. However, this method does not solve the problem of the weak posterior inguinal canal wall. With a large varicocele, the spermatic cord can be divided without risking testicular atrophy, as in these cases, collateral vascular circulation is well developed.

Excision of the cremaster muscle has been known, since Marcy (1892), to be important in exposing the deep inguinal ring. However, in the inguinal and scrotal course of the spermatic cord, dilated veins should be preserved as well as the surrounding fat in order to prevent testicular ischemia. This is contrary to what was proposed by Halsted.

In 35% of cases, the genital branches of the ilioinguinal and genitofemoral nerves run within the cremaster muscle fibers [Moosman 1977]. These branches should be looked for and preserved. Chevrel (1983) classified postoperative neuropathic sequelae which are usually caused by intraoperative nerve injury. He divided them into neuroma formation, somatic pain and referred pain. These will be discussed later.

"Parietalization" of the components of the spermatic cord, in the preperitoneal approach, eliminates risk of injury to nerves and spermatic vessels. The cord is often spread out laterally during herniorrhaphy. Other methods of spermatic cord and testis displacement - through the abdominal wall [Wolfler 1892], the rectus muscle [Leslie 1978] or the suprainguinal region [Ferrand 1952; Toupet 1963] should be abandoned, as they damage the abdominal wall and the testicular blood supply - have not been shown to be effective.

Any handling of the spermatic cord beneath the pubis should be avoided so as to preserve the testicular venous return [Wantz 1982] and the testicular artery.

3. Management of the Hernial Sac

Before the development of surgical asepsis, and because of the risk of peritonitis, the hernial sac was replaced within the abdominal cavity without excision. Czerny (1877) was the first to resect and ligate the peritoneal sac.

Since Bassini (1887), high ligation and excision of the sac have been considered as important elements in the repair of inguinal hernia by the anterior approach. However, Shouldice (1953), Ryan (1953), Lytle (1961), Glassow (1963) and Welsh (1964) concluded that this procedure was unnecessary for small direct hernial sacs, and dangerous for the intestines and the spermatic cord in sliding hernias. They demonstrated, in large series, that adequate dissection of the sac from the spermatic cord and up into the preperitoneal space of Bogros was most important in preventing recurrence. Opening an indirect sac allows inspection of its contents and the detection of associated unknown hernias by palpation. The "Huguet maneuver" transforms a direct hernia sac into an indirect one, by exerting traction on the direct hernia sac in order to place it laterally, outside the inferior epigastric vessels. In the same way, upward traction on a femoral hernial sac could place it in the inguinal region [McLure 1939]. Eskleand (1964), Ellis (1965), Smedberg (1984) and Wantz (1989) stated that ligation of the sac was irrelevant, and for sliding hernias, it is safer to verify their contents and then to push them back into the abdominal cavity. Shulman (1993) reported several thousands of patients operated on without hernial sac ligation. He concluded that there was less postoperative pain in this series. Finally, Levy (1951), Fruchaud (1965) and Wantz (1982) recommended that long indirect sacs should not be dissected distally in order to avoid

damage to testicular vessels. That is what I believe as well, in spite of higher rates of postoperative intrasaccular seromas which may need repeated needle aspiration.

4. Reconstruction of the Inguinal Canal

Reconstruction of the posterior inguinal wall in order to resist high abdominal pressures and prevent peritoneal protrusion, would heal inguinal hernias. This goal is achieved by two radically different methods.

a) The "Tissue Repair Technique"

The "tissue repair technique", which reconstructs the posterior wall by sutures or myoplasties, utilizes for this the fibrous structures of the myofascial layer, excluding red muscular fibers. This may impose some tension on the suture line, so that a relaxing incision is also performed to avoid tension. Operations which are limited to the reconstruction of the deep inguinal ring, thus leaving the rest of the posterior inguinal without further reconstruction, may lead to side recurrences in this area.

Some authors, such as McVay, stress the importance of complete closure of the "myopectineal orifice", which leads to high tension on the suture line. Postoperative pain rates and recurrences are higher unless a relaxing incision is performed at the same time.

We agree with the Shouldice school that herniorrhaphy should be carried out with a synthetic monofilament nonabsorbable suture. In a recent series, Deroide et al (1996) demonstrated the superiority of nonabsorbable sutures over steel wire in the Shouldice type hernia repair. There were 5.22% of recurrences using absorbable sutures, versus 0.5-3% of recurrences in other series which used nonabsorbable sutures. It should be emphasized, however, that all the operations performed by the anterior approach disturb the critical balance of physiological mechanisms which protect the inguinal canal.

b) "Mesh Repairs"

"Mesh repairs", utilizing synthetic prosthetic materials, can be performed via an anterior or posterior approach, conventionally or laparoscopically.

The advantages of prosthetic materials will be discussed later. In general, prostheses are composed of large pieces of mesh, including patches and plugs which can be cylindrical, conical or umbrella-shaped, and help to reinforce the weak posterior inguinal wall. Simply stated, patches are used to repair the direct component of hernias, while plugs repair the indirect component. This could be described as the "belt and braces" approach. Many materials have been developed since the Second World War. They are all well tolerated. The differences in physical, mechanical and morphological properties between different kinds of polymer are useful for their varied surgical applications.

The most useful prostheses in surgical practice are the semi-rigid polypropylene prosthesis (Marlex, Prolene) and the supple Dacron mesh (Mersilene). Its elasticity makes Dacron mesh suitable for packing of irregular tissue surfaces. Semi-rigid prostheses are more effective in reinforcing the abdominal wall. They are easily molded and hence are popular for laparoscopic herniorrhaphy. Coarse macroporous meshes (with large interstices) are usually preferred to smooth microporous ones because of their rapid integration into scar tissue and their good tolerance in an infected milieu. The microporous (EPTFE) or impermeable (Silastic) prostheses become surrounded by a linear arrangement of fibroblasts, and are never incorporated into the host tissue. They should be securely sutured in order to prevent migration. Absorbable meshes (polyglactine 910), which are gradually absorbed over a period of six weeks, should only be used in septic conditions. This was confirmed by the experiences of Tyrell (1989) and Alexandre (1983). The polyglactine pads proposed by Lierse (1987) and Bremer (1988) have been abandoned. As will be seen later, surgeons can place these prosthetic meshes in many anatomical regions, such as between the external oblique muscle and the deeper layers, or behind this layer. However, we believe that it is more logical to insert the prosthetic mesh into the deepest layer, so as to fulfill the hydrostatic principles of Pascal, which are independent of physiological, degenerative and other aggravating factors. This positions the mesh directly between the weak abdominal wall and the abdominal pressure thrust, rather than in a limited space. These prosthetic repairs are the only tension-free herniorrhaphies, can even be performed without sutures (sutureless repair of Gilbert, giant prosthesis repair of Stoppa).

In conclusion, the results of herniorrhaphy depend on the quality of the inguinal structures, which should be correctly evaluated, and the surgical procedure. Careful operative technique will avoid the development of hematomas, seromas and infections, and every effort should be made to prevent such complications. Hernia surgery is particularly prone to complications because it is frequently performed and considered as "minor" surgery.

5. Anesthesia in Hernia Surgery

There is a tendency, nowadays, towards more ambulatory surgery and shorter hospitalization. Intramuscular premedication is often replaced by an intravenous infusion of sedative, anxiolytic and analgesic agents which can be managed by the patient himself. This technique improves patient satisfaction and reduces drug dosage.

The instructions given to the patient during the preoperative interview with the anesthetist are of the most importance. A well informed patient can participate in the choice between local, general and spinal anesthesia. Young's review (1987) comparing different anesthetic methods in surgical hernia repair is an interesting update on this subject.

a) Anesthesia and Laparoscopic Herniorrhaphies

Laparoscopic herniorrhaphy has modified anesthetic techniques. The pneumoperitoneum produces a decrease in cardiac output due to lowered venous return and raised peripheral resistance, and hypercapnia due to the modification of the pulmonary ventilation/perfusion ratio. In long-standing pneumoperitoneum, a decrease in renal and mesenteric blood perfusion occurs, as well as an increase in intracranial and intraocular pressure. Gas insufflation into the retroperitoneal spaces produces hypercapnia. This is proportionate to the pressure and to the amount of insufflated CO_2. Thus, anesthetic monitoring and technique are more complex in laparoscopic hernia surgery than in traditional repairs.

Epidural anesthesia for laparoscopic surgery is possible. However, it should block all dermatomes from T4 to S5 levels in order to effect peritoneal and abdominal wall analgesia. Its hemodynamic effects, added to those of the pneumoperitoneum, limits its use to rapid surgical procedures in young patients.

b) Local Anesthesia Performed by the Surgeon

Carl Koller, a Viennese ophthalmologist who sought for celebrity, used locally applied cocaine solution in ocular anesthesia. He was informed by Sigmund Freud, another Viennese doctor who was not, however, interested in surgery. Halsted from Baltimore (1884) confirmed the efficiency of truncal anesthesia in general surgery. Paul Reclus from Paris (1895) and Schleich (1894) from Berlin diluted the cocaine solution used for local anesthesia, in order to reduce its toxicity.

Local anesthesia is now largely used for primary herniorrhaphy by the inguinal approach, even when a prosthesis is to be inserted (more than 90% of patients operated on in major hernia institutions in the USA). It offers numerous advantages. The preoperative premedication as well as the physiological consequences (headache, intestinal ileus, nausea, retention of urine and respiratory complications) are markedly reduced compared with other forms of anesthesia. Return to normal physical activity is more rapid (this is important for the prevention of DVT), and patients more often leave hospital on the same day of operation. Anxiety and noncooperation (which are common in young patients) are reasonable contra-indications to local anesthesia.

Advocates of local anesthesia often mention the satisfaction felt by the surgeon in applying his anatomical knowledge, the possibility for him to converse with the patient during the operation and the possibility for the patient to choose the background music and to collaborate actively in the operation. Usually the surgeon asks the patient to cough or to strain in order to identify the hernia sac and to check the soundness of the repair.

Many local anesthetic agents are now available. We use 0.5% lidocaine combined with 0.84% semi-molar sodium bicarbonate solution (40 ml of lidocaine and 2 ml of sodium bicarbonate). This solution, which has a pH of 7.5%, is painless during local infiltration. Lidocaine is also presented in combination with adrenaline. This is useful for the superficial layers. However, it has an acid pH which necessitates the addition of 2.5 ml of the same sodium bicarbonate to each 20 ml of mixture.

It has been suggested that the presence of an anesthetist is not required during an operation performed under local anesthesia. This, together with the elimination of unnecessary laboratory tests, still further reduces medical costs. However, recommendations from Harvard Medical School (1986) suggest the need for monitored care for all anesthetic techniques. In day surgery, many surgeons perform the local anesthesia in association with an intravenous administration of a sedative (e.g. Diprivan) in order to enhance the patient well-being. This implies that an anesthetist should be present during the operation (Amid, Gilbert), a procedure known as ambulatory or standby anesthesia.

We believe that the presence of an anesthetic assistant who has special training in standby anesthesia is important in case of (fortunately rare) anesthetic morbidity (anaphylaxic, syncope and CNS problems). This

Table 9.4. Toxic doses of local anesthetics

Anesthetics	mg/kg	ml
Procaine	18	100 (1%)
Novocaine	22	50 (2%)
Lidocaine	7	100 (0.5%)
Bupivacaine	1.5	150 (0.25%)

Table 9.5. Duration of action of local anesthetics (min)
(N = without adrenaline, A = with adrenaline, 1/200,000)

Anesthetics	%	Local		Peridural		Rachis	
		N	A	N	A	N	A
Procaine	0.5	30	120	30	90	-	-
Lidocaine	0.5	90	240	-	-	-	-
	1	120	300	60	180	-	-
	2	Toxic		90	-	-	-
	5	Toxic		-	-	-	60
Bupivacaine	0.25	180	400	360	180	-	-
	0.5	Toxic		> 90	180	180	-

assistant can also supervise the postoperative analgesia.

Local anesthesia still involves some intraoperative discomfort. This depends on the surgeon's dexterity, the design of the operating table and the duration of the operation. It is essential to record all agents administered (Table 9.4) and the overall time of the operation (Table 9.5).

In conclusion, local anesthesia can be widely used for primary noncomplicated hernia repair if it is performed by experienced teams in psychologically well prepared, nonobese and nonallergic adults. Many controlled studies show the same results in patients operated on under local anesthesia as in those receiving other anesthetic techniques [Flanagan 1981; Britton in Hernia 3 1989; Royal College of Surgeons of England 1993].

C. Classical Herniorrhaphy by the Inguinal Approach

The first herniorrhaphies were performed before the era of aseptic surgery at the end of the last century. After excision of the hernia sac, the external inguinal ring was narrowed (Czerny, Lucas-Champonnière, Mc Ewen, Halsted, Ferguson, Andrews). This technique is no more practiced. Marcy (1892) stressed the importance of the closure of the deep inguinal ring. At the same time, Bassini (1887) suggested reconstruction of the myofascial layer which was often deficient. This forms the basis of surgical hernia repair in Europe. However, it is not always well executed. In contrast to the retrofunicular repair of Bassini, Forgue (1909) suggested the totally prefunicular repair. This proved ineffective and has now been abandoned. Shortly before the Second World War, McVay (1939) described the solid anatomical structures of the inguinal region. These structures, which are very important for the surgeon, are the pectineal ligament (or ligament of Cooper) and the iliopubic tract (or bandelette of Thomson). He proposed his "posterior reconstruction" of the groin. In 1945, Shouldice developed a surgical procedure that was principally based on the Bassini concept (still unknown in North America). He introduced many modifications and was concerned about every detail. The postoperative follow-up of his patients was meticulous.

Many publications followed. These include the different editions of the Hernia textbook by Nyhus et al. in 1964, 1978, 1989 and 1995, the articles of Rives et al., those of Houdard et al. in the Encyclopédie Médico-Chirurgicale in France, the report of the 86th Congrès Français de Chirurgie by Houdard and Stoppa, and the last edition of "Chirurgie de la paroi abdominale" by Chevrel et al., which has been translated into English and Japanese. These publications contain the technical details of all hernia repairs mentioned in this chapter, and other classical herniorrhaphies as well

1. The Marcy Operation (1871)

This achieves adequate closure of the deep inguinal ring. It was recommended by McVay for small indirect inguinal hernias associated with a moderate enlargement of the deep inguinal ring and no defect in the inguinal floor. The technique was described again by Griffith in "Hernia" (1964, 1985, 1995).

Marcy's operation can be performed under local anesthesia (Fig. 9.4). Good exposure of the deep inguinal ring is obtained after thinning of the spermatic cord and opening of the cremaster muscle. The spermatic cord is displaced laterally as far as possible and the external spermatic (or cremasteric) vessels divided if necessary. Nonabsorbable sutures are then placed progressively from medial to lateral in order to close the medial end of the deep inguinal ring. These sutures take up the conjoint tendon above and the iliopubic tract and the femoral sheath inferiorly. The deep inguinal ring is, thus, closed snugly around the sper-

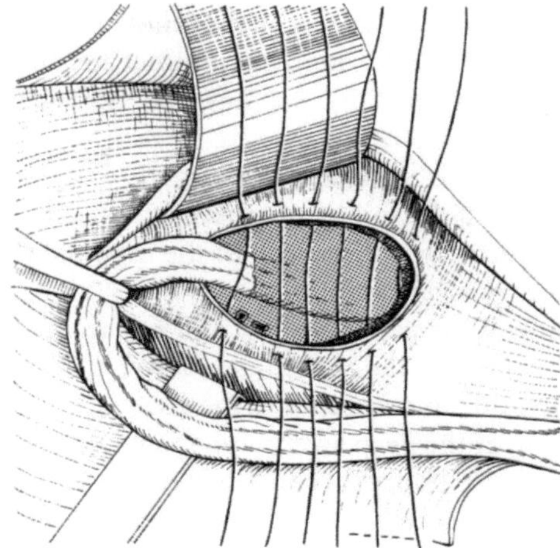

Fig. 9.4. The essential step in Marcy repair is the closure of the deep inguinal ring. The cremaster m. has been resected and the hernial sac resected and closed via the inguinal approach. The fascia transversalis is sutured transversely, medial to the spermatic cord (adapted from Griffith 1964)

matic cord, admitting only the tip of the little finger laterally. The external oblique aponeurosis is then closed with a continuous suture of slow absorbable material, over the spermatic cord.

In a series of 580 herniorrhaphies, McVay (1958) performed this procedure in 59.3% of patients with 3.2% of recurrences. Of the 13 recurrences in this series, 11 occurred after the Marcy operation.

This operation is not commonly practiced in France. Nyhus believes that it is indicated in type II indirect inguinal hernias associated with an intact inguinal floor. No recent series have been published.

The advantages of Marcy's operation are many. It is simple and does not include division of the myofascial layer which is thus preserved if it is solid and intact.

As in all other procedures performed by the inguinal approach, complications such as injuries to superficial nerves and spermatic cord elements, can occur.

2. The Bassini Operation (1887)

This important innovation was incorrectly reproduced by many generations of surgeons, even the Italians. Catterina (1931), who was one of Bassini's disciples, recalled the original steps of the operation in his publications. These are (Fig. 9.5):

- low oblique inguinal incision parallel to the line of Malgaigne;
- incision of the external oblique aponeurosis;

- dissection and isolation of the whole spermatic cord, the cremaster and the indirect hernia sac together "en bloc" by the finger or the scalpel handle;
- excision of the cremaster muscle;
- dissection of the indirect hernia sac;
- exposure and wide opening of the inguinal floor and the transversalis fascia;
- opening of the peritoneal sac and replacement of its contents into the abdominal cavity;
- high ligature and excision of the sac;
- suturing of the deep layer with 6 to 8 interrupted sutures of a nonabsorbable material, beginning medially, and placed carefully. They include the tendinous insertion of rectus abdominis and the aponeurotic portions of the internal oblique and transversus muscles (falx inguinalis) as well as the transversalis fascia and the inguinal ligament. While suturing, the spermatic cord is placed in contact with the inguinal floor, and the external oblique aponeurosis is then sutured anterior to it.

This original technique underwent many modifications. Some of them resulted in completely different techniques, such as those of Andrews, Ferguson and Coley which were used for a long time in the USA.

Other variations performed in Europe have also not followed the Bassini's principles. The transversalis fascia was not divided in these techniques.

Some other variations are, however, more in keeping with the Bassini operation. The Shouldice operation (1945-1952) was a return to the Bassini method, although Shouldice was unaware of Bassini's publications. The Houdard (1973) and Chevrel (1983) modifications also deserve mention.

Houdard proposed some interesting technical modifications. He stressed the need to ligate the external spermatic vessels in order to displace the spermatic cord laterally, and he performed a two layered instead of a one layer repair of the inguinal wall. The first layer brings together the transversalis fascia and the iliopubic band, and the second joins the conjoint tendon to the inguinal ligament (of Poupart). Houdard used his procedure for both direct and indirect inguinal hernias.

In his original works, Bassini (1887) published a recurrence rate of 3.2%. At the same time, Berlinger reported a 11.5% recurrence rate in 720 operations and Belanger published a 25% recurrence in 1,102 cases.

The advantages of the original Bassini operation are its simplicity, the absence of significant distortion of the inguinal region and the repair being performed on

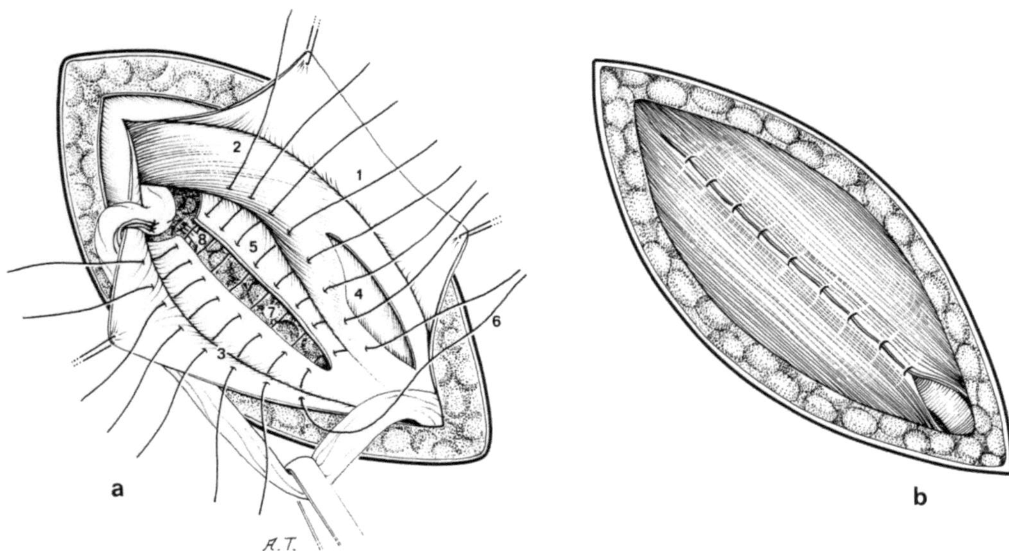

Fig. 9.5. Bassini repair. **a** Note the correct method of performing this procedure: the fascia transversalis is incised widely to allow suturing to the deep layer. The sutures take up the inguinal ligament and the fascia transversalis below, and the fascia transversalis and falx inguinalis above. *1* Aponeurosis of external oblique; *2* internal oblique; *3* inguinal ligament; *4* relaxing incision of the falx inguinalis with exposure of the fleshy fibers of the rectus abdominis; *5* fascia transversalis; *6* abdominal wall repair achieved with gauge 000 nonabsorbable interrupted sutures; *7* subperitoneal fat. **b** The aponeurosis of the external oblique is repaired by interrupted sutures in front of the conjoint tendon

Table 9.6. Rate of recurrence after Bassini's operation (inguinal hernias)

Authors	# Cases	% Follow-up	Years Follow-up	% Recurrences
Madden (1993)	2,374	-	-	1.9
Marsden (1962)	367	-	-	4
Houdard (1984)	46	69.6	-	6.2
Vayre (1965)	305	-	-	7.2
Callum (1974)	186	-	5 to 12	7.5
Chevrel (1983)	119	50	-	8.4
Magnusson (1981)	305	-	6 to 7	9.6
Hay (1995)	1,706	-	8	11
Berliner (1978)	720	-	4 to 9	11.5
Piper (1969)	246	67.7	1 to 6	15.8

the myofascial layer. Local anesthesia is also appropriate for this operation, although it was originally carried out under general anesthesia.

The risks of injuries to the superficial nerves and spermatic cord are the same as in other repairs.

We believe that the routine division of the deep inguinal layer is not necessary in type I and type II inguinal hernias. In many direct type III hernias, weakness of the deep layer persists in spite of partial excision and reconstruction of the transversalis fascia, so that recurrence rates are higher in this group.

Thus, it seems reasonable to state that the Bassini operation is indicated in direct type II hernias and in small type III hernias. We think that it is inadequate for large type III and recurrent hernias. It is not indicated in femoral hernias.

A review of all published series of the Bassini operation is shown in table 9.6.

a) The Houdard Procedure

Houdard has put forward some interesting modifications of the technique (Fig. 9.6). The neck of the sac is divided so as to allow lateral displacement of the cord; the muscle and fascia are repaired in two layers behind the cord, the first joins the transversalis fascia to the iliopubic band, the second joins the conjoint tendon to the inguinal ligament. Houdard uses this

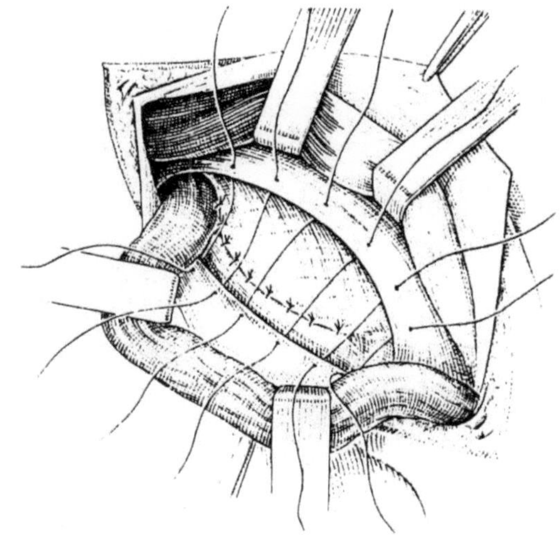

Fig. 9.6. Houdard's procedure resembles Shouldice repair in the mantle-like suturing of the fascia transversalis and the suturing of the muscle arch to the inguinal ligament

technique for both direct and indirect inguinal hernias.

b) The Chevrel Procedure

Founded on the Bassini principle, the technique proposed by J. P. Chevrel has three advantages over the original proposal of the Master of Padua. These are:

1) insertion of a tension free stitch between the conjoint tendon and the inguinal ligament, thanks to a relieving incision in the conjoint tendon;
2) reinforcement of the posterior wall of the canal by the aponeurosis of the external oblique, which is the procedure of choice in direct hernias;
3) reconstruction of the deep inguinal ring, thus minimizing the risk of a recurrent direct hernia.

The skin incision is low, starting at the pubic tubercle. The external oblique aponeurosis is incised at the external ring for three or four centimeters in the direction of the anterior-superior iliac spine. After isolating the spermatic cord and identifying the ilioinguinal and iliohypogastric nerves, the cremaster is incised longitudinally, without resecting it, which uncovers the peritoneal sac in the case of an indirect hernia. In most cases the sac is resected and its stump tucked under the transversus muscle and its fascia, as described by Barker. The dissection of the deep aspect of the two layers of the external oblique aponeurosis exposes the inguinal ligament below and the anterior aspect of the conjoint tendon above, in front of the

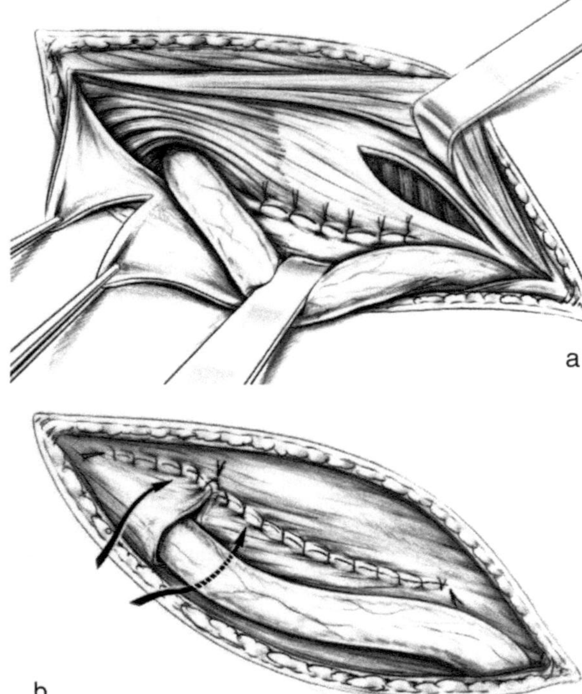

Fig. 9.7. The Chevrel procedure. **a** First layer of suture, lowering the falx inguinalis to the inguinal ligament after a relaxing incision on the rectus sheath. **b** The aponeurosis of the external oblique m. is sutured behing the cord after making a vertical incision on the inferior flap

lower end of the rectus abdominis muscle. A curved relieving incision is then made, similar to that described in the McVay operation for the repair of femoral hernias. The transversalis fascia is then incised from the deep ring medially, part of it being resected in the case of a direct hernia. Finally the lower leaf of the external oblique aponeurosis is incised at right angles to its free border at the medial edge of the deep inguinal ring, but not as far as the inguinal ligament. The repair is carried out in two layers, using interrupted sutures of oo nonabsorbable material.

The sutures of the first layer take up the transversalis fascia and the inguinal ligament below, and the transversalis fascia and the conjoint tendon above (Fig. 9.7a). Due to the relaxing incision, they can be tied without tension. The second layer lies behind the cord, joining the upper leaf of the external oblique aponeurosis to the medial part of the lower leaf of that muscle, as far as the deep ring. The suture on the lateral part of this aponeurosis, lateral to the deep ring, allows one to fashion the caliber of the ring to fit the spermatic cord, following the Marcy principle, but in

a more effective way. The superficial fascia is closed with a running stitch of absorbable material, in front of the cord. This operation can be used for indirect as well as direct hernias. It gives protection against medial suprapubic recurrences, as are often seen following repairs by the inguinal route. The recurrence rate reported by Chevrel is below 2%.

3. The Shouldice Operation

R. Bendavid

The plethora of surgical techniques available for the treatment of inguinal hernias is enough to baffle the brightest and most conscientious of newcomers to the surgical field. Unfortunately, students will mimic or emulate their preceptors who may have a dedicated if not biased view of a certain technique. What we inherit from our predecessors must always be evaluated openly and objectively against the wider spectrum of what others do. The final outcome in the choice of a technique must never be what is most challenging to us as technical wizards. Instead, one should be influenced by the Hippocratic tenets of what is safest, least harmful and most affordable for the patient.

The Shouldice operation, properly understood and carried out, goes a long way towards satisfying those requirements.

The most important asset of the Shouldice repair is that it compels the acquisition of anatomical knowledge that is an absolute necessity if one is to be a competent hernia surgeon. Every surgeon will be faced at some time, with a situation where laparoscopic surgery cannot be resorted to or one where mesh cannot be used (emergencies, need for bowel resection, multiple abdominal operations, pediatrics, pregnancies, etc.). It becomes imperative, therefore, for each and every one of us to master a technique that can handle all groin hernias, regardless of the clinical constraints.

a) Evolution of the Technique

The Shouldice repair incorporates the most significant contributions of Bassini (1889) (ligation of the cremasters and division of the inguinal floor from internal ring to pubis); the inclusion of the ligament of Poupart [Bassini 1889; Halsted 1893] in the repair; the overlapping of the myoaponeurotic layers [Lucas-Champonnière 1908] to provide a substantial posterior wall.

Shouldice added the inclusion of the iliopubic ligament (Thomson's bandelette) in the repair, and an incision of the cribriform fascia to reveal unsuspected femoral hernias. The use of stainless steel wire as a suture eliminates the chronic sinuses which were observed with silk and cotton sutures.

The major contribution however was the institution of local anesthesia for all groin hernias. Though Cushing (1900) and Halsted (1893) reported the use of cocaine anesthesia in selected patients, Shouldice established the use of Procaine Hydrochloride for all patients, thus providing the largest and safest series ever studied.

As practiced today, the Shouldice operation includes several aspects which will lead a patient through to uneventful recovery. These are: weight control, local anesthesia, dissection, reconstruction, active convalescence and an assiduous follow-up.

b) Weight Control

Obesity has always been the bane of surgery. Ideal weight facilitates surgery, requires less infiltration anesthetic, allows earlier and easier ambulation and hence, a lesser incidence of pulmonary problems and deep vein thrombosis. Whether weight loss will lessen the recurrence rate in groin hernias has been a controversy which was taken up extensively by Abrahamson (1995) without convincing conclusions. In incisional hernias however, weight loss is of paramount importance.

c) Local Anesthesia

The fear engendered by general anesthesia is well anchored in many patients' minds. This fear is betrayed by a sign of relief when they learn that surgery can be done under local anesthesia. The advantages are many: a) patients will readily submit to surgery electively rather than delay until an emergency imposes an operation; b) with advancing age, pathologies develop and anesthetists are reluctant to administer a general anesthetic; c) a review in 1994 at the Shouldice Hospital revealed that 52.1% of the patient population was over the age of 50 and the associated vascular problems were seen to be: anticoagulation (Coumadin, ASA, Anturan) in 12% of the patients; history of a myocardial infarct (15%); history of angina (15%); active treatment for congestive heart failure (17%); hypertension (20%); cardiac arrhythmias (50%) [Bendavid 1995]; d) local anesthesia eliminates the need for expensive preoperative investigations and consultations; e) on the operating table, the patient's cooperation can reveal the more discrete hernias as well as test the repair.

All patients receive sedation consisting of diazepam 10 to 20 mg and pethidine hydrochloride 50-100 mg 90 and 45 minutes preoperatively respectively. The local anesthetic is Procaine Hydrochloride (Novocaine) 1% up to 200 ml.

d) Surgery

The surgery for inguinal hernia can be divided into two clear cut components: the dissection and the reconstruction.

(1) Dissection

Procaine is first infiltrated along a line joining the anterior-superior iliac spine to the pubic crest, in order to raise a weal 5 cm wide. An incision is made along the same line extending medially over the pubic spine. The external oblique aponeurosis is divided in the direction of its fibers from the superficial inguinal ring to a point 2-3 cm lateral to the deep inguinal ring. The two resulting flaps are freed from all underlying structures. The ilioinguinal and iliohypogastric nerves will be clearly identified and protected. The cremaster muscle can now be clearly seen and is incised in the direction of its fibers from the pubic crest to the internal ring.

This step results in two flaps of cremaster, medial and lateral. The medial flap which is invariably flimsy is resected from the level of the pubis to the internal ring. The lateral flap of the cremaster which includes the external spermatic vessels and the genital branch of the genitofemoral nerve is doubly clamped and cut between the clamps. Each stump is doubly ligated with a resorbable tie. Each of these stumps will later serve a purpose. At this time any indirect and direct hernia, if present will become evident. An indirect sac is dissected from the spermatic cord and freed at its base from the loose adhesions of the transversalis fascia to beyond the level of the internal ring. If it appears safe to do so, the sac may be opened, ligated and resected. If there is doubt because of the possibility of a sliding hernia, the sac is simply reduced into the preperitoneal space.

The next step consists in incising the floor of the canal from the medial aspect of the deep inguinal ring to the level of the pubis. This incision must cut through the transversalis fascia and its posterior lamina to enter the preperitoneal space of Bogros. This is confirmed by the appearance of the glistening fatty tissue of the preperitoneal space. When the incision is complete one can observe medially the internal oblique, transversus abdominis and the lateral edge of the rectus muscle. The lateral edge of the newly incised posterior wall, as it proceeds towards the inguinal ligament is the iliopubic tract or bandelette of Thomson. At this stage, the cribriform fascia which lies lateral to the inguinal ligament, is incised from the level of the pubis to the level of the femoral vessels. This maneuver will allow inspection of the femoral ring from above and the femoral orifice from below. Care must be taken not to injure the iliopubic vein situated on the deeper aspect of the iliopubic tract.

(2) Reconstruction

Reconstitution of the floor of the inguinal canal is carried out with stainless steel wire (gauge 32 or 34: Ethicon). Two strands are used. Each strand passes back and forth, providing two lines of suture. The first strand is inserted, from a lateral approach, into the iliopubic tract near the pubis, then crosses over to be inserted through the transversalis fascia, the lateral edge of the rectus, the transversus and internal oblique. A knot is tied (Fig. 9.8a). The short end is held with a hemostat, the longer end proceeds towards the internal ring, repeating the suture which approximates the two borders of the incised floor. At the midportion of the floor the rectus becomes too medially placed and is omitted. Near the internal ring, the suture picks up the lateral stump of the cremaster and carries it deeply within the newly formed internal ring (Fig. 9.8b). The suture now reverses its course as line #2, to proceed toward the pubic crest by incorporating the inguinal ligament (Fig. 9.8c). The two ends of this strand are now tied at the level of the pubis.

Strand #2 is now used, beginning at the internal ring and picks up the internal oblique and transversus, then crosses to incorporate the inner aspect of the external oblique aponeurosis along a line parallel and superficial to the inguinal ligament (Fig. 9.8d), proceeding towards the pubic crest, where it reverses its course, to return towards the internal ring, incorporating along its way, a more superficial layer of the external oblique aponeurosis. At the internal ring, a knot is tied, thus completing the four lines of the repair (Fig. 9.8e). The medial cremasteric stump is anchored near the pubic crest, to prevent eventual drooping of the testicle. The spermatic cord is then replaced in its normal anatomic bed and the external oblique aponeurosis is approximated over it with a running strand of absorbable suture. The subcutaneous tissue is approximated with absorbable sutures and the skin sealed with Michel clips. Half of these clips are removed in 24 h, the remainder at 48 h. The surgery terminated, the patient stands, walks to a wheelchair and returns to his room. Following four hours of bedrest to allow for the premedication to dissipate, the patient is encouraged to ambulate. On the morning of the following 24 to 72 h, all patients participate in a class of light exercises.

e) Follow-up

The follow-up of patients at Shouldice Hospital is assiduous if not tenacious. Over 100,000 letters are mailed yearly to determine the status of the operation. From 1952 to 1992, the recurrence rate has varied between a low of 0.177% (1991) to a high of 1.535% (1973) [Bendavid 1995].

Since 1983 when prosthetics were introduced at Shouldice Hospital, 1,600 out of 80,225 patients have benefited from their use (2%).

Table 9.7 illustrates what type of hernias required mesh in 1993. Table 9.8 identifies results as reported by various authors.

f) Complications

Complications following the Shouldice repair are uncommon and invariably of a benign nature. Thanks to local anesthesia and early ambulation, pulmonary and venous complications are rare. A mortality of 30 out 230,000 operations is convincing evidence of the safety of the procedure. The deaths have occurred in elderly patients and have been of cardiac and cerebrovascular nature [Bendavid 1992].

(1) Infections

The incidence varies from 0.5 to 1% from year to year. This low incidence is due to the fact that no contaminated surgery is performed in our theaters. These infections are invariably subcutaneous, and may require antibiotics and drainage. There is no record of a deep seated infection requiring a takedown of the repair.

(2) Hematomas

Hematomas represent a minor problem which may require exploration of the incision (1 to 5 a year).

(3) Hydroceles

Postoperative hydroceles have been identified in one of the largest series ever reported, by Obney (1956) and of the order of 0.7% out of 14,442 operations.

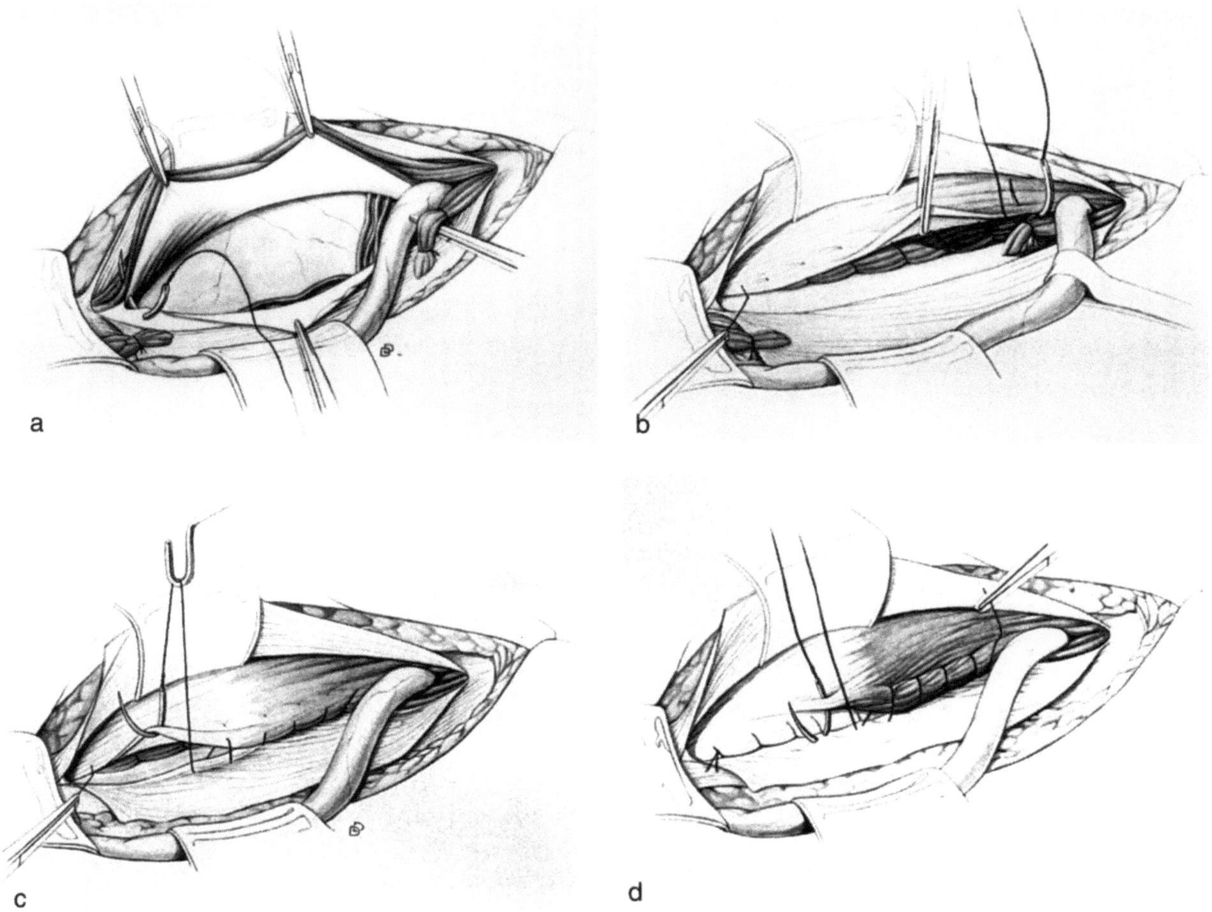

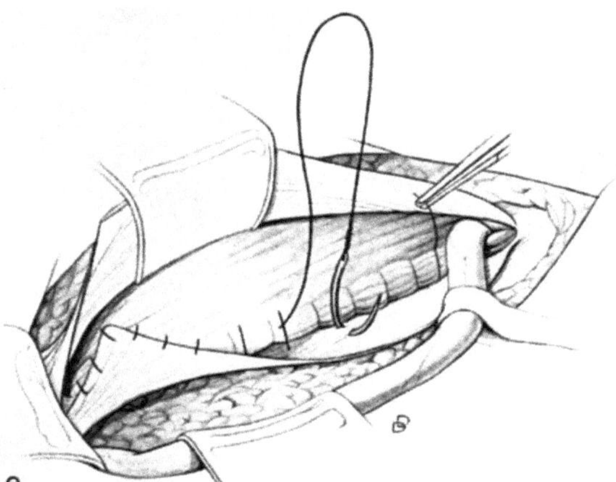

Fig. 9.8. Shouldice's procedure. **a** First line of suture: iliopubic tract laterally then across through transversalis fascia, lateral edge of rectus, transversus abdominus, internal oblique. **b** Continuation of line 1. The last stitch incorporates the lateral cremasteric stump and carries it deep within the new internal ring. **c** Line 2 now incorporates the inguinal ligament all the way to the pubic crest. **d** Line 3 begins at the internal ring, includes the internal oblique and transversus laterally then crosses over to include the inner aspect of the lower end of the external oblique aponeurosis, creating a pseudo-inguinal ligament. **e** The 4th line returning towards the internal ring. A portion of the lateral crus of the external oblique covers the medial portion of the new floor of the canal

Table 9.7. Operations where mesh was used (1993)

Type	Primary	Recurrences	Total	%
Inguinal hernias	7	52	59	1.03
Femoral hernias	15	18	33	0.58
Inguinofemoral hernias	1	21	22	0.39
Indirect /direct/ femoral hernias	9	16	25	0.44
Paravascular	-	3	3	0.05
Others	1	3	4	0.07
TOTAL	33	113	146	2.56

Table 9.8. Results of the Shouldice repair from various authors

Authors	# Cases	% Follow-up	Years Follow-up	% Recurrences
Shearburn & Myers	550	100	13	0.2
Volpe & Galli	415	50	3	0.2
Wantz	2087	-	5	0.3
Myers & Shearburn	953	100	18	0.7
Devlin	350	-	6	0.8
Flament	134	-	6	0.9
Wantz	3,454	-	1 to 20	1.0
Bocchi	1,708	80	7	1.16
Welsh	2,748	-	35	1.46
Moran	121	-	6	2.0
Berliner	591	-	2 to 5	2.7

(4) Testicular Atrophy

In a study published in 1995 [Bendavid et al. 1995] from the Shouldice Hospital, reviewing 59,752 cases, 52 patients were identified who had suffered testicular atrophy, an incidence of 0.08%. However, atrophy following a primary repair is of the order of 0.036% (19 of 52,583) while following the repair of recurrent hernias, the incidence is 0.46% (33 of 7,169).

g) Activity

Following surgery, no limitation is imposed on activity. I have known patients to have played tennis in 10 days and ski in 11 days.

h) Cost

A subject that is becoming more significant today because of the introduction of prosthetics and laparoscopy is cost. For the Shouldice operation, the cost of all disposable equipment (caps, masks, IV fluids, drugs, needles, syringes, dressings, local anesthetic, tubings, etc.) amounted to US$ 17.45, a figure which could never be matched by any other method of herniorrhaphy.

i) Conclusion

The introduction of prostheses and laparoscopic equipment in an attempt to improve the results obtained by a classical, open, pure tissue repair has not been convincing in terms of lesser recurrences, safety or cost. It behooves each surgeon to be competent in the performance of the open technique for he will assuredly need to resort to it at some critical future time.

References

Abrahamson J (1995) Factors and mechanisms leading to recurrence. Problems in general surgery, vol 12. Lippincott-Raven, p 59

Bassini E (1889) Nuovo metodo operativo per la cura dell 'ernia inguinale. R. Stabilimento Prosperini, Padova

Bendavid R, Andrews DF, Gilbert AI (1995) Testicular atrophy: incidence and relationship to the type of hernia and to multiple recurrent hernia. Problems in general surgery, vol 12. Lippincott-Raven, pp 225-227

Bendavid R (1995) The merits of the Shouldice repair. Problems in general surgery, vol 12. Lippincott-Raven, pp 105-109

Bendavid R (1992) The Shouldice method of inguinal herniorrhaphy. In: Nyhus LM, Baker RJ (eds) Mastery of surgery, 2nd edn. Little Brown & Co., Boston, pp 1584-1594

Cushing H (1900) The employment of local anesthesia in the radical cure of certain cases of hernia with a note upon the nervous anatomy of the inguinal region. Ann Surg 31: 1

Glassow F (1978) The Shouldice repair for inguinal hernie. In: Nyhus LM, Condon RE (eds) Hernia, 2nd edn, Lippincott, Philadelphia, p 163-178

Halsted WM (1893) The radical cure of inguinal hernia in the male. The Johns Hopkins Hospital Bulletin #29

Hay JM, Boudet MJ, Fingerhut A, et al (1995) Shouldice inguinal hernie repair in the male adult: the gold standard? A multicenter controlled trial in 1578 patients. Ann Surg 222: 719

Lucas-Champonnière M (1908) Traitement de la hernie inguinale. Acts of the second international congress of surgery, Brussels, pp 374-377

Obney N (1956) Hydrocoeles of the testicle complicating inguinal hernias. Can Med Assoc J 75: 733

Shouldice EE (1945) Surgical treatment of hernia. Ontario Med Rev 12: 43

Shouldice EE (1953) The Treatment of hernia. Ontario Med Rev 20: 670

Wantz GE (1989) The Cadanian repair: personal observations. World J Surg 13: 516

4. The McVay Operation

While the previously described techniques are in their original form only applicable to inguinal hernias, this operation can be used for both inguinal and femoral hernias. It consists in suturing the conjoint tendon and transversalis fascia to the pectineal ligament. This is the first principle of the operation. Its second principle is to relieve any excessive tension on the deep suture whenever necessary, by a counter incision in the anterior rectus sheath, which involves its deep layer [McVay 1966].

In 1939 McVay and Anson, in a review of the anatomy of the groin (500 dissections) emphasized the essential weakness of the transversalis fascia and its lower insertion into the pectineal ligament and not the inguinal ligament. In 1942 McVay suggested repairing inguinal and femoral hernias by the use of the pectineal ligament as a solid anchorage point for the suture of the fibrous arch of the deep inguinal region, thus effecting a complete reconstruction of the posterior wall of the inguinal canal. Soon afterwards it was discovered that Ruggi (1892) and later Lotheissen (1898) had already made use of the pectineal ligament. My teacher Goinard, in Algiers, also used it and published a short account in French in 1939.

As regards the other important principle of the McVay operation, that is to say the relieving incision in the anterior sheath, Wolfler (1892) seems to deserve credit for this idea, which claims to reduce tension on the suture line whenever it is required, without involving Cooper's ligament. He was imitated by Halsted, Bloodgood, Fallis, Rienhoff, and Tanner, who antedated McVay in this regard, though McVay's contribution was of much greater importance, because of the combination of the two essential operative maneuvers.

The operation is carried out wherever possible under local anesthesia via an inguinal incision, and comprises exactly the same steps up to and including the incision of the transversalis fascia. Cooper's ligament is then fully mobilized. The exposure of the femoral vascular sheath deserves a detailed description. The incision in the transversalis fascia is prolonged laterally passing between the vessels and the spermatic cord, which is retracted upwards. The fascial sheath in front of the vein is held in a forceps and drawn upwards and medially, which reveals the orifice of the femoral canal, and allows one to estimate the strength of the vascular sheath and of the fascia, at the point where it is reinforced by the iliopubic band. At this stage the suprapubic vessels are secured and if present the accessory obturator artery is divided. The deep aspect of the conjoint tendon is separated from the preperitoneal fatty tissue. The relaxing incision in the anterior rectus sheath is now carried out 1 cm from the lateral border of the rectus muscle, running vertically from the pubic tubercle for 6-8 cm (Fig. 9.9a). This allows the edge of the sheath to be brought downwards without creating a weak point, as at this point the posterior sheath, which is composed of the transversalis fascia, is thickened. The cremaster muscle is opened and removed with any associated lipomas, the external spermatic vessels are divided and ligated, so that the spermatic cord can be delivered. Any associated hernial sacs are now dealt with. Small indirect sacs are ligated and resected, large ones are carefully separated from the cord, transfixed and ligated, whereas the majority of direct sacs are simply invaginated with a purse-string suture. Sliding hernias are reduced en masse. The repair is then begun (Fig. 9.9b-d). As a retractor we use a simple soup spoon inserted under the pubic ramus and held there by the abdominal pressure: the concavity of the spoon facilitates the incision of curved needles through the pectineal ligament, but a broad right-angled retractor may serve the same purpose. The sutures are of inabsorbable material and should take up the pectineal ligament and the transversalis fascia. As the femoral vessels are approached, a finger protects the vein, which must not be retracted too far laterally so as to avoid compressing it (Lataste and Helenon illustrated this in 1960). Two or three further sutures are placed through the femoral vascular sheath, the last of which takes up the inguinal ligament in front of the vessels. This is the "transition point" of McVay (1968) which must be handled with care and under direct vision. The sutures, which should be of nonabsorbable monofilament 0 or 1, can then be drawn taut without difficulty and with no excessive tension.

It will now be seen that the musculo-tendinous layer has been brought down to the pectineal ligament between the pubic spine and the femoral vessels, obliquely and laterally, from behind and below, which displaces the iliopubic band some 2 cm to 3 cm posteriorly. The operation is terminated by closure of the external oblique in front of the spermatic cord, and finally by closure of the skin.

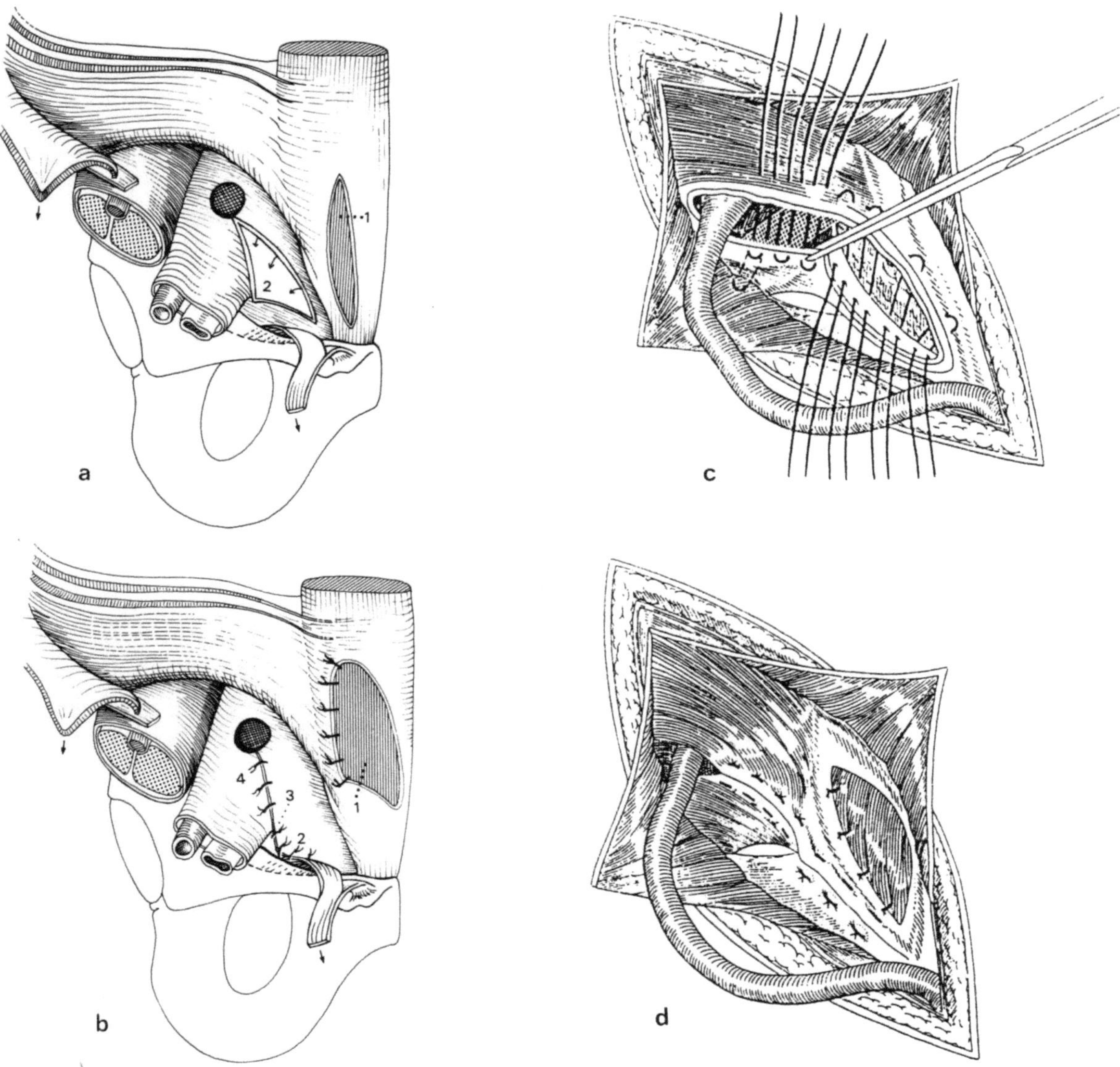

Fig. 9.9. Principles of McVay repair. **a** *1* Relaxing incision of the anterior lamina of the rectus sheath; *2* incision of the fascia transversalis from the pubic tubercle out to the deep inguinal ring. **b** *1* Suturing of the lateral margin of the relaxing incision to the rectus abdominis; *2* lowering of the fascia transversalis to Cooper's ligament; *3* the transitional suture; *4* lowering of the fascia transversalis to the vascular sheath. **c** and **d** McVay repair (according to Rives et al. 1974). **c** Deep repair and the essential "transitional suture"; note the forceps required to identify the vascular sheath and protect the femoral vessels. **d** Another essential step in McVay repair is the relaxing incision of the anterior lamina of the rectus sheath prior to repair of the external oblique

There are a few variations to this operation, which can be used for the treatment of inguinal hernias as well as femoral hernias, provided that the tissues sutured to the pectineal ligament are sufficiently solid and do not pull out. If the conjoint tendon or the fascia transversalis are weak, there is a risk of the deeper layers tearing through. When the femoral sheath is thin one may be obliged to place several sutures on to the pectoneal ligament in the neighborhood of the vessels, in a fan-shaped manner pointing upwards, but the result is not as satisfactory [Rives & Hibon 1974].

All in all this operation is anatomically correct, easy to carry out and gives a satisfactory impression to the surgeon. McVay does not recommend this type of posterior reconstruction for all groin areas but reserves it for direct hernias and indirect hernias of large size.

Complications include a certain number of cases of injury to the femoral vein occurring through the passage of sutures through its sheath. Bleeding usually stops after a few minutes of compression. This complication can be avoided by passing sutures very carefully and always under direct vision. As regards the forward transposition of the spermatic cord following downward displacement of the conjoint tendon to the pectineal ligament, this is corrected by freeing up of the deeper elements of the cord behind the abdominal wall and a careful reposition of the testicle in the lower part of the scrotum at the end of the operation. Postoperative pain is frequent, probably resulting from traction on the lower part of the musculo-fascial layers. There is also the risk of iliofemoral thrombosis resulting from compression of the vein by a suture which is placed too far laterally, or by a stitch which transfixes the vein.

The McVay operation using the pectineal ligament is a carefully controlled anatomical procedure. It is the only type of anterior repair which results in complete closure of the musculo-pectineal orifice, and can be used to treat all types of groin hernia. Its disadvantages include postoperative discomfort over the first few days which interferes with early ambulation. According to Rutledge (1995) who has a large experience of the procedure, return to work is delayed as compared with other types of surgery. The effectiveness of the relieving incision in the rectus sheath has been evaluated by Read (1981) who measured the tension at the suture line. In a few score of cases he concludes that the tension remains higher in the McVay than the Bassini type of operation. However, in the McVay group the same author found the relieving incision to be more effective in direct hernias. These conclusions have recently been confirmed by Cimpeanu in Bucharest (1995). However, one should bear in mind the view of Rutledge 1995 in this important matter, who states that when the tension remains high one should enlarge the incision. Bilateral hernias can be operated at the same session unless the first operation has proved difficult or has led to much tension. In 20% of cases Rutledge advises reinforcement of the procedure by a patch of polypropylene mesh.

As regards the indications for this type of repair, the pectineal ligament may be absent in certain recurrences. Goinard has encountered two such cases and Neidhardt one. McVay did not use the procedure for small indirect hernias which did not displace the inferior epigastric vessels, but solely for large indirect hernias, direct hernias and femoral hernias. Rutledge fur-

Table 9.9. Rate of recurrence after McVay's operation (inguinal hernias)

Authors	# Cases	% Follow-up	Years Follow-up	% Recurrences
Rutledge (1995)	572	80	9	0.13
Flament (1991)	135	-	6	1.5
Rutledge (1988)	906	97	9	2
Izard (1996)	1,332	85	5	3
Halverson (1970)	1,211	91	22	3.5
Lubeth (1979)	800	52	-	3.9
Barbier (1984)	1,140	70	9 to 17	4.7
Asmussen (1983)	270	91	1 to 5	7.5
Hay (1995)	1,706	-	8	8.6
Warlaumont (1982)	373	85	1 to 10	15.5
Panos (1992)	269	76	5	8.8

ther uses it routinely in all primary or recurrent cases whatever the type of hernia. Table 9.9 illustrates the published results.

5. The Nyhus Operation

This consists in closure of the hernial orifice by the preperitoneal route. Nyhus in 1959 described and classified a method of repair of inguinal and femoral hernias via the preperitoneal route, using the iliopubic band. One should not confuse the preperitoneal approach with the transabdominal intraperitoneal method, which has little place in hernia surgery. The posterior approach to hernias has been thoroughly reported in the four editions of "Hernia" by Nyhus and Harkins, and later by Condon. The concept was originally put forward by Annandale of Edinburgh in 1876. Lawson Tait of Birmingham (1891) described the advantages of the midline transperitoneal approach for closure of the hernial orifice. Bates of Seattle (1913) also went through the peritoneal cavity for suture of the transversalis fascia. Cheatle (1921) was the first to use the preperitoneal route. He limited himself to ligating the sac whereas Henry (1936) was the first to close the musculo-fascial layer through the same approach.

These two surgeons used the method for the treatment of inguinal, but not for femoral hernias.

Nyhus records the names of the many authors (1964 to 1995) who have repaired inguinal and femoral hernias in this way. He began to explore the possibilities of the preperitoneal route in 1955, and since 1959 has used it for closure of the orifices of direct and indirect inguinal hernias and femoral hernias, reinforcing the transversalis fascia with the iliopubic band, the fibrous rim of the deep inguinal ring and the pectineal ligament. In the four editions of "Hernia", Nyhus continues to distinguish between the preperitoneal repair of inguinal hernias and that of femoral hernias, although the incision is the same and the iliopubic band is used in each case. These observations justify our adherence to a unitary concept of groin hernias and our use of one paragraph to describe the Nyhus operation in for the two types of hernia.

The incision is made horizontally two fingers' breadths above the symphysis pubis (Fig. 9.10a-d). The musculo-aponeurotic layers are incised above the deep inguinal ring, the transversalis fascia is exposed and then incised transversely, taking care not to open the peritoneum, which is swept away together with the preperitoneal fat, by gauze dissection. At this stage the "hernial pedicle" is easily identified. A direct hernia reduces easily by simple preperitoneal dissection and an indirect or femoral hernia can be reduced by gentle traction assisted by blunt dissection. The sac is then dealt with either by ligation excision, or by invagination with a purse-string suture, bearing in mind, in the case of a direct hernia, the proximity of the bladder.

A direct hernia is repaired by closing the defect in the transversalis fascia with interrupted sutures, the lower edge of which merges into the iliopubic band. When this band is stretched by a large direct hernia the transversalis fascia must be sutured to the pectineal ligament. In the case of an oblique external hernia the upper and lower margins of the defect are sutured horizontally, either in front of or behind the cord. With large indirect hernias the distal part of the sac may be left open at the base of the scrotum, having reduced its contents. The cord is then drawn laterally and the defect is sutured medial to it, the cord is then drawn medially and the repair of the hernial defect completed on its lateral side. In the case of a femoral hernia, the sac is usually easily reduced by traction unless the hernia is incarcerated, in which case it is necessary to incise the medial part of the iliopubic band or the reflected ligament (of Gimbernat). The

femoral canal is closed by suturing the medial part of the iliopubic band to the pectineal ligament. In this approach there is no problem with identifying the external iliac vein, which is easily protected during precise closure of the femoral canal. An aberrant obturator artery is also easily seen and safeguarded.

Nyhus advises a relieving incision in the anterior rectus sheath in type IIIA (direct), IIIB (large indirect) and IV (recurrent) hernias according to his classification. The suprainguinal incision approach greatly facilitates the use of the pectineal ligament for the repair, which puts the inguinal structures under some tension. Lampe [in "Hernia" 1978] goes so far as to suggest a double vertical incision in the anterior rectus sheath, one above and one below the suprailiac incision.

Having for a long time resisted the use of prosthetic material in the preperitoneal position to reinforce the repair, Nyhus is now in favor of this when there is no risk of sepsis and the hernia is recurrent. He describes a number of procedures which can be combined with this technique including prostatectomy, cystoprostatectomy, orchidopexy, vascular procedures and appendectomy. Although the results of these combined procedures appear satisfactory, we personally are in principle opposed to the combination of a potentially septic operation with a hernia repair, particularly if the suprainguinal route is used, which may result in postoperative eventration if sepsis occurs.

Results. In a series of 1,200 primary repairs (1993) Nyhus reports a very low morbidity in particular as regards testicular complications or postoperative neuralgia. The five year recurrence rate is 1% for femoral hernias, 3% for indirect and 6% for direct inguinal hernias, as against 2% in the case of prosthetic repairs.

Other North American surgeons have reported similar results. But some who have had good results following primary repair on indirect hernias have been disappointed by those in direct hernias, as the following recurrence rates will show:

    28% [Margoles & Brown 1971]
    16% [Harris 1971]
    17% [Robertson 1966 & Ljungdahl 1978]
    21% [Gaspar 1971]
    35% [Dyson 1965] and 18% [Skeie 1971]

This is one reason why Nyhus has suggested reinforcing the repair with a polypropylene patch (6 × 14 cm) fixed to the pectineal ligament and stretched out behind the abdominal wall.

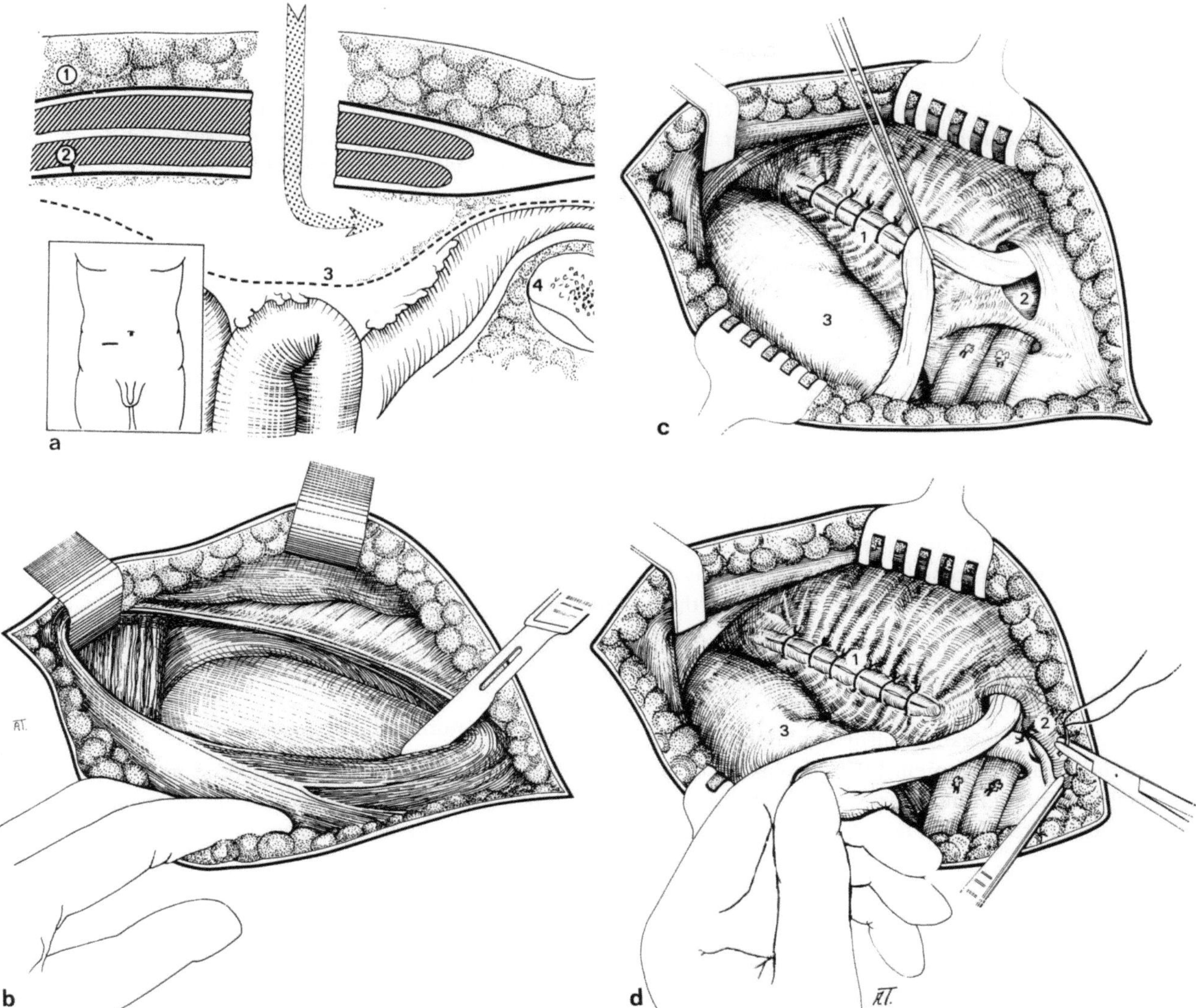

Fig. 9.10. Nyhus repair. **a** Approach via the preperitoneal space. *1* Subcutaneous areolar tissue; *2* fascia transversalis; *3* peritoneum; *4* horizontal ramus of pubis. **b** The incision of the fascia transversalis is begun flush with the deep inguinal ring. **c** Endoparietal view; *1* closure of the direct, inguinal hernia by interrupted sutures; *2* deep inguinal ring; *3* peritoneum (displaced at the beginning of the operation by blunt dissection). **d** Endoparietal view; *1* reduction of the direct hernia; *2* narrowing of the deep ring lateral to the spermatic cord; *3* peritoneum (adapted from Nyhus and Condon 1978)

6. General Observations on Suture Repairs

Although this type of operation has been the longest to be practiced, suture repairs present a certain number of disadvantages. Wide experience and a fair degree of skill are required to estimate the quality of the structures employed. Classical suture methods are of uncertain benefit for the repair of recurrent hernias, and there is always an excessive degree of tension on the suture line which is responsible for postoperative pain and a number of early recurrences.

Weakening of the scar tissue is an unavoidable fact which is not taken into consideration. There will always be patients with degenerated tissues (connective tissue disorders are an extreme example), and one can add the risks of involvement of the superficial nerves and the elements of the spermatic cord, particularly in the case of recurrent hernias re-repaired via the inguinal route. Finally, mention should be made of the unnecessary disruption of the posterior wall in hernias type I and II.

These criticisms have resulted in a tendency to restrict the indications for suture repair. The Marcy operation should be reserved for hernias type II or I (though theoretically unsuitable for this latter) and the Bassini procedure for hernias type II or III (but the weakness of the posterior wall is ignored in the last type). The McVay operation should be reserved for hernias type II and III (ignoring the considerable tension which results from it). For any type of recurrent hernia the present tendency is virtually always to use synthetic material.

D. Tissue Transfers via the Inguinal Route

These are not often used today, except possibly the Berger-Orr procedure. We will mention them briefly in order to include them within the therapeutic armamentarium. When the deeper layers are so weakened that no suture is possible without tension, this it would seem logical to close the hernial defect by the use of neighboring muscles and aponeuroses.

1. The Berger-Orr Procedure

Berger (1902) began by suturing the conjoint tendon to the inguinal ligament, as in the Bassini operation. He then incised the anterior rectus sheath a finger's breadth parallel to its lateral border (Fig. 9.11a). The resulting flap was then brought down across the canal and sutured so as to reinforce its deep layer. Vayre and Petit-Pazos (1965) suggested some further details: the incision in the rectus sheath must be as medial as possible and curved laterally, measuring 5 to 7 cm, without detaching the lateral layer before passing nonabsorbable sutures taking up the inguinal ligament and the free edge of the aponeurotic flap. The sutures are then successively tied from below upwards, so as to turn the flap downwards, resulting in a tension-free plasty around the external edge of the rectus (Fig. 9.11b).

Two supplementary maneuvers are advised, namely the careful reconstruction of the posterior layer and its reinforcement by a synthetic prosthesis. This procedure, which reinforces the inguinal triangle, at the same time creates a weak spot at the lateral border of the rectus, close to its medial angle, giving rise to a possible Spigelian type of recurrence, as the posterior rectus sheath at this point is often extremely weak. Vayre and Petit-Pazos state that they have frequently used this technique and are completely satisfied with it.

2. The Hindmarsh Procedure

A similar procedure is that of Hindmarsh [in Detrie 1967]. The rectus sheath is incised parallel to the inguinal ligament and sutured to it, rather as in the

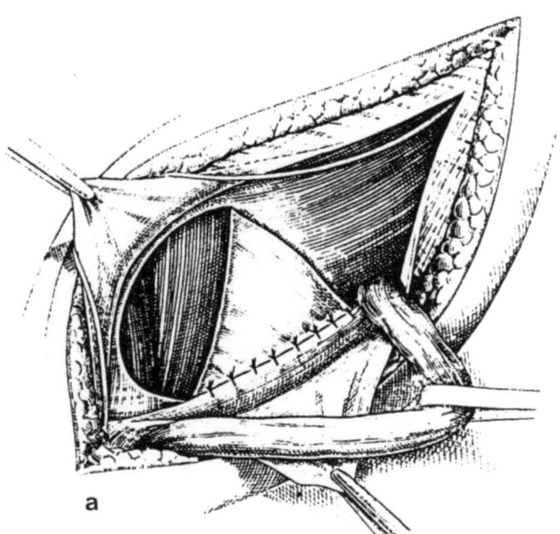
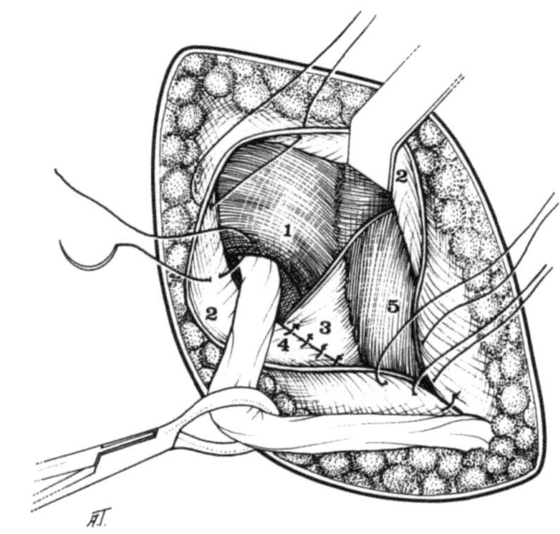

Fig. 9.11. a Berger-Orr autoplasty [Quénu and Perrotin 1955]. **b** The technique, according to Vayre. Repair is done using a flap (3) derived from the aponeurotic covering of the terminal part of the rectus abdominis (5). This covering is formed by the blending together of the aponeuroses of the internal oblique and transverse. The flap is sutured to the inguinal ligament (4). The lateral suture, positioned above and lateral to the spermatic cord, and between the inguinal ligament below and the internal oblique and transverse above (1), is designed to avoid external recurrence. The aponeurosis of the external oblique (2) can be sutured either in front of or behind (as shown) the spermatic cord

preceding technique. In order to cover the defect so created the inferior layer of the external oblique aponeurosis is incised vertically at the level of the emergence of the spermatic cord and the aponeurotic flap thus created is sutured to the upper and medial edge of the incision in the rectus sheath.

3. Transposition of the Spermatic Cord

Without necessarily approving the principle, and bearing in mind the absence of recorded results, the concept of transposition of the cord and testicle should be mentioned, if only for the sake of completeness. In this technique the cord and the testicle are completely freed throughout their scrotal course, and re-introduced into the preperitoneal space through the deep inguinal ring. This creates a "button hole", through the groin either across the rectus [Wolfler 1892] or at its lateral border [Leslie 1978] or above and lateral to the inguinal canal [Ferrand & Pellissier 1955; Toupet 1963] through which the testis can be replaced in its scrotal site. We strongly disadvise this technique because of the high risk of ischemic orchitis and testicular atrophy. Furthermore it does not resolve, or may even exacerbate, the problem of the weakness of the inguinal structures.

4. Transfer of Fascia Lata or Skin

Lattices constructed by strips of autogenous fascia lata or skin [Suire 1966; Gosset 1972] have not been widely used. A strip of skin cut from the edge of the incision, 5 mm across, is carefully freed from fat. A traction stitch is inserted at each end and a lattice is then constructed from below upwards from the inguinal ligament to the conjoint tendon, with the aid of a Reverdin needle into which the traction stitch is laid [Detrie 1967] (Fig. 9.12). We have no knowledge of any published series of hernias repaired in this way.

Ménégaux (1965) and Pautet (1969) used a free skin graft taken from the outer part of the thigh and carefully freed of fat, then sutured to the inguinal ligament below and the conjoint tendon above, to compensate for the loss of abdominal wall structure. It is important to stretch this piece of skin "tight as a drum" so that the epithelial elements degenerate and it behaves as a source of collagen [Detrie 1957]. Once again we have no knowledge of published series using this approach.

5. General Criticism of Tissue Transfer

All these procedures which use neighboring structures have the disadvantage of still further weakening these structures, which are already abnormal either congenitally or through acquired factors. This applies equally to the Berger-Hindmarsh operation as to the complimentary techniques such as additional suture lines and movement of flaps. The use of skin lattices is a relatively complex method which requires training in plastic surgery and one cannot be certain that it does not carry the same disadvantages as the suture methods, and the risk of late eventration through the scarred area. The use of skin patches goes some way to answering the problem of replacement of loss of sub-

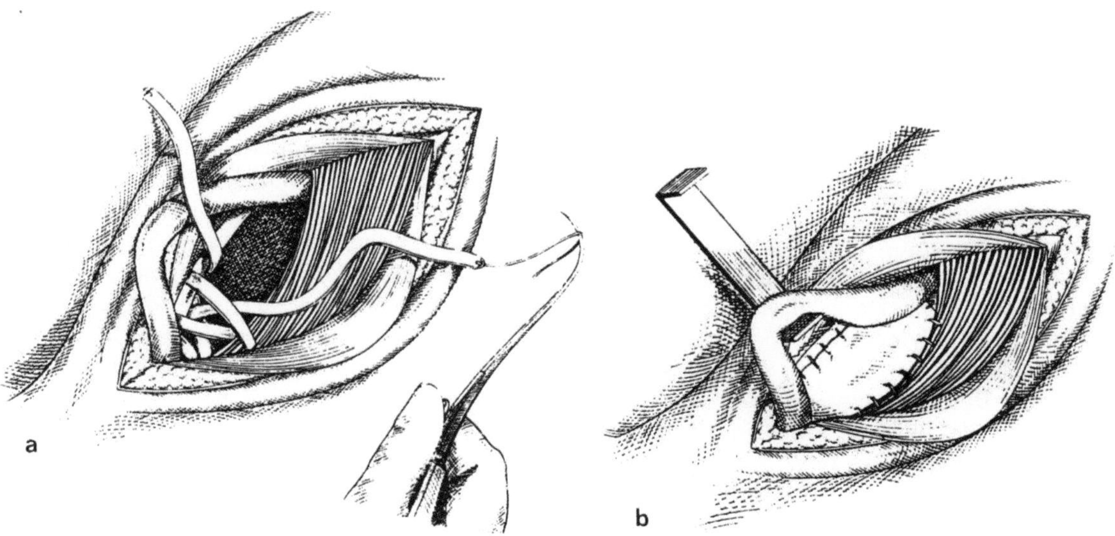

Fig. 9.12. a Autoplasty with skin lacing [J. Gosset]. **b** Inguinal skin grafting [Detrie 1967]

stance of the abdominal wall, but these techniques are relatively "heavy" and depend for success on the resistance of the edges of the musculo-pectineal orifice to which the sutures are applied. This probably explains the small number of surgeons who use skin, which has practically disappeared from the repertoire of hernia repair, while the use of prostheses is so much simpler.

E. Techniques Involving the Use of Prosthetic Material

This type of repair has acquired a major place in hernia surgery. Various synthetic materials are used as patches of different sizes, or as plugs, in order to reinforce sutures and also to replace the transversalis fascia. This enthusiasm for prosthetic repair has been stimulated by the publication of good results. The fact that septic complications are far less of a risk than was the case 20 years ago, has meant that in order to overcome the problem of widespread tissue degeneration which is so often found in acquired hernias, the surgeon can make extensive use of prosthetic materials. Although much of this activity is the result of the promotional efforts of the manufacturers of quality prostheses, their use has nonetheless allowed us to repair even the most difficult cases.

The idea of using foreign material in surgery of the abdominal wall is not new. In 1889 Witzel used a primitive type of silver mesh, and this was followed by Göpel (1900). In 1901 Busse used plates of gold, aluminum, copper and various alloys (Dural, Elektron), with bad results due to their rigidity and dangerous weight. Rubber sponges [Fieschi 1913] and patches [Delbet 1914] produced such severe complications that they were rapidly abandoned. Metallic meshes reappeared with titanium and stainless steel which were quite frequently used for several years around the 1940s, then abandoned around 1950 because of the discomfort produced by their rigid nature, their tendency to migrate and invade higher organs and finally their rapid fragmentation.

Following the Second World War, the chemical industry came up with a variety of surgical products which were commonly known as "plastics", but should probably be termed polymers.

Synthetic meshes for hernia repair were introduced into Europe by Don Acquaviva in 1948, who used nylon, and in the USA by Koontz who since 1959 used polypropylene. Nowadays the main synthetic materials used are polyester meshes (Dacron) or polypropylene, which are well tolerated and because of their macro porosity are rapidly incorporated by ingrowth

of scar tissue. Impermeable materials such as silastic or Teflon are rapidly encapsulated and have been abandoned. The same applies to expanded PTFE, which is microporous and not easily incorporated.

Numerous studies have been conducted in order to determine the features of good prosthetic materials [Policard & Fullbringer 1950; Cumberland 1952; Scales 1953; Usher 1959-1962; Koontz 1959-1962; Petit & Stoppa 1973; Arnaud & Adloff 1976-1977; Minns & Tinkler 1976; Stoppa & Soler 1992; Rath & Chevrel 1996]. A "good prosthesis" should be resistant, supple, easily penetrated by connective tissue, solid after incorporation in the body, radiolucent, easily sterilized and cheap.

The materials which best fulfill these criteria are polypropylenes, widely used in Britain and America and polyesters (Dacron) which are favored in France.

Here is a brief account of one of these experimental studies. With Petit (1974), we studied the behavior of Dacron implanted into guinea pigs. We measured the reaction to the material, the density of that reaction, the fibroblastic activity and the development of scarring in the interstices of the material. These studies led us to favor Dacron mesh, which became fixed in the tissues from the tenth day onwards. Arnaud and Adloff (1976-1977) have emphasized the importance of the ratio between fibroblasts and inflammatory cells which is high when tolerance and resistance is increased. The practical result of this is that macroporous prostheses function better than those which are impermeable. With Soler (1992) we tested various materials in the rat model, of varying permeability, both absorbable and nonabsorbable, and confirmed the importance of this ratio, confirming also that all materials, whether absorbable or nonabsorbable, placed within the peritoneal cavity, generate adhesions. Rath and Chevrel (1996) re-examined the biological tolerance of several synthetic materials used in surgery of the abdominal wall and carried out further studies estimating the resistance induced after incorporation of macroporous materials. They found that all the different materials in present use, in particular polypropylenes and polyesters, give adequately strong support, but experimentally the abdominal walls which are re-enforced with polypropylene are somewhat more solid, in the face of tensions which are certainly higher than those encountered in the clinical situation.

Absorbable prostheses (polyglactine 910, polyglycolic acid) are hydrolyzed within six weeks and cannot be recommended in hernia repair where a strong scar only develops after completion of the maturation and re-modeling process which lasts for at least one year [Tyrell 1989]. Finally, composite materials such as mixtures of polyester and polyglactine or carbon fiber and polyglycolic acid are well tolerated and produce more fibrosis, but clinical trials give varying results and these materials are considerably more costly than the existing prostheses.

These prostheses can be used in various ways such as the Lichtenstein and Gilbert patches and plugs, and the variations (Rutkow, Trabucco, Dudai) representing the "patch plug method" which uses a limited inguinal approach and the simultaneous and separate insertion of a patch and a plug. The Bendavid umbrella and the "fletching" prosthesis are more complex in design, as is the Rives operation through the inguinal route. Prosthetic repair via laparotomy can be done through the midline preperitoneal approach (Rives) by enveloping the visceral sac in a large bilateral preperitoneal prosthesis (Stoppa) or by wrapping the visceral sac through the suprainguinal route (Wantz).

1. Prosthetic Repair by the Inguinal Route

a) The Rives Operation

A Mersilene prosthesis which is considerably larger than the musculo-pectineal orifice is carefully fixed and stretched out, in order to promote its incorporation in granulation tissue. The size of the prosthesis may be reduced somewhat in order to reduce the risk of infection. The principles of the operation are as follows.

General or local anesthesia may be used (epidural in the young patient or spinal in the elderly), the choice of anesthetic being made together with the patient at the preoperative consultation. The incision runs parallel to and about 1 cm above the inguinal ligament and reaches the pubic spine. The external oblique aponeurosis is opened along its fibers and the superficial inguinal ring cleared, avoiding the cutaneous nerves. The cremaster muscle is then resected and the spermatic cord retracted with a loop. The sac is dissected and removed in the normal manner and indirect sacs are ligated as high as possible with removal of excess peritoneum. The transversalis fascia which is now exposed is opened along the length of the posterior wall of the canal, from the deep inguinal ring to the pubic spine, protecting the inferior epigastric vessels. The extraperitoneal fat is swept upwards with a spoon, the pectineal ligament is exposed as far as the external iliac vessels laterally. It is often necessary to divide bet-

ween ligatures a large vertically running communicating vein or some small horizontal vessels above the pubis. The deep aspect of the muscles is then cleared upwards by dissection with the finger or gauze swab.

(1) Preparation of the Prosthesis (Fig. 9.13)

A piece of Mersilene mesh 10 cm across is laid out and a notch cut in its inferolateral edge to allow passage of the iliac vessels. The prosthesis is first fixed below to the pectineal ligament, using four or five no. 3 Flexocrin sutures, at least 1 cm apart, constructing a large lower hem 3 to 4 cm long, which will be folded over the iliopubic ramus when the sutures are tied. The prosthesis is then fixed to the deep aspect of the broad muscles, as far up as possible, by a series of mattress sutures tied in front of the muscles but behind the aponeurosis of the external oblique, usually from within outwards. A slit is then constructed, of which the medial angle is strengthened by a stay suture of Flexocrin, in order to avoid tearing. The two limbs of the slit allow passage of the spermatic cord, which should be brought upwards and laterally as far as possible, so as to restore its curved course. The two limbs of the prosthesis are fixed in the same way beneath the muscles laterally by mattress sutures. The orifice thus constructed should not be too wide, as it might otherwise form the site of a recurrent indirect hernia. Finally, the prosthesis is fixed by a few sutures below to the vascular sheath and the inguinal ligament so as not to leave a vascular defect. In this manner the prosthesis should lie without any fold, but should bulge gently in response to abdominal pressure. It only remains to remove the excess Mersilene, corresponding to the upper flange.

A continuous suture taking up the two edges of the transversalis fascia in front of the prosthesis reunites the conjoint tendon to the inguinal ligament. This suture seals off the prosthesis which is thus separated from the superficial layers. The external oblique aponeurosis is sutured in front of the cord. Drainage is not usually necessary. The superficial fascia and skin are closed in two layers. The dressing is usually removed after 24 h and the wound left open to allow inspection. The course is usually uncomplicated and the patient leaves hospital on the fourth or fifth day with no special postoperative regime such as anti-coagulation. The patients are advised to limit their physical activities for some three weeks, during which time the prosthesis is becoming incorporated.

The results of this operation have recently been reported by J. Rives and his successors J. B. Flament and J. P. Palot in a series of 720 hernias treated from

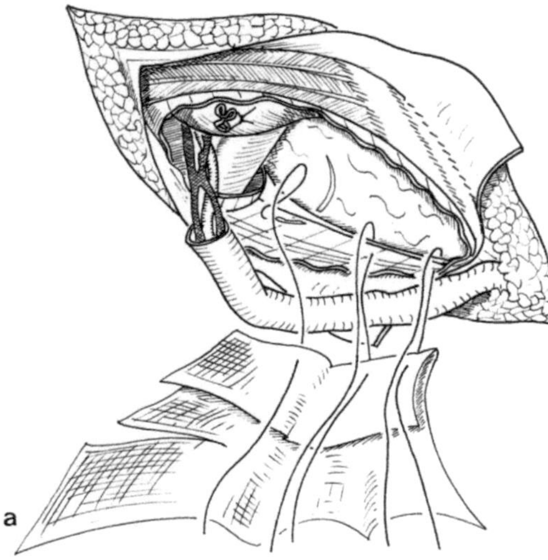

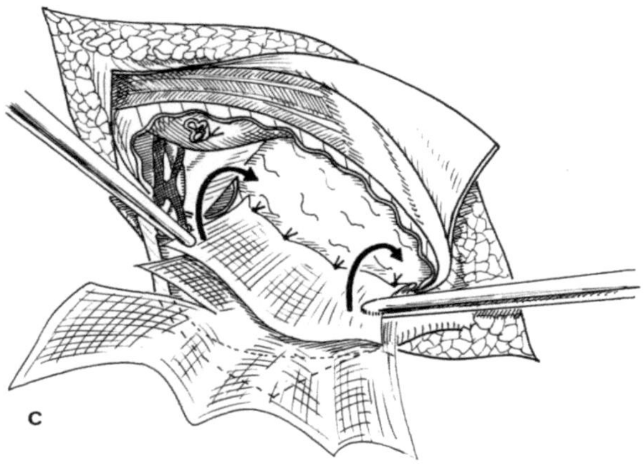

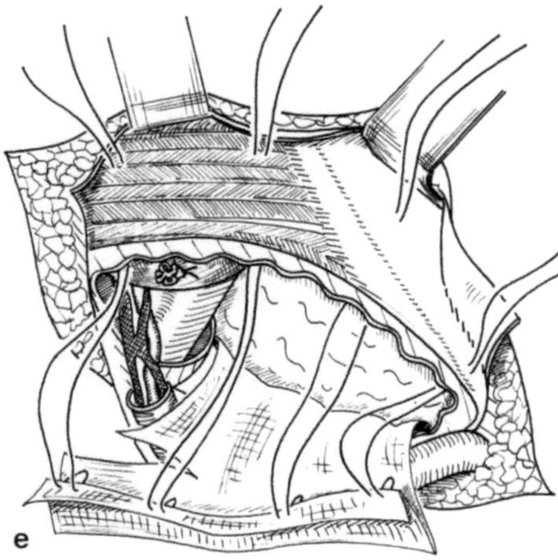

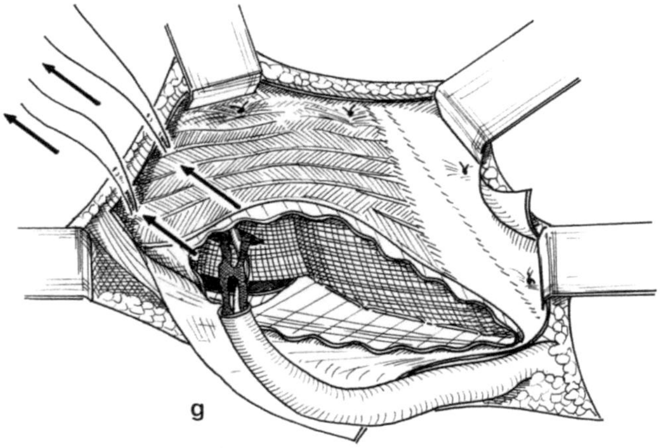

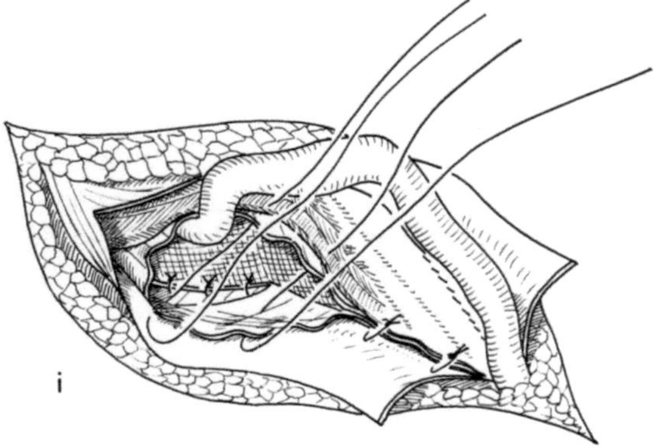

Fig. 9.13. Rives' technique of prosthetic repair (photos courtesy of Rives). **a** The mersilene mesh (containing a lateral slit to allow passage of the spermatic cord) is presented close to the operative field. The retropubic part is folded over like a hem and the mesh is attached to Cooper's ligament. **b** Operative view. **c** The sutures are tied off, after which the fold is turned down behind the horizontal ramus of the pubis, thereby hiding the sutures in Cooper's ligament. **d** Operative view. **e** The upper margin of the prosthesis is anchored to the deep surface of the flat abdominal muscles. A small (0.5 cm) fold ensures solid fixation. **f** Operative view. **g** Appearance of the implanted prosthetic mesh. h Operative view. **i** Operation is terminated by Bassini-like suturing of the flat abdominal muscles and fascia transversalis above to the fascia transversalis and inguinal ligament below. **j** Operative view

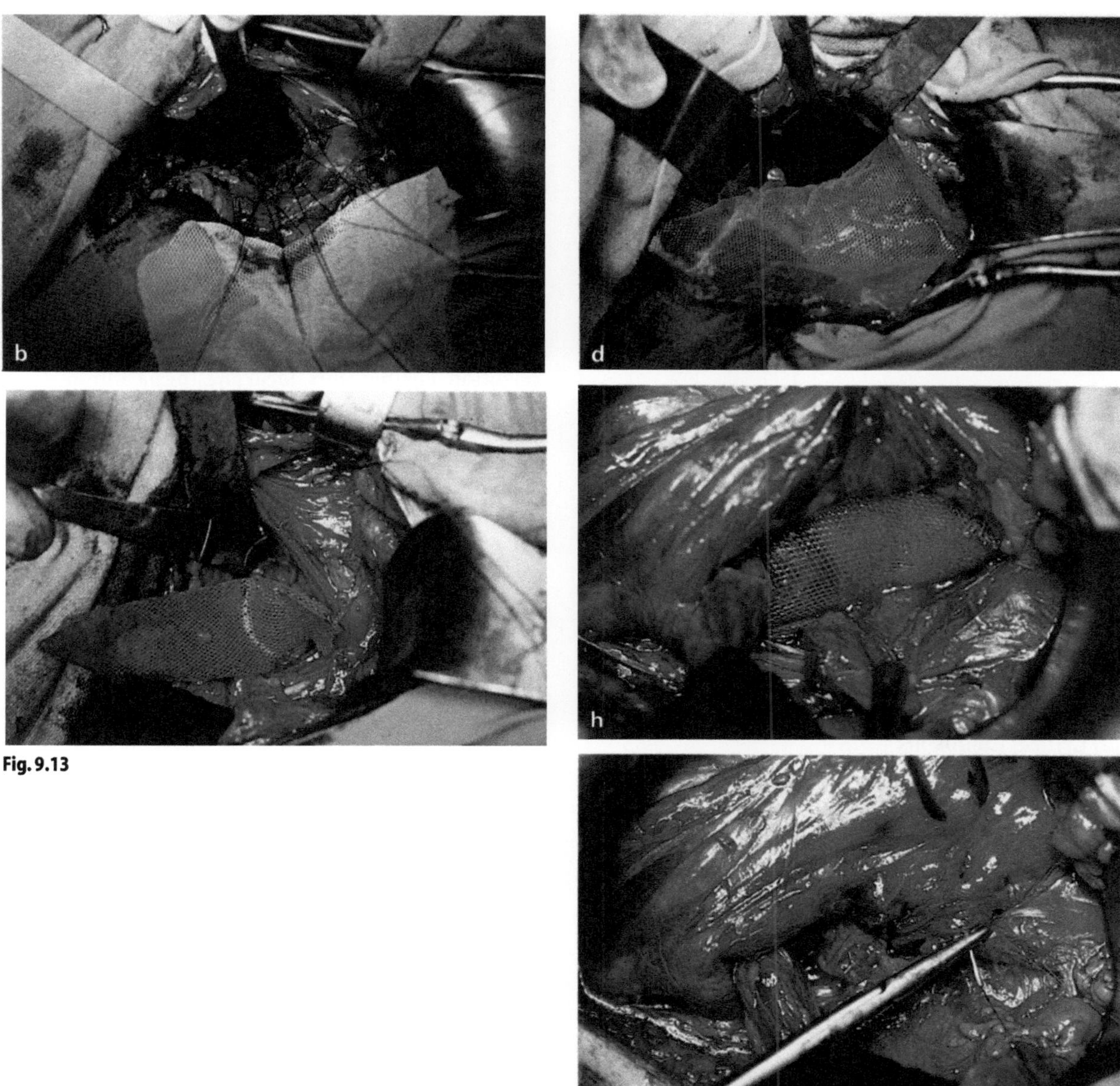

Fig. 9.13

1970 to 1994. This comprises some 20% of an overall series of 2,235 hernias. Infection rate was 1.6%, a figure comparable to that occurring following the classical operation (1.5%). This usually resolves when the wound is laid open and the prosthesis exposed. It is best to avoid removing the prosthetic material which is prone to produce a recurrence. Over the last seven years no septic problem has been observed. There were 13 recurrences (1.9%): in primary cases the rate was 1.3%. Recurrence is usually the result of poor technique such as incomplete removal of the sac, too wide an opening between the two limbs of the prosthesis,

sutures inadequately taking up the pectineal ligament, too small an inferior flange, or inadequate lateral fixation.

The authors of this series suggest the following indications: direct hernias in the presence of transversalis fascia which is of poor quality, or where there exist risk factors for recurrence including strenuous occupations, chronically raised abdominal pressure and a history of recurrent herniation.

The surgery must be carried out in a carefully controlled manner. The rules of asepsis in every type of surgery using prosthetic material must be carefully

Table 9.10. Rate of recurrence after Rives' operation (inguinal hernias)

Authors	# Cases	% Follow-up	Years Follow-up	% Recurrences
Alexandre (1993)	117	77	3.5	1.1
Rives (1973)	183	66.1	1 to 9	1.6
Flament (1983)	586	80	5	1.7
Flament (1991)	135	-	6	1.9
Palot (1995)	720	85	-	1.9
Galeone (1991)	118	75	5	5.5

respected, the operating theater must be disinfected on the day proceeding surgery, the skin must be carefully prepared, no touch technique used with liberal use of povidone iodine, the number of people entering and leaving the theater must be limited as also must be the movement of the operating light and the use of the sucker.

(2) Critical Comments

The operation requires a solid and firm pectineal ligament, which is not always the case with multiple recurrence, particularly following the McVay operation. This technique carries a risk of wounding the spermatic cord if a recurrence is approached by the inguinal route. Additionally, the incision in the prosthesis to allow passage of the spermatic cord creates a weak point in the layer of greatest resistance, in spite of taking every precaution to suture the two limbs separately on to the muscular wall. Rives himself recognizes that this operation is not simple and should be reserved for experienced surgeons, an opinion already advanced by Usher in 1959. However it is an excellent modern procedure, the success of which is apparent from the published results illustrated in Table 9.10.

b) The Lichtenstein
Open Tension-free Hernioplasty

P. K. Amid

For more than a century, the measure of the success of hernia repair was its recurrence rate. In 1966, for the first time, the importance of the postoperative disability period was brought to the attention of surgeons by Lichtenstein (1966). With the aims of decreasing post-

operative pain, recovery period, and recurrence rate, the tension-free hernioplasty project was started at the Lichtenstein Hernia Institute in June 1984 [Amid et al. 1996 (I)]. The concept is based on: a) the degenerative origin of inguinal hernia which results in destruction of the inguinal floor [Read 1992], b) the fact that traditional repairs are associated with undue tension at the suture line [Amid et al. 1996 (I)].

The procedure is performed under local anesthesia, which is our preferred choice for all reducible adult inguinal hernias. It is safe, simple, effective, economical, and without any side effects or risk of urinary retention. Furthermore, local anesthesia administered before making the incision produces a prolonged analgesic effect by preventing the build-up of local nociceptive substances. Several safe and effective anesthetic agents are currently available. Our choice, however, is a 50:50 mixture of 1% lidocaine (Xylocaine) and 0.5% bupivacaine (Marcaine).

(1) Techniques of Anesthesia

Some 45 ml of this mixture is usually sufficient for a unilateral hernia repair and is administered as follows.

Subdermal infiltration. About 5 ml of the mixture is infiltrated along the line of the incision with a 5 cm long 25 gauge needle inserted into the subdermal tissue parallel with the skin surface. Infiltration continues as the needle is advanced. Movement of the needle reduces the likelihood of intravascular injection because even if the needle penetrates a blood vessel, the tip will not remain there long enough to deliver a substantial amount of the anesthetic agent. This step blocks the subdermal nerve endings and reduces the discomfort of the intradermal infiltration which is the most uncomfortable stage of local anesthesia.

Intradermal injection (making the skin weal). The needle in the subdermal plane is withdrawn slowly until its tip reaches the skin. Without withdrawing the needle completely, the dermis is infiltrated by slow injection of about 3 ml of the mixture along the line of the incision.

Deep subcutaneous injection. A total of lo ml of the mixture is injected deep into the subcutaneous fat with the needle inserted perpendicular to the skin surface at points 2 cm apart. Again, the needle is kept moving during injection to reduce the risk of intravascular infusion.

Subaponeurotic injection. About lo ml of the anesthetic mixture is injected immediately beneath the aponeurosis of the external oblique muscle through a window created in the subcutaneous fat at the lateral corner of the incision. This injection floods the inguinal canal and anesthetizes all three major nerves in the region while the remaining subcutaneous fat is incised.

It also separates the external oblique aponeurosis from the underlying ilioinguinal nerve, reducing the likelihood of injuring the nerve when the aponeurosis is incised.

Occasionally it is necessary to infiltrate a few milliliters of the mixture at the level of the pubic tubercle, around the neck and inside the indirect hernia sac, to achieve complete local anesthesia.

The local anesthesia can be further prolonged by spraying 10 ml of the mixture (with added adrenaline) into the inguinal canal before closure of the external oblique aponeurosis, and into the subcutaneous space before skin closure [Bays et al. 1991].

Epidural anesthesia is preferred for repair of irreducible or bilateral inguinal hernias in obese patients. Sedative drugs given by the surgeon, or preferably by an anesthetist as "conscious sedation" via infusion of rapid short-acting, amnesic and anxiolytic agents such as propofol, reduce both the patient's anxiety and the amount of local anesthetic agents required, particularly for bilateral inguinal hernia repair.

(2) Technique of Operation

A 5 cm skin incision, which starts from the pubic tubercle and extends laterally within the Lange's line, gives an excellent exposure of the pubic tubercle and the internal ring. After skin incision, the external oblique aponeurosis is opened and its lower leaf freed from the spermatic cord. The upper leaf of the external oblique is then freed from the underlying internal oblique muscle and aponeurosis for a distance of 2-3 cm above the inguinal floor. The anatomical cleavage between these two layers is avascular and the dissection can be done rapidly and atraumatically. High separation of these layers has a dual benefit, as it visualizes the iliohypogastric nerve and creates space for insertion of a wide sheet of mesh that overlaps the internal oblique by at least 3 cm above the upper margin of the inguinal floor. The cord with its cremaster covering is separated from the floor of the inguinal canal and the pubic bone for a distance of about 2 cm beyond the pubic tubercle. The plane between the cremasteric sheath and the aponeurotic tissue attached to the pubic bone is avascular, so that there is no risk of damaging the testicular blood flow. When lifting the cord, care should be taken to include the external spermatic vessels and the genital nerve with the cord. This ensures that the genital nerve, which is always in

juxtaposition to the external spermatic vessels, is preserved (Fig. 9.14a).

Cutting or ligating the genital nerve can cause long-term incapacitating neuralgia [Lichtenstein et al. 1988]. The ilioinguinal and iliohypogastric nerves should also be preserved.

To explore the internal ring, for an indirect hernia sac, the cremasteric sheath is transversely or longitudinally incised at this level (Fig. 9.14a). The latter prevents disturbance of testicular retractibility. Complete stripping and excision of the cremasteric fibers is unnecessary, and can result in injury to the nerves, small blood vessels, and vas deferens.

Indirect hernial sacs are freed from the cord to a point beyond the neck of the sac and inverted into the abdomen without ligation. Ligation of the highly innervated peritoneal sac leads to mechanical pressure and ischemic changes, and is a major cause of postoperative pain [Smedberg et al. 1984; Amid et al. 1995 (I)]. It has been shown that avoiding ligation of the indirect sac does not increase the chance of recurrence [Smedberg et al. 1984; Shulman et al. 1993]. To minimize the risk of postoperative ischemic orchitis, complete scrotal hernia sacs are transected at the midpoint of the canal, leaving the distal part in place, but incising its anterior wall in order to prevent the formation of a hydrocele.

Large direct hernias are inverted with an absorbable suture. A thorough exploration of the groin is necessary to rule out the coexisting intraparietal (interstitial) or femoral hernia.

The femoral ring is palpated through a small opening in the canal floor. A precut mesh of 8 × 16 cm is used. We prefer monofilament polypropylene meshes (such as Atrium, Marlex, Prolene and Trilex) because their surface texture promotes fibroplasia and their monofilament structure does not promote or harbour infection [Amid et al. 1994; Amid et al. 1992]. The medial end of the mesh is rounded to the shape of the medial corner of the inguinal canal. With the cord retracted upwards, the rounded corner is sutured, with a running suture of a nonabsorbable monofilamented material, to the aponeurotic tissue over the pubic bone, overlapping the bone by 1.5 to 2 cm (Fig. 9.14b). This is a crucial step in the repair because failure to cover this bone with the mesh can result in recurrence. The periosteum of the bone is avoided. This suture is continued to attach the lower edge of the patch to the shelving margin of Poupart's ligament up to a point just lateral to the internal ring. Suturing the mesh beyond this point is unnecessary and could injure the femoral nerve. If there is a concurrent femo-

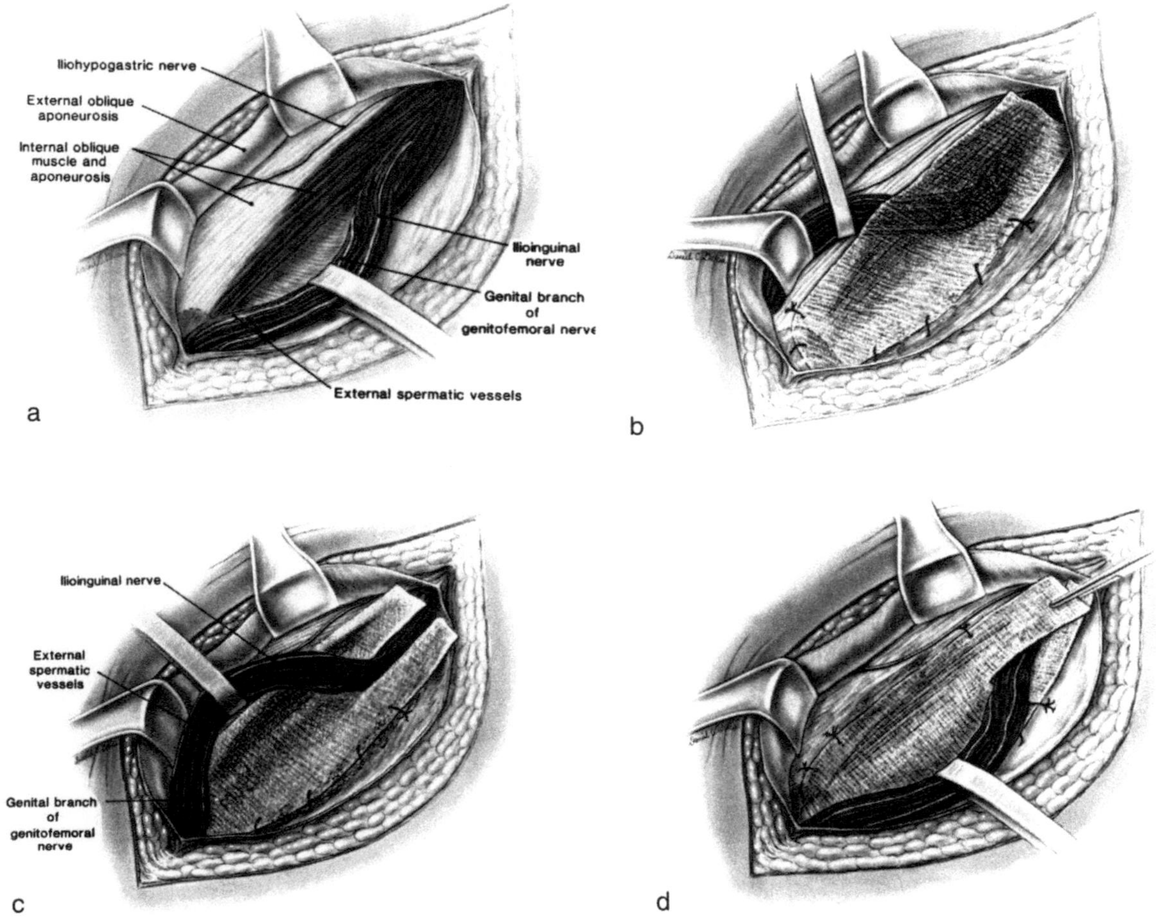

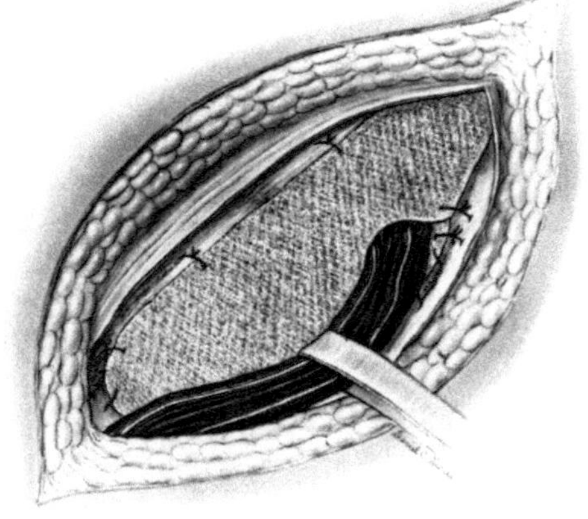

Fig. 9.14. Lichtenstein's operation. **a** The spermatic cord together with its cremasteric covering, external spermatic vessels, and genital nerve is raised and the cremasteric fibers are cut transversely or longitudinally at the level of the internal ring. **b** The medial corner of the patch overlaps the pubic bone by 1-1.5 cm. **c** The spermatic cord is placed in between the two tails of the mesh. **d** Crossing of the two tails. **e** The lower edges of the two tails are sutured to the shelving margin for creation of a new internal ring made of mesh

ral hernia, the mesh is also sutured to Cooper's ligament 1-2 cm below its junction with the inguinal ligament, so as to close the femoral ring.

A slit is made at the lateral end of the mesh creating two tails, a wide one (two-thirds) above and a narrower (one-third) below.

The upper wide tail is grasped with a hemostat and passed towards the head of the patient from underneath the spermatic cord; this positions the cord between the two tails of the mesh (Fig. 9.14c).

The wider upper tail is crossed and placed over the narrower one and held with a hemostat (Fig. 9.14d). With the cord retracted downwards and the upper leaf of the external oblique aponeurosis retracted upwards, the upper edge of the patch is sutured to the internal oblique aponeurosis or muscle, whichever is available, with a few interrupted absorbable sutures avoiding injury to or entrapment of the iliohypogastric nerve. Firm retraction of the upper leaf of the external oblique during this phase of the repair is important because it achieves the appropriate amount of laxity for the patch [Amid et al. 1995 (I)]. As the retraction is released, the mesh buckles slightly, and this laxity assures a true tension-free repair and is taken up when the patient is asked to strain during the operation, or resumes an upright position.

Using a single nonabsorbable monofilament suture, the lower edges of each of the two tails are fixed to the shelving margin of Poupart's ligament just lateral to the completion knot of the lower running suture. This creates a new internal ring made of mesh (Fig. 9.14e). The crossing of the two tails produces a configuration similar to that of the normal transversalis fascial sling, which is assumed to be largely responsible for the integrity of the internal ring.

The excess patch on the lateral side is trimmed, leaving about 4-5 cm of mesh beyond the internal ring. This is tucked underneath the external oblique aponeurosis (Fig. 9.14e), which is then closed over the cord with an absorbable suture.

(3) Outcome Measures

5,000 primary inguinal hernias in 4,000 adult male patients were performed under local anesthesia by the authors from 1984 to 1995. The series included 1,000 bilateral inguinal hernias, which were repaired simultaneously under local anesthesia [Amid et al. 1996 (II)]. The age range of patients was 19 to 86 years. 44% of patients had indirect, 43.1% had direct, and 12.5% had a combination of indirect and direct inguinal hernias. 78% of patients were of normal weight or up to 10 kg overweight. 20% of patients were 10 to 20 kg

overweight, and 2% were more than 20 kg overweight. 27% of patients had bilateral inguinal hernias and 11.4% had sliding hernias. With regard to employment, 60.2% had sedentary jobs, and 38.8% performed hard manual labor.

99% of the patients underwent outpatient surgery and the hospital stay after the operation was two to three hours. One percent of patients were admitted to the hospital because of unrelated medical or personal reasons. Analgesic requirement for postoperative pain was 0 to 20 (mean of 8) tablets of Vicodin (hydrocodone bitartrate 5 mg and Acetaminophen 500 mg) for a period of one to four days. Postoperative unrestricted activity was encouraged. Patients returned to their usual work with no restrictions at between two to fourteen days. There was one chronic postoperative neuralgia and no patient developed a seroma that required aspiration. Early in the evolution of this technique, four patients developed recurrences as a result of technical errors.

Three hernias recurred at the pubic tubercle because of failure to overlap the bone with the mesh. One recurrence resulted from total disruption of the mesh from the inguinal ligament because the mesh was too narrow. There has been only one recurrence in those patients operated on within the last six years.

(4) Prevention of Recurrences

Reported recurrence rates by individuals or institutions are scientifically meaningless unless the method of follow-up is known and length of observation is sufficient. The only reliable method of follow-up is by physician examination. Written questionnaires and telephone inquiries are notoriously unreliable and up to 50% inaccurate [Abramson et al. 1978; Panos et al. 1992]. Short-term follow-up, particularly after mesh repair, only reveals the therapeutic value of the repair [Amid et al. 1995 (I)]. A long-term follow-up of 10 years or more is required to evaluate in addition its prophylactic effectiveness [Amid et al. 1995 (I)].

The use of a wide mesh to overlap the tissues for 3-4 cm outside Hesselbach's triangle is important in reducing the chance of recurrence. After incorporation is complete, this overlap results in a uniform distribution of intra-abdominal pressure over the whole surface of the overlapped area, rather than on to the line where the mesh joins to the tissue.

Because the mesh is placed behind the external oblique aponeurosis, the intra-abdominal pressure works in favor of the repair. The aponeurosis keeps the mesh tightly in place by acting as an external support when intra-abdominal pressure rises [Shulman et al.

1995 (I)]. Placement of the mesh underneath the transversalis fascia (such as the Rives procedure), although a sound concept, requires unnecessary dissection and increases surgical trauma. Proper fixation of the margins of the mesh to the groin tissue is another important step in the prevention of recurrence. In mobile areas such as the groins, there is a tendency for the prosthesis to fold, wrinkle, or curl around the cord. More importantly, in vivo, mesh prostheses lose approximately 20% of their size due to shrinkage. The slightest movement of the mesh from the pubic tubercle, the inguinal ligament, and the area of the internal ring, due to the above factors, is a leading cause of failure. Adequate laxity must be allowed during fixation to eliminate tension and compensate for the increased intra-abdominal pressure that results when the patient stands or strains. A mesh which has no ripple when the patient is sedated and lying down, will be subject to tension in the standing position and with straining.

Use of the tension-free technique in conjunction with local anesthesia has drastically reduced the hospital stay, postoperative discomfort, recovery period, recurrence rate and the cost of hernia surgery. Since its introduction, the open tension-free hernioplasty has been employed by many surgeons worldwide with outcome measures identical to ours [Rutten et al. 1992; d'Ambrosi 1995].

A survey of 70 surgeons with no special interest in hernia surgery, who had done 22,300 Lichtenstein open "tension-free" hernioplasties gave similar results [Shulman et al. 1995 (II)].

The fact that the results from surgeons with no special interest or expertise in hernia repair are identical to those with a special interest in this subject, is a testimony to the simplicity, safety, and effectiveness of the open "tension-free" hernioplasty. The procedure is simple and safe and achieves all the goals of modern surgery, such as a more comfortable postoperative course and rapid return to unrestricted activities, with a recurrence rate of virtually zero (0.1% from early operations). It also avoids the need for general anesthesia and invasion of the peritoneal or preperitoneal spaces and their associated complications.

(5) Isolated Femoral Hernia and Recurrent Inguinal Hernia: Concept of the Plug Repair

Femoral hernia. The unacceptable recurrence rate of tissue approximation, repair of femoral hernias (such as Bassini, Bassini-Kirshner, Moschowitz and Lotheissen McVay) prompted the concept of tension-free plug repair of femoral hernias in the late 60s. In this technique, which is performed under local anesthesia after mobilization and reduction of the femoral hernia sac through a small subinguinal incision, a plug made of a ribbon of monofilamented polypropylene mesh is inserted into the femoral canal.

The plug is secured in place by suturing it to the inguinal ligament superiorly, pectineus fascia inferiorly, and the lacunar ligament medially, using several interrupted monofilament nonabsorbable sutures. The plug occludes the entire femoral canal, providing a strong repair without tension. The success of this repair encouraged us to expand the concept to the repair of recurrent inguinal hernias consisting of a single defect measuring 3 cm or less in diameter.

Recurrent inguinal hernias. Under local or epidural anesthesia, a small transverse incision is made over the previously marked hernia bulge. The hernia sac is identified; its localization can be greatly facilitated by asking the patient to cough during the exploration. When located, the sac is dissected away from the spermatic cord and freed to the fascial level, where a firm ring of scar tissue is found. The sac is surgically reduced. The plug is then inserted snugly into the defect and secured in place by multiple monofilament nonabsorbable sutures. The advantage of plug repair of recurrent inguinal hernia is its simplicity and safety. The technique requires minimal surgical dissection, and is associated with minimal risk of testicular complications.

(6) Discussion

Plug repair of recurrent inguinal hernias is an excellent therapeutic operation; however, because the repair is limited to the location of the hernia defect without protecting the rest of the inguinal floor, it does not address the progression of the degenerative process to the rest of the inguinal canal. Therefore, in contrast to the plug repair of femoral hernia, which is both therapeutic and prophylactic, the plug repair of recurrent inguinal hernia is solely therapeutic, and provides no prophylactic repair. The operation is most suitable for older patients with a single defect of 3 cm or less. Currently, our recommendation for recurrent inguinal hernias consisting of more than one defect, defects larger than 3 cm, or recurrent hernias in younger patients, is the same as to repair employed for the repair of primary inguinal hernias.

A crucial step of plug repair for femoral and recurrent inguinal hernias is the construction of the plug. A simple way to construct a plug is to start with an 8×16 cm sheet of monofilament polypropylene mesh. When the sheet is folded twice along its longitudinal axis, it creates a strip of mesh equivalent to 2×64 cm. The edge of this strip is held with a straight hemostat and rolled into a firm plug of an appropriate size, based on the size of the hernia defect. The plug must be firm, because a soft plug that can be collapsed by pinching it between two fingers (the pinch test), would collapse as a result of the patient's own scarring process. This often leads to recurrence of the hernia [Amid et al. 1995 (II)].

References

Abramson JH, Gafin J, Hopp C, et al (1978) The epidemiology of inguinal hernia: a survey in Western Jerusalem. J Epidemiol Community Health 32: 59

Amendolara M, Perrl S, Breda E, Valenti G, Busso A, Gelmi G (1995) Inguinal hernioplasty: current trends. G Chir 16: 239-44

Amid PK, Shulman AG, Lichtenstein IL (1996 I) Open "tension-free" repair of inguinal hernias: The Lichtenstein technique. Eur J Surg 162: 447-453

Amid PK, Shulman AG, Lichtenstein IL (1996 II) Simultaneous repair of bilateral inguinal hernias under local anesthesia. Ann Surg (in press)

Amid PK, Shulman AG, Lichtenstein IL, Hakakha M (1995 I) The goals of modern hernia surgery. How to achieve them: open or laparoscopic repair? In: Problems in General Surgery. Lippincott-Raven, Philadelphia, 12: 165-171

Amid PK, Shulman AG, Lichtenstein IL (1995 II) Hernioplasty. In: Bendavid R (ed) Prosthese and abdominal wall hernias. R G Landes, Austin, pp 389-394

Amid PJ, Shulman AG, Lichtenstein IL, Hakakha M (1994) Biomaterials for abdominal wall hernia surgery and principles of their applications. Langenbecks Arch Chir 379: 168-171

Amid PK, Shulman AG, Lichtenstein IL (1992) Selecting synthetic mesh for the repair of groin hernia. Postgrad Genet Surg 4: 150-55

Amid PK, Shulman AG, Lichtenstein IL (1991) Femoral hernia resulting from inguinal herniorrhaphy - the "plug" repair. Contemp Surg 39: 19-24

Barnes JP (1987) Inguinal hernia repair with routine use of Marlex mesh. Surg Gynecol Obstet 165: 33-37

Bays RA, Barry L, Vasilenko P (1991) The use of bupivacaine in elective inguinal herniorrhaphy as a fast and safe technique for relief of postoperative pain. Surg Gynecol Obstet 173: 433-7

Bocchi DP, Amid PK, et al (1995) Opération "tension-free" de Lichtenstein pour hernie inguinale sous anesthésie locale. J Chir (Paris) 132: 61-66

Brown JH, Khaira HS (1995) Early results with the Lichtenstein tension-free hernia repair. Br J Surg 82: 419-410

Capozzi JA, Berkenfield JA, Cherry JK (1988) Repair of inguinal hernia in the adult with prolene mesh. Surg Gynecol Obstet 167: 124-28

Corlett MP, Pollock D, Marshall JE (1995) Early results with Lichtenstein tension-free hernia repair. Br J Surg 82: 418

D'Ambrosi GR (1995) Free tension in inguinal hernioplasty. Minerva Chir 50: 523-6

Davies N, Thomas M, McIlroy TB, Kingsnorth AN (1994) Early results with the Lichtenstein tension-free hernia repair. Br J Surg 81: 1475-78

Di Martino C, Celestre P, Conti, A, Caruso N, Iancampo M, Civitella A, Cristini F, Farina C, Stipa F (1995) L'intervento di Lichtenstein e varianti nel trattamento dell'ernia inguinale. Chirurgia (in press)

Evans WS (1994) Endoscopic inguinal herniorrhaphy vs open mesh repair. A comparison of cost and outcome in a community hospital setting. Endo Expo '94, Annual Endoscopic Exposition

Galasse S, Abbandonati M, Chiappa R, Dominici E, Gagliano F, Pinarelli E, Chiappa G (1994) Repair of inguinal hernia with prolene mesh. Preliminary results on 102 cases. Chirurgia Generale XV: 225-27

Gianesi R, Borgato F, Seraglio P, Ceoloni A, Pesavento S, Piccoli A, Faccin S (1994) Our experience in inguinal and femoral hernia treatment with Lichtenstein technique. Acta Chir 50: 151-55

Himal HS (1994) Inguinal hernia repair - laparoscopic vs open Marlex mesh technique. Surg Endosc 8: 478

Hinson EL (1995) Early results with Lichtenstein tension-free hernia repair. Br J Surg 82: 418-419

Horeyseck G, et al (1995) Early results with "tension-free" hernia repair, laparoscopic versus open. Surg Endosc 5: 597

Kark A, Kurzer M, Waters KJ (1995) Tension-free hernia repair: review of 1,098 cases using local anesthesia in a day unit. Ann R Coll Surg Engl 77: 299-304

Kux M, Fuchsjager N, Feichter A (1994) Lichtenstein patch versus Shouldice technik bein primaren Lestenhernien mit hoher Rezidivgefahrdung. Dermatol Chir 65: 59-63

Lichtenstein JL, Schulman AG, Amid PK, Montlor MM (1989) The tension free hernioplasty. Am J Surg 157: 188-193

Lichtenstein IL, Shulman AG, Amid PK, Montllor M (1988) Cause and prevention of post-herniorrhaphy neuralgia: a proposed protocol for treatment. Am J Surg 155: 786-90

Lichtenstein IL (1970) Hernia repair without disability. CV Mosby, St Louis

Lichtenstein IL (1966) Immediate ambulation and return to work following herniorrhaphy. Indust Med Surg 35: 754-759

Martin RE, Max CE (1984) Primary inguinal hernia repair with prosthetic mesh. Hosp Medica 1: 1

Mattocci A, Rezzo R, Comes P, Bergomi B, De Gregori M (1994) Il razionale del trattamento chirurgico dell "ernia inguinale" nostra esperienza e considerazioni (in press)

Notaras MJ (1994) Laparoscopic hernia repair. The Lancet 343

Panos RG, Beck DE, Maresh JE, Harford FJ (1992) Preliminary results of a prospective randomized study of Cooper's ligament versus Shouldice herniorrhaphy technique. Surg Gynecol Obstet 175: 315-18

Pinocy J, Koveker G, Busing M, Becker HD (1994) Lichtesntein alloplastic repair of inguinal hernia. Helv Chir Acta 60: 981-985

Read RC (1992) A review: the role of protease-antiprotease imbalance in the pathogenesis of herniation and abdominal aortic aneurysm in certain smokers. Postgrad Genet Surg 4: 161-5

Rutten P, Ledecq M, Hoebeke Y, et al (1992) Hernie inguinale primaire hernioplastie ambulatoire selon Lichtenstein: premiers résultats cliniques et implications économiques; étude des 130 premiers cas opérés. Acta Chir Belg 92: 168-71

Shulman AG, Amid PK, Lichtenstein IL (1995 I) Mesh between the oblique muscles is simple and effective in open hernioplasty. Am Surg 4: 326-27

Shulman AG, Amid PK, Lichtenstein IL (1995 II) A survey of non-expert surgeons using the open tension-free mesh repair for primary inguinal hernias. Int Surg 80: 35-36

Shulman AG, Amid PK, Lichtenstein IL (1993) Ligation of hernial sac a needless step in adult hernioplasty. Int Surg 378: 152-53

Smedgerg SGG, Broome AEA, Gullmo A (1984) Ligation of the hernia sac? Surg Clin North Am 64: 299

Tinkler LF (1985) Inguinal hernia repair using local anesthesia. Ann R Coll Surg Engl 67: 268

c) The Gilbert Operation

A. I. Gilbert and M. F. Graham

"The internal inguinal ring is Nature's window into the preperitoneal space - Why not use it?"

The aim of repair of an indirect inguinal hernia is to reduce all of the herniated peritoneum into the abdominal cavity and to prevent it from reherniation by restoring the competency of the internal ring. Satisfactory repair permanently prevents passage of bowel and omentum outside the musculoaponeurotic plane of the abdominal wall. That portion of hernia sac that protrudes through the internal inguinal ring into or through the canal must be fully reduced, or a larger sac may be divided and its proximal part ligated and reduced. This frees the true neck of the sac from its attachments at the musculo-fascial threshold of the internal ring. To complete the repair it is necessary to prevent passage of peritoneum through the internal ring. In the past, this was achieved by suturing the internal ring, as described by Marcy, Bassini and Shouldice. The technique we prefer uses a patch of polypropelene mesh to block the ring. A significant number of primary and recurrent hernias have been repaired and followed long enough to conclude that the results of this tension-free technique and its degree of patient satisfaction are excellent.

The Gilbert repair of inguinal hernia accomplishes these tasks with minimal tissue damage. In most cases it requires no sutures, thereby obviating pain-producing tension in the repair. This advantage is clearly appreciated by every patient who mobilizes in the recovery room, and continues to do so as usual activities are progressively resumed a day or two after surgery. Most patients return to regular work before the end of the first postoperative week.

The technique incorporates three principles: a) the internal ring is a convenient passageway to the preperitoneal retromuscular space, b) prosthetic mesh is an excellent permanent barrier to protect the internal ring, c) the intra-abdominal pressure (Pasqual's principle) is all that is necessary to fix the mesh permanently in position. The more the patient strains, thereby raising his intra-abdominal pressure, the more firmly the mesh becomes seated in place.

After dissection of the inguinal canal and determining that there is no direct hernia, the indirect peritoneal sac is invaginated completely through the internal ring. A full sized 2 × 4 in patch of polypropelene mesh (Prolene/Ethicon or Marlex/Bard-Davol) is folded four times to form an umbrella-shaped plug. The plug is inserted through the internal ring into the retromuscular preperitoneal space. Once in that plane the carrier-clamp is released and withdrawn allowing the mesh umbrella to open. Unfolded, the mesh barricades the peritoneum deep to the internal ring and most of the myopectineal orifice in the adjacent abdominal wall.

The initial version of this repair incorporated a second patch of mesh as an overlay graft, placed on the anterior aspect of the intact posterior wall to protect it from developing a direct hernia. In our latest series of more than a thousand types I, II and III hernias, subsequent direct hernia formation has not occurred (Gilbert). This change from the original version has reduced the incidence of wound seromas requiring aspiration from 5% to less than 1%, and it allowed a much simpler repair of type III hernias by the use of an umbrella-plug aided by a single Marcy suture. The surgeon can gain access to the space where the mesh will be implanted through the internal ring.

(1) Technique (Fig. 9.15)

For best results this procedure should be done under local or regional anesthesia. The patient who is able to cough and strain on request will give the surgeon the best chance of knowing the extent of the hernia. Also, once the repair has been completed the patient will be able to cough and strain to demonstrate that it is sound. To complement the local anesthetic, the patient is given a short acting intravenous sedative and an analgesic. The anesthetic solution is composed of 60 ml Bupivacaine 0.25% (Marcaine), 30 ml Cloroprocaine 3% (Nesacaine), and 9 ml sodium bicarbonate 8.4% (Neut). A field block of approximately 60 ml of the solution is infiltrated into the skin and subcutaneous tissues. A low inguinal incision is made, its average length is 7 cm. The subcutaneous layer is divided through Campa's and Scarpa's fasciae. The superficial epigastric vessels which lie between these layers are divided. The external oblique aponeurosis and the tissues lying immediately deep to it are anesthetized with 10-15 ml of anesthetic solution. If identifiable, the cremasteric branch of the ilioinguinal nerve is preserved. The cremasteric fascia is opened lengthwise and the spermatic cord lifted from it. The cord is retracted with a soft rubber drain. The thin internal spermatic fascia which covers the cord is opened. The posterior wall of the canal is inspected to exclude a coexisting direct hernia. When an indirect peritoneal sac is present it is usually evident. If not, the obliterated processus vaginalis, or a nub of peritoneum high in the cord should be identified to minimize the chance of overlooking a thin sac. If a lipoma is present it is ligated and excised. Dissection of the necks of the lipoma and the peritoneal sac is painful unless they are anesthetized. Another 10-15 ml of anesthetic solution is injected into these vulnerable areas. A small indirect sac is left intact and dissected free from the cord structures. A larger sac is best handled by leaving the distal portion undisturbed, dividing its mid or proximal portion, ligating it and reducing it back into the abdominal cavity. The proximal portion of the sac must be cleared from the threshold of the internal ring. This is done with sharp dissection to remove the vas deferens and other cord structures from the posterior wall of the sac; and by dividing the investing fibers of the transversalis fascia that encase the true neck. Once the sac is reduced it is helpful to continue its dissection by inserting an opened sponge through the internal ring. This further open up the potential retromuscular preperitonal space. The space created allows the umbrella to unfold deep to most of the myopectineal orifice including the internal ring. The insertion is done as follows: a) an index finger is inserted through the internal ring into the submuscular space, b) the pulsating iliac artery is palpated laterally, c) the unfolded umbrella-plug, on a clamp-carrier, is slid down the medial side of the index finger into the preperitoneal space, d) the clamp is released and removed, e) the patient coughs and strains to seat the mesh in place and to allow the surgeon to visualize the completed repair. In type III hernias, (internal ring greater than one fingerbreadth) when the patient coughs the plug may be extruded. To prevent failure, if only an umbrella-plug is used, a single 3-0 prolene suture is placed lateral to the cord to reduce the internal ring diameter to one fingerbreadth (size or a type II hernia). The suture is not placed through the graft. The patient tests the repair again by coughing and straining to prove that it is complete. In type I and type II hernias an umbrella-plug alone is sufficient, sutures are unnecessary. The repair is complete; now it remains only to reconstruct the canal. The cord and nerve are replaced in their bed. The external oblique aponeurosis is closed over them with a 3-0 vicryl suture. In closing this aponeurosis, minimal tissue bites are taken and approximation is done without tension to minimize postoperative discomfort. The subcutaneous layers are closed with two sutures of 3-0 plain catgut. The skin is approximated with a continuous 4-0 monocryl subcuticular suture. Adhesive strips support the closure. Telfa and a dry dressing are applied.

(2) Results

From September 1987 through December 1995 we repaired 1,981 indirect inguinal hernias with the sutureless technique. Two years ago we abandoned the overlay graft component of the original operation, and have successfully relied on the enlarged umbrella-plug graft alone for the repair. We have simplified our repair for type III hernias by using the larger umbrella graft and have added a Marcy suture, thereby avoiding the need to open the posterior wall in all pure indirect hernias, regardless of their size. This repair has been

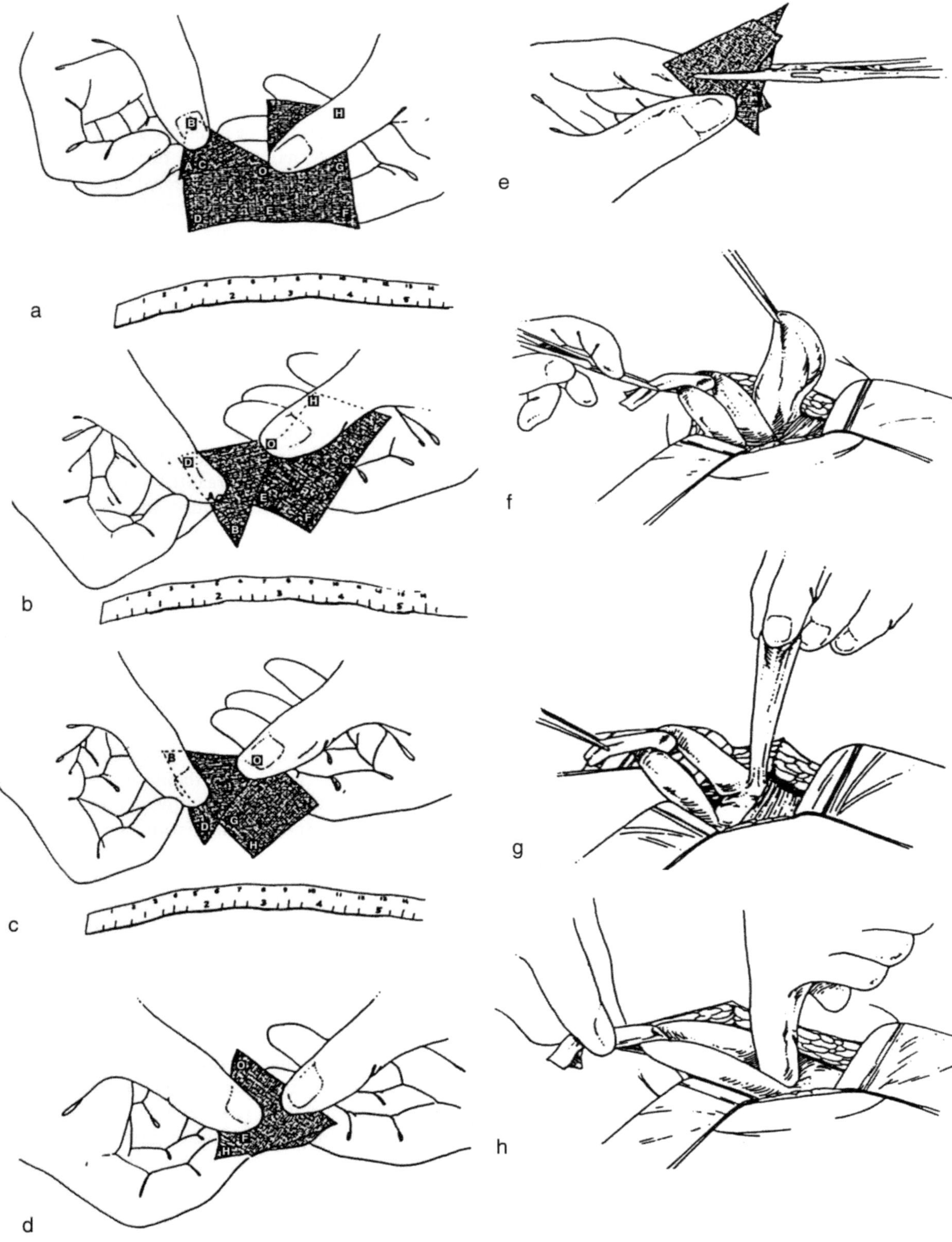

adopted as the operation of choice for indirect hernias at many surgical centers. It is simple to learn and to perform. Patients make a rapid and relatively pain-free recovery. At present, in two multicenter study-groups, it is being compared to certain other open and endoscopic repairs. It is usually carried out under local anesthesia and its effectiveness can be tested before the wound is closed. Recurrent indirect inguinal hernias are repaired in exactly the same manner, except that a regional anesthetic is preferred.

(3) Complications

Complications have been minimal with the improved technique. These have included: seroma needing aspiration (0.8%), hematoma requiring drainage (0.6%), infection requiring re-opening the wound and culture (0.2%), testicular swelling (0.2%), testicular atrophy (0%), short-term neuralgia (1%) and protracted neuralgia (0.1%).

One unusual complication has occurred related to the Gilbert repair. A 69 year old male had an umbrella-plug graft sutureless repair of a right recurrent type II hernia, from which he made a prompt and complication-free recovery. Six months later, while playing golf, he made a sudden movement to avoid being hit by a golf ball. Within minutes he began to develop acute left lower quadrant pain, and within two hours he was seen in the emergency room where he complained of diffuse pain and had peritoneal signs. Radio-

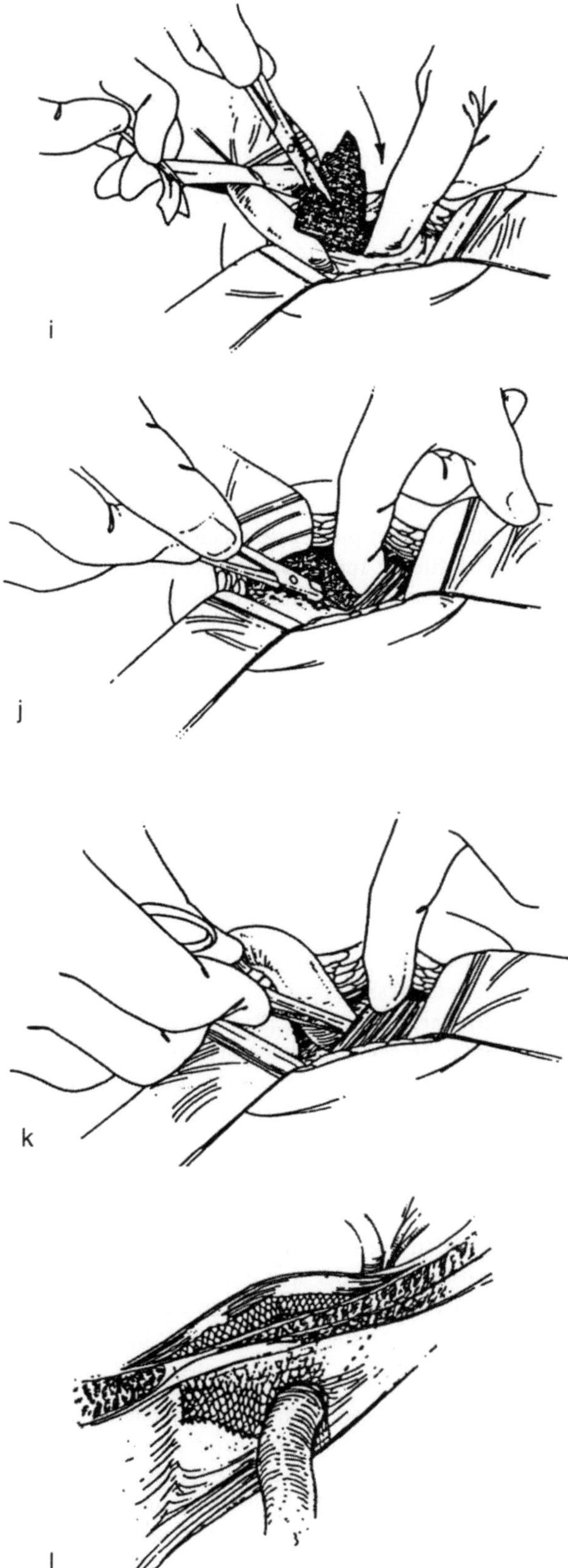

Fig. 9.15. Gilbert's operation. **a-d** Technique of forming the umbrella-plug: **a** move point A, the generator, to point C, rotate the graft 90° in the left hand; **b** move point B to point E, rotate the graft 90 degrees in the left hand; **c** move point D to point G, rotate the graft 90° in the left hand; **d** move point F to point H, completing the formation of the plug.

e-k The insertion maneuver: **e** grasp the folded umbrella-plug with a straight clamp; **f** separate the peritoneal sac from the spermatic cord and from the investing fibers of the transversalis fascia at the internal ring; **g** empty the peritoneal sac after high dissection and actualizing the potential submuscular preperitoneal space; **h** reduce the peritoneal sac; **i, j** insert the umbrella-plug into the preperitoneal space by sliding it along the index finger, which has been passed through the internal ring; **k** with the mesh plug in the preperitoneal space the carrier-clamp is removed.

l The unfolded umbrella graft remains in the preperitoneal space between the peritoneum and transversalis fascia. Here it protects the greater part of the myopectineal orifice. The repair is complete

graph showed free air under his right diaphragm. Emergency exploration revealed a 2 mm perforation in his terminal ileum where the bowel had pulled away from an adhesion to the mesh. The perforation was closed, the peritoneal cavity lavaged and antibiotics given. The mesh was not removed. He went home afebrile, on a regular diet five days later, resumed work in two weeks and has remained well ever since. This complication is unique. No others have been reported related to the umbrella-plug. We speculate that the invaginated peritoneal sac must have had a hole in it that allowed a loop of bowel to become adherent to the mesh. The loop pulled away and perforated when he made the sudden jerking motion. Incidentally, he has since returned for the repair of his recurrent left inguinal hernia which was also done with an umbrella-plug graft.

(4) Conclusion

Since adding the single suture for larger indirect hernias (type III) the repair obviously is no longer done sutureless, therefore we now refer to it as the Gilbert repair. As such, the Gilbert repair for type I and type II hernias continues to be done sutureless, while the type III uses a single suture. The essence of the Gilbert repair is that it uses the internal ring to gain access to the retromuscular preperitoneal space, for repair of all types of indirect inguinal hernia. This obviates the need to divide or suture the posterior wall, and minimizes the chance of creating a defect or undue tension, which may favor recurrent herniation.

d) The Plugs

J. P. Palot and J. B. Flament,
with the collaboration of
J. P. Cailliez-Tomasi and G. Greffier

Faced with the great variety of groin hernias, the surgeon has to choose the most appropriate procedure in every individual case. For many years we have made that choice according to the principles outlined by H. Fruchaud [Fruchaud 1956 I & II] (all hernias result from the rupture or the dissension of the transversalis fascia in the area of the myopectineal hole), and we have treated the hernias by either a deep repair including the transversalis fascia (Bassini; Shouldice; McVay) or a prosthetic repair using a Mersilene mesh placed in the preperitoneal space in most cases via an inguinal approach and less frequently by a midline approach [Rives et al. 1973; Rives et al. 1994]. More recently we were interested in the concept of "tension

free hernioplasty" and especially by the "plug repair". The great simplicity of the procedure and the very good results published by American authors [Gilbert 1992; Lichtenstein et al. 1989; Rutkow & Robbins 1995] and some French authors as well [Dieudonné 1992; Pelissier & Blum 1996] led us to investigate this operation.

(1) A Short History of the Concept

The first description of a "plug repair" was made by Lichstenstein and Shore (1974). The procedure was applied to femoral and some recurrent hernias: after identification and dissection the peritoneal sac was simply invaginated without resection or ligation and the fascial defect was closed by a "cigarette plug" created by rolling a piece of Marlex mesh. In spite of good results this procedure remained infrequent.

In 1989, Gilbert published a classification of groin hernias [Gilbert 1989] and described a "sutureless repair" of small and medium indirect hernias [Gilbert 1992].

The hernial sac was simply dissected and inverted though the internal ring. Then a piece of polypropylene was slit and fashioned in a cone shape and this "plug" was inserted into the internal ring. In addition a nonsutured onlay mesh was placed on the posterior wall of the inguinal canal. In this operation there was absolutely no modification of the normal anatomy.

More recently, I. M. Rutkow and A. W. Robbins extended the procedure to all types of hernias. In a first period, they used a hand made plug of polypropylene [Rutkow & Robbins 1993] and right now a flower shaped mesh plug of their conception (Perfix Plug* by Bard corporate) [Rutkow & Robbins 1995]. The plug is presented in two parts: the plug itself and a little onlay mesh with a lateral slit to accommodate the spermatic cord. We have been using this plug since 1995.

(2) Technique (Fig 9.16)

Anesthesia. In our department, this operation is currently performed under spinal (61%) rather than general (29%) or local (16%) anesthesia. The choice is generally given to the patients except in some particular indications.

Dissection. The dissection, in our experience, is more extensive than in the original procedure described by Rutkow and Robbins. A 5-6 cm horizontal incision is made 1 cm above the level of the inguinal ligament. Medially the incision reaches the level of the pubic tubercle. The external oblique aponeurosis is then

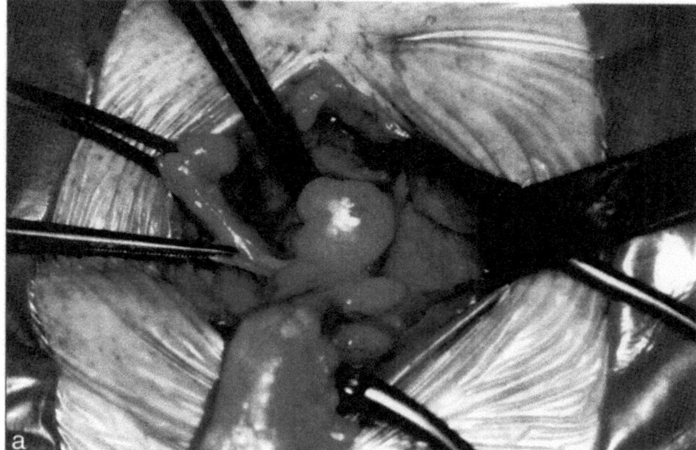

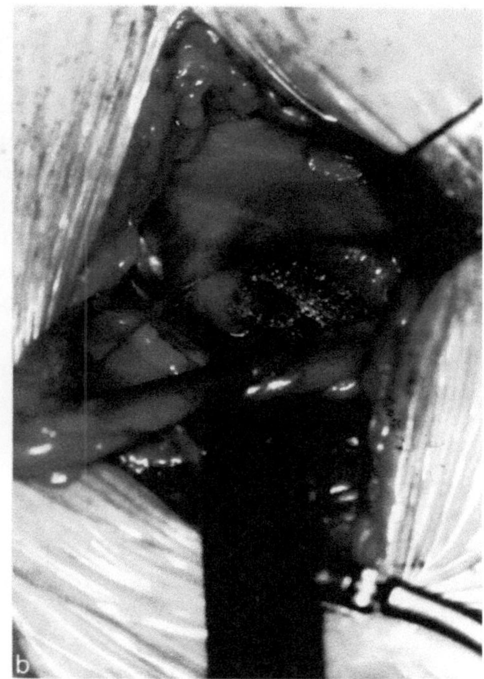

Fig. 9.16. a Treatment of an indirect hernia. The spermatic cord is taped. The sac is dissected and is being reintegrated in the internal ring. **b** Same patient. The plug is in place in the internal ring

incised down to the superficial ring while sparing the ilioinguinal and iliohypogastric nerves, and separated from the underlying structures of the inguinal canal by blunt dissection. The spermatic cord is then dissected and isolated on a tape and an assessment of the posterior wall is made to determine the final choice for the repair. Treatment of an indirect sac is made by division or only by longitudinal separation of cremasteric muscles. The sac is dissected up to the internal ring. Large sacs are resected and tied but in most cases the indirect sac is simply reduced in the preperitoneal space through the internal ring. Direct sacs are treated in the same way, being dissected free to the level of the transversalis fascia. Recurrent hernias and femoral hernias can also be treated in the same way.

The mesh plug repair. A plug of proper size is inserted through the internal ring (indirect hernia) or the fascial defect (direct hernia) and secured with 3 or 4 nonabsorbable sutures. When under spinal or local anesthesia, the patient is requested to cough in order to check the correct positioning and the efficacy of the plug. Reinforcement of the posterior wall of the inguinal canal can be obtained by placing the onlay mesh of Marlex from the pubic tubercle to above the internal ring. The lateral slit of the mesh is sutured around the cord. Generally the onlay mesh is secured by interrupted sutures to avoid slippage. The external oblique aponeurosis is then closed over the spermatic cord to recreate the inguinal canal. The operation ends with the closure of superficial layers (fascia and skin).

(3) Personal Experience

We have been using the mesh plug repair since 1995. From January 1995 to February 1997 we completed 306 hernioplasties and out of them 96 mesh plug repairs.

Evolution of our indications is presented in table 9.11. The operations were performed by four surgeons who were totally free concerning the choice of procedure. It is interesting to emphasize that mesh plug repairs represented 20% of our indications during the first year now represents 42% of our hernioplasties.

Among the 96 hernias treated by this technique there were 70% primary and 30% recurrent hernias; 60% were indirect and 35% were direct. In 5% of cases

Table 9.11. Evaluation of our indications

	1995	1996-1997
Shouldice	75 = 51.4%	60 = 37.5%
McVay	20 = 13.7%	17 = 10.5%
Inguinal mesh	18 = 12.0%	16 = 10.0%
(J. Rives operation)		
Midline mesh	4	0
Plug	**29 = 20%**	**67 = 42%**
Total	146	160

the hernias had an indirect and a direct component and necessitated two plugs. We used the plug alone in 30 cases and the plug and the onlay mesh in 66 cases. The mean age of the patients was 61 years (range 22 to 90 years). Seven patients had minor complications such as hematomas or seromas. Five of these patients had been operated on for recurrent hernias. There were 2 failures: we had to remove one plug for persistent neuralgia after 6 months. The plug repair was converted into a Rives' procedure with a good result. Another patient operated for a multirecurrent hernia after previous laparoscopic prosthetic repair had a re-recurrence after 6 months: so only one recurrence is known (1/96 = 1.05%) in this series.

(4) Discussion

This preliminary report is too recent to draw some definitive conclusions but our first impressions are rather favorable.

Mesh plug repair seems particularly interesting for treatment of indirect hernias of little and medium size. In these cases the transversalis fascia is very strong and a Shouldice operation, as we used to do, is probably too extensive a procedure. This type of repair is also of major interest for the treatment of recurrent hernias. The procedure needs minimal dissection and thus may avoid postoperative complications like ischemic orchitis. On the other hand, we don't think that all types of hernias should be treated in this way and we still use conventional prosthetic repair by an inguinal approach (Rives' operation) for large direct hernias where there is total destruction of the transversalis fascia.

(5) Conclusion

The plug repair is a very simple and reproducible operation which can be done with any type of anesthesia. The first results of this short experience are promising but further evaluation is needed to evaluate the long-term results and the tolerance of the material.

References

Dieudonné G (1992) L'oblitération de trajets herniaires par bouchon de tulle prothétique. Chirurgie 118
Fruchaud H (1956) Anatomie chirurgicale des hernies de l'aine. Doin, Paris
Fruchaud H (1956) Traitement chirurgical des hernies de l'aine. Doin, Paris
Lichtenstein JL, Shore JM (1974) Simplified repair of femoral and recurrent inguinal hernias by a "plug" technique. Am J Surg 128: 439-444
Pélissier EP, Blum D (1996) Le plug dans la hernie inguinale. Etude prospective de faisabilité. Ann Chir 30 (suppl.) 63
Rutkow IM, Robbins AW (1993) "Tension free" inguinal herniorrhaphy: a preliminary report on the "mesh plug" technique. Surgery 114: 3-8
Rutkow IM, Robbins AW (1995) Mesh plug hernia repair: a follow-up report. Surgery 117: 597- 598.

2. Prosthetic Repair via the Open Abdomen

a) The Rives Operation: Unilateral Prosthesis by the Preperitoneal Route

The preparation of the patient, both general and local, should be carried out with the same attention as in all prosthetic procedures. Anesthesia may be general, epidural or spinal. The surgeon stands on the opposite side to the hernia.

One begins with a midline subumbilical incision. The peritoneal sac is freed with a mounted sponge or with the finger. The "hernial pedicle" is soon seen and isolated as in all posterior approaches. Direct sacs are easily reduced and "interiorised", though with an adherent sac it may be necessary to open it at the neck and introduce a finger to aid the dissection. If necessary the base of the sac can be left and the neck divided flush with the deep aspect of the abdominal wall.

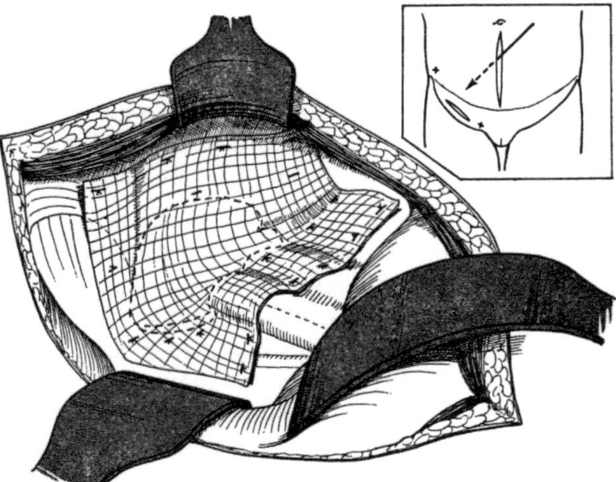

Fig. 9.17. Implantation of a dacron mesh prosthesis via the midline subperitoneal route. This procedure, derived from that of Mahorner and Goss (1962), can be done when Cooper's ligament cannot be used for repair [Rives et al. 1974]

Medium-sized sacs are resected, the peritoneum sutured with nonabsorbable material (Fig. 9.17).

The surgeon completes the retroperitoneal dissection and the entire groin region is then revealed with great clarity. The presence of the spermatic cord requires an incision to be made in the material either at its upper or its lateral border, the slit thus created being then closed around the cord, which helps to secure the patch in place. This is buried down in the area between the inguinal canal and the internal iliac fossa and its edges smoothed out. Rives fixes it with a few sutures placed in the most accessible parts, namely the psoas muscle, the posterior aspect of the rectus and the pectineal ligament. When the retractors are removed the peritoneal sac returns to its original position, thus completing the adherence of the patch to the abdominal wall. When the hernia is bilateral the same procedure can be carried out on both sides. The wall is then closed having inserted a suction drain. This technique, which was described by J. Rives in 1966, has not been employed to any great extent by the present authors, and its indications have been restricted [Palot 1995] to the treatment of those recurrent hernias in which it would be difficult to approach the spermatic cord via the superficial route, and those where there is destruction of the inguinal mechanism and disappearance of the pectineal ligament.

In the 1983 series there were five recurrences in 84 operations (6%), in the 1994 series 1 recurrence in 27 operations (3.7%). The use of medium-sized patches (10 cm across) may be criticized as follows. There is a risk of injuring important structures such as the femoral and obturator nerves and vessels, as they may be masked by the patch, at the moment it is fixed in place. This fixation is in fact the most critical stage in the operation. The gap for passage of the cord is a regrettable weak point. Incision of the midline raphé below the umbilicus carries a risk of postoperative eventration in subjects with a weakened abdominal wall. However, overall, the positioning of a patch from above greatly simplifies the dissection of the sac and the deep muscular ring, as compared with the same stages carried out by the direct inguinal route. The merits of the high approach have already been emphasized. Table 9.12 sets out the published results of this operation.

There are a number of variations in the per-peritoneal repair of the unilateral prosthesis. Rignault and Dumeige 1981 have suggested using a Pfannenstiel incision, arching across the suprapubic fold, for operation on these neighboring structures. The subcutaneous tissues, anterior rectus sheath and external oblique aponeurosis are incised at right angles to the skin incision. The anterior rectus sheath is detached from the fleshy bellies of the rectus and pyramidalis muscles, to reach the pubis below and the junction of the upper third and lower two-thirds of the umbilico-pubic line above. The preperitoneal space is opened in the midline and the operation continued by retroperitoneal mobilization so as to insert a unilateral prosthesis, slit for the passage of the spermatic cord, on to the pectineal ligament, iliac fascia and conjoint tendon. An identical procedure is carried out on the other side in the case of a bilateral hernia, and the layers are closed with a suction drain. Rignaud reports a very low infection rate (1.1% deep sepsis, 3% superficial sepsis). In a series of 134 operations, and eventration through the Pfannenstiel incision is unusual. The recurrence rate following an unspecified follow-up period is 1.5% [Thesis by C. Dubois, 1982].

b) The Stoppa Operation

This is a highly individual method which has nonetheless been developed using proven principles. Since 1968, sufficient clinical experience has been obtained both within and outside France, to render this procedure "a classic".

Principles of the method. The choice of Mersilene mesh will come as no surprise to the reader who is already aware that this material constitutes a "good prosthesis". Since its introduction into France by J. Rives we have used it to exclusion of all others. Its acceptance by the tissues allows the use of very large prostheses which completely enwrap the lower part of the parietal peritoneum, which thus becomes inextensible, so that no further herniation is possible in the groin region. Due to the close contact between the peritoneum and fascia transversalis, there can be no "deeper" method of reinforcement for the inguinal region. In spite of extensive dissection of the parietal structures this procedure renders unnecessary any attempt at repair of the hernia defect.

The use of the preperitoneal route brings many advantages which have already been mentioned, particularly important in the case of recurrent or multiply-recurrent hernias. The retroperitoneal dissection is quick and bloodless, proceeding logically from the (normal) midline region towards the inguinal area which may be site of scarring. There is excellent exposure of the hernial structures, and no sac can be overlooked. The anatomy and function of the groin structures is not disturbed, and it is possible to develop a very extensive retroperitoneal space for the insertion

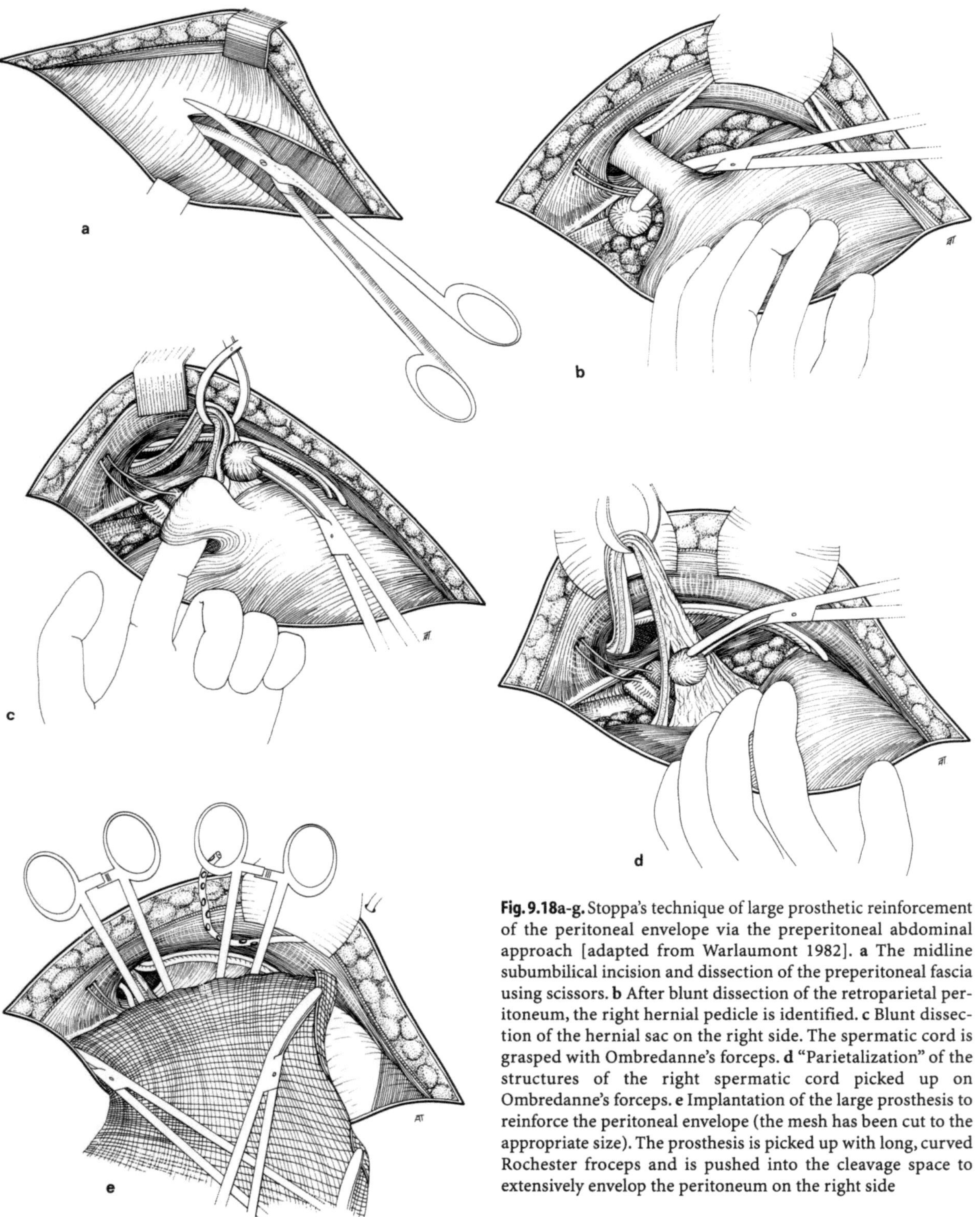

Fig. 9.18a-g. Stoppa's technique of large prosthetic reinforcement of the peritoneal envelope via the preperitoneal abdominal approach [adapted from Warlaumont 1982]. **a** The midline subumbilical incision and dissection of the preperitoneal fascia using scissors. **b** After blunt dissection of the retroparietal peritoneum, the right hernial pedicle is identified. **c** Blunt dissection of the hernial sac on the right side. The spermatic cord is grasped with Ombredanne's forceps. **d** "Parietalization" of the structures of the right spermatic cord picked up on Ombredanne's forceps. **e** Implantation of the large prosthesis to reinforce the peritoneal envelope (the mesh has been cut to the appropriate size). The prosthesis is picked up with long, curved Rochester froceps and is pushed into the cleavage space to extensively envelop the peritoneum on the right side

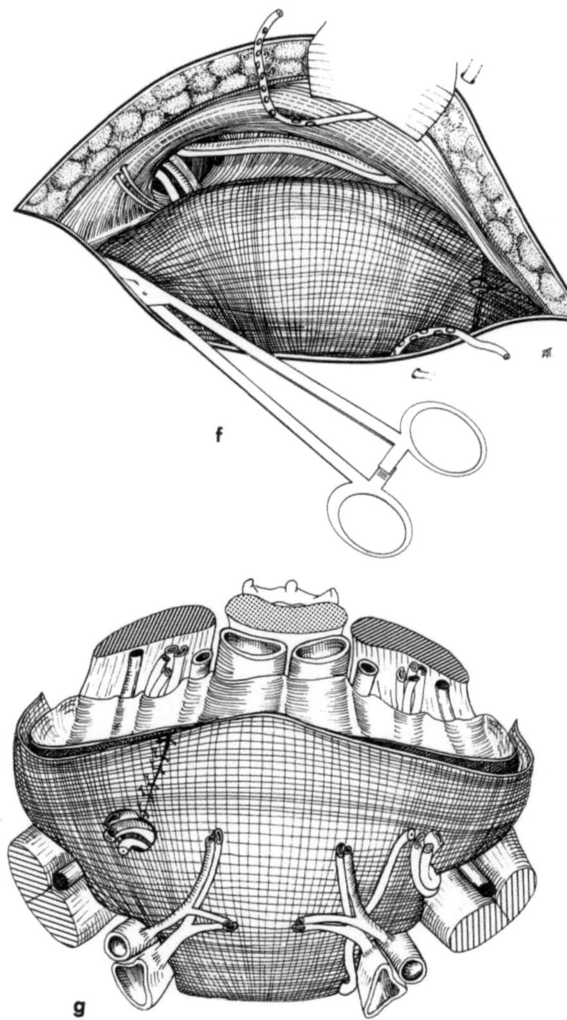

Fig. 9.18. f The large prosthesis has been implanted on both sides. Note the single suture joining the middle of the upper edge of the prosthesis to the lower margin of Richet's umbilical fascia (on the *right*). The inferior midline clamp is used to hold the mesh in front of the bladder. Two Redon tubes have been prepared for suction drainage of the cleavage space.

g Anteroposterior illustration of the finished operation. Note the large prosthesis enveloping and reinforcing the peritoneum, which is now inextensible. The abdominopelvic wall has not been drawn. Note also that the two spermatic cords have not been treated in the same way. The left spermatic cord (on the *right side* of the figure) has been treated by "parietalization", whereas the right cord (on the *left side* of the figure) passes through a slit in the upper margin of the prosthesis

and wrapping of the visceral sac in a large bilateral Dacron mesh prosthesis. The idea of a maximal dissection of the retrofascial preperitoneal and prefascial spaces led us to conduct an anatomical research exercise with B. F. K. Odimba in 1980. From this we were able to develop a clear and accurate description of this important anatomical space which gives such excellent access to the musculo-pectineal orifice, for the benefit of the practicing surgeon. The large size of the single prosthesis used for bilateral wrapping of the peritoneal sac also effectively protects the midline part of the approach, against any possible future eventration.

The "parietalisation" of the elements of the spermatic cord is another important technical principle which avoids slitting the prosthesis and preserves the integrity of the reinforcement. The idea of routinely exteriorising the elements of the cord occurred to us as a result of noting the compliance of the cord in cases of multi-recurrent hernias. We reported the idea in 1973 and have used it routinely since 1976 without any problems.

The last principle underlying this method is the hydrostatic principle of Pascal, that is to say to make use of the intra-abdominal pressure, which produced the hernia in the first place, to prevent its recurrence. It is in fact the intra-abdominal pressure exerted directly on to the prosthesis and the abdominal wall, via the peritoneal sac. This ensures the immediate firm fixation of the large prosthesis, which is followed by a further solidification as the interstices of the Dacron mesh are invaded by scar tissue. An original feature of the procedure is that it is not necessary to fix the prosthesis, which simplifies the technique considerably. This method is appealing in its originality, simplicity and radicality. In the most difficult cases, instead of having to struggle to repair an abdominal wall of poor quality, one simply renders the peritoneal sac inelastic, by wrapping it in material. This is the first published account of a method of repair of groin hernias which is without tension and without sutures. The local preparation of the operative area must be meticulous. Particularly in the case of massive hernias which have "lost their right of residence" in the abdominal cavity, and in patients with respiratory problems, a preoperative pneumoperitoneum as proposed by Goni-Moreno may very occasionally be required.

General or spinal anesthesia are preferred: local anesthesia is not advisable.

Technique (Fig. 9.18). The operation is usually complete within 20 to 45 minutes. The standard incision is a midline subumbilical. The preperitoneal space is easily freed by the finger or a mounted sponge. In the case of multi-recurrent hernias it may be useful to use the scissors to free the peritoneum from the scar. The dissection begins in the retropubic space of Retzius in front of the bladder and as far as the prostate. It is extended laterally behind the rectus muscle and epigastric vessels, in the retroinguinal space, as far as the iliopsoas muscle. The sac of a direct inguinal or femoral hernia is easily reduced by simple traction, and the spermatic cord drawn aside with a loop. With an indirect hernia, the sac and the spermatic cord compose a sort of "pedicle" whose elements need to be separated from each other. The retroperitoneal cleavage plane is extended to expose the deep aspect of the obturator region below, the iliac vessels laterally and the psoas major muscle. There is no need to extend the dissection upwards beyond the arcuate line of Douglas.

Direct hernial sacs, inguinal, femoral or rarely obturator are inverted with a purse-string suture. Indirect sacs are opened in order to simplify the dissection, with a finger introduced within. Small sacs are managed by resection-invagination, being careful not to dissect the sac below the level of the pubis, which carries the risk of ischemic orchitis, due to trauma in the distal part of the cord. The anterior aspect of the distal sac should be opened widely so as to promote drainage into the surrounding tissues, and a suction drain is placed within it. The contents of the spermatic cord are then parietalised separately from the peritoneum, while leaving them included in their fibrous sheath, which is triangular in its lower portion. This quick and simple maneuver greatly simplifies the positioning of the prosthesis and avoids the necessity of cutting it to allow passage of the cord.

When the first side has been completed, the surgeon and his assistant change places and carry out an identical operation on the other side. At the end of the procedure, all the hernial orifices are clearly seen, and there is no need to attempt to close them, which only leads to unnecessary complications. The Dacron prosthesis is then prepared, the chevron with the major stretch line transversely. Its overall breadth is equivalent to the distance between the two anterior-superior iliac spines, less by 1 cm or 2 cm (mean 24 cm) and its height is that of the umbilico-pubic line (mean 17 cm). The upper border of the chevron is 4 cm across and the lower one 6 cm. The prosthesis is rapidly soaked in povidone iodine and then grasped in eight long curved hemostats. It is positioned in the following manner. The preperitoneal space is opened up by lifting the abdominal wall opposite to the surgeon with a retractor, while the surgeon's left hand pulls up the

peritoneal cavity towards the midline. The middle and lower forceps then draw the prosthesis behind the pubis and in front of the prostate, while the lower lateral forceps is introduced as far as possible behind the corresponding obturator foramen. The middle lateral forceps is passed in towards the internal iliac vessels almost vertically, and the upper lateral forceps pull the patch as far as possible upwards and posteriorly. The final maneuver is to slide the upper midline forceps underneath the umbilical fascia. At this point the retractors and forceps are removed, being careful not to change in any way the position of the prosthesis. The surgeon and his assistant then once again change sides in order to close the prosthesis on the opposite side. When all the forceps are removed, it only remains to insert one suture at the upper extremity of the patch into the umbilical fascia so as to suspend it in a manner of a curtain, before closure. The musculo-aponeurotic layers are closed by a continuous number 1 suture.

The complete operation includes a wide retroperitoneal dissection on both sides, parietalisation of the elements of the spermatic cord and having dealt with the hernial sacs, a massive enwrapment of the visceral sac in a flexible mesh, with no attempt at direct repair of the hernial orifices. Clearly, handling of this prosthesis and its holding forceps requires scrupulous asepsis.

Postoperatively, the patient is encouraged to return to early activity, which is usually easy considering the absence of postoperative pain, and there is no necessity for routine antibiotics. The drains and dressing are removed on the second day, to allow inspection of the wound. Most patients are discharged between the second and fourth postoperative day.

Variations on the above technique include a horizontal type incision which has cosmetic advantages. On occasion a complimentary incision at the neck of the scrotum may be required in order to free the adherent contents of a scrotal hernia. Pelvic lesions can be dealt with at the same time as the repair, provided that there is no risk of sepsis. On occasion we have carried out this operation on a patient with a unilateral hernia, in view of the fact that 20% of contra-lateral hernias appear within the first five years following repair of a one-sided lesion.

The *complications* include hematomas 3%, hydrocele 5.5%, ischemic orchitis 0, sepsis 2.1% (all but three were superficial infections which did not involve the prosthesis). At present this operation is indicated in between 20% and 25% of groin hernias. We use it for

Table 9.12. Rate of recurrence after Stoppa's operation (inguinal hernias)

Authors	# Cases	% Follow-up	Years Follow-up	% Recurrences
Boucard (1982)	381	-	1 to 11	0
Van Damme (1985)	100	57	2	0
Stoppa (1986)	522	-	1 to 5	0.56
Beaten (1990)	150	-	1.5 to 5.5	0.66
Moutorsi (1991)	45	99	3	1.2
Stoppa (1982)	285	91.3	1 to 10	1.2
Cubertafond (1983)	399	75	1 to 10	1.6
Gross (1992)	35	-	-	2.8
St Julien (1983)	309	63	0.5 to 6	2.9
Stoppa (1974)	168	88	1 to 7	3.3
Rignault (1983)	568	-	-	4

all hernias with a high risk of recurrence, i.e. recurrent and multi-recurrent (type IV).

It is also used for primary prevascular femoral hernias, bulky hernias, multiple and bilateral lesions, hernias in obese patients with abdominal distension, chronic bronchitis or stressful occupations, and those in whom difficulties with healing could be foreseen. The method is also useful in patients in poor general state such as gross obesity, chronic respiratory problems and cirrhosis, where there is a high risk and a guaranteed satisfactory result is essential. Contra-indications to the use of the massive bilateral prosthesis are septic risks, a midline subumbilical scar, a history of ileocaval thrombosis and those rare cases where general or spinal anesthetic is impossible. However, Wantz (1993) will carry out a unilateral operation under local anesthesia.

Critical remarks on the bilateral prosthesis. It has been said that this operation is too extensive for general use, especially from the cosmetic point of view. Precise case selection is vital, and the method is of particular use and complex hernias with an adverse course, which will undoubtedly recur without a prosthetic repair. Crossing the lower midline theoretically risks postoperative eventration, but we have not encountered a single case of incisional hernia in several thousands of operations, because the bilateral prosthesis protects the relevant area. The risk of infection, which would be expected to correlate with the size of the prosthesis, has been a preoccupation for a long time, and certainly underlines the need for strict antisepsis before, during and after the operation. However, present day experience does not reflect these fears of 20 years ago, to the extent that we no longer prescribe routine prophylactic antibiotics. When infection supervenes it is important to diagnose it early and treat it along established lines, including opening and debridement of the wound, and wide exposure and irrigation, without removing the prosthetic material, which will be incorporated once the infection has been overcome.

In contrast, one would emphasize again the radical nature of this method, which gives an almost certain insurance against recurrence. The laparoscopic surgeons have adopted it as a model procedure. Its simplicity makes it an operation which is easy to reproduce and requires no special skill or experience. Vital structures are not threatened, and postoperative discomfort is minimal because of the lack of tension and of sutures in the abdominal wall. Indeed the repair of the superficial layers of the wound is protected by the presence of a large preperitoneal patch. Table 9.12 shows some of the published results.

c) The Wantz operation (G.E. Wantz)

This technique, published in 1989, represents a combination of the two preceding principles, namely prosthetic reinforcement of the visceral sac (Stoppa) and a transverse incision through the lower quadrant of the abdomen as originated by Nyhus and Read. Wantz has stated that the reason for developing this technique of unilateral reinforcement of the visceral sac was to devise a reliable procedure which was suitable for repair of all types of groin hernia on a day case basis. In selected cases, the operation can be carried out under local anesthesia.

The preperitoneal space is approached through a transverse incision extending outwards for 8 cm to 9 cm from the midline, and situated 2 cm to 3 cm below the iliac crests (Fig. 9.19). This gives direct access to the deep inguinal ring. The rectus sheath and oblique muscles are incised horizontally. The fascia transversalis appears at the lateral edge of the rectus covering the inferior epigastric vessels and the preperitoneal fat. Incision of the transversalis fascia along the border of the rectus allows one to retract the muscle medially, to enter the preperitoneal space and to expose the epigastric vessels, which need not necessarily be divided. The preperitoneal space is freed in all directions towards the midline. Upwards this is from the rectus and transversus abdominus, and below from the Cave of Retzius so as to expose the upper border of the iliopubic ramus, the obturator foramen, and the iliac vessels. Laterally, Wantz insists that the psoas major muscle has to be exposed. The hernial sacs are treated in the usual manner. Direct inguinal hernias and femoral hernias and other rare types are easily identified and dissected and are then either resected or invaginated into a purse-string, so as to flatten the visceral sac. The sac of an indirect hernia is divided and the proximal peritoneum closed. The distal part of an inguino-scrotal sac is left in place, attached to the spermatic cord. Naturally, the sac of a sliding hernia must be separated from the cord. In the case of a bulky hernia with incarcerated contents, a separate incision in the upper part of the scrotum

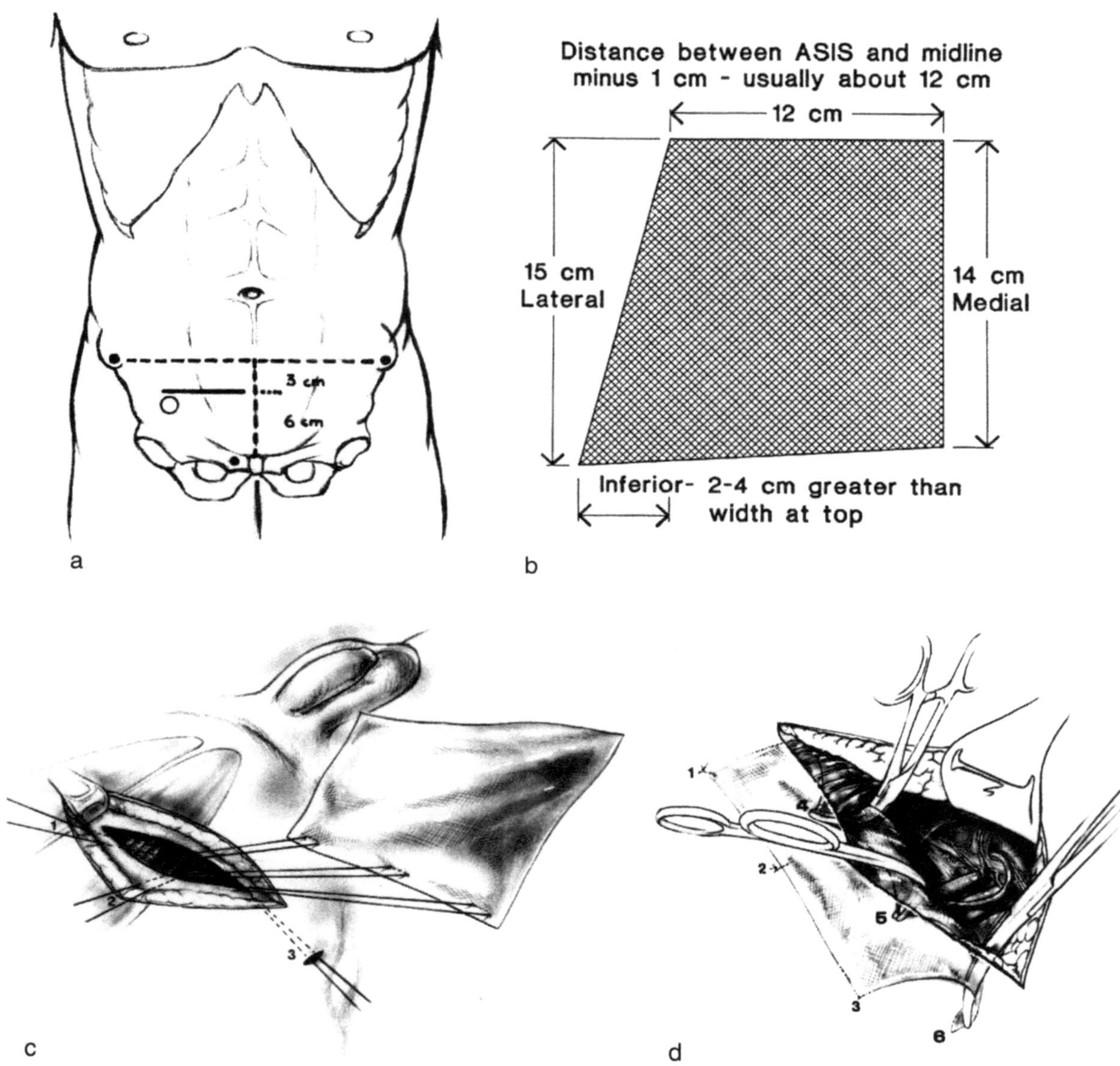

Fig. 9.19. Wantz' operation. a Incision for unilateral wrapping of the visceral sac. b "Diamond" shape of the prosthesis. c Insertion of the superior margin of the prosthesis. d Setting up of the inferior margin of the prosthesis [reproduced with permission from Wantz GE (1991) Atlas of hernia surgery. Raven Press, New York]

may be of help in securing reduction of the adherent contents. The spermatic cord is then paritealised as in the Stoppa operation. The hernial orifices are not closed. If necessary the dead space created by the reduction of the hernial sac can be obliterated by drawing across the transversalis fascia to the interior of the abdomen and fixing it by one stitch to the deep aspect of the abdominal wall. The Mersilene mesh should be arranged so that its elasticity is horizontal. The patch is roughly trapezoid, with a height of some 14 cm. It is placed in position under the rectus muscle and the upper part of the inguinal region with three traction sutures, of absorbable synthetic material, which transfix the abdominal wall and fix the patch 2 cm or 3 cm above the muscular incision. These sutures are inserted with the aid of a Reverdin needle. The lower part of the Mersilene patch is then placed with the aid of three long forceps which seize the two lower corners and the middle of the inferior edge and allow the lower part of the patch to be pulled into a good position behind the iliopubic ramus. A suction drain is inserted in order to deal with any oozing or if a large indirect sac has been left in place, and the incision is closed with loosely tied sutures. A dose of Cephazoline or Vancomycin is given intravenously immediately before the start of the operation.

In a recent series of 358 groin hernias, Wantz reports two deep hematomas, but no case of deep sepsis nor of testicular atrophy. The indications suggested by him are recurrent or re-recurrent hernias, primary hernias in patients with a collagen disease such as the Ehlers-Danlos or Marfan's syndrome, patients with abdominal distension due for example to ascites, and those who have already undergone an operation in the groin region and are therefore at risk of chronic neuralgia or testicular atrophy. As regards the long-term results, in his series of 358 groin hernias, Wantz reports 16 recurrences (4.4%) most of which resulted from technical errors.

3. Prosthetic Repair
via the Laparoscopic Route

a) The Extraperitoneal Route (TEP)

G. Champault

Although it is true that up to the present there is no firm evidence to show that laparoscopic treatment of hernias is superior to classical methods of repair [Houdart, Stoppa 1984], apart from reduced postoperative discomfort [Champault 1994] most particularly

in terms of recurrence, three laparoscopic techniques are at present in use:

- the preperitoneal approach [Dulucq 1991, Begin 1993];
- the "mixed" intra- and preperitoneal route [Leroy 1992] or transabdominal preperitoneal;
- the intraperitoneal route [Elhadad, Fourtanier 1993].

The preperitoneal route popularized in France by J. L. Dulucq (1991) and G. Begin (1993) and taken up in the USA by McKernon (1993) seems to us to have outstanding features. It is founded on the principles of the Stoppa operation 1989, which it closely resembles. A parietal route is used for treatment of a parietal abnormality. There is no need for a pneumoperitoneum, with all the accompanying risks of injury to viscera and vessels. The peritoneum remains intact between the prosthesis and the bowel.

We have chosen to use a fenestrated polypropylene (Prolene) mesh, without fixation, which while having the qualities needed for a sound repair, lessens costs and avoids the risks which accompany stapling. We will describe the different stages of this method and its variations, in order to define its role in the large range of available treatments for inguinal hernia.

(1) Technique

Preparation of the patient. The patient is under general anesthesia, intubated, with monitoring of oxygen and CO_2, the bladder is emptied by spontaneous micturition and a bolus of antibiotic is given intravenously at the moment of induction. The patient lies supine with sometimes a modest Trendelenburg tilt of 10-15°. A wide area of skin is prepared from the upper sides to the costal margin and including both flanks. The monitor is placed at the foot of the table with the diathermy apparatus, and a right-handed surgeon stands on the patient's left with his assistant opposite him, or vice versa.

Instruments required. A self-regulating CO_2 insufflator, a cold light source, a 0° axial telescope, two disposable 10 mm trocars and one or two 5 mm, a 10-8 mm cylindrical reducer, a Palmer Verres needle, a pair of coagulating scissors, a coagulating hook, two flexible grasping forceps (Bag), fine grasping forceps, a polypropylene prosthesis, one pair of Mayo scissors.

Puncture sites (Fig. 9.20). (1) A Palmer-Verres needle in the midline suprapubically, 1 cm above the bone. (2) Optical 10 mm trocar at the lower margin of the umbilicus. (3) A 5 mm operating trocar in the midline

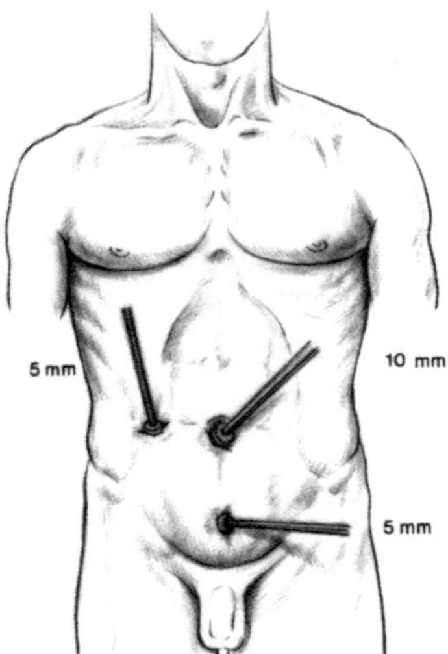

Fig. 9.20. Puncture sites

at the inferior third of the umbilico pubic line. (4) A second 10 mm operating trocar with a 5 reducer, 2 cm medial to the anterior-superior iliac spine on the side of the hernia (if unilateral). (5) A 5 mm trocar symmetrically placed on the opposite side, in the case of a bilateral hernia.

Insufflation of CO_2 into the retropubic space. (1) The function of the Palmer-Verres needle is checked. (2) Midline puncture 1 cm above the pubis, with the open needle inclined 30° behind the pubis. Two clear points of resistance are felt. The needle is aspirated to confirm the absence of blood or urine. (3) Insufflation of CO_2 is started first at a low flow then, progressively introducing 1.5 to 2 liters of gas.

The insufflation of CO_2 into the retropubic space is signaled by a visible forward projection of the rectus muscles in the subumbilical region in thin patients, an increase in size of a direct hernia in the groin area resonant to suprapubic percussion, and absence of resonance over the liver, confirming that there is no pneumoperitoneum. The pressure is stabilized at between 12 and 15 mmHg and remains at this level during the operation.

Placement of the optical trocar. A delay of 3 to 5 minutes is necessary after creation of the prepneumoperitoneum to ensure good mobilization of the peritoneal sac upwards to the level of the arcuate ligament. A 1 cm incision is made at the lower margin of the umbilicus and a 10 mm trocar introduced directed towards the pubis, piercing the aponeurotic layer tan-

gentially in the vertical axis, thus entering the freed-up preperitoneal space. The satisfactory position is confirmed by escape of gas when the mandrill is removed.

The optical trocar is introduced into the preperitoneal space which has been freed up by the gas dissection. It appears as a cellular area crossed by fine whitish fibrous bands and by a few vessels. The optical trocar is passed downwards into the midline so as to regain the vertical axis of the Palmer needle.

Preliminary dissection of the space is carried out with the optical trocar, firstly downwards and behind the pubic bone, which easily reveals the white and pearly pectineal ligament. Dissection is then carried laterally for 3 or 4 cm on either side of the midline in order to improve the access. These maneuvers which are carried out from above downwards, compress the peritoneal sac posteriorly and do not give rise to bleeding.

Placement of the first operating trocar. Having replaced the CO_2 insufflator in the sheath of the optical trocar and leaving in place the Palmer needle which acts as an axial landmark during dissection and is useful during placement of the prosthesis, a 5 mm trocar is inserted under direct vision in the midline, 4 to 5 cm above the pubis, directed towards the deep inguinal ring in the case of a unilateral hernia or perpendicularly in a bilateral case.

Dissection and creation of the preperitoneal space. This can be accomplished by scissors or sometimes by a hook, introduced via the 5 mm trocar and taken inwards and outwards, from below and above, progressively dividing the fibrous bands. The first landmark is the "inferior epigastric pedicle" which limits access laterally. This must be followed to its origin behind the rectus muscle. It must be carefully separated from the hernial sac and the components of the spermatic cord. The dissection is continued maintaining close contact with the muscular layer, with backward displacement of the parietal peritoneum. The dissection proceeds across the deep aspect of the anterior abdominal wall up to the psoas muscle in the internal iliac fossa, keeping in view the anterior-superior iliac spine. This lateral dissection requires division of the paramedian tissues in order to open up the entire preperitoneal space into a broad cone, the base of which is limited by the cord. In the case of a bilateral hernia, the same procedure is carried out on the second side, often aided by placement of a second operating trocar.

Placement of the second operating trocar. Two centimeters medially to the anterior-superior iliac spine a 10 mm trocar is inserted under direct vision, directed towards the deep inguinal ring. The muscles should be traversed at a point where the peritoneum has already been well detached. The use of a 10 to 5 reducer allows this stage of the operation to be carried out with two hands.

Dissection of the cord and hernial sac. A flexible forceps (Bag) is introduced into the midline with scissors and a hook or a second similar forceps, according to the side. Dissection begins in the region of the deep inguinal ring, the limits of which are freed up with scissors or a hook. Gentle traction on the cord will quite often reveal, particularly in the case of a direct hernia, one or more lipomas, which can be quite easily freed from the elements of the cord. These can either be left behind or removed via the 10 mm trocar.

Two or three structures must then be identified at the level of the muscular ring. These include the vas deferens which is seen as a whitish colored tube running downwards and medially across the external iliac vessels and which is easily followed to the brim of the pelvis. The testicular pedicle runs upwards and laterally, forming with the vas a triangle at the bottom of which, when the fatty tissue is freed, appear the external iliac vessels. The hernial sac, if present, appears at the origin of the cord as a whitish colored sheet, sometimes triangular, in continuity with the parietal peritoneum. It must be carefully separated from the vascular structures over a distance of 4 to 5 cm, and then displaced posteriorly. It may be quite small, and can be found only when the cord is dissected towards the peritoneum, or bulky, in which case it may occupy part of the inguinal canal. It is then necessary to dissect around the lower aspect of the cord so as to create a window between the cord and the iliac vessels. Gentle traction on the fibrous bands which fix it to the muscles, allows progressive reduction of the sac into the abdomen.

Anatomical check. The freed hernial sac is replaced backwards and the dissection of the cord completed over 4 to 5 cm. It is then necessary to check for a second or other associated hernial sac such as a femoral or obturator, and to check the landmarks including the pectineal ligament, iliac inferior epigastric and testicular vessels. The size of the deep ring must be checked with respect to the cord, and the extent of preperitoneal dissection verified in order to make sure that there is room for insertion of a large prosthesis.

Preparation of the prosthesis. This is a rectangular polypropylene mesh with an in-built memory which allows it to return to its original shape following stretching. Whether a 10 × 7 or 15 × 15 cm sheet is used depends on the local anatomical situation. After changing gloves, the prosthesis is prepared by reducing it to 15 × 12 cm according to the extent of the upper dissection. The corners are rounded off. A 60° slit is made at the lower edge, extending for 2 to 3 cm so as to create a gap of 1 to 1.5 cm, to allow passage of the cord components. Its position is determined by local anatomical considerations, in order to ensure that the entire weak area can be covered, at the same time making certain that there is a 3 cm margin all round the deep inguinal ring. A 5 mm fine toothed forceps is introduced into the reduction tube. It seizes the two ends of the slit in the prosthesis and wraps them around its long axis clockwise. The resulting prosthetic cylinder is passed into the sheath of the 8 mm reducer.

Placement of the prosthesis. The mesh is introduced via the lateral 10 mm trocar, rolled up in the reducing tube and passed into the preperitoneal space as near as possible to the wall. The end of the forceps which keeps the two edges of the slit together is positioned with regard to the deep ring, where the vas deferens and vessels are brought together. With the aid of the midline or contralateral forceps, the prosthesis is unrolled in an anticlockwise direction. It is kept open in front and above by a Palmer needle while the midline and lateral forceps guide the components of the cord into the central orifice of the slit. The lateral edge is passed under the vas deferens and vessels, and overrides the other edge in order to close the slit. The prosthesis, which is orientated by the orifice for the cord, is placed against the abdominal muscle wall. It should extend from the pectineal ligament to the psoas muscle and upwards to the iliac vessels as far as the extremity of the plane of dissection. It must in every case overlap the deep inguinal ring by 3 to 4 cm. It is manipulated into place by the aid of two forceps and a Palmer needle, but the slit is not sutured to itself.

Maintenance of the prosthesis. The mesh is not fixed. Its structure determines its inclusion into the abdominal wall and it is held in position by peritoneal pressure. Following hemostasis, cessation of insufflation and opening the valve of the trocar so as to evacuate the pneumoperitoneum under direct vision, it will be seen that the peritoneal sac becomes closely applied to the mesh.

Additional measures. The trocars are removed and the musculo-aponeurotic ports closed, together with the skin. Suction drainage is only rarely required.

Postoperative care. Low molecular weight heparin is given for prophylaxis against thromboembolism together with analgesics as necessary. The patient gets up at 24 h and leaves hospital at 48 to 72 h.

(2) Variations

Bilateral hernias. The principles of dissection are identical but are facilitated by the use of a fourth 5 mm trocar which may be inserted laterally, in symmetrical position to the first one. Two prostheses may be used of which the dimensions of the slit and the window are adapted to the local anatomical requirements. It is best to begin with the prosthesis which is on the opposite side to the 10 mm introduced trocar. The prosthesis is prepared in exactly the same way on both sides, because both slits are directed medially. It is difficult to insert one single large prosthesis, although a 30 × 12 cm patch with parietalisation of the cord can be used.

Anesthesia. General anesthesia with intubation is customary, but epidural or spinal techniques are possible when one uses the preperitoneal route [Begin 1993]. However, the risk of an inadvertent pneumoperitoneum occurring during the dissection may limit this type of anesthesia.

Direct approach to the preperitoneal space. This requires a horizontal 12 mm incision over the lower edge of the umbilicus, or 1 to 2 cm below it, or even a vertical cut [Begin 1993]. The subcutaneous tissues are dissected with the scissors under direct vision and the anterior rectus sheath is incised transversely. The muscles are drawn aside, exposing the posterior sheath. A blunt 10 mm trocar is introduced into the space tangentially to the cutaneous plane, which reveals the cobweb structure of the lamina propria. Insufflation is then begun.

Dissection of the preperitoneal space. This can be facilitated by the use of a 30 to 40° optical axis.

Balloon dissection. Having exposed the preperitoneal plane a plastic balloon, of either a round or oval shape, is introduced through the blunt trocar in order to follow the shape of the Cave of Retzius. It is inflated by 300 to 600 mm of normal saline every two or three minutes, or by air. The balloon separates the plane of the fascia propria and creates a large cavity at the peritoneal sac below and behind. The empty balloon is then withdrawn through the sheath and replaced by a 10 to 11 mm trocar for the insufflation of CO_2. Apart from their very high cost, these techniques have the disadvantage of lacerating small vessels in the space, and thus rendering subsequent dissection and identification of important structures more difficult.

Trocars. Two 10 mm and one or two 5 mm re-usable trocars are usually adequate, though some prefer the disposable type. If the prosthesis is to be stapled, a 12 mm port is necessary.

Prostheses. There is an enormous choice available for hernia repair, all of which have been tested or used in the laparoscopic preperitoneal approach. Dacron mesh, which is strong and light and is widely used in the Stoppa operation, is too supple for this procedure and lacks memory. It tends to ruffle up like a curtain and is difficult to maintain in place in spite of fixation. "Crinoplast" is cheap but dangerously rigid and also lacks memory. PTFE patches again are supple, opaque and difficult to use in this technique. They require extensive stapling. Apart from the high cost, their expanded structure hampers the construction of a slit. Furthermore, they do not adhere strongly to the muscle layer. Composite vicryl mesh which is a mixture of absorbable polyglycolic acid and nonabsorbable Dacron has no advantage here, as regards strength, safety and tolerance. Polypropylene is today widely used because of its texture and excellent memory. It has the disadvantage of being relatively rigid, particularly in contact with vessels. Its long-term tolerance is well known.

- The Dimensions. The prosthesis should not only cover the deep inguinal ring but also the surrounding area for at least 3 to 4 cm. In most cases a patch of 11 × 7 cm is sufficient. When the muscular defect is large it should either be narrowed by bringing the muscle down on to the ligament by two or three interrupted nonabsorbable sutures, or else a larger prosthesis (15 × 15 cm) should be used. Prolene is employed. It can be reduced in height to 12 cm or, in the case of Marlex, cut to fit. Too small a prosthesis runs the risk of being pushed out into the inguinal canal (prosthetic hernia).

- The Form. Certain authors such a Dulucq (1991) cut the inferomedial angle to form a 4 cm edge which can be stapled to the pectineal ligament.

- Should a window be used? Begin (1993) uses a slit prosthesis 14 × 14 cm with a 7 cm vertical incision from above downwards ending in a 5 mm orifice cut out of its central part. The prosthesis is accordion pleated or rolled onto itself and introduced into the preperitoneal space around the elements of the cord. When it unfolds (spontaneously or after cutting the thread) the two edges of the slit take up position on one and other side of the cord deep to the abdominal wall. This method requires closure of the slit by one to three endoscopic sutures, or by staples, in order to avoid a persistent weak area.

- Parietalisation. Dulucq (1991) places the polypropylene prosthesis on the deep aspect of the abdominal wall as a simple cover for the weak area, having mobilized the vas deferens and spermatic vessels over at least 5 cm. This "parietalisation" of the elements of the cord requires fixation of the prosthesis medially to the pectineal ligament and laterally on to the psoas, in order to avoid a low recurrence. An automatic expanding umbrella prosthesis has been described. Apart from its cost, it has disadvantages as regards structure and failure to adapt to the local anatomical conditions.

- Fixation. This is required for all prostheses which do not possess the rigidity and memory of polypropylene and in all cases where the cord is parietalised [Dulucq 1991]. It can be achieved by threads which are tied either inside or outside with the body with knots which are buried under the skin, or by automatic stapling devices such as the endo-hernia and endopap EMS. These necessitate the use of a special 12 mm trocar, and are thus very expensive. Fibrin glue can also be used. Fixation must take up the pectineal ligament below and medially, the psoas muscle laterally and the transversalis fascia in front. It carries risks of injury to the lateral cutaneous nerve of the thigh and sometimes the inferior epigastric vessels or their branches. Sepsis is rare [Kraus 1993].

Repair without prosthesis. This is technically achievable by bringing the conjoint tendon down on to the inguinal ligament and tensing the transversalis fascia. Mastery of the technique of laparoscopic knotting is required, and the indications are limited to hernias of Nyhus type I or II in young subjects.

(3) Complications

Complications peculiar to the technique. These include problems with insufflation such as hypercapnia. CO_2 is absorbed four times more readily in the preperitoneal space than from the peritoneal cavity, which occasionally gives rise to severe hypercapnia, and requires routine continuous monitoring of the PCO_2 and readiness to lower the insufflation flow as required, and induce hyperventilation.

Puncture accidents are unusual. It is important that the patient empties his bladder before the Palmer needle is introduced. A puncture of the bladder which is later detected by the safety checks is unimportant. The trocars occasionally cause bleeding, through damage to a muscular branch of the inferior epigastric vessels, which is easily controlled by means of a Foley catheter passed along the trocar sleeve. On the other hand, this approach excludes the risk of injuring the small bowel colon or major abdominal vessels.

Pneumoperitoneum may occur in three circumstances. It may arise during placement of the umbilical trocar, through direct puncture. One should wait three to five minutes before inflating the preperitoneal space, in order to ensure satisfactory detachment of the upper recess. This problem is avoidable if the opening is made under direct vision, as proposed by Begin (1993). In the lateral dissection, particularly on the right side in patients who have had an appendectomy, it is important to insufflate gently and carefully as near as possible to the deep aspect of the muscles. Care must be taken during dissection of the hernial sac in recurrent cases, particularly with unusually large or delicate sacs. Pneumoperitoneum occurs in some 10 to 15% of cases, particularly while experience is being gained. It is revealed by a sudden drop in PCO_2 and in pressure, a reduction in the field of vision due to restriction of the preperitoneal space and the development of hepatic resonance. Three remedial measures are required: namely, an increase in insufflation flow, evacuation of the pneumoperitoneum by placing a Palmer needle in the left hypochondrium, and identification of the defect. It is often very small and can be neglected but if this is not the case repair is essential.

Pneumoscrotum is sometimes discovered at the end of the operation (15 to 20%) particularly if the procedure has taken some time. Although the appearances are striking, they usually regress within one or two hours with no ill effects. Very occasionally surgical emphysema may extend up into the neck and mediastinum, following an inordinately high insufflation pressure.

Seromas are collections of serous fluid of variable degree which can present early on the 2nd to 5th day or as late as the 21st. They may cause confusion with an early recurrence of the hernia or even strangulation, although they are painless and have no cough impulse. They appear in 10 to 20% of cases for quite unknown reasons and almost always resolve spontaneously. If required, the collection may be aspirated to reassure the patient and hasten disappearance.

Nonspecific Complications. Graft sepsis is unusual. It should be prevented by rigorous aseptic technique and the routine use of antibiotics.

Occasionally a hematoma may collect in the retropubic space, usually the result of injury to the venous plexuses or to the veins of the spermatic cord, or if the wrong plane of dissection has been entered between the epigastric vessels and the abdominal wall. It usually accumulates after the counter-pressure of the insufflation has disappeared. Hematomas may be favored by the use of low molecular weight heparin as anti-thrombotic prophylaxis.

Injury to the spermatic cord is due to over-vigorous or rough dissection in an obese patient, and may be followed by later testicular atrophy.

Wounds of the bladder are most unusual using this approach.

Complications of variant techniques. Apart from rare cases of osteitis pubis [Ledquart 1994] stapling problems principally involve injuries to the inferior epigastric vessels and to the femoral and lateral cutaneous nerves. The diagnosis is immediate because of the recurrence of intense pain in the distribution of these two nerves. The offending staple must be removed without delay, usually via the laparoscopic approach. It is wise to identify the nerves before fixing the prosthesis though this may not always be easy, particularly in obese subjects. Once again, it must be emphasized that the best means of prevention is not to fix the prosthesis.

(4) Indications

The preperitoneal route is indicated for the treatment of uni- or bilateral inguinal hernias, direct or indirect, primary or recurrent, in the adult. This corresponds to types II, IIIa, and b and IV in the Nyhus classification (1991). The limits of this technique are as follows.

Age considerations. It would seem unwise to use prosthetic materials whose long-term behavior is unknown, in patients under the age of 40 to 45, who could be treated easily by an inguinal herniorrhaphy. It would seem equally unwise to use this technique in very old patients because of the risks of general anesthesia and hypercapnia. In the absence of specific physiological indications, patients older than 70 to 75 should be treated along conventional lines (Stoppa, Shouldice, Lichtenstein).

Physical condition. Patients with cardiac failure, unstable coronary disease, respiratory problems, alcoholic cirrhosis, clotting deficiencies and unoperated glaucoma, should be excluded from this form of treatment. A purely preperitoneal approach may be unsuitable for the obese patient, due to difficulties in creating a sufficiently large space of dissection, and the intra/pro-peritoneal route [Leroy 1992] may be preferred. Finally, patients whose concomitant disease may require an extraperitoneal pelvic approach in the future (arterial obstruction, prostatism) should be excluded because further surgery may be rendered extremely difficult by scarring around the prosthesis. In these cases a local approach is to be preferred.

Local pathology. Large inguino-scrotal hernias, prolapse of the groin tissues and sliding hernias are better managed by the Stoppa operation. Multiple recurrent hernias sometimes following a previous prosthetic repair may be treated by a Stoppa operation, the direct approach or a Spaw procedure [El Haddad, Fourtanier 1993], which constitutes one of its rare justifications, or possibly a plug.

The preperitoneal space may have been obliterated by previous surgery or previous prosthetic repairs.

Other local risks include a history of pelvic or regional sepsis which contra-indicates placement of a prosthesis, previous pelvic radiotherapy and a possible pregnancy.

b) The Trans-Abdominal Preperitoneal Route (TAPP)

C. Meyer

(1) Technique

The patient is placed supine with the arms by the sides. The surgeon stands on the opposite side to the hernia. Through a small umbilical incision (open laparoscopy) or by means of a Veress needle, the pneumoperitoneum is induced with a pressure of 14 mmHg. Two trocars are then introduced under visual control, on either side of the umbilicus and on the same horizontal line, using a 5 mm trocar on the hernial side and one of 12 mm opposite it to allow introduction of the graft. A 0° optical angle is used.

The peritoneum of the inguinal region is incised with diathermy scissors beginning above the deep inguinal ring, extending to the medial umbilical ligament medially, and to the anterior-superior iliac spine laterally. The pectineal ligament is identified and, in the case of an indirect hernia, the sac is dissected and separated from the elements of the cord, which are parietalised. This immediately reveals the conjoint tendon and the posterior aspect of the rectus muscle on the side of the hernia, which should be gently cleared of fat in order to facilitate stapling of the graft. The inguinal ligament is also seen but no staples should be inserted below it because of the presence of the external iliac vessels medially and the genitofemoral and lateral cutaneous nerve of the thigh laterally. For the same reason, no diathermy should be used in this area. With a direct hernia, the peritoneum is simply freed from the elements of the cord and the fascia transversalis, around the origin of the hernia.

The musculo-pectineal orifice is then covered by a prosthesis which is preferably of polypropylene. This material has the advantage of staying in position and its loose network allows the tissues to be visualized through the prosthesis, which aids accurate stapling.

Size is important, as too small a prosthesis carries a risk of recurrence. We recommend a graft 10-12 cm high and 10-12 cm across. The prosthesis is fixed to the pectineal ligament, to the posterior edge of the rectus muscle and to the conjoint tendon, usually by staples, but occasionally by infra-abdominal suture. It may be placed behind the spermatic cord or incised to allow its passage. In every case the prosthesis must be large enough to cover all the inguino-femoral orifices including the deep inguinal ring, the medial inguinal fossa and the femoral canal.

The peritoneum is then closed in order to isolate the prosthesis, either by a suture or by staples. This closure is aided by reducing the pneumoperitoneum pressure to 9 mmHg. This pneumoperitoneum is then evacuated and the fascial layers at the umbilicus and the 12 mm trocar orifice are sutured.

(2) Special Cases

Indirect hernias are simple to manage, as the components of the spermatic cord can be quickly and rapidly isolated. If there is much bulging of the transversalis fascia it may be helpful to evert it and fix it by staples or by suturing it to the inguinal ligament with the aid of an endoloop [Corbitt 1993].

With an indirect inguino-scrotal hernia dissection of the sac may be difficult and the elements of the cord are at risk. In these cases it is preferable to leave the distal part of the sac and only to resect its proximal portion.

In the case of a bilateral hernia the operation is repeated on the other side using a second prosthesis. Some authors prefer to use a single prosthesis extending from one iliac spine to the other and passing in front of the symphysis pubis, which is exposed by a preliminary short dissection.

(3) Advantages and Disadvantages

As with all operative techniques, TAPP carries certain advantages and disadvantages, some connected with laparoscopy in general, others peculiar to the transperitoneal route.

The laparoscopic approach, which achieves a tension-free repair of the hernia, must in principle alleviate postoperative pain and promote early return to full physical activity. This has been confirmed in several studies [Brown 1994; Taylor 1994; Kald 1995; Felix 1994]. However it carries the disadvantage of requiring general anesthesia whereas the inguinal operation can be carried out under spinal or local anesthesia, which is an important point for the frail patient. Among the available laparoscopic techniques, most surgeons seem to prefer the TAPP method [Estour 1995] no doubt because of its relative simplicity. In fact, the creation of a pneumoperitoneum provides excellent visualization of the structures, in a more extensive working area than can be obtained by the preperitoneal route, which aids dissection for the relatively inexperienced surgeon. Furthermore, the contralateral hernial orifice is clearly seen and any associated hernia on the other side can be treated at the same time. Also, this is the only route which allows a complete abdominal exploration and can confirm the viability of the bowel in the case of a strangulated hernia. TAPP is also readily adaptable to recurrent hernias.

However the creation of a pneumoperitoneum and access to the abdominal cavity carries certain disadvantages. Cardiovascular and pulmonary complications may be exacerbated by the tension induced by the pneumoperitoneum. The risk of injuring viscera or blood vessels during introduction of the trocar or entering an adherent loop of gut, although slight, must also be taken into consideration when comparing the complication rate with that of the purely preperitoneal approach.

Finally, if the peritoneum is not adequately closed, there is always the risk of a loop of small bowel becoming adherent to the prosthesis.

(4) Results

Intraoperative Complications

They are seen in from 0-5% of cases (Table 9.13). These include:

Hemorrhage. This may occur through wounding of the epigastric vessels during introduction of the lateral trocars, or during dissection. In general, the bleeding is controlled by the application of clips or hemostatic sutures, but may sometimes necessitate conversion to open surgery.

Injuries to the vessels of the cord, leading to a congestive orchitis in the case of venous involvement or testicular atrophy in the case of the artery.

Visceral injuries. These may involve the bladder, which can be closed laparoscopically, but also the sigmoid colon or an adherent loop of small intestine. These latter require open correction.

Injury to the vas deferens, in particular during dissection of the components of the spermatic cord.

Postoperative Complications

They are seen in from 0-10% of cases and vary in their nature and severity (Table 9.14).

Hematomas are the most frequent complication. They may occur in the inguinal region or in the cavities and usually require no treatment. For a large collection aspiration may be necessary.

Seromas and hydroceles usually resorb spontaneously but also may occasionally require aspiration.

Inguinal and testicular pain is usually slight and resolves spontaneously. It may occur through stapling around a nerve passing under the inguinal ligament or in the muscular layers. If persistent infiltration with

Table 9.13. Peroperative complications

Authors	# Cases	Hemorrhage	Visceral vesicle wound
Felix (1994)	326	-	0.6
Estour (1995)	7,340	3.4	0.12
Corbitt (1993)	1,994	2	0
Tetik (1994)	553	-	-
Kavic (1993)	101	-	0
McFadyen (1993)	186	-	1
Ramshaw (1992)	300	-	0.8
Van Steensel (1994)	254	2.3	1.18
Olgin (1994)	300	3.8	-
Personal series	225	0	0

Table 9.14. Postoperative complications

Authors	Hernia/infection on trocar	Hematoma	Seroma	Hydrocele	Inguinal pain	Testicular pain	Occlusion	Urinary Retention
Felix (1994)	0.6	-	4	0.3	0.3	-	0.3	0.3
Estour (1995)	0	3.4	3.9	0.5	2.1	2.3	0.2	0
Corbitt (1993)	0	2	-	-	2	-	0.3	1.3
Tetik (1994)	0.5	-	-	-	1.2	2	0	2.1
Kavic (1993)	-	-	-	-	2	1	0	1
McFadyen (1993)	0.5	-	-	1.6	1	-	-	0.5
Ramshaw (1992)	-	-	-	-	2.4	-	0.4	5.6
Van Steensel (1994)	0.8	2.3	-	-	-	0.3	-	0.4
Olgin (1994)	1.7	-	6	-	4	-	-	-
Personal series	0.4	2.7	3.1	-	1.3	1.3	0	0

Table 9.15. Rate of recurrence and of conversion (%)

Authors	# Cases	Conversion rate	Recurrence rate
Felix (1994)	326	-	0
Estour (1995)	> 7,000	-	0.9
Corbitt (1993)	1,994	-	1
Tetik (1994)	553	0.8	0.7
Kavic (1993)	101	0	2
McFadyen (1993)	186	-	3.2
Ramshaw (1992)	300	0.7	2
Van Steensel (1994)	254	-	1.9
Olgin (1994)	300	-	4
Personal series	233	2.6	2.7

lignocaine ± corticosteroids usually resolves the symptoms.

Hernias at the port sites occur in less than 1% of cases and can be avoided by closing these incisions at the end of the operation.

Postoperative obstruction is very rare and usually results from a faulty closure of the peritoneum allowing contact between the prosthesis and loops of intestine.

The conversion rate is of the order of 0.5-3% (Table 9.15). It may occur through wounding of a viscus or a blood vessel or because the presence of a long-standing bulky inguino-scrotal hernia creates difficulties with the dissection of the sac and endangers the components of the spermatic cord.

The mid-term recurrence rate (Table 9.15) is comparable to that of the inguinal route being from 0-5%.

(5) Personal Series

From 1st January 1994 to 31st December 1995, 225 groin hernias were operated upon via the TAPP method. The series included 209 men (93%) and 60 women (7%) the median age was 51 (range 22-86). There were 177 unilateral hernias (79%) and 48 bilateral hernias (21%). There were no intraoperative complications. Postoperative problems included six hematomas (2.7%), seven seromas (3.1%), three cases of testicular pain (1.3%) and three of ilioinguinal pain (1.3%), which regressed spontaneously in two months. The conversion rate was seven cases out of 225 (2.6%) and the recurrence rate, six out of 225 (2.7%).

(6) Discussion

The treatment of inguinal hernias is a master of controversy between the proponents of the classical methods [Houdart 1984; Stoppa 1989; Nyhus 1991] and those of the laparoscopic techniques [Dulucq 1991; Begin 1993; Corbitt 1991; Philipps 1993]. Controlled studies are as yet rare [Champault 1994] and too recent to provide firm conclusions. The introduction of new procedures immediately raises problems regarding feasibility and reproducibility. The three main laparoscopic techniques are now well defined in respect of their indications.

The pure intraperitoneal route (the Spaw operation) [El Haddad, Fourtanier 1993] combines the risks incurred by the use of trocars in the abdominal cavity with those of a prosthesis in contact with the viscera. Only PTFE can be used in this method. This requires fixation by stapling. These two factors involve considerable expenditure which limits the use of the technique, the results of which nonetheless seem to be quite good. This technique finds its true place in the treatment of multi-recurrent bulky hernias previously repaired prosthetically.

The infra- and preperitoneal route proposed by J. Leroy 1992 is by far the most frequently practiced at present. The operative field is much larger than that of the preperitoneal route and the visualization of all the hernia sites permits the detection of previously unsuspected or unusual herniations It carries the same risk as does the Spaw technique of trocar injuries and difficulties connected with peritoneal closure [Hendrickse 1993] notably the trapping of a loop of small bowel in a defect or adherence to the prosthesis [McFayden 1993]. Furthermore, the one year recurrence rate [McFayden 1993] is higher than with the preperitoneal route. These reservations should nonetheless not lead us to abandon the technique, the results of which have been shown to be excellent in many thousands of cases, both in terms of comfort and of effectiveness. It overcomes the contra-indications to the preperitoneal route (e.g. a previous history of subumbilical surgery) and bears comparison with conventional techniques such as that of Lichtenstein (1989), the results of which in terms of postoperative comfort are comparable.

The preperitoneal route [Dulucq 1991; Begin 1993; McKerman 1993; Read 1989] is that which most closely resembles the Stoppa operation and should in our view be preferred. The technical aspects are fully established with the exception of those involving parietalisation and fixation. Apart from the cost involved in the use of stapling devices and special trocars, stapling does carry certain specific risks. These include injuries to vessels [McFayden 1993], nerves [Kraus 1993] and more recently problems with infection [Letoquart 1994] including the rare but serious complication of osteitis pubis. This technique is necessary if one chooses parietalisation of the cord as recommended by Dulucq (1991). Splitting the prosthesis, as described by Champault (1994), following the technique originated by Stoppa (1989) allows one to dispense with stapling without risking displacement of the prosthesis, which is held in place by the elements of the cord. In our experience (480 cases in 1986) there were only three recurrences at four years [Champault 1994], figures which have been confirmed by Taylor (1993) and Van Steenel (1993) who used the same procedure. G. Begin (1994), one of the originators of this technique, also advises the use of a split prosthesis (see above). He has recently reported a series of 15/20 cases with no mortality and low morbidity comprising 47 seromas (3.4%), three trocar hematomas and no infection. The hospital stay was 1.6 days and the average time off work 17 days with one single recurrence (0.06%) at a late follow-up period of 29 months. These figures have been confirmed in our own practice [Champault 1994].

Whatever technique is chosen, a thorough apprenticeship is required, beginning with a review of laparoscopic anatomy of the hernia site [Rosser 1994] and complete mastery of the techniques of this new type of surgery.

(7) Conclusion

The purely preperitoneal approach for groin hernias seems to be by far the best adapted to the principles of hernial surgery, and its technique is well established. The use of a prosthesis constitutes a limiting factor in young patients. It furthermore seems that the use of a fenestrated prosthesis is preferable to parietalisation of the cord elements, in terms of risk, cost and efficiency. Although well described, this technique, like other laparoscopic procedures, requires to be evaluated in comparison with more conventional operations, which are recognized to be effective at low cost and little risk.

References

Arregui ME, Dulucq JL, Tetik C, Castro D, Davis CJ, Nagan RF (1994) Laparoscopic inguinal hernia repair with preperitoneal prosthetic placement. In: Bendavid R (ed) Prosthesis in abdominal wall hernias. R G Landes, Austin, pp 507-523

Begin GF (1993) Cure cœlioscopique des hernies de l'aine par voie pré-péritonéale. J. Coelio Chir 7: 23-9

Begin GF (1994) Traitement laparoscopique des hernies de l'aine par voie extrapéritonéale. A propos de 520 henies. J Coelio Chir 9: 33-6

Brown RB (1994) Laparoscopic hernia repair, a rural perspective. Surg Lap Endosc 6: 469

Champault G, Benoit J, Lauroy J, Rizk N, Boutelier P (1994) Hernies de l'aine de l'adulte: Etude randomisée contrôlée, 181 patients (résultats préliminaires). Ann Chir 48: 1003-1008

Corbitt JD Jr (1991) Laparoscopic herniorrhaphy. Surg Lap Endosc 1: 23-5

Corbitt JD (1993) Transabdominal preperitoneal herniorrhaphy. Surg Lap Endosc 3: 328-332

Dulucq JL (1991) Traitement laparoscopique des hernies de l'aine par mise en place d'un patch prothétique sous-péritonéoscopie. Cahiers Chir 179: 15-16

Elhadad A, Balique JG, Bégin G, Gillion JF, Fourtanier G (1993) Cure cœlioscopique des hernies de l'aine selon Spaw. Résultats préliminaires: 124 cas. Chir Endosc Suppl 13 (Abstract)

Estour E (1995) Revue de 9221 cures laparoscopiques de l'hernie de l'aine réalisées chez 7340 patients. J Coelio Chir 16: 42-48

Felix EL, Michas CA, McKnight RL (1994) Laparoscopic hernlorraphy; transabdominal preperitoneal floor repair. Surg Endosc 8: 100-104

Filipi CJ, Fitzgibbons RJ, Salerno GM, Hart RO (1992) Laparoscopic herniorrhaphy. Surg Clin North Am 72: 1009-1114

Hendrickse CW, Ewans DS (1993) Intestinal obstruction following laparoscopic inguinal hernia repair. Br J Surg 80: 1432

Himpens JM (1992) Laparoscopic hernioplasty using a self-expandable (Umbrella like) prosthetic patch. Surg Lap Endosc 2, 3: 12-16

Houdart C, Stoppa R (1984) Le traitement chirurgical des hernies de l'aine. Monographies de l'AFC, Masson, Paris

Kald A, Smedh K, Anderberg B (1995) Laparoscopic groin hernia repair: results of 200 consecutive herniorrhaphies. Br J Surg 82: 618-620

Kavic MS (1993) Laparoscopic hernia repair. Surg Endosc 7: 163-167

Kraus MA (1993) Nerve injury during laparoscopic hernia repair. Surg Laparosc. Endoscop 2: 342-5

Leroy J, Fromont G (1992) Hernies de l'aine de l'adulte. Prothèse sous-péritonéale sous contrôle cœlioscopique: 110 cas. J. Coelio Chir 1: 22-5

Letoquart JP, La Gamma A. Le Dantec P, Kunin N, Pawlotsky Y, Mambrini A (1994) Ostéoarthrite pubienne après réparation herniaire par voie coelioscopique. J Path Dig 2: 62 (abstract)

Lichtenstein IL, Shulman AJ, Amid DK, et al (1989) The "tension-free" hernioplasty. Am J Surg 157: 188-93

Mc Fayden BV, Arregui ME, Corbitt Jz JD, Filipi J, et al (1993) Complications of laparoscopic herniorrhaphy. Surg Endosc 7: 155-8

Mc Kernan JB, Laws HL (1993) Laparoscopic repair of infuinal hernias using a totally extra-peritoneal approach. Surg Endosc 7: 26-8

Nyhus LM (1991) Inguinal hernias. Current Probl Surg 6: 418-9

Olgin HA, Seid A, Doug T (1994) Laparoscopic herniorrhaphy-transabdominal preperitoneal floor repair: 300 cases. Surg Lap Endosc 4: 471

Phillips EH (1994) Complications of laparoscopically guided inguinal hernioplasty. In: Berndavid R (ed) Prosthesis in abdominal wall hernias. R G Landes, Austin, pp 524-529

Philipps EH, Carroll BJ, Fallas MJ (1993) Laparoscopic preperitoneal inguinal hernia repair without peritoneal incision : technique and early results. Surg Endosc 7: 159-62

Ramshaw B, Tucker JG, Conner T, Mason EM, Duncan TD, Lucas GW (1992) A comparison of the approaches to laparoscopic herniorrhaphy. Surg Endosc10: 29-32

Read RC (1989) Pre-peritoneal herniorrhaphy: A historical review. World J Surg 13: 532-40

Rosser J (1994) The anatomical basis for laparoscopic hernia repair revisited. Surg Lap Endosc 4: 36-44

Stoppa R, Warlaumont CR (1989) The pre-peritoneal approach and prosthetic repair of groin hernia. In: Nyhus LN, Condon R (eds) Hernia. J P Lippincott, Philadelphia, pp 199-255

Taylor RS, Leopold P, Loh A (1994) Laparoscopic hernia repair: preliminary results in 100 patients. Surg Lap Endosc 6: 473

Taylor RS, Fiennes A (1993) A tension free modification of the Dulucq pre-peritoneal laparoscopic hernioplasty. Chir Endosc, Suppl 19 (Abstract)

Tetik C, Arregui ME, Dulucq JL, Fitzgibbons RJ, Franklin ME, McKernan JB, Rosin RD, Schultz LS, Toy FK (1994) Complications and recurrences associated with laparoscopic repair of groin hernias. Surg Endosc 8: 1316-1323

Van Steensel CS, Weidema WF (1993) Laparoscopic inguinal hernia repair without fixation of the prothesis. Chir Endosc, Suppl 18 (Abstract)

F. Intraoperative Complications of the Classical Surgical Repairs

Because of the development of laparoscopic herniorrhaphy, many clinical studies have been conducted to account for the complications of classical herniorrhaphy, in addition to the already published reviews of Nyhus and Condon in the four editions of Hernia (1978-1995). The list of complications is long but, fortunately, their incidence is very low.

The problem is, however, significant if we consider the great frequency of hernia repair. In the United States, more than half a million repairs are performed every year. A 1% incidence of complications would thus affect about 6,000 patients, and a 10% incidence means that more the 60,000 patients would be subject to these unfortunate troubles.

1. Hemorrhage

Surgical anatomists have considered the "corona mortis" injuries, especially those involving an accessory obturator artery, as the most serious. However, injuries to the inferior epigastric or external iliac vessels are as unpleasant, especially when they occur at the principal pedicle during deep suturing on the prevascular segment of the inguinal ligament, close to the vascular sheath. A venous injury of the external iliac vein should be suspected and identified before knotting the suture, otherwise further venous laceration may occur. It is better in such cases to withdraw the suture material and manual compression. If the bleeding is not controlled with compression, the arterial or venous lesion should be widely exposed and then repaired under temporary vascular occlusion. Vascular clamps should be immediately available and hernia surgeons should be able to do vascular surgical procedures such as venous or prosthetic bypass. Femoral vein ligature should be abandoned as it results in dramatic complications. It is fortunately rarely necessary though may be useful as a temporary salvage procedure. Only a few series of serious vascular complications have been published including those of Natali, Gautier in 1972 and Meillière in 1980.

2. Spermatic Cord Lesions

Complete division of the spermatic cord could be performed intentionally in some special cases [Heifetz 1971]. However, this procedure is useless and never facilitates the repair of large hernial defects. Inadvertent spermatic cord division is a very rare complication which mainly occurs mostly in recurrent or multi-recurrent repair. Testicular necrosis only occurs when the spermatic cord is divided below the level of the pubis. Division of the cord in its inguinal course or behind the abdominal wall does not give rise to testicular atrophy.

Injuries of the spermatic veins in their funicular course during dissection of an indirect sac dissection are uncommon. They especially occur in cases of recurrent hernia repair or large scrotal sacs.

Thrombosis of these venous plexuses results in a great risk of ischemic orchitis.

There are two means of preventing injuries to the testicular vessels. First, an indirect sac should not be dissected below the pubic level. Second, multirecurrent hernias and all patients who have a history of previous operation on the same side should be operated on using the posterior abdominal approach [Wantz 1984].

3. Nerve Injury

The inguinal approach risks nerve injury since it passes through the layers in which run the sensory nerves of the region and those included into the cremaster muscle. The risk is maximum in recurrent hernia repair by the inguinal approach. By contrast, the posterior abdominal approach does not cross the path of any nerve, which is an important advantage. To prevent nerve injury, the surgeon should be familiar with their inguinal course in order to recognize and preserve them. There is no advantage in attempting surgical repair of these nerves, since neural anastomoses and accessory pathways will ensure sufficient sensory innervation. However, compression of one of them by a suture may lead to persistent symptoms. Femoral nerve injury is the most serious, because it is usually associated with motor signs. It is fortunately rare. We are aware of two femoral nerve injuries in two patients who were operated on elsewhere which resulted from the suturing of a Dacron prosthesis to the psoas major sheath by the inguinal approach. To avoid such complications deep sutures should only be inserted under direct vision.

4. Injury to the Vas Deferens

This complication must not be overlooked in young adults. Immediate repair, with the help of a magnifying lens, should be performed. A steel probe is used to support the anastomosis which is done using very fine monofilament thread. This probe passes through the wall of the vas and the skin at some distance from the injury and is pulled out on the tenth day. This classical technique restores patency in about 50% of cases. Microsurgery gives even better results (80-90% of patency). Stenosis of the vas, even in the absence of complete obstruction, results in hypofertility or sterility due to increased serum antisperm antibodies. Friberg (1979) revealed that up to 7% of adult patients suffering from azoospermia or hypozoospermia without testicular atrophy had undergone a hernia repair during childhood.

5. Bladder Injury

This may occur when the sac is opened in direct femoral or inguinal hernias associated with sliding of the bladder. The injury is not unduly serious. The defect should be identified and sutured in two-layers using slowly absorbable synthetic material, while the bladder is filled with water. Accidental injury of the bladder excludes the use of prosthetic material because of the risk of infection.

6. Injury to an Abdominal Organ

The intestines, bladder and ureter may be damaged during herniorrhaphy. All injuries should be immediately identified and properly treated. Special attention must be paid during high ligation of the hernial sac to avoid injuries to the abdominal organs. In repair of sliding hernia, direct or vascular injuries of the caecum or sigmoid colon may occur. To avoid such complications, the sac need not be entirely resected and the abdominal viscera should not be freed from their peritoneal attachments. The whole sac with its sliding contents should be pushed back into the abdominal cavity. According to the type of colic injury, the colon is sutured in one or two layers. Vascular intestinal injuries are more difficult to evaluate. Their management depends on the extent of the ischemia (partial resection, colectomy with immediate anastomosis or colostomy). Intestinal defects, which are often small, should be also sutured immediately. These complications are very serious and usually precludes the use prosthetic material.

Appendicectomy should also be avoided during herniorrhaphy as it also predisposes to septic complications. However, the appendix is sometimes found in the peritoneal sac of a right indirect hernia, in which case it may be removed provided that it can be delivered into the operative field. The ureter may lie close to a large direct or indirect sac. If it is divided, immediate repair is indicated. Many surgical procedure have been proposed including end to end anastomosis with interrupted absorbable sutures, supported a double J catheter, or reimplantation into the bladder, if the injury lies close to that structure.

G. The Postoperative Period

Hernial repair is in the great majority of cases a straightforward operation, and postoperative care simply involves the comfort of the patient and the avoidance of complications. The effectiveness of treatment can only be assessed by long-term follow-up, taking into account the recurrence rate observed over a period of up to ten years.

1. Postoperative Analgesia

Over the first 24 hours the patient requires some relief, usually achieved by oral or parenteral analgesics. Buprenorphine chlorhydrate (Temgesic) is administered sublingually, intramuscularly or intravenously (0.3 mg six to eight hourly). Propacetamol chlorhydrate (Pro-dafalgan) is given in a dose of 1 g eight hourly. Occasionally subcutaneous morphine (20-40 mg over 24 h) may be required. Sinclair has suggested the use of a lignocaine spray before closing the wound, in order to reduce postoperative analgesic requirements. Epidural Fentanyl has the major disadvantage of preventing early ambulation. For children, Hinkel has suggested a percutaneous inguinal nerve block.

2. Prevention of Thromboembolism

This is best achieved through early ambulation, but anticoagulants are indicated if there is a preceding history of thromboembolism, varicosities or oral contraception. Prophylaxis begins on the eve of operation for high risk subjects, two hours postoperatively for the others. Calcium heparin or low molecular weight heparin are the usual agents, as they require only three injections in 24 hours. In patients who are already anticoagulated, heparin is injected continuously by an infusion pump, in order to calculate the exact dosage. This treatment does not in our experience increase the rate of hemorrhagic complications. Patients with no history of thromboembolism do not require anticoagulation provided that they ambulate early, as is the case with all those undergoing day surgery.

3. Antibiotics

Routine antibiotic cover is unnecessary if the conditions for operation are good, in a healthy patient, even if prosthetic material is used. A prosthetic repair in a patient with a risk of sepsis, with an artificial heart valve or a prosthetic joint replacement, should be covered by a preoperative bolus dose of a cephalosporin or vancomycin. Incidental risks occurring during operation such as opening the GI tract or the bladder require postoperative wide spectrum antibiotic protection against gram negatives and anaerobes.

4. Ambulation and Length of Hospital Stay

When the operation is carried out under local anesthesia the patient can walk back to his room and go home the same evening. Every patient is advised to get out of bed on the day of surgery. Oral feeding is recommended according to the type of anesthesia and requires no special consideration in hernial repair. Hospital stay varies with national custom, but the overall tendency is to reduce it to a minimum. Since the Board of Regents of the American College of Surgeons reported on "Out-patient or office surgery as an alternative to operations in hospital" most American surgeons have adopted a day surgery policy. In "hernia institutes" up to 95% of patients are treated in this way (Amid, Gilbert). The guidelines of the Royal College of Surgeons of England (1993) estimate that 30% of hernia repairs can be carried out on a day surgery basis. This early discharge policy has not yet become widely adopted in France but is already being practiced in a number of private clinics.

As in all types of day surgery, the time of discharge is decided jointly by the surgeon and the anesthetist. The patient leaves with a supply of analgesics. In certain cases he/she may prefer to stay in a recovery unit near to the hospital. The surgical team must be available by telephone 24 hours in the day during the first postoperative days because the contractual responsibility of the surgeon is the same as with patients who are admitted for longer. The patient and his relatives must be fully informed of the circumstances. Many publications (Farquharson, Bellis, Lichtenstein, Teasdale, De Bruin, Mejdahl) have shown that day hernia surgery, which is now almost the rule in the United States and Britain, has no adverse effects either as regards postoperative morbidity or the quality of results. At the same time the new ideas in patient management require rethinking of traditional care, and the personal involvement of the surgical team, as well as re-education of the patient.

It goes without saying that the stay in hospital may be prolonged under certain circumstances. These include suction drainage, (which reduces the frequency, number of and duration of drains), intestinal resection, the elderly, unfit or anxious patient, and unsatisfactory home circumstances. Local factors include the type of operation (in particular the length of the incision) the size of the prosthesis and whether or not the procedure has been bilateral. In France the mean hospital stay has been shortened over the last ten years. In our personal practice it has been reduced from seven days for herniorrhaphy and 10.3 days for large bilateral prostheses (in 1980) to one or two days for herniorrhaphy and two to four days for prostheses (in 1993). The use of intradermal absorbable sutures avoids the need for a consultation on the eighth day.

Staples may be loosened on the first postoperative day and removed between the third and sixth day. Skin stitches are removed at around the eighth day.

At the beginning of the modern era of hernia surgery Halsted (1889) kept his patients in bed for 21 days and even questioned whether they should be allowed to walk at that time. In 1945 the publications from the Shouldice Hospital produced a radical change of policy by recommending early return to activity for all patients, but in 1990 their patients were hospitalized for three days after a unilateral repair and five days after bilateral surgery. Kux (1994) reports hospital stays of six to eight days in Austria, eight days in Germany, six to eleven days in France. Since then however these periods have been sharply reduced and in specialist units do not exceed two to three days.

5. Resumption of Activities and Work

This is the question most often put by the patient. As far as resumption of activity is concerned we should repeat that it can be as early as the comfort and mental attitude of the patient allow. We feel that a hospital stay of two or three days allows the patient to resume a number of daily activities under medical supervision and encouragement, in a supportive environment, whereas immediate discharge, even with written recommendations, does not perhaps encourage such a rapid return to independence. As regards return to work we feel, as do most surgeons, that it should be related to the patient's profession, bearing in mind that it will depend very much on the advice and medication supplied by the general practitioner and occupational physician. In a controlled study by Adler (1978) a short hospital stay was associated with a short period off work. In the United States office work is resumed at the end of 48 hours to two days and more strenuous activities at between the 15th and 30th postoperative day.

The Shouldice Hospital patients go back to work between the eighth day and the fourth week [Bendavid 1994]. In the U.K. [Barwell 1981] salaried employees returned to work 35 days postoperatively while manual workers returned between the seventh and twenty-first day. In France, the mean time off work in 1975 was 60.9 days [Sournia]. It seems reasonable to adapt the period of unemployment to the patient's requirements and to advise sedentary workers to be off work for ten to fifteen days and manual workers for 30 to 45 days. Semmence (1980) gives a list of the socio-economic factors which prolong time off work. These include strenuous work, an incapacitated or weak patient, family problems, among the most notable. One should also mention a study by Bourke in 1981 which showed that recurrences are no more frequent when work is resumed early. In conclusion, and to argue scientifically in favor of early resumption of work, we should recall that following herniorrhaphy the inguinal structures regain 70% of their strength immediately, which continues up to the eighth week, which is then followed, according to Lichtenstein, by a period of weakness.

6. Early Postoperative Complications

The overall morbidity rate including all types of surgery and all local and general complications, lies at around 6 and 7%.

a) Hematomas

Their frequency is at around 2%. They are prone to occur following extensive dissections by the inguinal route, for a bulky hernia. In contrast, dissection of the abdominal wall and anticoagulant prophylaxis do not seem to increase the risk. Certainly, careful hemostasis should always be maintained.

Small collections may lead to disruption of the skin incision, with delayed healing. True inguinal hematomas, the frequency of which was 1.9% in the AFC inquiry of 1984 (Houdard and Stoppa) if they are large, require removal of clots under general or local anesthesia, with careful aseptic precautions. Scrotal hematomas appearing two or three days after surgery are extremely conspicuous and unsightly when large, and aspiration or removal of clot is disappointing as the collection frequently recurs. They may eventually lead to excision of redundant scrotal tissue due to functional problems and discomfort. Some surgeons have advised elective resection of very distended scrotums, in order to lessen the risk of these sero-sanginous collections.

The posterior preperitoneal route occasionally gives rise to a hematoma in the abdominal wall, usually of no significance but which may lead to displacement of an inadequately fixed prosthesis. Salinier (1983) advises following these intraparietal hematomas by means of serial ultrasonography.

b) Wound Infection

This varies in frequency from 0.7 to 6% of patients, according to circumstance. Its incidence is 1.4% in the AFC Series [Houdard & Stoppa 1984]. It may follow a hematoma, certainly its frequency rises with emergency operations or when other procedures are carried out simultaneously. Marsden (1962) observed a 6% incidence of infection when appendectomy was combined with hernia repair. It is favored by diabetes or immuno-suppressed states. The use of prosthetic material does not increase the risk of infection but makes it more difficult to treat. The degree of severity of sepsis is determined by the extent of its spread and its future course. Following an inguinal herniorrhaphy, infection is usually easy to control by debridement of the wound. The problem usually resolves in a few weeks, but there is a risk of late recurrence of the hernia. When infection follows the use of prosthetic material, a distinction must be made between superficial sepsis, which usually subsides as in the previous case, and infection of the prosthesis itself, which carries the risk of septicemia. Precise diagnosis and early treatment is crucial in both cases, but particularly in the second. Drainage of any collection of pus is essential, associated with systemic antibiotics and prolonged maintenance of local care of the wound. A good means for early diagnosis of deep sepsis is to monitor the progress of the intraparietal collection by means of ultrasound. It is usually unnecessary to remove the prosthetic material, whatever route was used to introduce it, but simply to expose it widely, to irrigate the wound and to encourage progressive incorporation of the prosthesis, although this may require a prolonged stay in hospital. Because of the risk of infection, prosthetic material should not be used in patients who are poorly prepared for operation or operated on as emergencies, or if there is any associated septic procedure such as resection of the bowel or prostate.

c) Hydrocele

This is promoted by dissection of the distal spermatic cord or by leaving the lower part of an indirect sac within the scrotum. Serous collections in the scrotum or groin have been reported following the use of a polypropylene prosthesis. Houdelette has described the same problem with a bilateral Mersilene prosthesis, although this is something we have not encountered. These collections may be aspirated, or if they recur may require more definitive surgery.

d) Ischemic Orchitis

This presents between the second and fifth day as a testicle which is increased in volume and sensitivity. Palpation of the testis, epididymis and spermatic cord reveal loss of elasticity, with testicular retraction. The symptoms last for a variable time and may develop over several months either by a return to normal or by progress towards complete atrophy, as occurs in half the cases, particularly after repair of a recurrent hernia. The frequency reported by Wantz in several publications (1982 to 1991) is around 1% but rises to 3% after treatment of a recurrent hernia. However Schumpelick (1984) reports a frequency of 2% after primary repair and 2 to 10% after repair of recurrent hernias. Ischemic orchitis never leads on to septic necrosis. It is an aseptic process which both clinical examination and Doppler flowmetry show to occur because of trauma to the lower part of the pampiniform plexus, much more often than from injury to the testicular artery.

There is no known treatment for ischemic orchitis. Antibiotics and steroidal and nonsteroidal anti-inflammatory drugs have no proven effect. Prevention consists essentially in avoiding all traumatic dissection of the cord, particularly below the level of the pubis. Blunt dissection must in particular be avoided as it is particularly traumatic for the veins. Use of the preperitoneal route does not give rise to this trauma and should be used in multi-recurrent cases or in patients with a past history of a scrotal operation such as vasectomy or resection of the tunica vaginalis. Arising from these principles, it is probably wise to avoid repairing a bilateral indirect inguinal hernia if an indirect sac has been excised as a first stage, for fear of producing bilateral testicular atrophy. It is better to delay the contralateral operation for a year, because late testicular atrophy has been reported (Wantz). It should be remembered that the preperitoneal abdominal route completely obviates this complication.

e) Urinary Complications

Postoperative retention of urine, signaled by complete anuria for more than six hours in the presence of an enlarged bladder, seems to be more frequent following spinal anesthesia, the use of atropinelike drugs and over zealous postoperative analgesia. In patients over 60 retention is frequently due to prostatic enlargement, which should have been detected by the history and rectal examination before the operation. Prevention consists in anti-prostatic medication or elective resection before the hernia is treated. Treatment of established acute retention includes administration of drugs such as dihydro-ergocryptine (Vasobral) 2-4 mg by mouth, in minor cases. If the problem persists then a urethral catheter should be passed and left in place for at least 24 h, covered by antibiotics, because of the considerable risk of iatrogenic urinary infection. Retention of urine particularly complicates hernia repair by the anterior route, in elderly men, in some 30% of cases [Haskill 1974].

f) Thromboembolism

The femoral vein risks injury because of transfixing sutures, contusion or constriction, in any operation in the neighborhood of the pectineal (Coopers) ligament, or the femoral sheath (for example in the McVay operation 1.2%). The risk is considerably less when a prosthesis is inserted by the posterior route. Phlebography has demonstrated a number of overlooked cases of venous constriction following the McVay operation [Lankau 1975]. Established femoral thromboses may extend into the iliac veins or inferior vena cava and be complicated by a pulmonary embolus. They need to be treated with full anticoagulant doses of heparin. Marsden (1960) reports a mortality of 0.5% in the 1% of thromboembolic complications seen in a series of 2,254 hernia repairs. Several other series report similar figures.

g) Respiratory Complications

Broncho-pulmonary infection may follow hernia repair much as in any surgical procedure involving an incision in the abdominal wall. Those most at risk include aged patients and those with chronic respiratory problems. Massive inguino-scrotal hernias impose an additional risk. Re-introduction into the peritoneal cavity of a large visceral mass interferes with diaphragmatic movement and raises intra-abdominal pressure. In the case of a complicated hernia, induction of a preoperative pneumoperitoneum as described by Goni-Moreno may be considered. Physiotherapy is of great use in preventing these complications.

h) Gastrointestinal Complications

Postoperative intestinal obstruction is almost unknown following hernia repair by the inguinal route. With a posterior repair, loosening of the peritoneal suture of the hernial neck may on rare occasions be followed by entrapment of an intestinal loop in the peritoneal breach thus created. We have only seen one such case.

Postoperative peritonitis is above all seen after operations for strangulated hernia, and particularly following the highly dangerous procedure of reducing a loop of doubtful viability, which subsequently undergoes necrosis. Peritonitis may also result from leakage from an intestinal anastomosis.

i) General Complications and Mortality

As in all types of surgery the preoperative risk may be assessed by using the ASA classification, which takes into account the age and circumstances of the emergency surgery (e.g. strangulation). Above 65, the overall complication rate is higher [Barbier 1989; Nehme 1983] infections are commoner [Nichelsen 1982], and mortality increases with the same ASA grade. The lethal risk of strangulated hernia is twenty times higher after the age of 60 than before. A study from the US Army Heydorn (1990) showed that mortality was related to age. Other series emphasize the problems posed by emergency surgery for strangulation in respect to complications and death [Stoppa 1989; Lewis 1989]. The size of the hernia [Stoppa 1989], the presence of strangulation and above all the need to resect necrosed intestine raise the risk of death from 20 to 40%, as against 5.2 to 8% where no resection is required. Death usually occurs due to pre-existing problems or cardiac respiratory and thromboembolic complications, in elective repairs. Published mortality figures vary from 0 to 1% and underline the necessity for careful preoperative assessment of these patients.

As regards the anesthetic risks, local anesthesia is certainly safer. Spinal anesthesia carries a high incidence of urinary and thromboembolic complications [Guillen 1970]. The risks of general anesthesia have been greatly reduced by careful selection of patients and the introduction of newer anesthetic agents (see above).

H. Late complications

1. Sequelae

a) Testicular Atrophy

Testicular atrophy may occur at any stage after repair of an inguinal hernia. It is the most frequent cause for legal actions for damages, as quoted by the medical defense organizations. One case of ischemic orchitis out of two leads to late testicular atrophy. The operation causing the problem has always been via an anterior inguinal approach, no case of testicular atrophy has yet been reported following repair via the abdominal route. The problem has been intensively studied by Wantz, who reports an incidence of 0.9% in a personal series of 2,240 primary repairs by the Shouldice method (1982). In another series he reports a 3% incidence for recurrent hernias. Wantz attributes the problem to trauma to the spermatic veins in the lower part of the cord during dissection of a scrotal hernial sac. He feels that division of the testicular artery is much less important and that compression of the cord by the reconstituted inguinal ring is an impossibility. The higher frequency of testicular atrophy following repair of recurrent hernias is explained by difficulty in freeing up the cord from the scar tissue. Some cases of bilateral testicular atrophy have been reported, which lead to legal actions against the surgeon of a punitive nature. Prevention of testicular atrophy is achieved by avoiding dissection of the cord below the level of the pubis, leaving behind the distal portions of indirect sacs within the scrotum (as already advised by Fruchaud 1956) and the use of a posterior abdominal approach in all patients who have had a previous scrotal operation [Wantz 1982]. Testicular atrophy which is painful or is suspected of having undergone malignant change should be treated by orchidectomy and insertion of a testicular prosthesis, following full discussion with the patient.

b) Chronic Postoperative Pain

A century ago, the condition known as "meralgia paraesthetica", in the distribution of the lateral cutaneous nerve of the thigh, was independently put forward by three German surgeons namely Roth, Bernhardt and Freud (1895) as a sequela of a repair operation carried out through the groin. The initial enthusiasm for neurectomies and neurolyses has diminished to the point where such operations are only very occasionally practiced. The frequency of postoperative pain of neurological origin has been assessed at 5% following repairs through the inguinal route at 3% in the AFC series [Houdard & Stoppa 1984] and 5% independently by Gilbert Moosman and Wantz. While herniorrhaphy via the inguinal route, particularly in recurrent cases, predisposes to this problem, the use of prosthetic material seems not to affect the issue. In certain cases a psychological problem has been unearthed, hence the recommendation to carry out a full neurological examination of the complaining patient, to make an unbiased differential diagnosis and to be very cautious in electing to carry out a further surgical operation. Recent reviews of the question include those of Wantz (1986), Chevrel and Gatt (1991) and Starling (1994). We should bear in mind Chapter 1 of this work, which describes the nerve supply of the region represented by the branches of the genitofemoral, ilioinguinal and iliohypogastric nerves. From the differences between the observations of Moosman (1977) and those of Chevrel

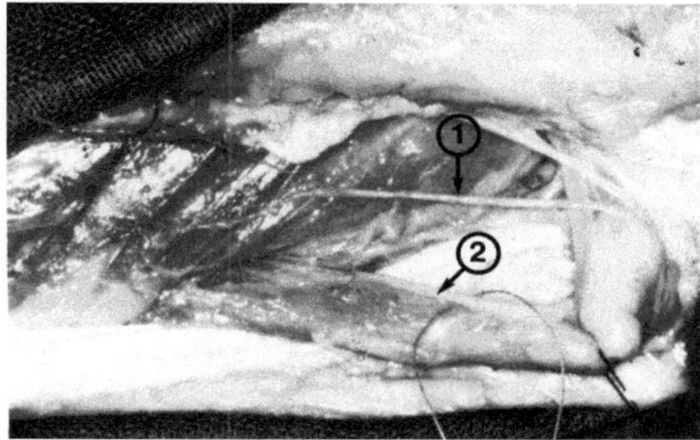

Fig. 9.21. Postmortem dissection of the genital nerves. The abdominopelvic branch of the iliohypogastric nerve *(above)* (1) pierces the internal oblique and then joins the spermatic cord. The genitofemoral nerve can be seen to enter this region via the deep ring of the inguinal canal (2) (courtesy of J. P. Chevrel and J. Salama)

(1982) there arise important variations in the topography of the superficial nerve plexuses, which luckily have the capacity to compensate over time for loss of a particular branch (Fig. 9.21). But these anatomical variations oblige the surgeon to take great care to isolate and protect these fine filaments during the course of the superficial dissection. The inguinal approach inevitably involves passing through the superficial network of nerves in order to reach the hernial defect and there are certain stages in this approach at which the nerves are at risk. These include the incision and subsequent repair of the external oblique aponeurosis (iliohypogastric nerve), the division of the cremaster muscle bundles and the internal spermatic fascia and funicular artery (genital branch of the genitofemoral nerve), and the dissection of an indirect sac (ilioinguinal nerve). These nerves may be cut, coagulated, stretched, included in a ligature, secondarily involved in scar tissue, or irritated by contact with an infected focus.

According to Chevrel (1982) there are four types of neuralgia which in most cases are accompanied by thymic troubles and disorders of behavior such as absenteeism and familial isolation, depending on the psychological type.

Pain from a neuroma, which is the one best recognized by surgeons, is due to proliferation of nerve fibers around the neural sheath, after partial or total division of the nerve. They present as hyperesthesia or hyperpathia, either fixed or transitory, clinical examination reveals an exquisite shooting type of pain in the region of the neuroma, resembling that of an electric shock.

Complete or partial section of a nerve, or inclusion in a ligature, may produce a deep deafferentation type of pain, which is a burning sensation in the corresponding distribution, constant but with paroxysms, appearing after a latent period of several weeks. Examination initially reveals an area of anesthesia in the corresponding territorial distribution, surrounded by a hypoesthetic zone, which is progressively replaced by hyperesthesia. There is no sharp pain produced by contact but some degree of dysesthesia which becomes spontaneously painful.

Some reported pains are due to irritation of a nerve without interruption of its continuity, because of involvement in a fibrous mass or a ligature. This produces a type of permanent hyperalgesia without reported paroxysms, in the corresponding cutaneous zone.

The third pain is due to a lesion at some distance from the nerve concerned. This can be muscular because of the inflammatory granuloma (visceral intestinal adhesions in the stump of the peritoneal sac). Reference to the particular zone of skin affected is explained by a failure of integration of the centripetal stimuli to the spinal cord, because of superimposed messages from one dermatome or "viscerotome". It produces a fixed hyperalgesia without paroxysms in an area which may affect various dermatomes. On examination the hyperesthesia or hyperpathia may be accompanied by contractions.

Apart from neuromas, the diagnosis and treatment of which are the concern of the surgeon, the clinical picture of these types of pain should be discussed with a specialist in pain relief where the various components of this symptom complex can be better sorted out and analyzed.

Intraoperative prevention involves the careful identification of the three nerves at risk of injury, and protecting them. This is not always easy in the case of recurrent or re-recurrent hernias.

Postoperative pain should not be ignored and early treatment with analgesics such as paracetamol, amidopyrine, and nonsteroidal anti-inflammatories, should be provided, supplemented if necessary with anxiolytics and muscle relaxants. There are some who advocate that this treatment should be given prospectively rather than on demand. Medication should be adapted to the type of pain experienced by the individual patient.

Neuromas respond to infiltration of local anesthetic and steroids. When the diagnosis is clear, early operation to divide and coagulate or to free up the proximal segment may be indicated. Deafferentation

pain is relieved by TNS or anticonvulsants for paroxysmal attacks. Injections of anesthetics and steroids may also be useful. Referred pain may require chemical neurolysis of the peripheral nerve, nerve trunk or root, guided by local anesthesia. TNS again may be indicated.

It should be remembered that apart from those rare cases where a neuroma can be diagnosed early and with confidence, surgery is on the whole contra-indicated. It is essential to look at the problem as a whole, because central mechanisms may sustain and prolong the physiopathology of the pain, which will then persist even after successful treatment of the peripheral lesion. This situation will require specialized medical measures [Ochs 1987].

In the series of 47 patients reported by Chevrel (1991) eleven were cured, 22 were 50-85% improved, five patients with deafferentation pain were failures and three depressed patients were lost to follow up. Only six patients required reoperation for a neuroma, with five successes and one failure. It was noteworthy in this series that the patients who were cured and improved were younger than the others, that depression increased the difficulties of treatment, that accidents at work did not seem to predict a poor result and that hasty and ill-considered re-operation often resulted in failure. This latter point is confirmed in the literature [Siegfried 1984; Lewis 1987; Demierre 1989]. In spite of the multidisciplinary approach recommended by Chevrel and Gatt, abolition of neurogenic postoperative pain, particularly of the deaferrentation type, can never be guaranteed, and this problem often leads to difficulties in the relationship between the surgeon and his patient.

c) Painful Ejaculation

This is a syndrome recently described from the Shouldice Hospital by Bendavid (1992). The author reports some 30 patients who experienced burning pain along the spermatic cord lasting for several seconds, following hernia repair by the inguinal route. No treatment was really helpful, and the pains continued for from two months to five years. The probable explanation is reflux of ejaculate up the vas deferens with distension proximal to a stenosis or a kink due to scarring. According to Bendavid the incidence of the syndrome is around 0.04%.

d) Migration of the Prosthesis

Together with Warlaumont (1982), we reported two cases of late intravesical migration of prosthetic material following combined hernia and prostatic surgery. This has led us to advise very firmly against this type of combined surgery, advice which is confirmed by the observations of Chevalier (1987) and Lauriere (1991).

e) Late Infectious Complications (fistulae)

These were common up to the 1970s, when silk and other absorbable materials such as braided nylon, were in use. They are practically never seen today, as we now use slowly absorbed monofilament materials.

The extent to which plugs, sometimes of considerable size, are tolerated, seems quite inexplicable, as these are foreign bodies which are never completely incorporated, particularly as regards the central portion of cylindrical plugs. A late and serious type of infectious complication, fortunately rare, is osteitis pubis, which is probably the result of deep sutures passing through the pubic spine, which should always be avoided. The pain resulting from osteitis pubis is severe, and can be confirmed by the characteristic radiological signs.

Treatment is difficult and is liable to end up in extensive destruction of the pubic bone with weakening of the surrounding inguinal area, which may be followed by progressive eventration.

2. Problems with Re-operation Following Retromuscular Prosthetic Repair

The efficacy of these materials depends on their incorporation in scar tissue, which leads to the almost total disappearance of the retroparietal spaces of Bogros and Retzius over their whole extent. This fibrosis may make subsequent dissection difficult if it becomes surgically necessary, the difficulties varying with the type of prosthesis, whether it is uni- or bilateral, and the type of re-operation required. However, these difficulties do not cause problems when the further surgery involves an intraperitoneal organ.

a) Surgery for Benign Prostatic Hypertrophy

Access to the retropubic space may be prevented by fibrosis in the cave of Retzius. We have encountered two cases of fibrosis in this area following dislocation of the pubic symphysis complicated by suprapubic herniation, and had recourse to subperiosteal dissection in order to insert a retromuscular prosthesis. Access to the prostate by the transvesical or endoscopic routes, which are nowadays the usual method, is unimpaired.

b) Surgery for Prostatic or Vesical Malignancy

Total cystectomy or prostatectomy is usually carried out transperitoneally, and a supplementary subperiosteal retropubic dissection will resolve most of the problems. It should be noted that when a unilateral prosthesis is inserted via the inguinal, suprainguinal or midline subumbilical route, these subsequent difficulties in dissection of the cave of Retzius can largely be avoided.

c) Surgery of the External Iliac Vessels

Insertion of a large uni- or bilateral prosthesis may lead to a considerable degree of perivascular sclerosis, which may seriously hamper subsequent vascular surgery, heterotopic organ transplant or clearance of iliac lymph nodes. Founded on our operative experience, and confirmed by cadaveric dissections, our advice is to suggest combining the transperitoneal and paraperitoneal routes of access, beginning the dissection of the vascular pedicle in its proximal, undisturbed segment. The other solution, clearly, is to use an extra-anatomic form of bypass, when possible. We would also emphasize the need to foresee and avoid the difficulties involved in subsequent surgery. Thus when considering candidates for the insertion of a large prosthesis, it is necessary to eliminate those at high risk for subsequent surgery, such as patients with prostatic hypertrophy, bladder tumors, high levels of PSA, occlusive or aneurysmal disease of the aorto-iliac segment, etc. This list of contra-indications is founded upon simple common sense. Attention to one technical detail may obviate the development of perivascular sclerosis. There is a constant sheath of tissue surrounding the retroperitoneal segment of the elements of the spermatic cord, and if the integrity of this sheath is preserved in order to protect the external iliac vessels from direct contact with the prosthetic material, then this may keep them free from subsequent fibrosis. To achieve this, however, it is important not to cut a slit in the prosthesis to allow passage of the elements of the cord, because this involves direct contact between the foreign material and the vessels. As regards fibrosis in the cave of Retzius, it should be possible to foresee and at least partially prevent this by preserving the integrity of the fascia between the umbilicus and the bladder, during the subumbilical median approach, which will allow one if necessary to dispense with the retrofascial plane of cleavage.

I. Special Problems

The aspects of the problem which should prompt the surgeon to re-examine his technique, are as follows. They bear witness to the broad variation between the types of groin hernia.

1. Irreducibility

Irreducibility is a fairly common finding in indirect inguinal and femoral hernias (between 10 and 20% according to Condon and Nyhus 1995). Irreducibility is an important feature because a considerable proportion of these patients will proceed to obstruction and strangulation, with a increasing risk of morbidity and mortality. Manual reduction should be attempted very gently, but is useful in distinguishing between complete and partial irreducibility. In the first case, even if the hernia is small, and particularly if it is of the femoral variety, the signs of strangulation must be carefully sought. In the second case, and particularly if there is a bulky hernia, the findings suggest a sliding hernia, not necessarily incarcerated. A persistent cough impulse is helpful in excluding the diagnosis of strangulation. Successful reduction of an incarcerated hernia is of benefit, because it allows operation to be carried out 24 hours later, when the condition of the patient is improved. Sudden disappearance of an incarcerated mass without the characteristic gurgling sound is an alarming finding, that may represent a "reduction en masse", which requires immediate laparotomy.

2. Bruising around the Hernial Site

This is a rare complication, confined to inguinal hernias. It must be recognized because of its potentially serious significance, which can be avoided by a well performed operation. It may result from various injuries including a visceral hematoma, perforation or complete rupture of the intestines, a tear in the omentum, rupture of the hernial sac or of the spermatic cord. Bruising resulting from traumatic attempts at reduction should be a thing of the past. In practice, there are two clinical pictures.

One represents a pseudo strangulation, which may lead to re-exploration via the inguinal route, later extended into a laparotomy, and the other is a picture of generalized peritonitis where the need for laparotomy is obvious in order to diagnose and treat the lesion.

3. Problems with Trusses

Provision of a truss may be justified in certain cases such as in the control of an easily reducible hernia, as a short term measure, where operation has been delayed for some reason such as correction of co-morbidity, or during the third trimester of pregnancy, or as a long-term measure in the case of an elderly patient. This latter is not a credible policy, because nowadays procedures are available which are suitable for all ages and all degrees of frailty, that can provide permanent comfortable containment of the lesion, whereas a truss can never guarantee permanent reduction. It must also be emphasized that wearing a truss increases the risk of complications which may lead to emergency surgery [Nyhus 1995]. A truss increases the risk of strangulation by compressing the lymphatics and veins in a small sac whose contents may be difficult to reduce, while at the same time the pressure exerted on the margins of the hernial orifice may cause it to swell. Any increase in the volume of the hernia makes subsequent repair more difficult.

4. Strangulation

This implies interruption of the blood supply of the contents of the sac. The usual strangulating agent is the neck of the sac, whether inguinal or femoral. Any sudden increase in the volume of the contents leads to

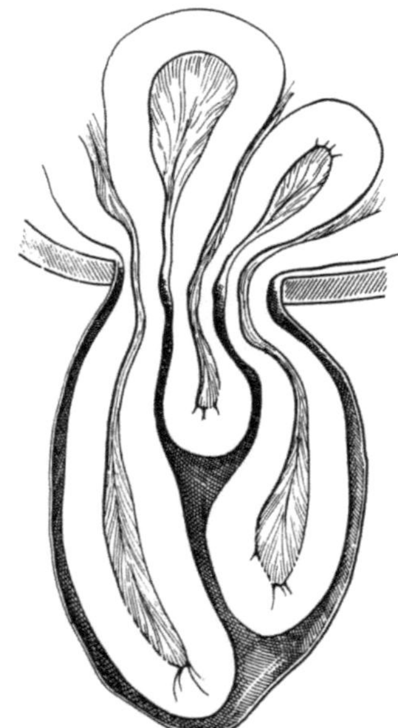

Fig. 9.22. Strangulated hernia with W-shaped arrangement of the involved bowel segments [Quénu & Perrotin 1955]

stasis in the lymphatics and veins, and thus increases the pressure at the neck. This is followed by arrest of the arterial circulation.Strangulation may be partial and lateral (Richter's hernia) or total, which completely obstructs the lumen of the bowel and produces early signs of intestinal obstruction (Fig. 9.22).

The percentage of strangulated hernias was 8% of those operated upon in the French Association of Surgeons series (1984) and 8.9% in my personal series reported by Warlaumont (1982).

The guidelines laid down by the Royal College of Surgeons of England (1993) report that the annual incidence of strangulation of inguinal hernia was estimated at 0.3 to 2.9%, with a higher risk during the first three months following appearance of the hernia. Femoral hernias presented to the surgeon as a case of strangulation in 34 to 51% of cases, as against 10% for inguinal hernias. Direct inguinal hernias strangulate ten times less often than do indirect, but the clinical distinction between direct and indirect hernias is rarely possible. Even among experts there is only a 69% accurate correlation.

The timing of strangulation is very difficult to establish because of the frequent absence of clinical signs, particularly in the case of femoral strangulations. Diagnosis is especially difficult in the case of a Richter's hernia, where there are no signs of obstruction.

These facts should discourage attempts at manual reduction, even in young patients, in order to avoid reduction en masse, returning a necrotic loop of intestine to the peritoneal cavity or bruising the contents of the sac. Patients suspected of strangulation should be operated upon as a matter of urgency.

However, the urgent situation does not absolve the surgeon from careful preoperative preparation and choice of anesthesia, in conjunction with the anesthetist.

Operative Technique

The incision is made along the long axis of the hernial protrusion for both inguinal and femoral hernias. The essential steps of the operation include identification of the sac and its opening, being careful to protect the wound from any septic contents. The neck must be freed up, taking care to avoid damaging the epigastric vessels, dividing the inguinal ligament or the iliopubic band. The contents are examined, which may include omentum (this can be removed if it is infarcted) or small intestine, which should be widely exposed in order to evaluated its state. Estimation of intestinal viability is extremely important and a loop should

only be returned to the abdomen if it recovers its color and peristalsis. Otherwise, a wide resection and end to end anastomosis, carried out through healthy bowel, is the wiser course. Once the sac and its contents have been dealt with, the abdominal wall should be repaired by the simplest possible means, bearing in mind the potentially infective nature of the operative field and the state of the patient.

There is much to be said in favor of leaving the skin open. Stewardson [in Nyhus 1978] reported a 60% incidence of wound infection following intestinal resection. Recently published short series, however, suggest that there is now no increased mortality or morbidity following the use of a prosthesis, so that prosthetic materials should perhaps be more extensively used in strangulated hernias, although this was previously regarded as an absolute contra-indication. In a recent open discussion in the French Academy of Surgeons, following a paper by Henry (1994), we suggested that prostheses should only be used in the treatment of strangulated hernia when there was complete absence of identifiable sepsis, the surgeon was well experienced, small amounts of prosthetic material were used, and the supporting services were of high quality.

Surprising situations may occur. The sac may contain normal intestine. Before reducing the loop one should carry out a wide exploration of the intestine in order not to miss a retrograde strangulation, (W-shaped hernia or a double sac, i.e. an external sac containing a normal loop of intestine and a preperitoneal sac with strangulated contents). Preperitoneal hernial strangulation is rare but is almost always followed by reduction "en masse" of the sac and its contents, which remain strangulated by the rigid peritoneal ring. Under these circumstances, one should not hesitate to convert the herniotomy into a "hernio-laparotomy", if necessary via a separate laparotomy incision. In practice, the physical findings should be carefully assessed, and no reduction undertaken without total understanding of the situation. The situation has a grave prognosis because of the element of intestinal resection; also the average age of the patients is higher and overall management more difficult because of the emergency circumstances. The adult mortality for strangulated hernia has scarcely changed over the last 60 years and remains at around 13% [Frankau 1931; Vick 1932; Requarth 1948; Hjaltason 1980; Andrews 1981; Flament 1987].

Hernial phlegmon represents a late stage of strangulation which nowadays is rarely seen (0.6% in the French Association of Surgeons Study). It represents a feco-purulent mass, which occasionally breaks out through the skin, but more often leads to death. Three methods of treatment have been proposed [Detrie 1970]. Wide incision of the phlegmon does not lead to a cure and is no longer defensible. An alternative is to carry out a bypass anastomosis which excludes the necrotic loop. This is accomplished in two stages, a preliminary laparotomy followed later by debridement of the phlegmon. Although some success has been reported, the postoperative course is prolonged and beset with problems. The most radical solution, which has nonetheless given one or two successes, consists in an abdominal approach which divides the intestine and restores continuity, followed by an inguinal incision which removes the necrotic loop and cleans up the infected area, leaving in place a large drain, with no attempt to repair the abdominal wall. The mortality of feco-purulent hernial phlegmon was 66% in the series reported by Warlaumont in 1982.

5. Femoral Hernias

This type of groin hernia represents some 5% of the total, or 11% according to Devlin (1988). They are surgically important because of their tendency to strangulate, which is higher than with inguinal hernias, and still carries a mortality. Classical herniorrhaphy gives poor results, so that it is appropriate to review briefly the pathological anatomy.

The classical anatomical description states that femoral hernia is a direct hernia through the femoral ring in the transversalis fascia, medial to the femoral vessels, under the iliopubic band and the inguinal ligament. The femoral septum maintains the integrity of the deeper layers, together with fatty and lymphatic tissue. Logically, therefore, repair should involve the tendino-fascial structures, which are approached with equal ease via the femoral or the inguinal route. According to Lytle (1953) the true hernial orifice is not at the femoral ring but lies considerably more distally, at the lower end of the femoral canal, near to the termination of the long saphenous vein (Fig. 9.23). Femoral hernias are therefore of the indirect type, crossing the abdominal wall through the femoral canal, as a result of the double structure of Gimbernat's ligament, which has both tendinous and fascial origins.

This concept results in simplification of surgical treatment of femoral hernia, by an approach to the superficial femoral orifice, which is the structure responsible for strangulation and need only be repaired by simple suture, if necessary under local anesthesia. Fruchaud considers that the femoral ring is a compartment of the "musculo fascial hole" and the femoral canal forms part of the abdomino-femoral investing fascia. He considers that, in common with all other groin hernias, total repair of the musculo-pectineal orifice in the deep part of the inguinal area is essential, for example by the McVay operation.

From these conflicting anatomical concepts there has arisen a degree of uncertainty as to the principles, the choice and the method of carrying out a surgical repair. The mechanism of the ordinary type of femoral hernia is multi-factorial, particularly when com-

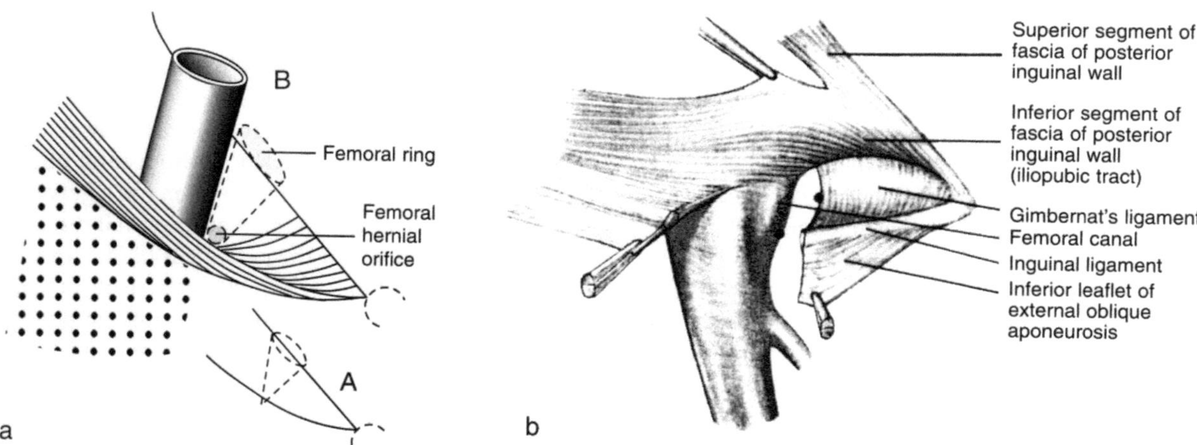

Fig. 9.23. Lytle's concept (femoral hernias). **a** The femoral hernial orifice; A femoral canal without hernia; B femoral canal containing a hernia with the distal hernial ring medially bordered by the Gimbernat's ligament [Lytle (1961) Proc R Soc Med]. **b** Duality in the constitution of the Gimbernat's ligament [Madden (1989) Saunders, Philadelphia]

paring the differences between men and women. The broader pelvis in the female gives rise to an enlargement of the vascular compartment beneath the inguinal ligament and the increased frequency in elderly women is explained by the senile atrophy of the iliopsoas muscle, coupled with the ageing of the ligamentous structures such as the iliopubic and ileopectineal bands. In certain cases there is added the traction effect of a lipomatous mass in the peritoneal cul-de-sac. As in all abdominal hernias, this passive mechanism is increased by factors which raise intra-abdominal pressure such as obesity or severe emaciation, and abdominal distension resulting from conditions already described. The usual type of femoral hernia lies within the femoral canal, but occasionally weakness of the vascular sheath leads to the emergence of atypical varieties. These include lateral femoral hernias which come out beside the femoral vessels ("Hesselbach hernias" 1906). These are found essentially in men, and have a short sac with a wide neck, often associated with a lipoma, and appear beneath the femoral fascia, and occasionally through it (Camera). Prevascular femoral hernias [Teale 1846; Fabricius 1895] are contained within the femoral vascular sheath in front of the vessels, and are thus of small size. Moschowitz (1912) and Turner (1953) described quite large hernias taking a deep course between the peritoneal cavity and lateral to the inferior epigastric vessels. A few very rare types of hernia should be included such as the medial femoral hernia, the bisaccular hernia of Astley Cooper, the diverticular hernia of Hesselbach (the sac is contained within the femoral canal and emerges through a gap in the cribriform fascia) the pectineal hernia of Cloquet which crosses the pectineal aponeurosis, and the hernia of Laugier or medial hernia of Velpeau which crosses Gimbernat's ligament sometimes very far medially and beside the umbilical artery. Additional types include the femorogenital hernia of Cooper which develops within the labium majus and finally Serafini (1917) described a retrovascular hernia the existence of which, already cited in the literature, had been denied by Moschowitz.

The existence of these atypical forms of femoral hernia still further complicates the diagnosis which is often already rendered difficult because these hernias are of small volume and occur in obese patients, often without a cough impulse and irreducible. Spangen [in Hernia 1995] advocates the use of herniorrhaphy in obese women complaining of pain in this area, but in whom no hernia is palpable. He finds this method sensitive and reliable. In the same clinical circumstances Deitch (1981) finds little use for ultrasound, but in contrast Truong and Schumpelick (1994) defend its use in patients with a palpable tumor, and also in those who have pain of obscure origin with no obvious swelling. They find that this method not only gives a reliable diagnosis of hernia, but also distinguishes it from other swellings and causes of local pain. However there are certain limitations to the technique, particularly in the case of suspected recurrence, where false echoes are common. These overall difficulties suggest the wisdom of employing an inguinal approach for femoral hernias in order better to identify the lesion and cope with any unexpected features. The preperitoneal route is equally effective from that point of view. The diagnosis of small hernias is difficult, but in the case of large femoral hernias with a long history, there is always the risk of the bladder being included, and if there are any urinary symptoms a preoperative cystogram is advisable. However the possibility of bladder en glissade is one that should be borne in mind in every case of femoral hernia.

The classical surgical treatment of femoral hernias can be carried out through three routes.

The low, femoral, route allows one to define the sac up to its neck to verify its contents. This narrow route of access does not allow one to deal with chronic incarceration nor to close the sac accurately at its neck. Clearance of the neck should preferably be carried out on the medial side towards the reflected part of the inguinal ligament, in order not to injure the obturator artery. Closure of the femoral ring is often difficult and sometimes inadequate, and tends to take up the pectineal fascia and inguinal ligament rather than the pectineal ligament and iliopubic band. The Lytle method of closing the distal, superficial femoral orifice is, however, much simpler. We therefore advise this approach as often as possible for small hernias, if necessary under local anesthesia, an alternative method being the use of a Lichtenstein type of cylindrical plug.

The inguinal approach is better adapted for treatment of bulky femoral hernias with a neck broader than two fingers breadths. Following the usual superficial dissection, the transversalis fascia is incised and the neck of the femoral hernia can be found within the extraperitoneal fat, and drawn upwards, if necessary having cleared the lacunar ligament of Gimbernat. Any bladder involvement is more easy to identify and control via this route. Having dealt with the sac, the repair is carried out on the deep femoral ring, approached from above. This can be done either by interrupted nonabsorbable sutures between the iliopubic band and the medial part of the pectineal ligament, or else by the McVay technique, completely closing the musculo-pectineal orifice, if necessary using a conical plug in the femoral canal.

The suprainguinal route described by Nyhus and Reid, or the midline preperitoneal route in the case of bilateral hernia, makes possible the suturing of the deep femoral ring or the placement of a large prosthesis which can be fixed (Rives) or free (Stoppa). Unusual varieties of femoral hernia are much more easily identified from above and are generally treated by a prosthesis. Prosthetic repair is, in particular, the only possible method for prevascular femoral hernia or bulky recurrences. In a personal series of 185 uncomplicated femoral hernias, of which 171 have been followed up from between two and twelve years, the suture operations and McVay procedure gave poor results (15% of recurrences), the Lytle operation 6% and Lichtenstein plugs 3%, whereas prostheses inserted via the inguinal or midline subumbilical route gave consistently good results. Our experience confirms that of the Shouldice Hospital, where femoral recurrences following suture had a mean recurrence rate of 22%, and there were 75% re-recurrences in six cases. The reader will find in Tables 9.16 and 9.17 the results of the prosthetic techniques.

a) An Umbrella for Femoral Hernias

R. Bendavid

(1) The Source of the Problem

The difficulties which beset femoral hernia repairs are due to the rigid anatomic configurations of the femoral canal. Posteriorly the femoral canal is limited by

Table 9.16. Rate of recurrence of femoral hernias after non-prosthetic repair [Schumpelick & Wantz, 1995, according to Bendavid]

Authors	Procedure	# Cases	% Follow-up	Years Follow-up	% Recurrences
Ponka	Bassini	44	-	6	2.3
Bendavid	Bassini-Kirschner	251	84.6	1 to 8	6.1
Butters	Bassini-Kirschner	178	-	1 to 8	3.3
Glassow	Bassini-Kirschner	1,143	-	-	2
Ponka & Bush	Bassini-Kirschner	216	92	1 to 8	6.5
Nyhus & Harkins	Preperitoneal	113	-	-	0.8
Bagot & Walters	Preperitoneal	114	79.8	2 to 21	0.9
Halverson	McVay	96	-	22	3.1
Barbier	McVay	23	-	12	0

Table 9.17. Recurrences of femoral hernias after prosthesis repair [Schumpelick & Wantz 1995, according to Bendavid]

Authors	Procedure	# Cases	% Follow-up	Years Follow-up	% Recurrences
Wantz	Unilateral Stoppa	7	-	-	0
Wantz	Stoppa	16	-	-	0
Lichtenstein	Plug	168	-	14	0.61
Trabucco	Plug	27	98	2.5	0
Bendavid	Umbrella	70	-	5 to 8	0
Shouldice Hosp.	Umbrella	280	-	9	1.1

the pubic ramus and the overlying ligament of Cooper. Anteriorly, the inguinal ligament is tense if not rigid and cannot be easily brought near to the ligament of Cooper. Medially, the lacunar ligament of Gimbernat and its overlying transversalis fascia are also rigid and unyielding structures. Laterally, the femoral vein represents a structure that cannot be transgressed without dire consequences.

Approximation of the conjoint tendon to the ligament of Cooper, despite making a generous relaxing incision as in the McVay repair, produces an inordinate amount of tension.

The pectineus muscle and its fascia have no place in the treatment of a femoral hernia. This practice resulted from an erroneous interpretation of Bassini's text on the repair of femoral hernia, where he mentions the use of "the pectineal fascia at its crest". The key word is crest, meaning the ligament of Cooper [Bassini 1893].

(2) The Femoral Umbrella (Fig. 9.24a, b)

The femoral umbrella consists of an 8 cm disc of polypropylene (Marlex, Prolene, Trelex).

A suture is brought through the center of the disc to act as a stem for easier handling. The femoral hernia

can be repaired from below the inguinal ligament if the defect is large enough to identify the ligament of Cooper adequately and safely. If not, the repair can be done via the preperitoneal space, after dividing the posterior wall of the inguinal canal to gain access to the space of Bogros. When the exposure is complete, a Kelly forceps is inserted from below the inguinal ligament, to grasp the stem of the umbrella and pull it down until the disc covers the femoral defect. Prolene sutures are inserted in the ligament of Cooper (usually 4 to 6). I usually begin by inserting these sutures into the ligament from the level of the femoral vein to the pubic crest; then, when the disc is lowered into place, the ends of each suture are threaded through the grid of the mesh. Medially, a single suture anchors the mesh to the lacunar ligament. Anteriorly two to four sutures anchor the umbrella to the iliopubic and inguinal ligaments. Laterally, the disc lies against the femoral vein and is kept in place by suturing (from below the inguinal ligament) the femoral sheath to the disc. The decision to carry out the operation from below or above the inguinal ligament should be guided by the presence or absence of an inguinal hernia and the ease of access through the femoral defect.

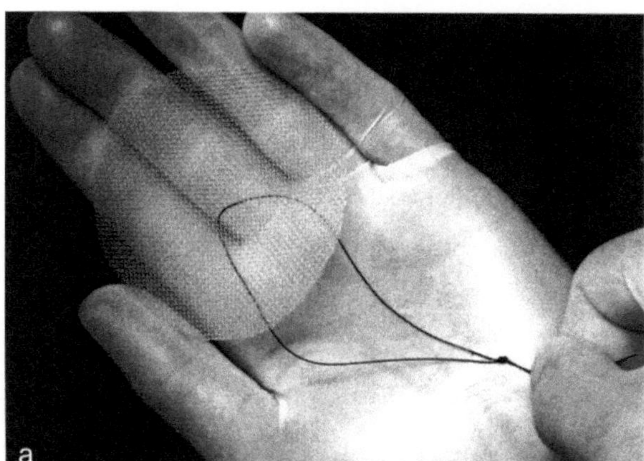

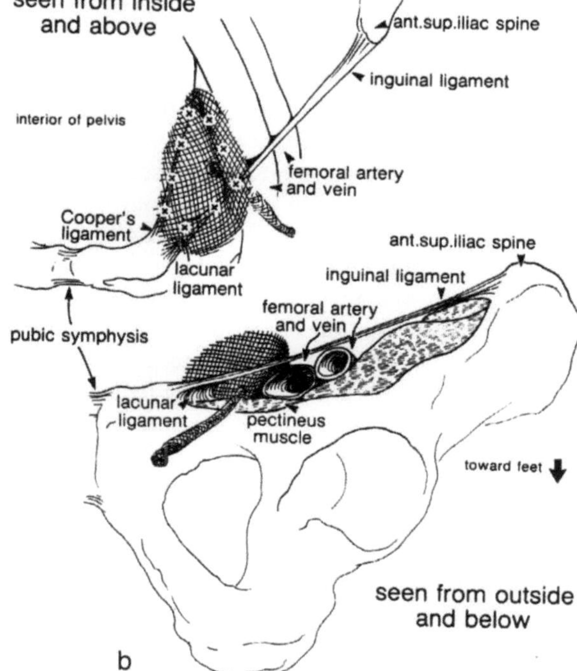

Fig. 9.24. a The umbrella. An 8 cm disc of polypropylene with a suture threaded through the center of the disc. **b** Schematic representation of placement and attachment of umbrella mesh

(3) Results

The use of prosthetic materials was introduced at the Shouldice Hospital in November 1983. The years 1983 and 1984 are eliminated from the study as the umbrella had only just been evaluated experimentally. From 1985 to 1995, the use of the umbrella became routine, though at the discretion of the operating surgeon.

During that period 1,476 femoral hernias were corrected. There were 836 primary femoral hernias and 640 recurrent femoral hernias. Of the 836 primary femoral hernias, 94 were repaired with an umbrella while 742 were corrected by some other method, without any prosthesis. Of the 640 recurrent femoral hernias, 266 were repaired with an umbrella, while 376 were repaired with no prosthetic material.

In total, 360 (94 + 266) femoral hernias (primary and recurrent) were treated with an umbrella while 1,116 (primary and recurrent) were treated without an umbrella. The results were as follows:

- 2 recurrences out of 360 femoral hernias repaired with an umbrella were recorded, an incidence of 0.55%;

- 89 recurrences, out of 1,116 femoral hernias repaired without an umbrella were recorded, an incidence of 7.9%.

(4) Discussion

Femoral hernias, to my mind, represent the most delicate abdominal wall hernias to correct. One has to be alert to the possibilities of injury to the femoral vein, the iliopubic vein, the aberrant obturator artery and vein, and also the inferior epigastric vessels which may be masked by scar tissue from previous operations and which can be seen over a length of 1-2 cm between the internal ring and the potential space between the femoral vein and the protruding femoral sac. The most tedious part of the operation is the reduction of the femoral hernia into the preperitoneal space, carefully separating the sac while leaving femoral sheath intact. The identification of the ligament of Cooper is usually a simple matter, though on occasion it may dip into a postero-medial direction rather than posterolaterally making the insertion of sutures a little more difficult.

The decision to use a prosthesis should be encouraged, more often than not. At the Shouldice Hospital, the use of prostheses in femoral herniorrhaphies has increased exponentially. The results of the present analysis may encourage surgeons to use umbrellas in most femoral defects, and the case seems sound. There has been no single case of an infected repair in this series.

(5) Conclusion

Femoral hernias remain the most challenging of all abdominal wall hernias. It is therefore important at the first operation to use the most reliable method available. The femoral umbrella has eminently served that purpose.

References

Barbette P (1676) The surgical and anatomical works of Paul Barbette. Moses Pitt Printer, London

Bassini E (1893) Nuovo metodo operativo per la cura radicale dellíernia crurale. Angelo Draghi Libraio Editore

Bendavid R (1994) Prosthesis and abdominal wall hernias. R G Landes, Austin

Bendavid R (1989) New techniques in hernia repair. World J Surg 13: 5

Bendavid R (1989) Femoral hernias. Primary versus recurrence. Int Surg 74: 99-100

Butters AG (1948) A review of femoral hernias with special reference to recurrence rate of low operations. Br Med J 2: 743-745

Cooke RV (1958) Discussion of small bowel obstruction. Proc R Soc Med 51: 503-508

David T (1967) Strangulated femoral hernias. Med J. Aust 1: 258-261

Dunphy JE (1940) The diagnosis and surgical management of strangulated femoral hernias. JAMA 114: 394-396

Jens J (1943) Strangulated femoral hernias. Lancet 1: 705-707

Lawson RS (1949) Strangulated hernia. Alfred Hospital Clinic Reports 1: 51

McClure RD, Fallis LS (1939) Femoral hernias. 90 operations. Ann Surg 109: 987-1000

O'Dell A. Personal communication. Administrator, Shouldice Hospital

Ponka JL, Brush BE (1971) The problem of femoral hernia. Arch Surg 102: 417-423

Temple CO (1958) Incarcerated and strangulated femoral hernia. J Int Coll Surg 30: 1-11

Welsh DRJ (1974) Inguinal hernia repair. Mod Med 42: 49-54

b) Strangulated Femoral Hernia

The diagnosis is often made late, or missed, because of the absence of symptoms (only half of the patients complain of local pain) or of physical signs (obesity).

Additional aggravating risk factors are frequent and can be age, obesity and a partial pinched off occlusion of the loop (Richter's hernia - 15-90% of Richter's hernias are of the femoral variety). Nonetheless, a high index of suspicion must be maintained, because false negative diagnoses are far more frequent than are false positives. Important points in differential diagnosis should be emphasized. These include the fact that acute inflammation of a femoral lymph node (Cloquet's node) only occurs with a port of entry of infection, and that any tender red swelling in this area can always represent a local intestinal necrosis through femoral strangulation. These difficulties lead to delay in diagnosis, which often involves a subsequent resection of the bowel. This determines the prognosis, which, in my personal series (1988) comprises a mortality of 8.8%, the same as that reported by Champault (1986).

We urge surgeons to pay more attention to defining the anatomy of femoral hernia, from which should emerge more effective treatment. The risks of strangulation indicate routine repair of this lesion, whatever the physical state of the patient, which in any case can usually be proved by suitable preparation.

Femoral hernias have conventionally been treated by suture via the femoral route (Bassini, Kirschner, Lytle), the inguinal route (McVay, Moschovitz) or the suprainguinal route (Nyhus). Unfortunately all these techniques share the disadvantage of closing the femoral ring under tension, which cannot totally be compensated by relaxation incisions. For this reason repairs involving the use of prosthetic material seem to me to deserve wider consideration, except for very small femoral hernias. The plug proposed by Lichtenstein and its variations (Trabucco or Rutkow) gives good results in hernias of less than 1.5 to 2 cm in diameter. More bulky hernias require synthetic devices of which there are several types ranging from the umbrella (Bendavid) to large prostheses which envelope the entire visceral sac in the case of bilateral defects. At the Shouldice Hospital, for many years, prosthetic material has been used in 60.3% of femoral hernias and 91% of inguino-femoral hernias (1995).

6. Richter's Hernia

This implies lateral strangulation of the intestine, which may in fact lead to total obstruction and in which local physical examination may be very deceptive, because of the small volume of the strangulation. In all series, Richter's hernias are predominantly of the femoral type [Treves 1887; Frankau 1931; Jens 1943; Lyall 1948; Gillespie 1956] but they can also be obturator, inguinal, umbilical or incisional in origin. In all, Richter's hernias represent 5 to 15% of strangulated hernias of all types, in the major series.

One may say that the diagnosis of a Richter's hernia is best made when one thinks of it, because the clinical picture of obstruction is insidious and usually incomplete. Usually it is a small femoral hernia which is the cause, and physical examination may be negative or of doubtful significance. Because of late diagnosis (more than 48 h in 60% of Frankau's patients) the mortality remains at over 20%. Gillespie has described three clinical pictures. In one-third to one-half of the patients there is obvious obstruction and operation is carried before necrosis or strangulation. In another third there is no obstruction and there is partial necrosis of the gut found at operation so that intestinal resection carries a high mortality. 15% of the patients form a fistula between the bowel and the skin, as was described by Fabricius Hildanus in 1598, which heals in a number of weeks.

Modern methods of resuscitation allow one to improve the condition of the patient whatever the presenting clinical picture, but should not be allowed to delay operation, as soon as the diagnosis has been made. W. A. Tito (1995) advocates a suprainguinal incision and a preperitoneal approach when the diagnosis is made, because this not only allows one to evaluate the contents of the sac, but also to extend the approach into the peritoneum, in case of necessity.

7. Bulky Hernias

When a groin hernia is greater than the volume of the fist, it is usually no longer well tolerated, even when the patient is self-neglectful. 88% of large groin hernias are of the indirect variety [Rives 1974]. Progressive enlargement of the inguinal canal is paralleled by a loss of substance in the deeper tissues, through superimposition of the deep and superficial inguinal rings. The disappearance of the obliquity of the inguinal canal promotes prolapse of the viscera and leads to an increase in the volume of the sac which becomes divided by adhesions and scar tissue between the viscera. There thus forms a type of "direct" hernia complicated by loss of substance of the abdominal wall and intrasaccular adhesions. To these are frequently added other abnormalities such as sliding of parasaccular organs including the bladder and the elements of the spermatic cord, which are often found at the lower pole of the sac in front of the abdominal wall. Eventually, the enveloping scrotal layers are involved and add to the difficulties during and after the operation. Recurrent scrotal hematoma is an example of these.

This condition frequently affects frail and elderly patients in whom a large hernia has caused difficulties because of its volume, weight and problems with local hygiene. Additional problems include envelopment of the penis and subacute obstruction due to the visceral adhesions and the total or partial irreducibility of the contents of the sac. When this stage is reached, the long neglected bulky hernia necessitates surgical treatment, emphasizing the advantages of operation at an earlier stage when the hernia is relatively uncomplicated. Together with other types of complex hernia, the bulky hernia constitutes a major argument in favor of the personal approach to these problems. Large groin hernias can become complicated by intestinal obstruction, occasionally because of strangulation at the neck, but much more often because of intrasaccular bands.

The frequency was 22.7% in our study carried out in 1984 for the AFC. In a personal series presented by Warlaumand (1982), it was 14.1%, with no predilection for size. The proportion of the sexes are 20% in men and 9.3% in women.

Once the decision to operate has been made, together with the anesthetist, careful preparation of these patients who were often elderly and either obese or emaciated, is essential. These operations are of a major nature, but may well serve to improve the patient's functional status and independence. Surgery, however, is the only answer. Advantage is taken of the preoperative preparation period to prepare the local tissue area.

The repair of choice is undoubtedly that which uses a retromuscular prosthesis which one can place in position by the inguinal approach. This allows freeing up of the adherent contents of the sac and placement of the prosthesis, bearing in mind the above mentioned difficulties, either by the suprainguinal or preperitoneal route, with unilateral or bilateral wrapping of the visceral sac. An additional high scrotal incision may on occasion be required in order to liberate adherent contents, but placement of the prosthesis by the preperitoneal route is certainly simpler. Scrotal sacs are not fully resected: the distal part is left in place, with adequate drainage.

Giant hernias present particular problems. The inguinal canal is transformed into a large gaping ring which allows passage of a mass of viscera constituted in the main by small bowel but which also may contain right or left colon "en glissade". The visceral mass has often "lost its right of domicile" in the abdo-

men. The reduction of the contents must be carefully prepared for by slimming, pulmonary physiotherapy, and the use of a preoperative pneumoperitoneum as described by Goni-Moreno (1964) perhaps lasting two or three weeks. This requires a scrotal retaining device in order to prevent air distending the scrotaml sac. The preparatory pneumoperitoneum is important not only because it increases the capacity of the abdominal cavity for acceptance of the contents of the large hernia, but also because it helps to break down the adhesions and free up the contents of the hernia. It would be useful to make a preoperative diagnosis of sliding viscera, as suggested by a hernia which is both bulky and partially irreducible, but this is not usually possible clinically (20% of cases in the report by Piedad (1973). The contents of the hernial sac can sometimes be made clear by conventional contrast radiological examinations.

Certain operative details should be mentioned. In the obese patient, the Trendelenburg position helps to reduce the contents during the operation. A separate incision in the upper part of the scrotum is useful for identifying the sliding nature of the hernia, and the degree of adherence. In bulky sliding hernias, we advise dissecting the sac and its contents together, and reducing them en masse into the abdomen, without freeing the contents of the sac. Reduction of the sac and its contents may exceptionally require enlargement of the hernial orifice, or even division of the tendon of the rectus muscle as suggested by Chevrel (Fig. 9.25a-c).

It is our practice to treat these giant hernias with a large reinforcing prosthesis introduced via the midline preperitoneal route.

In nonsliding hernias the part of the sac which is left behind may accumulate a large serosanguinous collection of fluid, which should be aspirated rather than re-explored. The choice must be made between preserving the distal sac and risking a hematoma, or else resecting the sac with the corresponding risk of ischemic orchitis. We prefer the first alternative. Very large scrotums, following reduction of a sac with a massive en glissade element often form recurrent seromas, which may become infected as a result of multiple aspirations, removal of clots or surgical drainage. This sometimes results in an elephantiasis-like change in the scrotal coverings, a disfiguring infolding of the skin, or painful scars at the drainage sites. Surgeons who frequently encounter this type of pathology (tropical Africa, Egypt, Madagascar) often eventually resort to a plastic resection of the scrotum, in order to resolve the hematoma problem and to prevent recur-

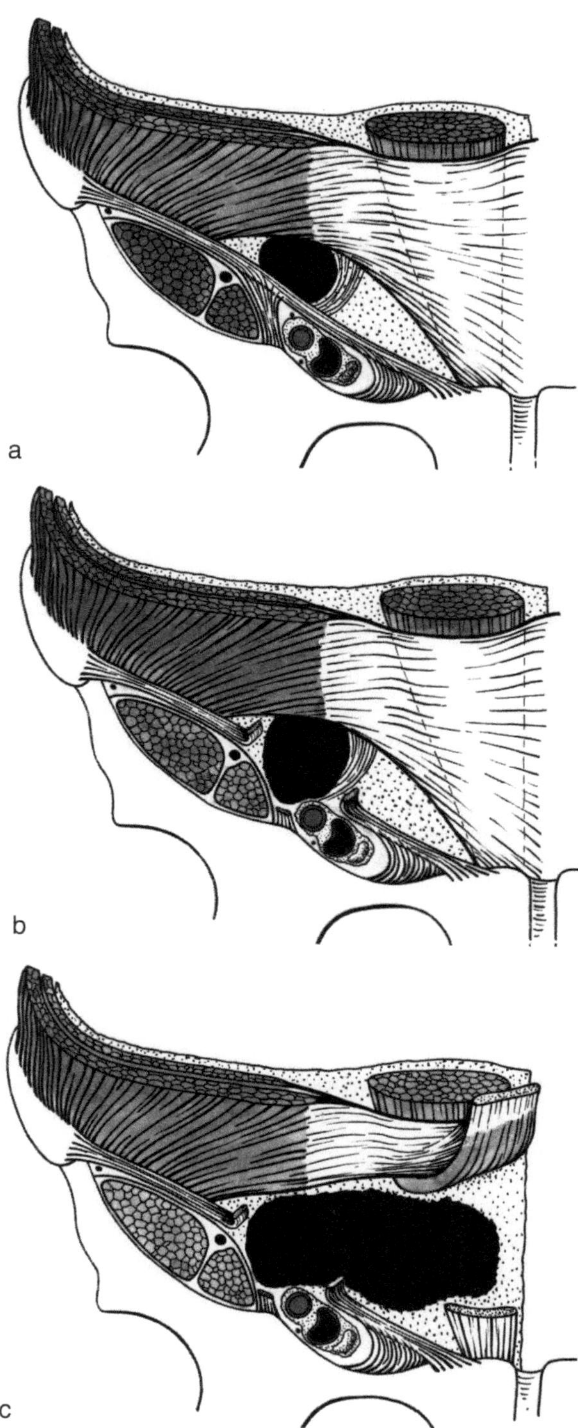

Fig. 9.25. Enlargement of the hernial orifice: Chevrel's procedure.
a Enlarged hernial orifice, peritoneal sac and spermatic cord are
not shown. b First step: section of the inguinal ligament. c If this
is not enough, section of the rectus abdominis tendon. After
replacing the peritoneal sac in the pelvic cavity, the rectus abdominis tendon and the inguinal ligament are repaired by interrupted sutures (0 or 00 nonabsorbable monofilament)

rence. We have no personal experience of the "hitch
titch" procedure of suspending the scrotum on to the
abdominal wall, as advocated by Joseph O'Boyle
(1989).

Results. In 1984 we operated upon 230 bulky groin
hernias out of a total of 1,628. 25% of the patients were
over 60 years and 42% of the bulky hernias were bilateral. The recurrence rate at two to five years was 3.4%,
as against 1% for the other hernias in the series managed with a prosthesis, and 25% after the Bassini-
Shouldice operation carried out on frail patients with
large hernias.

8. Adherent Hernias. Sliding Hernias

Adherent hernias seem to have been commoner in
the past, probably explained by the prolonged use of
a truss. Omental adhesions can be dealt with quite
simply by resecting them with the sac. Intestinal
adhesions should be freed with care in order to avoid
deperitonising the bowel, if necessary by resection a
portion of the sac. With extensive bowel adhesions it
is better to proceed as with a sliding hernia. In these
cases, the descent of the peritoneum is accompanied
by that of one or more attached viscera, which lie
within or beside the sac. These may be the bladder or
the cecum on the right and the pelvic colon on the
left.

The percentage of sliding hernias is from 3 to 6% of
the total number [Glassow in Hernia 1978]. The left
side is affected 4.5 times more frequently that the right
and males more than females. The incidence increase
with the duration and the size of the hernia. Hernias
in small girls often contain some adnexa such as a
Fallopian tube, or a broad ligament with or without an
ovary. Rayan divides sliding hernia into three types:
parasaccular (the viscus forms one part of the sac
from which it can be separated: 95% of cases), intrasaccular (a free viscus is connected to the sac by the
mesentery) and extrasaccular (rare); here the viscus
lies completely outside the sac, as for instance the
bladder. Preoperative diagnosis of sliding hernia is
unusual (25% of 86 cases of Piedad 1973). The suspicion should arise in the presence of a large inguinoscrotal hernia with a broad neck and contents which
are nonetheless only partially reducible. A poorly
functioning truss is also suggestive. A barium enema
showing colon within the hernial sac is not diagnostic, because the colon may occupy the sac without
being fixed within it. The diagnosis of sliding hernia is
thus usually made at the time of operation. Clumsy

opening of the sac can lead to serious accidents, so that the sac must be carefully entered from above and in front, whenever there is a suspicion of adherent contents.

The suprainguinal approach of Laroque (1932) provides access to the sac intraperitoneally, after dissection of the muscles. Reduction of the contents may cause problems to the surgeon, as shown by the large number of complicated and ingenious procedures which have been described in the past (Hotchkiss, Moschowitz). Because high ligation of the sac is no longer considered an essential procedure, and carries high risks, I advise, together with surgeons such as Fruchaud and Wantz, verifying the contents of the sac and reducing it en masse, as already described. We suggest the following strategy. A scrotal incision is made and the sac opened, then freed together with its adherent contents, and reduced into the abdomen if possible. The second stage of the operation, which is carried out through the midline subumbilical preperitoneal or suprainguinal preperitoneal approach, completes mass reduction of the bulky sac, and then proceeds to the prosthetic repair. We personally always employ a large bilateral type of prosthesis.

Given the present status of laparoscopic hernia repair, it would seem that this should be used as a video assisted technique where very large hernias are concerned.

9. Bilateral Hernias

The major series report a variable frequency from 15% to 50%, bearing in mind the time relations. Glassow (1969) reports 17%. Sawagushi (1975) 25%, a personal series reported in Walraumont's thesis (1982): 27%. Kingsnorth (1993) reports that bilateral direct hernias are four times commoner than indirect hernias. Watson, Jason, observed the appearance of a contralateral hernia in 25% to 30% of cases in the years following a unilateral repair and Rutledge (1995) 46%. Simultaneous repair does not increase the recurrence rate, as cited by Miller [Mayo Clinic 1991, in "Inguinal Hernia" by A. Gaynant]. As regards children, 20% to 25% of contralateral hernias appear after unilateral repair, at the end of the growth period. This is probably due to persistence of the communicating canal on the side opposite to the hernia, 40% at birth, 22% at two years of age. The same applies to 58% of girls in respect of the canal of Nück.

The existence of bilateral groin hernias is explained by a certain symmetry of the congenital abnormalities such as persistent processus vaginalis in boys and variations in muscular insertions.

In the presence of one patent hernia, examination of the other side may reveal signs which are difficult to interpret. Dilatation of the inguinal ring is not enough to confirm the presence of the hernia and is necessary to discover a cough impulse or to feel the upper border of the pubis through the dilated inguinal ring, when a direct hernia is involved, or there may be a contralateral dilatation associated with a major scrotal hernia. Special investigations are quite frequently used in children. These include herniorrhaphy in the very young patients, ultrasound scan (accepting its degree of subjectivity) and occasionally diagnostic laparoscopy [Johanet 1995]. It must be borne in mind that the insufflation pressure of the peritoneum may procure artifacts and a falsely raised rate of bilateral hernia (48.2% as against 37.2% clinically, in Johanet's series). A contralateral "hernia point" which is asymptomatic and overlooked is not necessarily a threat to the patient.

Although it is not mandatory, the two sides may be dealt with a the same operative session. If it is chosen to operate in two stages, it is best to begin with the larger hernia and to decide a policy for the other side according to how the first operation evolves. This is the policy adopted by the Shouldice Hospital, where operation is carried out in two stages at an interval of 48 h, partly in order to reduce the dosage of local anesthesia. The advantages of simultaneous repair include a reduction in the length of hospital stay, avoidance of a second hospitalization, and also the local complications are no more frequent [Serpel 1990] as it is in the case for respiratory complications [Devlin 1993]. Certain drawbacks include an increased frequency of urinary retention, an increased risk of suppuration in the operative wound and a few cases of bilateral ischemic orchitis. This last complication has been particularly studied in Wantz (1984 to 1991) and is notable in cases of bulky hernias (1.5%). The author advises, where ischemic orchitis follows the first operation, to defer the second procedure for at least one year (because testicular trophy may occur late) and then to choose the preperitoneal route.

Which operation should be chosen for simultaneous repair? The approach may be horizontal, for a few centimeters on either side of the midline, or may include two inguinal or suprainguinal incisions, or a midline preperitoneal approach or laparoscopy. Whatever procedure is chosen, it should plan to avoid any element of lateral traction (for example the McVay operation) as relaxation incisions are not only ineffective but also introduce yet another weak point. Prostheses are a much better answer, as they can be introduced without tension and with no limit to the extent of the reinforcement, particularly in large hernias. In particular cases, unilateral strangulation of one of two hernias poses no great problem provided that there is no intestinal necrosis or anesthetic difficulty. The use of prosthetic material is particularly indicated in multiple bilateral hernias of combined types.

10. Hernial Lipomas

Fatty collections in or around the spermatic cord in the neighborhood of the deep inguinal ring have long been known, and interpreted differently. McGregor (1929) felt that such lipomas dilate the deep inguinal ring and prevent efficient working of the sphincter mechanism. Connor and Peacock (1973) feel that the fatty cushion prevents passage of intestine into the scrotum (at least in the case of the rat) before testicular descent. In practice, when one approaches the inguinal canal and the spermatic cord from the front, one can deal with such lipomas by carefully dissecting them away with the points of the scissors, sparing the veins, arteries and nerves of the cord. Using the posterior approach, we push back the fatty mass into the retroperitoneum, in order to avoid "false recurrences", through postoperative protrusion. When prosthetic material is used, the nature of any perivascular lymphatic or fatty masses should be ascertained and they should, if necessary, be resected between two ligatures, in order not to increase the risk of sepsis. It is useless and dangerous to excise fatty collections in the "Space of Bogros".

11. Associated Lesions

a) Patent Processus Vaginalis

There is no true neck, as the sac communicates directly with the tunica vaginalis. These congenital hernias are seen in children and young adults. The operation for the inguinal approach does not differ as regards dissection and treatment of the sac. Henri D [in Detri 1967] opens the upper part of the sac and sews it from the inside with a nonabsorbable stitch, and in order to prevent accumulation of serous fluid in the lower part of the processus, the serous tunica is folded back around the cord, as in certain types of operation for hydrocele.

The other method, which we prefer, consists in separating the cord from the upper part of the sac by an incision in the serous layer, dissecting with a damp swab in order to preserve the elements of the cord,

then freeing the proximal part of the sac up to the deep inguinal ring where it is tied off. The lower part is left behind or folded back around the cord as described above. When operating via the preperitoneal abdominal route, it is preferable to leave the lower part of the sac in the scrotum, having separated the elements of the cord from it. It may be left open on its anterior aspect, so as to avoid serous collections and assist drainage.

b) Hernias with Ectopic Testis

In the adult the ectopic testicle is usually trophic, functionless and carries a risk of neoplasm, points which are in favor of removing it during an operation for hernia repair. In the absence of testicular atrophy it is justified to bring down the testicle using one of the classical techniques. In cases of bilateral ectopia, bilateral orchidopexy in one stage by the Ombredanne method is not advised, as it carries a risks of urethral compression. It is better to fix the testicle to the skin of the thigh. Using the preperitoneal route, it is a very simple matter to free up the cord, the testicle can then be brought down into the scrotum via a small high counter incision.

c) Hernia and Hydrocele

Communicating hydroceles are treated in the same way as a patent processus. An independent hydrocele is treated at a second stage in the same operation, preferably by a separate scrotal incision, using one of the accepted methods (eversion or better resection) leaving a suction drain in the appropriate operative space.

d) Hernia with Varicocele

During inguinal repair, one may resect the bundles of the dilated veins between ligatures, and eventually suspend the testicle to one of the pillars of the external inguinal ring, having verified by phlebography that there are no abnormal veins in the "Space of Bogros", which require ligation. Ligation of abnormal veins is much simpler via the preperitoneal route, following their identification by phlebography.

e) Hernias with Malformation of the Processus Vaginalis

Inguinosuperficial hernias, inguinointerstitial or preperitoneal hernias are better identified and recognized by the inguinal approach. In these conditions a wide incision of the inguinal canal followed by opening up the sac allows the relations of the sac and its diverticula to be explored both digitally and visually, and to reconstitute the abdominal wall according the chosen method. Ectopic testes are frequently found in these situations, and are dealt with as described above. In case of strangulation, a deeper sac should be ignored while the superficial sac may contain an intact loop of intestine. This emphasizes the importance of wide exploration of the small intestine in operations for suspected strangulated hernia. This important step is rendered easier by the preperitoneal abdominal approach.

12. Inguinal Hernias in Women

Glassow (1973) published a series of 1,784 cases of which 1,548 indirect and 124 direct inguinal hernias were in females, giving an incidence of 1/25. This relative rarity in the female is partly due to the smaller inguinal triangle associated with the female pelvis and also to the more solid transversalis fascia which is found in women. The round ligament has the same relation to the sac as does the spermatic cord in men. Any difficulty in dissection of the sac should be unhesitatingly resolved by resecting the round ligament together with it. "Desaxation of the uterus", can be avoided by using Barker's maneuver.

Inguinal hernias in women are usually quite small, and as there is no concern regarding passage of vital structures, repair is easily carried out by a small low-place incision, the scar of which will be concealed by the pubic hair. Glassow follows the practice of the Shouldice Hospital by making use of the firm transversalis fascia found in women, with a recurrence of 1.3% over ten years.

However, the relatively higher frequency of femoral hernia in women has led us to prefer attachment of the conjoint tendon to the pectineal ligament, in order to avoid the possibility of femoral recurrence following the Bassini or Shouldice operation. In small hernias in elderly women we use a conical plug of the Gilbert or Rutkow type.

13. Hernias in the Elderly

These have a bad reputation because of the risk of strangulation, of respiratory and cardiovascular problems following repair, and of the high incidence of recurrence. They are frequently neglected for some time, until their size produces problems by reduction in physical activity and also their psychological effects [Monod-Broca 1969].

An elderly patient who requests urgent operation for his hernia should also prompt the clinician to consider other causes of an increase in intra-abdominal pressure such as obstructive uropathy, respiratory failure, colonic cancer or cirrhosis. In general, the correct therapeutic decision will be made on the basis not only of life expectancy, but also because of the increased mortality from postoperative complications. The three important reasons for operating on an elderly patient with a hernia are to increase comfort, to avoid the possibility of an emergency operation for strangulation, and to give an opportunity of a full evaluation of the patient in the preoperative phase.

Williams and Hale [in Hernia I, Nyhus 1978] reported a mortality of 13% following emergency operations as against 1.3% of elective operations in their series of 270 hernia repairs carried out in patients over 60. In a personal series reported by Warlaumont in 1982, approximately one in four men and four in ten women of over 70, emergency surgery for strangulated carried a mortality of 9% as against 0.5% for elective procedures. According to Condon and Nyhus (1978) many elderly patients wear trusses, however a truss does not control an inguinal and still less a femoral hernia, and increases the risk of strangulation, at the same time leading to atrophy of the fascial and aponeurotic structures in the groin, rendering subsequent repair more difficult.

Operative strategy therefore requires taking into account the general state of the patient and the local fragility of the tissues. The surgeon will choose the technique with which he is most familiar, but in the case of a massive inguinoscrotal or bilateral hernia, a large prosthesis containing the entire peritoneal sac is a swift and sure solution, which has afforded us regularly satisfactory results. However, in these cases, disappointment is frequent, and the surgeon should be prepared for this.

In conclusion, elective hernia surgery can be undertaken even in octogenarians of ASA grade III, provided that adequate preoperative preparation has been carried out, and that the patient is capable of walking up one flight of stairs, where local anesthesia is envisaged. For general anesthesia, more extensive preparation is required. Epidural techniques provide an excellent solution in cases of respiratory insufficiency. The preperitoneal route which provides rapid access to all hernial lesions is the only one guaranteed not to overlook any associated hernia, and provides access to the peritoneal cavity in order to reduce an incarceration. It is also suitable for recurrent hernia and many authors (Greenburg, Condon, Niehuss) have, like our-selves, been very satisfied with it. Nowadays, elderly patients are enabled to buy an elective operation to recover their independence and security, and at the same time to escape the high mortality associated with strangulation and all the risks of intestinal resection.

14. "Incidental" Hernias

It sometimes occurs during the course of a laparotomy that patent hernial orifices are discovered by the surgeon, which may represent a risk of later strangulation. When the approach is below the umbilicus, and provided that there is no sepsis, the hernia should be treated by resection of the sac and closure of the defect by modification of the Nyhus 1960 technique. When the approach is above the umbilicus, if it is considered essential to repair the hernia, then this is better done by a separate inguinal incision, provided always that consent has been obtained from the patient or from his family. When the main operation involves sepsis, it is even more important to repair the hernia through a separate incision, without, if possible, opening the sac.

15. Recurrent Hernias

A recurrent hernia, or one reappearing on the same side of a previous operation, poses a special problem for the surgeon. Recurrent hernias carry the same complications as do all other groin hernias, but with some difficult added problems. The anatomy will have been distorted by one or more previous interventions; there may be necrosis of the muscles and aponeurosis, planes of cleavage will have disappeared and the peritoneal sac is of variable thickness, and may be so delicate that it seems almost like a covered eventration. A previous preperitoneal approach will have obliterated the retroparietal spaces. Recurrences vary in size from a small partial recurrence (often around the pubis) to a total recurrences with disappearance of all inguinal structures including the conjoint tendon or even Cooper's ligament.

a) Frequency

The frequency of recurrent hernias in major series varies from 10% [Borgeskow 1970] 12% [Ljundahl 1973] 19% [Warlaumont 1982; Read 1979] to 30% [Koontz 1960; Zimmerman 1978]. Long term follow-up of the major series of operations show recurrence rates of less than 1% from the Shouldice Hospital [Glassow 1970] and in the Stoppa (1986) series, 3.5% in the McVay series (1989), 6.8% after three years in the Marsden (1962) series and 8.6% after ten years in the series of Palumbo (1971). These series comprise expert teams, and the same operations carried out in other places could well produce higher figures. The Shouldice Hospital series (1979) illustrates the virtues of experience. The recurrent figures were 18.8% in 1945, 12% in 1946, 6% in 1947, 4% in 1948, and less than 1% since 1951. In my personal series, the recurrence rate following the use of large reinforcing prostheses via the abdominal route, have been 3.3% in 1974, 1.2% in 1983 and 0.56% in 1986, as regards primary repairs.

b) Delay in Presentation

The delay period varies and may be as long as 25 years after the first operation [Holes 1979]. Retrospective analysis of our own series comprising various techniques shows some 5.6 recurrences appearing during the first postoperative month. 39.1% in the first year, 23.5% after the 10th year, in the group repaired without prostheses. Following introduction of prosthetic repair all of the recurrences appeared during the first postoperative year, indicating technical errors. Halverson and McVay (1970) put forward a formula for calculating the predicted recurrence rate at the 25th postoperative year, by multiplying the figures for the first year by 5, those of the 2nd year by 2.5, those of the 5th year by 1.5 and those of the 10th year by 1.2. This formula appears only applicable to techniques involving herniorrhaphy.

c) Anatomical Types

Of 459 recurrent hernias reported by Glassow from the Shouldice Hospital (1970), 60% were inguinal and 40% femoral. These latter recurred more often in men (2.2%) than in women (1.3%). Thereafter came hernia en glissade (1%). These remarkable recurrence figures are equaled in an inquiry carried out by the French Association of Surgeons [Houdard & Stoppa 1984] where femoral hernias had by far the highest recurrence rate (8.2%), followed by complicated inguinal hernias (7.9%). Some series show that recurrence is more frequent following second or subsequently operations than following primary intervention. Marsden recorded that the first recurrence (7%) recurred in 90% of cases. Clear (1976) recorded a 39% rate of re-recurrence. Thus recurrent hernias may be considered as new lesions, in part produced by preceding operations. The usefulness of prosthetic repair in these cases have been recommended by the surgeons of the

Shouldice Hospital [Bendavid 1987] when dealing with recurrent femoral hernias.

d) Mechanism

The mechanical aspects of recurrence are difficult to identify when they are late and when a complete account of the first operation is lacking. The problem continues with subsequent surgery. We have, together with Houdard, classified the risk factors for recurrence into three types, namely faults in technique, degenerated supporting structures, and sundry others (1984). Among the technical faults which may lead to recurrence during the first postoperative year are sacs which are either not found or badly dissected [Glassow 1970], leaving a long peritoneal stump [Rayan 1953], incomplete closure of the hernial orifice resulting in recurrence of indirect hernia, and suture carried out under tension, particularly in the case of direct recurrences [Postlethwaite 1985]. Certain techniques are more prone than others to lead to recurrence such as the pre- or retrofunicular operation, and the sutureless McVay operation. Hernias with a large defect recur twice as frequently as small ones and simple suture in these cases is a technical mistake. Too extensive a dissection, sutures which are too large or tightly placed may transform the contractile inguinal wall into a fibrous area which is prone to progressive breakdown [Iason 1964]. Other risk factors are independent of the quality of the operation and more related to age or to the general condition of the patient. These include weakness of the anatomical structures and obesity [Borgestorm 1951]. Other dangerous factors are postoperative sepsis and chronic cough. In contrast, early resumption of activities and work is no longer considered a risk factor for recurrence. 80% of recurrent hernias are unrelated to hard work [Ryan 1953]. Sedentary workers have a higher recurrence rate (18.6%) than manual workers (9%) according to Postelsthwaite (1985) Marsden (1962) Rives (1974) and Houdard (1971). Recurrence following prosthetic repair is always the result of faulty technique and for this reason appears during the first postoperative year. In the immediate postoperative period a serosanguinous collection in the fascial space of a direct hernia must be distinguished from a true recurrence, if necessary making use of ultrasound to confirm the physical signs.

Technical faults which may lead to recurrence following preperitoneal repair include an insufficiently large prosthesis to allow passage of the cord, which we prevent by parietalisation. Abrahamson (1995) has made a review of all the factors leading to recurrence, according to which he divides them into early recurrences (experience of the surgeon, tension on the suture line, infection, suture material, suture technique and other local factors) and late recurrences (mainly biological factors), placing on one side the recurrences which recur after use of prosthetic material.

e) Treatment

The treatment of choice for recurrent hernias will be summarized briefly here. Partial recurrences which are usually found at one or other end of the previous repair present as a small localized protrusion. The previous inguinal scar is excised and the cord widely exposed, before incising the external oblique. One can then fairly easily assess the nature of the previous operation and the strength of the deeper layers. The hernial sac must be resected high up. Repair of the defect can be effected locally, but more often is achieved by resorting to a deeper and more solid procedure such as repairing onto the pectineal ligament after a Bassini or Shouldice operation. However the Shouldice surgeons advocate repeating the same technique.

A femoral recurrence after inguinal hernia repair is often treated by bringing the conjoint tendon down to the pectineal ligament. An inguinal recurrence after a femoral repair by the femoral route (occasionally an overlooked "pantaloon hernia") is treated by the McVay operation or better still by a prosthesis. Small partial recurrences, most often found around the pubis, can be managed by the used of a Lichtenstein plug. Total recurrences must be totally repaired, bearing in mind the reason for the failure. This is almost always due to suture under tension or to the use of absorbable material. The usual management is the McVay operation or prosthetic procedure.

In the case of multirecurrent hernia, the anatomical layers are often unrecognizable, the sac is stretched out under the coverings of the groin and the lesion is similar to the types of abdominal eventration. As the patient is usually an aged or obese female, treatment by simple suture is difficult because there is no lower point to which sutures can be fixed. The best means of closing the orifice is to use a prosthesis via the inguinal or abdominal route. This approach carries advantages including an easy progress from normal to abnormal tissues, easy identification of the hernial pedicle, easy reduction of the contents and elective closure of the hernial orifice. By inserting prosthetic material, the repair can be as extensive and secure as necessary. Additionally, the upper route does no further damage to the weakened inguinal structures and avoids all risk to the testicular blood supply or to the nerves, which is particularly high in repair of recurrences by the inguinal route. Repair through the inguinal route is not always easy because the previous operation will have fused together the anatomical layers and granulomas occurring around the sutures promote sepsis. Moreover, one frequently discovers more than one area of recurrence; having said this, however, one is occasionally surprised by finding, following a difficult dissection, deeper structures which are intact and of good quality. With much reservation we very occasionally do reoperate through an inguinal exposure, which must always be wider than the previous one, but in practice we prefer the upper route, either suprainguinal (Nyhus) or midline preperitoneal, using a modified Pfannenstiel incision.

Recurrence following prosthetic repair. If the prosthesis has been inserted by the inguinal route it is better to reoperate from above via a median or suprainguinal approach. When the previously inserted prosthesis is too small, we advise the inguinal or suprainguinal approach, either to fix the displaced edges of the prosthesis of the pectineal ligament or laterally to the abdominal wall, or else to extend the reinforcement with additional material. It is better to avoid reoperating through the midline preperitoneal route because the prosthetic material will be found closely adherent to the visceral sac and the back of the abdominal wall. We have no experience with recurrences following patch plugs, and there is little literature on the subject, but we would imagine that recurrences are closely similar to those occurring after an inguinal repair.

Very late recurrences (ten years or more). Some authors consider these to be true recurrences for the sole reason that they appear at the same place. However this raises the question of the true purpose of hernia repair: if this aims at restoring a normal anatomy and physiology then recurrences at later than ten years are really due to change much more due to the normal ageing in structures which are already weakened. If on the other hand the aim of the repair is to prevent the recurrence of a further hernia and to provide a lifelong correction of the vulnerable groin area, then the wide use of prosthetic material seems logical. This is not simply theoretical discussion but has important implications from the ethical and medicolegal points of view.

Certain unusual types of recurrence are characterized by an extreme degree of destruction of the abdominal wall following necrotising sepsis or severe pelvic trauma such as fracture dislocation of the symphysis. Trivellini (1991) has approached the question of repair of these lesions, which are unusual but exceedingly difficult to treat. Because of the disappearance of the planes of cleavage it is impossible to reenter the preperitoneal space and the presence of stitch granulomas and prosthetic material previously implanted, together with visceral adhesions are additional difficulties. The author suggests entering the peritoneal cavity through the midline, then incising

Table 9.18. Rate of re-recurrence following various surgical techniques (inguinal hernias)

Authors	Type of operation	% Re-recurrences
Peacock (1984)	Fascia lata autoplasty	0
Van Damme (1985)	Posterior prosthesis	0
Pietri (1986)	Posterior prosthesis	0
Glassow (1976)	Shouldice	0.6
Rignault (1986)	Posterior prosthesis	1.2
Lazarthes (1984)	Shouldice	1.5
Nyhus (1988)	Posterior prosthesis	1.7
Nyhus (1989)	Posterior prosthesis	< 2
Stoppa (1986)	Posterior prosthesis	2.1
Rutledge (1988)	McVay	2.4
Read (1979)	Posterior prosthesis	7
Wantz (1989)	Shouldice	7.2
Marsden (1988)	Various	9.4
Chevalley (1988)	Bassini	10
Holm (1985)	McVay + autoplasty	29

the parietal peritoneum at the edge of the adherent area, and leaving it in place as part of the abdominal wall. Following careful freeing of adhesions, the edges of the peritoneum are separated from the abdominal wall, creating a large loss of substance of parietal peritoneum which it is possible to cover over with some absorbable material, in order to close the visceral sac. The sac is then wrapped in a large bilateral prosthesis of prosthetic nonabsorbable mesh. A series of seven cases published in 1995 reports uniformly satisfying results.

f) Results of Repair of Recurrent Hernias

In a personal series (1989) of 349 recurrent hernias, four techniques were employed, namely Bassini (2 cases), use of the pectineal ligament (30 cases; 8.5%) and inguinal patch (39 cases; 11.2%) and a large bilateral prosthesis via the midline (270 cases; 77.4%). The results were as follows. One out of two of the Bassini operations recurred, five of the McVay operations, four after the inguinal patch (10.3%) and three after the large midline prosthesis (1.1%).

In a series of 193 recurrent hernias [Mongolfier 1982] the recurrence rate was 10% following simple suture, and the authors now routinely use a preperitoneal approach and prosthesis for such cases. Nyhus (1989) in a summary of the series of twelve authors, reports recurrence rates from 0.6% to 29% with a nonprosthetic repair, as against 0 to 1.7% when a prosthesis is used. Gaynant and Cubertafond (1991) collected various series from the literature and report new recurrence rates from 1.5% to 20% after suture, and less than 2% after prosthetic repair. These results all agree in indicating the routine use of prosthesis in recurrent or multirecurrent hernias.

References

Acquaviva DE, Bourret P, Corti F (1949) Considérations sur l'emploi des plaques de nylon, dites crinoplaques, comme matériel de plastie parietale. 52ème Congrès Français de Chirurgie. Masson, Paris, p 453

Alexandre JH, Bouillot JL (1996) Classification des hernies de l'aine. J Coelio Chir 19: 53-59

Alexandre JH (1983) Traitement des hernies et des éventrations. Utilisation du treillis resorbable de polyglactine 910. Presse Med 12: 644

Alexandre JH, Bouillot JL (1983) Traitement des hernies et des éventrations: utilisation du treillis résorbable de polyglactine 910. Presse Med 12: 395

Allaires F (d'), Contiades J (1936) Technique de réparation des muscles grands droits de l'abdomen. J Chir (Paris) 47: 922

Allen PIM, Zager N, Goldman M (1987) Elective repair of groin hernia in the elderly. Br J Surg 74: 987

Annandale T (1876) Case in which a reducible oblique and direct inguinal and femoral hernia existed on the same side and were successfully treated by operation. Edimb Med J 21: 1087

Arnaud JP, Eloy R, Weill-Bousson M, Grenier JF, Adloff M (1977) Résistance et tolérance biologique de 6 prothèses "inertes" utilisées dans la réparation de la paroi abdominale. J Chir (Paris) 113: 85-100

Barbier J, Carretier M, Richer JP (1989) Cooper ligament repair. An update. World J Surg 13/5: 499

Barwell NJ (1981) Recurrence and early activity after groin hernie repair. Lancet ii: 985

Bassini E (1887) Sulla cura radicale dell' ernia inguinale. Arch Soc Ital Chir 4: 380

Bassini E (1889) Nuovo metodo per la cura radicale del' ernia inguinale. Prosperini, Padova

Bates VC (1913) New operation for the cure of indirect inguinal hernie. JAMA 60: 2032

Belenger J, Flamand JP, Goldstein M (1967) Bilan de 14 années de cures de hernies. Acta Chir Belg 4: 283

Bendavid R (1986) The "Fletching: a new implant for the treatment of inguinofemoral hernies. Int Surg 71: 248

Bendavid R (1987) A femoral "umbrella" for femoral hernie repair. Surg Gynecol Obstet 165: 153

Bendavid R (1992) "Dysejaculation": an unusual complication of inguinal herniorraphy. Postgrad Gen Surg 4: 139

Bendavid R (1994) Prosthesis and abdominal wall hernias. R G Landes, Austin

Bendavid R (1995) The TSD classification: a nomenclature for groin hernies. In: Schumpelick V and Wantz GE (eds) Inguinal hernia repair. Karger, Basel

Berger G (1902) Traitement chirurgical des hernies inguino-crurales. Rev Chir 25: 1-9

Berliner S, Burson L, Katz P, Wise L (1978) An anterior transversalis fascia repair of adult inguinal hernias. Am J Surg 135: 633-636

Bogros AJ (1823) Essai sur l'anatomie de la region iliaque. Thèse Mèdecine, Paris

Brenner J (1988) Vieryl Kissens bei der Herniotomie. Bereich-Quartal, Hamburg

Britton BJ (1989) Local anesthesia for hernie repair. An aid or an hindrance to cure? In: Nyhus LM, Condon RE (eds) Hernia, 3rd edn. Lippincott, Philadelphia

Callum KG, Doig RL, Kimmonth JB (1974) The results of nylon dam repair for inguinal hernia. Arch Surg 108: 25-27

Cameron AEP (1994) Accuracy of clinical diagnosis of direct and indirect inguinal hernia. Br J Surg 81: 250

Campanelli G, Cavagnoli R, Bottero L, de Simone M, Pietri P (1996) Hernies recidivées de l'aine. Propositions de classification et de tactique chirurgicale. J Chir (Paris) 133: 270

Campling EA, Devlin HB, Hoyle RW, Lunn JN (1994) Report of the National Confidential inquiry into postoperative deaths. London Royal College of Surgeons of England

Celsus AC (1938) De Medicina. English translation by Spencer. Harvard University Press

Cheatle GL (1920) An operation for the radical cure of inguinal and femoral hernia. Br Med J 2: 68-69

Chevalier C, Hardy JC (1987) Complication vésicale d'une cure de hernie par prothèse. Acta Urol Belg 55: 387

Chevrel JP, Gatt MT, Sarfati E, et al (1982) Les névralgies résiduelles après cure de hernie inguinale. Groupe de Recherche et d'Etude de la Paroi Abdominale (GREPA), 4e Réunion, St Tropez, Bruneau, Boulogne-Billancourt: 29

Chevrel JP, Duchene P, Sarfati E (1983) L'opération de Bassini. Monographie GREPA 5: 9-12. Laboratoires Bruneau, Paris

Chevrel JP (1984) L'opération de Bassini: technique, indications résultats. Symposium, 86e Congrès Français de Chirurgie

Chevrel JP (1985) Chirurgie des parois de l'abdomen. Springer-Verlag, Paris, 288 p

Chevrel JP, Perez M, Lumbroso M, Morice P (1991) Récidives herniaires. Presse Med 20: 1543-1547-

Chevrel JP, Gatt MT (1992) The treatment of neuralgias following inguinal herniorrhapy. A report of 47 cases. Postgrad Gen Surg 4: 142

Cimpeanu I, Constantinescu V (1992) Hernille inguinale si femurale. Editura Militara, Bucarest

Clinical Guidelines on the management of groin hernies in adulte (1993). Royal College of Surgeons of England

Cloquet JG (1819) Recherche sur les causes et l'anatomie des hernies abdominales. Mequignon-Marvis, Paris

Condon RE (1995) Incisional hernia. In: Nyhus LM, Condon RE (eds) Hernia, 4th edn. Lippincott, Philadelphia, p 319

Corcione F, Cristinzio G, Maresca M, Cascone U, Titolo G, Califano G (1997) Primary inguinal hernia: the held-in mesh repair. Hernia 1: 37-40

Czerny V (1877) Studien zur radikalbehandlung der hernien. Wien Med Wochenschr 27: 497

Deroide JP, Reigner G, Deroide G (1996) Utilisation d'un fil à résorption lente dans le traitement par voie inguinale des hernies de l'aine. Ann Chir 50/9: 741

Détrie Ph (1967) Nouveau traité de technique chirurgicale, T IX. Masson, Paris, pp 51-111 and 133- 153

Dubois C (1982) Cure chirurgicale des hernies de l'aine. Thèse Médecine Lyon l

Ekberg O, Blomquist P, Olsson S (1981) Positive contrast herniography in adult patients with obscure groin pain. Surgery 89: 532

Ellis H, Harrison W, Hugh TB (1965) The healing of peritoneum under normal and pathological conditions. Br J Surg 52: 471

Farquaharson EL (1955) Early ambulation with special reference to herniorraphy as an outpatient procedure. Lancet 2: 517

Ferrand J, Pélissier G (1955) Une technique de cure des hernies inguinales. Presse Med 63: 6

Flament JB, Avisse C, Palot JP, Rives J (1995) Treatment of groin hernies with a Mersilene mesh via an inguinal approach (The Rives' Technique). Probl Gen Surg 12: 111

Flanagan L Jr, Bascom JU (1981) Herniorraphies performed upon ouf-patients under local anesthesia. Surg Gynecol Obstet 153: 557-560

Forgue H (1909) Choix du procédé dans la cure radicale de la hernie inguinale, chez l'adulte. Thèse Médecine, Paris

Friberg J, Frittjofsson A (1979) Inguinal herniorraphy and sperm-agglutinating antibodies in infertile men. Arch Andrology 2: 317

Fruchaud H (1956) Anatomie chirurgicale des Hernies de l'Aine. Doin, Paris

Gatt MT, Chevrel JP (1991) Traitement des névralgies après cure de hernie inguinale. Chirurgie 1: 96

Gautier R, Bonneton G, Natali J (1972) Deux observations de lésions artérielles au cours de la cure de hernie inguinale. Chirurgie 8: 722-723

Gilbert AI (1992) Sutureless repair of inguinal hernia. Am J Surg 163: 331-335

Gilbert Al (1991) Inguinal hernia repair: Biomaterials and sutureless repair. Perspectives in General Surgery 2: 113-129

Gilbert Al (1989) An anatomic and functional classification for the diagnosis and treatment of inguinal hernie. Ann Surg 157: 331

Glassow F (1963) Inguinal hernia in the female. Surg Gynecol Obstet 116: 701

Goinard P (1939) Cure radicale de certaines hernies inguinales par fixation du tendon conjoint au ligament de Cooper. Presse Med 44: 1586

Goni Moreno I (1964) The rational treatment of hernies and voluminous chronic eventrations with progressive pneumoperitoneum. In: Nyhus LM, Harkins HN (eds) Hernia, 1st edn, Lippincott, Philadelphia, pp 688-703

Gosset J (1972) La cure des hernies inguino-crurales récidivées avec effondrement de l'aine (Laparotomie médiane et prothèse sous-péritonéale en velours siliconé). J Chir (Paris) 104: 493-504

Griffith CA (1964) Indirect inguinal hernie. With special reference to the Marcy operation. In: Nyhus LM and Harkins HN (eds) Hernia, 1st ed. Lippincott, Philadelphia, pp 97-114

Griffith CA (1995) The Marcy repair of indirect inguinal hernie. In: Nyhus LM and Condon RE (eds) Hernia, 4th edn. Lippincott, Philadelphia

Gullmo SG (1995) Herniography. In: Nyhus LM and Condon RE (eds) Hernia, 4th edn. Lippincott, Philadelphia, p 525

Hahn-Pedersen J, Lund L, Hansen-Hojhus J (1994) Evaluation of direct and indirect hernia by computed tomography. Br J Surg 81: 569

Halsted WS (1889) The radical cure of hernie. Bull Johns Hopkins Hosp 1: 12

Halverson K, Mc Vay CB (1970) Inguinal and femoral hernioplasty: a 22 year study of the author's method. Arch Surg 101: 127-135

Heifetz CJ (1971) Resection of the spermatic cord in selected inguinal hernies: 20 years of experience. Arch Surg 102: 36-39

Henry AK (1936) Operation for femoral hernie by a midline extraperitoneal approach; with a preliminary note on this route for reducible inguinal hernie. Lancet 1: 531

Henry X, Randriamanantsoa V, Verhaeghe P, Stoppa R (1994) Le materiel prothétique a-t-il une place raisonnable dans le traitement des urgences herniaires ? Chirurgie 120: 123

Heydorn WH, Velanovitch V (1990) A five years US Army experience with 36250 hernia repairs. Ann Surg 56: 596

Hoguet JP (1920) Direct inguinal hernie. Ann Surg 7: 671

Houdard C, Berthelot G (1966) Traitement chirurgical des hernies inguinales de l'adulte. J Chir (Paris) 92: 627

Houdard C (1973) Traitement des hernies inguinales récidivées. Entretiens de Bichat. Expansion Scientifique, Paris

Houdard C (1980) Hernies inguinales récidivées de l'adulte. Rev Prat (Paris) 15: 701

Houdard C, Stoppa R (1984) Le traitement chirurgical des hernies de l'aine. Monographies de l'Association Francaise de Chirurgie. Masson, Paris

Huguier J, Huguier M (1963) Hernie crurale externe. J Chir (Paris) 86: 5-12

Hureau J, Agossou-Voyeme AK, Germain M, Pradel J (1991) Les espaces interpariétaux postérieurs ou espaces rétropéritonéaux; 1ère partie: anatomie normale. J Radiol 72: 101

Iles J (1979) The management of elective hernie repair. Ann Plast Surg 6: 538

Izard G, Guilleton R, Randrianasolo S, Houry R (1996) Traitement des hernies de l'aine par la technique de Mc Vay. A propos de 1332 cas. Ann Chir 50: 755

Johanet H, Cossa JP, Benhamou G (1995) Utilité de la coelioscopie pour le diagnostic de hernie de l'aine. Presse Med 24: 1161

Joseph MG, O'Boyle PJ (1989) The "hitch-stitch" and drain technique for the prevention of inguino-scrotal hematoma following complicated inguinoscrotal surgery. J Roy Coll Surg Edimb 34: 104

Keith A (1924) On the origin and nature of hernie. Br J Surg 11: 455

Kingsnorth AN (1995) Epidemiology, pathogenesis and natural history. In: Schumpelick V and Wantz GE (eds) Inguinal Hernia Repair. Karger, Basel

Koontz AR, Kimberley RC (1960) Tantalum and marlex mesh (with a note on marlex thread): an experimental and clinical comparison. Preliminary report. Ann Surg 151: 796-804

Kux M (1994) Return to activity after groin hernie repair in europe. In: Schumpelick & Wantz GE (eds) Inguinal Hernia repair. Karger, Basel, p 307

Lagrot F, Salasc J (1957) Eventrations. Encycl Med Chir Paris 2013 A10: 1

Lampe EW (1978) Cooper ligament repair. In: Nyhus LM and Condon RE (eds) Hernia, 2nd edn. Lippincott, Philadelphia

Lankau CA, Beachley MC (1995) Mc Vay Herniorraphy. The transition suture and femoral vein injury. Milit Med 64: 641

Laroque GP (1919) The permanent cure of inguinal and femoral hernias. A modifcation of the standard operative procedures. Surg Gynecol Obstet 29: 507

Lauriere R, Poinsot Y (1991) Migration asymptomatique intravésicale 14 ans après mise en place d'une plaque inerte pour cure de hernie. J Chir (Paris) 128: 31

Leslie DR (1978) The yo-yo operation for hernie in men. Aust NZ J Surg 48: 447

Levy AH, Wren BJ, Friedman AN (1951) Complications and recurrences following hernia repair. Ann Surg 133: 533

Lierse W (1987) Vicryl Kissens bei der herniotomie. In: Schumpelick "Hernien" (1). Verlag, Heidelberg

Lotheissen G (1898) Zur Radikaloperation der Shenkelhernien. Zbl Chir 25: 548

Lucas-Championnière J (1892) Cure radicale des hernies. Rueffet, Paris

Lytle WJ (1961) Operative treatment of hernie. Proc R Soc Med 54: 967

Mahorner H, Goss GM (1962) Herniation following destruction of Poupart's and Cooper's ligaments: a method of repair. Ann Surg 155: 741

Marcy HO (1891) The cure of hernie by the antiseptic use of animal ligature. Trans Int Med Congr 2: 446

Marcy HO (1892) A new use of carbolized catgut ligatures. Boston Med & Surg J 85: 315

Marsden AJ (1962) Inguinal hernia. A three year review of 2000 cases. Br J Surg 49: 384

McVay CB (1939) A fundamental error in the Bassini operation for direct inguinal hernie. Univ Hosp Bull, Ann Arbor 5: 14

McVay CB, Anson BJ (1940) Aponeurotic and fascial continuities in the abdomen, pelvis, and thigh. Ann Rec 76: 213

McVay CB, Anson BJ (1940) Composition of the rectus sheath. Anat Rec 77: 343

McVay CB, Anson BJ (1942) A fundamental error in current methods of inguinal herniorraphy. Surg Gynecol Obstet 74: 746

McVay CB, Anson BJ (1949) Inguinal and femoral hernioplasty. Surg Gynecol Obstet 88: 473

McVay CB (1954) Hernia. The pathologic anatomy of the more common hernies and their anatomic repair. Charles C. Thomas, Springfield

McVay CB, Chapp JD (1958) Inguinal and femoral hernioplasty. Evaluation of a basic concept. Ann Surg 148: 499

McVay CB (1966) Pre-peritoneal hernioplasty. Surg Gynecol Obstet 123: 349

McVay CB (1974) The anatomic basis for inguinal and femoral hernioplasty. Surg Gynecol Obstet 139: 931

McVay W, Morris R, Mushlin P (1987) Sodium bicarbonate attenuates pain on skin infiltration with lidocaine, with or without epinephrine. Anesth Analg 66: 572

Mellière D, Dermer J, Danis RK, Becquemin JP, Renaud J (1980) Complications artérielles de la chirurgie inguinale. J Chir (Paris) 117: 531

Ménégaux G (1965) Manuel de pathologie chirurgicale, Tome II, 2nd edn. Masson, Paris

Mertl P, Diarra B, Foulou P, Stoppa R, Laude M (1996) Le fascia uro-génital. Bases anatomiques et applications chirurgicales. Communication à la Société Anatomique de Paris, 28 juin 1996 (in press)

Moosman DA, Oelrich TM (1977) Prevention of accidentel trauma to the ilio-inguinal nerve during inguinal herniorraphy. Ann J Surg 133: 146

Munshi IA, Wantz GE (1996) Management of recurrent and perivascular femoral hernias by giant prosthetic reinforcement of the visceral sac. J Am Coll Surg 182: 417-422

National Research Council. Postoperative wound infections (1964) Ann Surg 160/S1: 192

Nicoll JH (1909) The surgery of infancy. Br Med J ii: 753

Nyhus LM, Stevenson JK, Listerud MB, Harkins HN (1959) Peritoneal herniorraphy: a preliminary report on fifty patients. West J Surg Obstet Gynecol 67: 48

Nyhus LM, Harkins HN (1964) Hernia,1st edn. Lippincott, Philadelphia

Nyhus LM, Klein MS, Rogers FB (1991) Inguinal hernie. Current Prob Surg 28: 405

Nyhus LM, Condon RE (1995) Hernia, 4th edn. Lippincott, Philadelphia

Odimba BFK, Stoppa R, Laude M, Henry X, Verhaeghe P (1980) Les espaces clivables souspariétaux de l'abdomen. J Chir (Paris) 117: 621-627

Palot JP, Flament JB, Avisse C, Greffier D, Burde A (1996) Utilisation des prothèses dans les conditions de la chirurgie d'urgence. Etude rétrospective de 204 hernies de l'aine étranglées. Chirurgie (Paris) 121: 48-50

Palumbo LT, Shape WS (1971) Primary inguinal hernioplasty in adult. Surg Clin North Am 51: 1293-1307

Panos RG, Beck de Maresh JE, Harford FJ (1992) Preliminary results of a prospective randomized study of Cooper ligament versus Shouldice herniorraphy technic. Surg Gynecol Obstet 175: 315

Panou de Faymoreau T (1976) Les plasties locales par plaques de nylon dans la cure chirurgicale des hernies inguinales et des éventrations. Thèse Médecine, Nantes

Pautet HJ (1969) Utilisation de la peau totale dans la cure chirurgicale des hernies et des éventrations. Thèse Médecine, Paris, n° 120

Peacock EE, Madden JW (1974) Studies on the biology and treatment of recurrent hernie; II: Morphological changes. Ann Surg 179: 567

Petit J, Stoppa R, Baillet J (1974) Evaluation expérimentale des réactions tissulaires autour des prothèses de la paroi abdominale en tulle de Dacron. J Chir (Paris) 107: 667-672

Piedad OH, Stoesser PN, Wels PB (1973) Sliding inguinal hernia. Am J Surg 126: 106-107

Piper JV (1969) A comparison between whole thickness skingraft and Bassini methods of repair hernia in men. Br J Surg 56: 345

Ralps DNL, Brain AJL, Grundy DJ, Hobsley M (1980) How acurately can direct and indirect inguinal hernias be distinguished? Br Med J 280: 1039

Rath AM, Zhang J, Amouroux J, Chevrel JP (1996) Les prothèses pariétales abdominales. Etude biomécanique et histologique. Chirurgie 121: 253

Ravitch MM (1969) Repair of hernias. Year Book, Chicago

Read RC (1968) Preperitoneal exposure of inguinal herniation. Ann J Surg 116: 653

Read RC (1970) Attenuation of rectus sheath in inguinal herniation. Am J Surg 120: 610

Read RC (1979) Bilaterality and the prosthetic repair of large recurrent inguinal hernias. Am J Surg 138: 788

Read RC, Mc Lead PC (1981) Influence of a relaxing incision on suture tension in Bassini's and McVay's repairs. Arch Surg 116: 440

Read CR (1984) Historical survey of the treatment of hernia. In: Nyhus LM, Condon RE (eds) Hernia, 3rd edn. Lippincott, Philadelphia

Read RC (1984) The development of inguinal herniorrhaphy. Surg Clin North Am 64: 185

Read RC (1989) Historical survey of the treatment of Hernia. In: Nyhus LM and Condon RE. Hernia 3rd edn. Lippincott, Philadelphia

Read RC (1989) Preperitoneal herniorraphy: a historical review. World J Surg 13: 532

Reclus P (1895) L'anesthésie locale par la cocaïne. Masson, Paris

Rignault D, Dumeige F (1981) Pose de deux plaques par voie de Pfannenstiel pour hernie bilatérale. J Chir (Paris) 118: 673-676

Rives J, Nicaise H, Lardennois B (1965) A propos du traitement chirurgical des hernies de l'aine. Orientation nouvelle et perspectives thérapeutiques. Ann Med Reims 2: 193

Rives J, Nicaise H (1966) A propos des hernies de l'aine et de leurs récidives. Sem Hop 31: 1932

Rives J (1967) Surgical treatment of the inguinal hernie with Dacron patch. Principles, indications, technic and results. Int Surg 47: 360-361

Rives J, Stoppa R, Fortesa L, Nicaise H (1968) Les pièces en Dacron et leur place dans la chirurgie des hernies de l'aine. Ann Chir 22: 159-171

Rives J, Lardennois B, Flament JB, Hibon J (1971) Utilisation d'une étoffe en dacron dans le traitement des hernies de l'aine. Acta Chir Belg 70: 284-286

Rives J, Lardennois B, Flament JB, Convers G (1973) La pièce en tulle de dacron, traitement de choix des hernies de l'aine de l'adulte. A propos de 183 cas. Chirurgie 99: 564-575

Rives J, Hibon J (1974) Hernies de l'aine. Encycl Med Chir, Paris, Estomac-Intestin, 9: 90095- 10

Rives J, Lardennois B, Hibon J (1974) Traitement moderne des hernies de l'aine et de leurs récidives. Encycl Med Chir Paris. Techniques Chirurgicales. Appareil digestif 3: 40090-40125

Rives J, ForteSA L, Drouard F, Hibon J, Flament JB (1978) La voie d'abord abdominale sous-péritonéale dans le traitement des hernies de l'aine. Ann Chir 32: 245-255

Rives J, Flament JB, Delattre JF, Palot JP (1982) La chirurgie moderne des hernies de l'aine. Cah Med 7: 1205-1218

Rives J, Flament JB, Palot JP (1994) Treatment of groin hernies with a Mersilene mesh via an inguinal approach (The Rives' Technique). In: Bendavid R (ed) Prostheses of the abdominal wall. R G Landes, Austin, pp 435

Ruggi G (1892) Metodo operativo nuovo per la cura radicale dellternia crurale. Bull Scienze Med di Bologna 7: 223

Russel RH (1906) The saccular theory of hernia and the radical operation. Lancet 2: 1197

Rutkow IM, Robbins AW (1994) Classification of groin hernias. In: Bendavid R (ed) Prosthesis and abdominal wall hernias. R G Landes, Austin, pp 106-112

Rutledge RH (1995) The Cooper ligament repair of groin hernies. In: Nyhus LM and Condon RE (eds) Hernia, 4th edn. Lippincott, Philadelphia

Ryan ER (1953) Recurrent hernies. An analysis of 369 consecutive cases of recurrent inguinal and femoral hernias. Surg Gynecol Obstet 96: 343-354

Salama J, Sarfaff E, Chevrel JP (1983) The anatomical bases of nerve lesions arising during the reduction of inguinal hernie. Anat Clin 5: 75-81

Scheich CL (1894) Schmerzlose operationen. Globus, Berlin

Schumpelick V, Treutner KH (1994) Inguinal hernia repair in adults. Lancet 344: 375

Semmence A, Kynch J (1980) Hernia repair and time off work in Oxford. J Roy Coll Gen Pract 21:90

Shulman AG, Amid PK, Lichtenstein IL (1993) Ligation of hernial sacs: a needless step in adult hernioplasty. Int Surg 78: 152

Smedberg SGG, Broome AEA, Gulmo A (1984) Ligation of the hernial sac? Surg Clin North Am 64: 299

Smedberg SGG, Broome AEA, Gullmo A (1985) Herniography in athletes with groin pain. Am J Surg 149: 378

Soler M, Verhaeghe P, Essomba A, Sevestre H, Stoppa R (1993) Le traitement des éventrations post-opératoires par prothèse composée (polyester-polyglactine 910). Etude clinique et expérimentale. Ann Chir 47: 598

Sournia JC, Zaria T (1975) Une journée de Chirurgie en France. Enquète statistique nationale. Chirurgie 101: 662

Stoppa R (1969) Technique de cure de certaines hernies de l'aine par voie médiane extrapéritonéale. Film. 71e Congrès Francais de Chirurgie

Stoppa R, Quintyn M (1969) Les déficiences de la paroi abdominale chez le sujet âgé. Colloque avec le praticien. Sem Hop Paris 45: 2182-2185

Stoppa R, Petit J, Abourachid H (1973) Procédé original de plastie des hernies de l'aine. L'interposition sans fixation d'une prothèse en tulle de dacron par voie médiane sous-péritonéale. Chirurgie 99: 119

Stoppa R, Petit J, Henry X (1975) Unsuturated Dacron prosthesis in Groin Hernias. Int Surgery 60:411

Stoppa R, Henry X, Verhaeghe P, Odimba BFK, Warlaumont C (1981) La place des prothèses réticulées non résorbables dans le traitement chirurgical des hernies de l'aine. Chirurgie 107: 333-341

Stoppa R, Warlaumont C, Verhaeghe P, Odimba BFK, Henry X (1982) Les prothèses dans le traitement des hernies de l'aine. Pourquoi? Comment? Quand?

Entretiens de Bichat. L'expansion Scientifique Française, Paris

Stoppa RE, Rives JL, Warlaumont CR, Polot JP, Verhaege P, Delattre J (1984) The use of dacron in the repair of hernies of the groin. Surg Clin North Am, 64: 269

Stoppa RE, Warlaumont CR (1989) Repair of recurrent hernias by the insertion of giant mesh prostheses through the midline preperitoneal approach. In: Madden JL (ed) Abdominal wall Hernias (an Atlas of Anatomy an Repair). Saunders WB, Philadelphia, p 242

Stoppa RE, Warlaumont CR (1989) The preperitoneal approach and prosthetic repair of groin hernia. In: Nyhus LM, Condon RE (eds) Hernia, 3rd edn. Lippincott JB, Philadelphia

Stoppa R, Henry X (1990) Classification des hernies de l'aine. Proposition personnelle. Chirurgie 119: 132

Stoppa RE, Warlaumont CR (1992) The midline preperitoneal appoach and the prosthetic repair of groin hernia. In: Nyhus LM and Baker RJ (eds) Mastery of Surgery, 2nd edn. Little Brown, Boston

Stoppa R, Boudouris O (1994) Groin hernie repair by extraperitoneal bilateral mesh prosthesis and midline subumbilical approach. In: Arregui ME, Nagan RF (eds) Inguinal Hernia. Radcliffe Medical Press Oxford, p 195

Stoppa R, Soler M, Verhaeghe P (1994) Polyester (Dacron) mesh. In: Bendavid R (ed) Prosthesis and Abdominal wall Hernias. R G Landes, Austin, p 268

Stoppa R, Soler M, Verhaeghe P (1994) Treatment of groin hernie by giant bilateral prosthesis repair. In: Bendavid R (ed) Prostheses and Abdominal wall Hernias. R G Landes, Austin, p 423

Stoppa R, Soler M (1995) Chemistry, geometry and physics of mesh materials. In: Schumpelick V, Wantz G (eds) Inguinal Hernia repair. Karger, Basel, p 166

Stoppa R (1995) The peritoneal approach and prosthetic repair of groin hernias. In: Nyhus LM, Condon RE (eds) Hernia, 4th edn. Lippincott, Philadelphia, p 188

Stoppa R, Henry X (1995) Stoppa GPRVS procedure. In: Schumpelick V, Wantz G (eds) Inguinal Hernia repair. Karger, Basel, p 212

Stoppa RE (1995) Errors, difficulties and complications in hernia repairs using the GPRUS. Prob Gen Surg 12: 139

Stoppa R (1996) The giant prosthesis for the reinforcement of the visceral sac in the repair of groin and incisional hernias. In: Nyhus LM, Baker RJ, Fischer JE (eds) Mastery of Surgery, 3rd edn. Little Brown, Boston

Suire P, Laffitte H, Pavy B (1966) Le laçage de peau totale pour les hernies inguinales volumineuses ou récidivées et les éventrations post-opératoires. Mem Acad Chir 92: 844

Tait L (1891) A discussion on treatment of hernia by median abdominal section. Br Med J 2: 685

Toupet A (1963) Procédé de cure radicale de hernie inguinale par transposition du cordon. Mem Acad Chir 89: 734

Trivellini G, Danelli PG, Cortese L, Sollini A, Rossi R (1991) L'impiego di due protes in contemporanea nella riparazione celle grosse perdite di sostanza reale della parete addominale. Chirurgia 4: 601

Truong SN, Pfingsten F, Dreuw B, Schumpelick V (1994) Value of ultrasound in the diagnosis of undetermined findings in the abdominal wall and inguinal region. In: Schumpelick V and Wantz GE (eds) Inguinal Hernia Repair. Karger, Basel

Tyrell J, Silberman H, Chandrosoma P, Nyland J (1989) Absorbable versus permanent mesh in abdominal operations. Surg Gynecol Obstet 168: 227

Usher FC, Ochsner JL, Tuttle LL jr (1958) Use of Marlex mesh in the repair of incisional hernias. Ann Surg 24: 969

Usher FC, Hill JR, Ochsner JL (1959) Hernia repair with marlex mesh. A comparison of techniques. Surgery 46: 718-724

Usher FC (1962) Hernia repair with marlex mesh. An analysis of 541 cases. Arch Surg 84: 325

Vayre P, Petit-Pazos C (1965) Utilisation d'un lambeau de la gaine du grand droit pour la cure chirurgicale de la hernie inguinale directe chez l'homme. Chirurgie 90: 63-74

Wantz GE (1982) Testicular atrophy as a risk of inguinal hernioplasty. Surg Gynecol Obstet 154: 570

Wantz GE (1984) Complications of inguinal hernial repair. Surg Clin North Am 64: 287

Wantz GE (1989) Giant prosthetic reinforcement of the visceral sac. Surg Gynecol Obstet 169: 408

Wantz GE (1989) The operation of Bassini as described by Attilio Catterina. Surg Gynecol Obstet 168: 67

Wantz GE (1991) Atlas of hernia surgery. Raven Press, New York

Wantz GE (1993) The technique of giant prosthetic reinforcement of the visceral sac performed through an anterior groin incision. Surg Gynecol Obstet 176: 497

Wantz GE (1996) Experience with the tension-free hernioplasty for primary inguinal hernias in men. J Am Coll Surg 183: 352-356

Warlaumont C (1982) Les hernies de l'aine. Place des prothèses en tulle de dacron dans leur traitement (A propos de 1236 hernies opérées). Thèse Médecine, Amiens

Welsh DRJ (1964) Sliding inguinal hernias. J Abdom Surg 6: 41

Whitmann DH, Schein M, Condon RE (1995) Antibiotic prophylaxie in Abdominal Wall Hernia Surgery: Never, always, or selectively. Prob Gen Surg 12: 47

Wolfler A (1892) Zur Radikaloperaffon des freien Leistenbruches. Beitr Chir (Festchr Geuidmet Theodor Billroth). Stuttgart: 552

Young DV (1987) Comparison of local, spinal and general anesthesia for inguinal herniorrhaphy. Am J Surg 153: 560

II. Other Hernias

A. Epigastric Hernias

These include hernias through the upper part of the linea alba, but exclude umbilical hernias. The first reliable description was in the middle of the 18th century by Le Dran. Arnauld de Villeneuve (1285) and de Garengeot (1743) attributed certain vague abdominal pains to the existence of such hernias, followed by Gunz (1744) who termed them "gastroceles", a concept contested by Richter at the end of the 18th century. It was Léveillé (1812) who introduced the term epigastric hernia. Detailed descriptions were provided by Bernitz (1848) and Cruveilher (1849). The first successful operation was attributed to Maunior (1802), but the procedure was abandoned because of postoperative peritonitis until Terrier (1886) reintroduced it following the advent of aseptic techniques. Luecke (1887) pointed out the frequent co-existence of intra-abdominal pathology with epigastric hernias, and recommended a complete exploration of the abdomen during the process of repair. At the beginning of the 20th century, it was thought that they were the cause of a gastric ulcer, to the extent that epigastric hernias were experimentally induced in dogs, in order to confirm this. The modern view is that the co-existence of an epigastric hernia and gastrointestinal symptoms is an indication for further investigations of the GI tract.

1. Frequency

The exact frequency of epigastric hernia is difficult to establish, because many asymptomatic lesions are not diagnosed. Autopsy studies indicate a prevalence of 0.5 to 10% in the general population. They are rare in children and males predominate in a ratio of 3:1, the greatest frequency being from the third to the fifth decade. Although congenital epigastric hernias are rare they occur with some frequency in the Indian population. Epigastric hernias represent 0.5 to 5% of all hernias operated on the older series (Jason, Lindenstein, Peters). The US Army reports [Heydorn

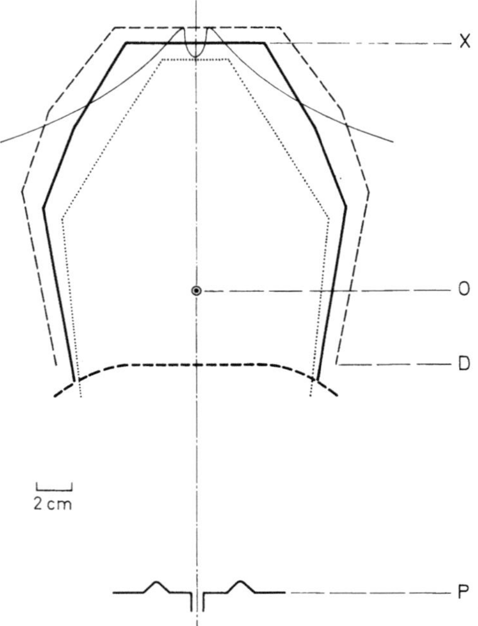

Fig. 9.26. The plane of the prefascial and retromuscular space, based on measurements in 20 dissections. The *heavy line* shows the mean dimensions of this space, the *dashed line* the maximum dimensions, and the *dotted line* the minimum dimensions. *X* xiphoid process; *O* umbilicus; *D* Douglas' line; *P* pubis [Odimba et al. 1980]

1990] reveal a slightly higher operation rate, perhaps because of the inclusion of asymptomatic hernias discovered on routine examination.

2. Pathological Anatomy

The linea alba is formed of interdigitated aponeurotic fibers which unite the rectus sheaths into a fibrous band perforated by a number of neurovascular bundles. Its posterior aspect lies in contact with the endoabdominal fascia and preperitoneal fat, the umbilical ligament and the parietal peritoneum. Divergence of the two recti at their upper ends produces a broadening of the linea alba which may attain 5 cm. For a detailed study of the anatomy, reference should be made to the works of Askar (1977-1984) and the studies by Rath and Chevrel (1996). For the radiological anatomy see the section on diastasis of the recti, at the end of this chapter. The anterior rectus sheath is adherent to the muscle at the level of the fibrous intersections, whereas the posterior sheath is free. A plane of cleavage exists behind the muscle on either side of the midline, which can be used for the insertion of prosthetic material (Fig. 9.26).

The diameter of the hernial defect varies from a few millimeters to several centimeters. The size of the hernia varies from that of a pea to a fist. Small hernias are frequently irreducible as they are composed only of preperitoneal fat. Larger hernias have a sac which in one third of cases is empty but in others contains omentum and, less often, small intestine. Epigastric hernias are multiple in 20% of cases.

It should be remembered that accurate reconstruction of the linea alba after it has been divided is practically impossible, because of the complex crossing pattern of its constituent fibers, which is usually in three layers.

These hernias are generally considered as acquired lesions, with a certain "congenital" element in respect of the perforating neurovascular bundles (Pollack, Moschowitz). Askar, who ascribes a respiratory function to the upper abdominal wall (as opposed to the lower part, which is a restraining mechanism) has observed that patients with epigastric hernias have only one layer of fibrous decussation, which promotes their appearance. The same author assigns a role to certain diaphragmatic fibers which perforate the upper part of the linea alba, which can exert traction upwards and laterally, promoting herniation.

3. Clinical Picture

Three quarters of all epigastric hernias are asymptomatic. It is often the smaller hernias, even if not incarcerated, which seem to cause pain or other rather inconstant symptoms. Epigastric pain which is worse on effort and relieved by lying down, seems to be typical.

Physical examination discloses a midline mass of variable size, with or without a cough impulse. The smaller hernias are often irreducible, whereas those of greater volume are usually easily reduced. Strangulation of the extraperitoneal fat or omentum is unusual, and strangulation of a viscus is exceedingly rare. In the obese subject it may be difficult to palpate the midline epigastric swelling, even on coughing. This maneuver may be useful in distinguishing hernias from other swellings of the abdomen or its wall.

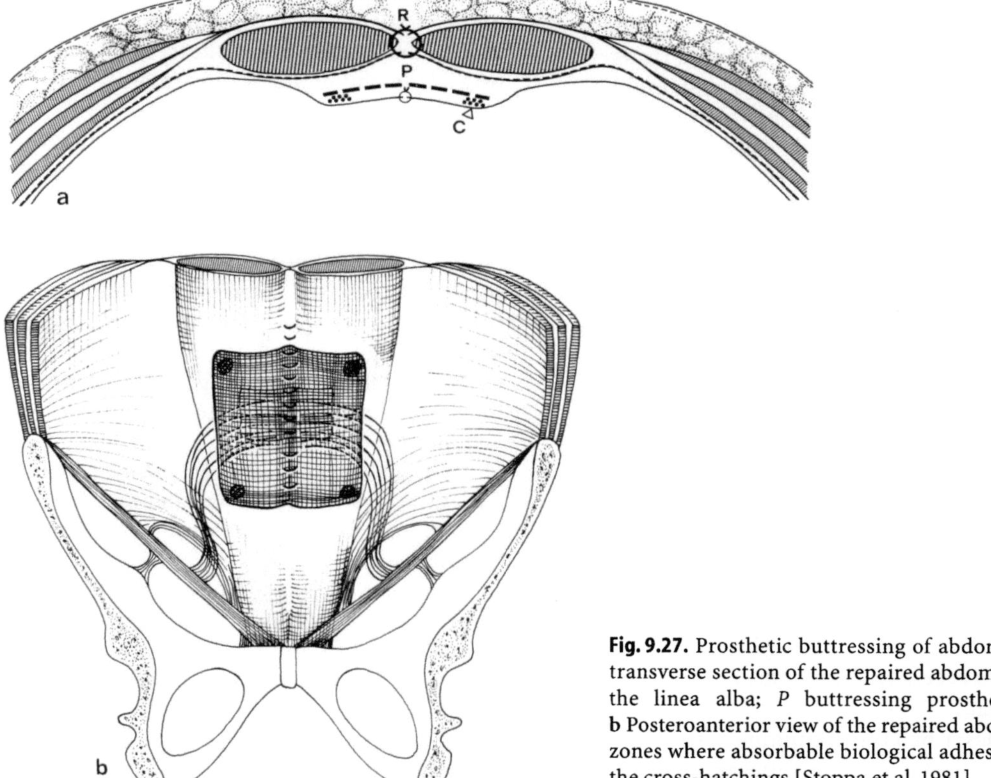

Fig. 9.27. Prosthetic buttressing of abdominal wall repair. **a** *A* transverse section of the repaired abdominal wall. *R* Suture of the linea alba; *P* buttressing prosthesis; *C* peritoneum. **b** Posteroanterior view of the repaired abdominal wall; note the zones where absorbable biological adhesive is used, shown by the cross-hatchings [Stoppa et al. 1981]

Yeh et al (1984) described the sonographic signs, which include a loss of substance of part of the fibrous abdominal wall, the volume of which varies with straining, and rarely peristalsis if the sac contains intestine. Where there are prominent GI symptoms, appropriate investigations should be carried out.

4. Treatment

The choice of treatment will depend on the type and severity of the symptoms. Children up to the age of six or seven should be managed conservatively [Pentney 1960]. Asymptomatic hernias in adults should be left alone when they are less than 10 to 15 mm in diameter. Hernias less than 25 mm across are usually treated by resection of the herniated extraperitoneal fat and simple suture of the linea alba which is all that is necessary, using nonabsorbable material. This may be carried out under local anesthesia. However, more extensive surgical treatment may be justified, bearing in mind that these lesions are frequently multiple. A midline exposure allows complete examination of the linea alba and excludes the presence of other unsuspected defects. Fatty hernias are resected without opening the peritoneum. The most frequent method of repair is simple suture using nonabsorbable material mounted on atraumatic needles. The paramedian Leriche type of incision across the rectus sheath is inadvisable, as it is unnecessarily destructive. The "wrapover" or Mayo type of repair involving transverse enlargement of the hernial orifice as in an umbilical hernia, has been advised for lesions 7 cm across, but seems to us to be unnecessarily invasive and to create tension on the suture lines. Berman (1945) used a type of plasty with overlap of the anterior and posterior rectus sheaths. Askar uses an autograft of strips of fascia lata in a lattice fashion, applying the principles of his observations on the biochemical properties of the anterior abdominal wall. He is the only surgeon to use this complex procedure.

In cases where the orifice is greater than 15 mm across, my personal preference is to debride it in a vertical fashion and then to close with a patch of synthetic mesh behind the muscle and in front of the sutured posterior sheath, before closing the anterior sheath (Fig. 9.27). I term this "the prosthetically reinforced suture repair". This method is particularly useful when there are a number of superimposed hernial defects which become united when the tissues are freed up, as it gives access to the whole area and simplifies the approach.

Chevrel (1979) described this technique in the treatment of epigastric diastasis, using a pre-aponeurotic synthetic patch, which seems a good solution for this particular problem (see Chapter on incisional hernia). The use of prosthetic material is always indicated in recurrent cases of epigastric hernia.

5. Results

Complications of epigastric hernia repair are not peculiar to this type of lesion. Infection (3-5%) may lead to suture failure even after insertion of a deep prosthesis. Local treatment of the complication without removing the synthetic material is usually successful. The reported long term results are less favorable than are those of the repair of groin hernia: Glenn (1936) 15% recurrences; McCauchan (1956) 9.4% recurrences; and Askar (1984) 7% recurrences. The factors predisposing to recurrence include obesity, infection and the presence of an overlooked associated hernia. My experience of reinforced suture was of one recurrence in 67 cases treated by retromuscular prosthesis and 30 of those treated by simple suture.

References

Askar OM (1978) A new concept of the aetiology and surgical repair of paraumbilical and epigastric hernias. Ann R Coll Surg Engl, 60: 42

Askar OM (1994) Aponeurotic hernias: epigastric, umbilical, paraumbilical, hypogastric. In: Bendavid R (ed) Prosthesis in abdominal wall hernias. R G Landes, Austin, pp 59-68

Boissonnault JS, Blaschak MJ (1988) Incidence of diastasis recti abdominis during the childbearing year. Phys Ther 66: 1082

Bursch SG (1987) Interrater reliability of diastasis recti measurement. Phys Ther 67: 1077

Champault G (1996) La pariétoscopie abdominale. Technique et indications. Résultats préliminaire. Ann Chir 50: 445-448

Chevrel JP (1979) Traitement des grandes éventrations médianes par plastie en paletôt et prothèse. Nouv Presse Med 89: 695-696

Chevrel JP, Dilin C, Morquette H (1986) Traitement des éventrations médianes par autoplastie et prothèse prémusculo-aponévrotique. 50 observations. Chirurgie 112: 612

Condon RE (1995) Incisional Hernia. In: Nyhus LM, Condon RE (eds) Hernia, 4th edn. Lippincott, Philadelphia, p 319

Detrie PH (1967) Nouveau traité de technique chirurgicale, T IX, Masson Paris, p 154

Heydorn WH, Velonowitch V (1990) Army experience with 36250 hernia repairs. Ann Surg 56: 596

Lagrot F, Salasc J (1957) Encycl Med Chir Laffont, Paris. 2013 A10: 1

Odimba BKF, Stoppa R, Laude M (1980) Les espaces clivables sous-pariétaux de l'abdomen. J Chir (Paris) 117: 621

Ramey B (1990) Diastasis recti and umbilical hernia causes, recognition and repair. SDJ Mde, 43/ 10: 5

Rath AM, Attali P, Dumas JL, Goldlust D, Zhang J, Chevrel JP (1996) The abdominal linea alba: an anatomo-radiologic and biomechanical study. Surg Radiol Anat 18: 281

Robin AP (1995) Epigastric hernia. In: Nyhus LM, Condon RE (eds) Hernia, 4th edn. Lippincott, Philadelphia, p 372

Testart J, Bismuth H (1971) Hernies de la ligne blanche. Hernies de la ligne de Spiegel. Hernies lombaires. Encycl Med Chir Paris Techniques chirurgicales, T1, fasc 40150

B. Diastasis of the Rectus Muscles

This represents a particular example of spontaneous hernia of the linea alba, appearing through broadening of the interlaced aponeurotic fibers. It has received little attention in the literature [Lagrot & Salasc 1957; Condon 1995]. A study by Bursch (1987) emphasizes the unreliability of clinical assessment of diastasis as seen in 40 pregnant women examined by four clinicians. An anatomical, radiological and biomechanical study of the linea alba by Rath and Chevrel (1996) is relevant here. This study defines diastasis of the rectus muscles in terms of the age of the subject, by relation to normal variants as seen on ultrasound. Diastasis may be defined as a separation of 10 mm above, 20 cm at, and 9 mm below the umbilicus, is subjects below the age of 45. Above 45 the respective values are 15, 27 and 40 mm (see chapter 1 linea alba).

Although recognized since the days of Avicenna, Malgaigne (1841) Cruveilher (1849) Quenu in Cange's thesis (1898) at the present time diastasis is of most relevance to obstetricians and plastic surgeons. It is most often found in multiparous women, who suffer a generalized loss of resilience in the abdominal wall, sometimes resulting from too early resumption of activity. The diastasis of pregnancy is a normal consequence of that state. In the past much emphasis was given to "ptosis" of various organs, but in fact no specific symptoms can be attributed to diastasis, apart from the cosmetic aspects. An associated umbilical hernia is mentioned by Ranney (1990) in 97 out of 673 cases of postpartum diastasis, in a series of 1,738 pregnancies.

Examination of the patient while supine reveals only a stretched out and striate abdomen, but when the patient sits up a longitudinal swelling appears extending usually from the xiphoid to the pubis, which again disappears on lying down. The palpating hand passes easily between the rectus muscles, of which the medial edges are easily felt and may lie as much as 10 cm apart at the level of the umbilicus. There is a tendency towards spontaneous correction, perhaps assisted by regular abdominal exercises, however these are rarely carried out as most patients are happy to wear an abdominal support. The indications for surgery must be critically assessed, because the extensive connective tissue degeneration often promotes recurrence. Physical and mental preparation of the patient is very important. In particular it should be made clear that there will be a midline scar from xiphoid to pubis, as a result of the procedure. The only cases which really merit treatment are those of major symptomatic diastasis. Surgery may comprise resection of the weakened portion of the linea alba followed by suture of the edges of the rectus sheaths, or may formally follow the technique described by D'Allaines and Contiades (1936) whereby by the enlarged part of the linea alba is reconstructed without opening the peritoneum by suturing the intact rectus sheaths following excision of excessive skin. This is a simple procedure suitable for moderate-sized defects. All major lesions require prosthetic reinforcement of the suture line, either in front or behind the muscle. Recently, endoscopic suture of the muscles has been described [Champault; Marchac 1996] (see the end of the following paragraph).

C. Spigelian Hernias

These occur through the aponeurotic area at the lateral edge of the rectus muscle, medial to the line of Spiegel, who was a Flemish anatomist well known in Padua during the 16th century. "Ruptures" in this area were first described by Le Dran (1742) and attributed by Klinkosch (1764) to herniation.

1. Frequency

Most publications report a few score cases observed by the same team. Spangen [Nyhus in Hernia 4 1995) collected a thousand of these cases.

2. Pathological Anatomy

The lateral linea alba runs a very gentle outward convex course. It contains no muscle fibers and is

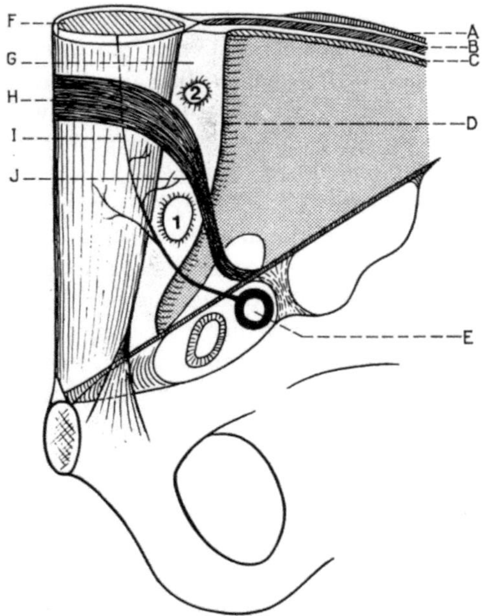

Fig. 9.28. Deep area of weakness in cases of Spigelian hernia: *1* between Hesselbach's ligament and the inferior epigastric artery (75% of cases); *2* above Hesselbach's ligament (25% of cases). *A* external oblique; *B* internal oblique; *C* transverse; *D* Spigelius line; *E* external iliac artery; *F* rectus abdominis; *G* lateral groove of the abdomen; *H* arcuate line; *I* inferior epigastric artery; *J* Hesselbach's ligament [Guivarc'h et al. 1974]

made up of the fused aponeuroses of the internal oblique and transversus muscles, passing in front of the rectus below the arcuate line of Douglas. At this point the inferior epigastric pedicle pierces the transversalis fascia in order to penetrate the rectus sheath, and the posterior aponeurosis of the transversus is often defective over several centimeters above the line of Douglas, where most Spigelian hernias occur (Fig. 9.28).

The hernial orifice lies below the epigastric vessels, the hernia is limited below. At this level the fused aponeuroses of the transversus and internal oblique produce a solid layer, which explains the comparative rarity of low Spigelian hernias. British and American authors describe a "Spigelian hernia belt", over an area lying between the infra-umbilical interspinous line and the horizontal line passing through the umbilicus, delineating a belt-like area 5 or 6 cm across, where most of these hernias occur. These hernias are interstitial and covered either by the aponeurosis of the external oblique or by those of both oblique muscles. Occasionally they pass through the external oblique to lie beneath the skin. The hernial sac is usually mushroom-shaped, and covered by a lipoma-like layer of

extraperitoneal fat. The defect is usually oval with rigid aponeurotic edges, varying in diameter from 1 to 6 or 8 cm. The sac may contain omentum, colon or at times the stomach.

Most of these hernias are acquired, though there may be a background of weakness in the area which lacks striped muscle fibers. The usual factors common to all hernias apply including age, degeneration of fibrous tissue, obesity, smoking, chronic intestinal distension, and more recently peritoneal dialysis. Thus these hernias may be combined with umbilical epigastric or inguinal defects. They are uncommon, particularly in the infra-umbilical form, and are equally distributed between the two sexes.

3. Clinical Picture

Small hernias (less than 2 cm across) are usually painful, but difficult to feel. The pain is the result of entrapped tissues. It is made worse by a rise in intra-abdominal pressure and relieved by lying down. Large hernias are more easy to feel. The symptoms vary according to their contents. The diagnosis is straightforward as soon as the swelling is noticed, and is signaled by reducibility and the presence of a cough impulse. Differential diagnosis includes intra-abdominal tumors, lipomas and desmoids, or occasionally an intramuscular hematoma. In difficult cases, investigations such as ultrasound and tomodensitometry may be of use, as they show variation in the volume of the sac within it, and occasionally peristalsis of the contained bowel. Herniorrhaphy may also be of use, in identifying the contents.

In any obese patient with a clinical history of abdominal pain, one should bear in mind the possibility of a complicated Spigelian hernia, particularly as a number of Richter type strangulations have been reported. Diagnostic laparoscopy in investigation of abdominal pain will help to reveal the situation, but for the time being a high index of suspicion should be maintained, as illustrated by a publication from Gabon [Diané 1978] which reported a series of 30 cases seen over a number of years.

These hernias require surgical treatment. When the hernial mass is palpable incision of the aponeurosis of external oblique as far as the anterior rectus sheath gives good exposure of Spiegel's fascia and allows treatment of the sac and its contents, followed by repair of the defect which is usually quite small. When there is no hernial mass palpable, having demonstrated the defect by ultrasound scan, a midline or paramedian incision gives access to the preperitoneal retromuscular space, and permits suture of the orifice with no damage to the muscle layers. Very occasionally an exploration is made by a midline transperitoneal approach when the internal oblique muscle appears normal on scanning. This route is also of course used for exploration of a strangulated Spigelian hernia. Prosthetic reinforcement is not usually necessary, except in lowly-placed hernias where the treatment is very similar to that of a high groin hernia, and if the orifice is large it can be dealt with as described above in connection with groin hernias. If there is an associated umbilical epigastric or inguinal hernia, there should be no hesitation in inserting a prosthesis. The prosthesis may either be sandwiched between the external oblique muscle in front and the internal oblique behind (J.P. Chevrel). Spangen [in Nyhus - Hernia 4 1995] in his survey of 1,000 cases reported only six recurrences, which supports a policy of surgical treatment of Spigelian hernias.

In certain circumstances Spigelian and epigastric hernias can be treated laparoscopically [Champault 1996]. The principle consists in insufflating carbon dioxide into the pre-aponeurotic layer and dissecting up this space under direct vision as far as the origin of the lesion. The insufflation can be carried out by a suprapubic subumbilical trocar. The two 5 mm trocars are lateralised in order to permit dissection and repair of the abdominal wall defect. One can make use of a pre-existing appendicectomy scar for insertion of the right lateral trocar. The aponeurotic defect can be closed either by nonabsorbable endoparietal sutures or by using a Reverdin needle introduced under direct vision via the umbilicus. This latter procedure has obvious advantages. It can also be used for the treatment of divarication of the rectus muscles and placement of a reinforcing prosthesis in the pre-aponeurotic layer.

References

Diane C, Mbumbe-King A, Balde I, Vinand P, Goudotte E (1978) Notre expérience de la hernie de Spiegel; à propos de 27 observations. Bull Med Owendo 1: 4

Guivarc'h M, Martinon F, Mouchet A (1974) La hernie dite de Spiegel (à propos de 6 observations). J Chir (Paris) 108: 87

Read RC (1978) Spigelian hernia. In: Nyhus LM, Condon RE (eds) Hernia, 2nd edn. Lippincott, Philadelphia, p 375

Spangen L (1995) Spigelian hernia. In: Nyhus LM, Condon RE (eds) Hernia, 4th edn. Lippincott, Philadelphia, p 381

Testart J, Bismuth H (1971) Hernies de la ligne blanche, de la ligne de Spiegel, hernies lombaires. Encycl Med Chir Paris, Techniques chirurgicales, T1, 40150

D. Lumbar Hernias

These arise in the lumbar region where they traverse the abdominal wall either in the superficial intermuscular triangle of Petit (1774) limited by the iliac crest below, the latissimus dorsi medially and the external oblique laterally, or else in the deep intermuscular quadrangle of Grynfeld (1866) which lies between the twelfth rib, the posterior and inferior serratus, quadratus lomborum and internal oblique. Some of these hernias are diffuse when they follow a surgical incision, and if the boundaries are of bone or cartilage this may create difficulties in repair. Swartz emphasizes that among the most difficult to treat are those which follow the removal of a vein graft from the iliac crest and those which are the result of gunshot wounds. The majority of lumbar hernias are incisional, and are commoner than those arising spontaneously.

The first description of these hernias is attributed to Barbette (1672). Ravaton (1750) reduced a strangulated lumbar hernia in a pregnant woman and in 1783 Jean-Louis Petit reported a case of strangulation and described the anatomical limits of the lower lumbar triangle. In 1866 Grynfeld described the upper lumbar quadrilateral. Before that it was assumed that all lumbar hernias passed through the triangle of Petit. In 1916 Goodman and Spence, Ravdin (1923), Virgillio (1925), Watson (1948), Thorek (1950) and Swartz (1978) have reported series of lumbar hernias.

1. Pathological Anatomy

These hernias have been classified as either congenital or acquired, spontaneous, post-traumatic or postoperative. Apart from the areas of Petit and Grynfelt, the vessels and nerves of the region can occasionally be the site of a hernia. Much more often incisional hernias emerge through the classical lumbotomy sites. Spontaneous hernias are comparatively rare (a few hundred published cases), congenital variations in the abdominal wall predispose to their appearance. A sac is almost always present but hernias of the kidney and perirenal fat without a sac have been reported. When there is a peritoneal sac it usually contains omentum, often colon, more rarely kidney or small intestine. Congenital lumbar hernias in children are often associated with other malformations whereas acquired hernias occur in the middle-aged adult, often with a background of obesity or cachexia, respiratory problems or chronic intestinal obstruction. One cause which has now become rare was tuberculous abscess of the spine, whereas one which is now much more frequent is postoperative eventration following surgery on the kidney (30% of cases). The sex ration is 2/1 in favor of the male according to Swartz.

2. Clinical Picture

There may be no symptoms, otherwise pain may occur as a result of incarceration. The hernia is usually a bulky and reducible mass, the contents of which can be ascertained on clinical examination. A cough impulse is present, but is lost where there is incarceration or strangulation. The mass is often resonant to percussion. Postoperative lumbar hernias are often very bulky (up to 25 cm in diameter) and deform the outline of the patient. Congenital hernias which are often seen at or shortly after birth, are large depressible bulky masses which markedly increase in size when the baby cries.

The pain may be interpreted in various ways including fatigue, displaced vertebrae, referred pain, all of which emphasize the importance of not attributing the symptoms to the hernia before carrying out a careful assessment of the musculo-skeletal system. In one reported series incarceration was not unusual (8-24%) whereas strangulation is less frequent than in other types of hernia because of the large dimensions of the hernial orifice. The differential diagnosis includes all other types of soft tissue swelling in the area, and does not require detailed elaboration.

3. Treatment

Although lumbar hernias rarely strangulate, they nonetheless require surgical action because of their increasing volume, which renders them symptomatic and cosmetically unacceptable. However, surgery for congenital lumbar hernia should be delayed until the child reaches the age of six months.

Before operation the appropriate radiological investigations should be carried out (upper GI series, barium enema, IVU) together with a CT scan. If the sac contains large bowel, the colon should be suitably prepared. These patients should be persuaded to lose weight. Careful preparation is essential because the treatment of a large lumbar hernia is complex and should be carried out in a specialized center.

The usual incision runs obliquely from the 12th rib above and behind towards the anterior part of the iliac crest. The hernial mass is separated from the subcutaneous fat and the sac identified, bearing in mind the possibility of its containing colon en glissade, with a consequent risk of injury to the mesocolon. When a sac is present it should be opened in

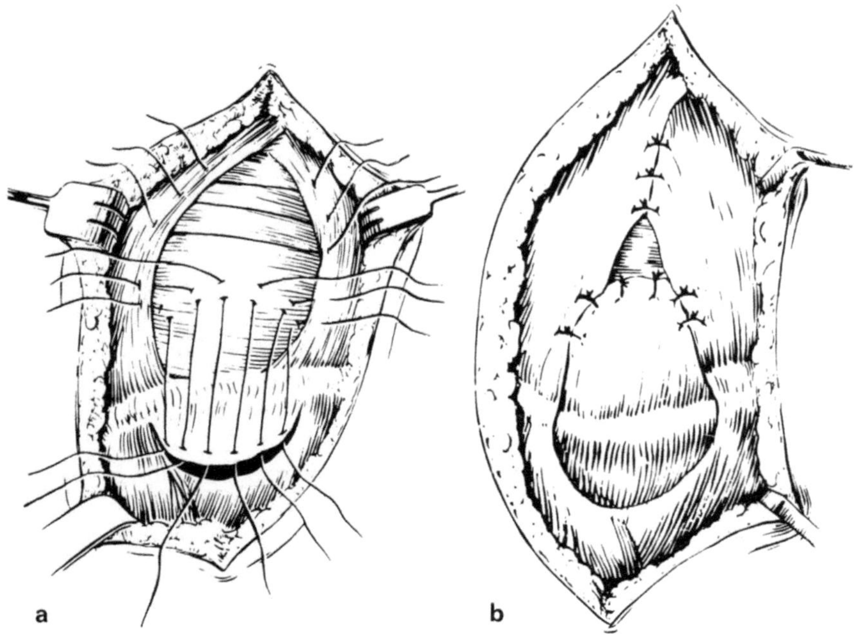

a   b

Fig. 9.29a, b. Dowd's technique, with mobilization of a flap of gluteus maximus and fascia lata and reinforcement of the remaining defect with a fascial flap from the latissimus dorsi

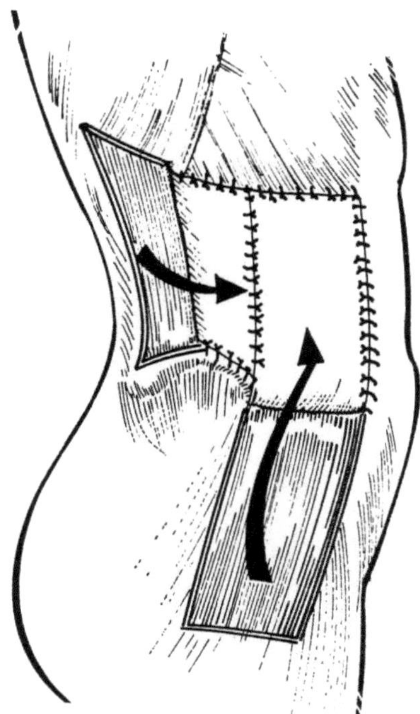

Fig. 9.30.

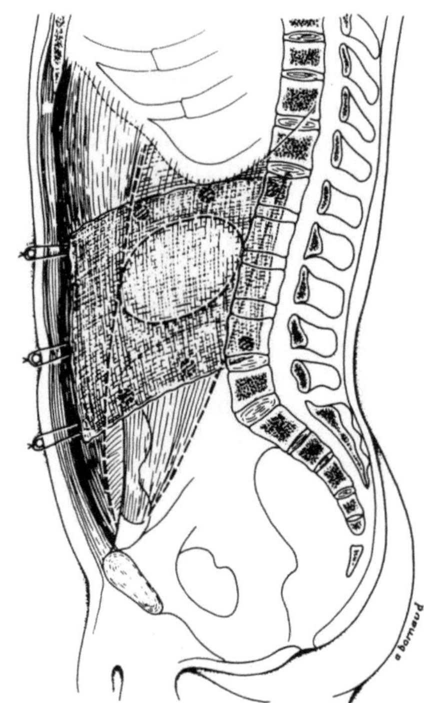

Fig. 9.31.

Fig. 9.30. Koontz's technique, using two flaps from the lumbar fascia and gluteal aponeurosis [Testart & Bismuth 1971]

Fig. 9.31. Illustration (from within and looking out) of a large prosthetic reinforcement of the visceral sac without abdominal wall repair in a case of voluminous lumbar hernia. The prosthesis is partially attached, anteriorly, by transfixing sutures of the abdominal wall and partially with adhesive (above, below, and posteriorly). The zones of adhesive are shown by the cross-hatchings [Stoppa et al. 1981]

order to check the contents and identify any separate locules. Complete sacs are unusual. When the base of the sac is too large to be controlled by a simple ligature, the sac may be inverted or plicated and sutured, to eliminate the bulge. Any dead space should be drained. The choice of repair for the abdominal wall will depend on the size and position of the hernia. With moderate sized hernias of the congenital or spontaneous type, it is sometimes possible to carry out a wrap over repair of the aponeurotic layers which will narrow the hernial orifice, using interrupted sutures of strong nonabsorbable monofilament material, and constructing two superimposed solid layers. With very large hernias, Ponka (1980) advises the use of musculo-aponeurotic reinforcement flaps, either a tailored flap composed of the aponeurosis of gluteus maximus together with fascia lata brought upwards [Dowd 1907] (Fig. 9.29) or else using the Koontz technique (Fig. 9.30), which combines a flap of gluteus and fascia lata brought upwards with one of latissimus dorsi which is swung forwards. Ravdin (1923)

suggested the use of free grafts fascia lata, Koontz uses skin, Thorek (1950) tantalum mesh and Hafner (1963) polypropylene. Overall, the most commonly used techniques are those of Dowd for hernias through the upper triangle and of Ravdin for hernias of the lower triangle.

With postoperative hernias, these procedures may be difficult because of scarring. The most difficult defects to repair are those which follow removal of an iliac bone graft. Various solutions include wide resection of the ilium [Bosworth 1955], bone graft [Oldfield 1945], and transposition of the iliopsoas muscle [Lewin & Bradley 1949]. We personally favor the use of a nonabsorbable prosthetic mesh placed extraperitoneally beneath the muscles (Fig. 9.31), and fixed at the edges, wherever there is a loss of substance of more than 5 cm in diameter. The results of surgical treatment of lumbar hernias are impossible to summarize here because of the multiplicity of the techniques used, the lack of consensus on the indications and the limited experience of the authors.

References

Detrie PH (1967) Nouveau traité de technique chirurgicale, T IX. Masson, Paris

Geis PW, Hodakowski GT (1995) Lumbar hernia. In: Nyhus LM, Condon RE (eds) Hernia, 4th edn. Lippincott, Philadelphia, p 412

Jamal L, Hillebrant JP, Bugnon P, Fazel A (1996) Hernie lombaire du quadrilatère du Grynfelt. A propos d'un cas. J chir (Paris) 133: 233-235

Stoppa R, Henry X, Odimba BFK (1981) Prothèses de paroi abdominale, Forum Chirurgical, 21: 28

Testart J, Bismuth H (1971) Hernies épigastriques, hernies de Spiegel, hernies lombaires. Encycl Med Chir Paris, Techniques chirurgicales, T1, fasc 40150,

Thorek M (1950) Lumbar hernia. J Int Coll Surg 14: 367-370

E. Pelvic Hernias

The orifices of these hernias lie below the level of the pelvic brim. They are rare and can be divided into three types: anterior or obturator hernias which emerge through the obturator foramen and appear in the anterior aspect of the thigh, posterior or sciatic hernias which emerge through the greater sciatic notch and appear in the buttock or the back of the thigh, and perineal hernias of which only the lateral types will be discussed here (excluding rectoceles, cystoceles and others which pass through the pelvic floor). Although rare, pelvic hernias are of importance because of their tendency to strangulate, which is often overlooked with serious results, especially in the case of obturator hernias.

1. Obturator Hernias

The surgeon should be aware of this rare hernia which is difficult to diagnose, but frequently strangulates, with serious results. Arnaud de Ronsil (1723) and later Croissant de Garangeot (1743) reported the first cases. Dupuytren described it at the beginning of the 19th century, so that Nyhus (1964) termed it the "French Hernia". Hilton (1848) was the first to attempt surgical repair under chloroform anesthesia, and the first successful operation was carried out by Obre in 1851. Howship (1840) described the characteristic pain on the inner side of the thigh, due to compression of the obturator nerve. This was independently described by Romberg in 1848. The most recent review is that of Skandalakis et al. (1995) in the fourth edition of the Nyhus book on hernia.

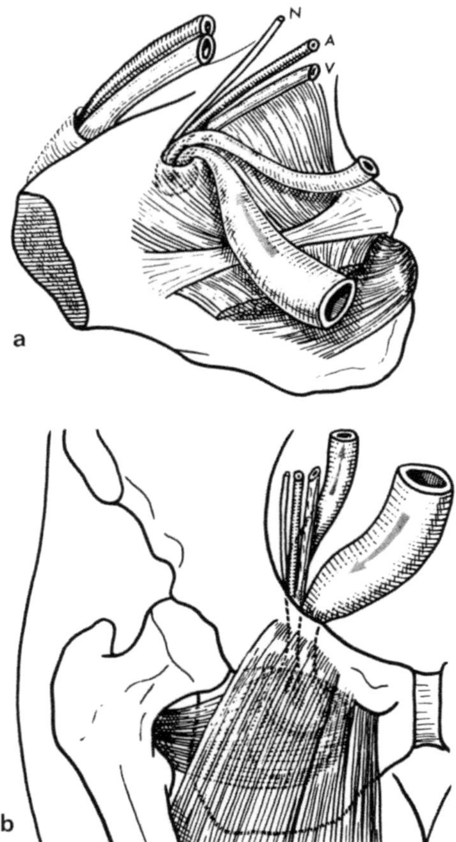

Fig. 9.32. Strangulated obturator hernia. a Endopelvic view showing the small bowel engaged in the internal ring of the subpubic canal, medial to the obturator neurovascular bundle. b Anterior view showing the pectineus covering the hernial sac [Guivarc'h & Houssin 1970]

The obturator canal is limited above by the horizontal ramus of the pubis and below by the upper edge of the obturator membrane. It is 10-15 mm across and 3 cm long. Running obliquely downwards, forwards and medially, the margins of this canal are rigid, resulting in its tendency to strangulate. The anterior end of the canal opens into the femoral triangle. The obturator canal transmits the neurovascular bundle composed of, from above downwards, the nerve, artery and vein. The hernial sac, often accompanied by a lipoma, is usually small. It often contains small bowel (hence the frequency of Richter type strangulation) but rarely may contain the appendix, Fallopian tube, Meckel's diverticulum, omentum or bladder.

a) Frequency

The hernia is found six times more often in women than men, because of the greater diameter of the obturator foramen in females. The usual presentation is during the eighth decade. Malnutrition, respiratory problems and chronic intestinal distension are frequent predisposing factors. The hernia is found more frequently on the right than on the left, and is bilateral in 6% of cases. It is often associated with a groin hernia.

Skandalakis (1995) has collected more than 450 published cases from the world literature. Rogers (1964) in a series of 3,000 mechanical obstructions encountered twelve obturator hernias (Fig. 9.32). Manning (1966) reports four obturator hernias in an overall series of 539 hernias operated in a Nigerian hospital. Bjork (1988) recorded eleven cases in more than 15,000 hernias repaired at the Mayo Clinic, and Persson (1987) 15 cases out of 850 herniorrhaphies. The exact frequency of obturator hernia is thus still unknown.

b) Clinical Picture

The usual presentation is of acute strangulation, often with a background of recurrent episodes which may extend over ten years. Skandalakis (1995) describes the prominent features which are intestinal obstruction (70 out of 79 cases), pain on the medial side of the thigh and the knee, and the "hip and knee pain" sign of Howship and Romberg in 41 patients out of 79. The absence of this symptom does not exclude the diagnosis but its presence indicates compression of the obturator nerve, which the surgeon should be aware of. A palpable mass (15 cases out of 79) which is more easily found when the patient lies down with the thighs flexed, abducted and externally rotated, at the upper part of the inner side of the thigh, is typical. It is sometimes palpable laterally on rectal or vaginal examination. In 28 out of the 79 patients in the Skandalakis' series, there were repeated episodes for between six months and ten years before surgery. Plain radiographs do not usually reveal the diagnosis, because air and fluid levels are only seen with a complete obstruction. Champault et al. have recently reported good visualization of a Richter's hernia of the small bowel by the use of water soluble contrast medium. There is some evidence that the diagnosis of strangulated obturated hernia is aided by the use of abdominal tomodensitometry, an examination which is receiving increasing interest in the investigation of small bowel obstruction, and is recommended by Farthouart (1996) as the examination of first choice in all cases of suspected obstruction. The Howhip Romberg sign is virtually pathognomonic, whereas the palpation of a tumor is the best objective sign.

However the best way of making the diagnosis is always to bear it in mind, and to operate early in order to avoid the necessity of resection, as was the case in 49 out of Skandalakis' 79 operations.

c) Treatment

(1) Route of Access

The difficulties resulting from the deeply placed location of the hernia are increased by the fact that the operation is usually carried out for obstruction. Reduction is difficult. The abdominal approach gives poor access to the sac, whereas identification of the neck and resection of intestine is virtually impossible via the femoral route. In most cases a lower midline incision will have been made, because the cause of the obstruction will not have been diagnosed. Exploration of the peritoneum discloses a strangulated loop in the obturator canal, and gentle traction should be used in order to disimpact the bowel without rupturing it. It may be necessary to free up the deep orifice of the obturator foramen, always bearing in mind that the neurovascular bundle lies immediately above the sac. When in spite of this the loop cannot be reduced, a separate approach through the thigh must be made in order to gain better access.

The femoral or obturator approach comprises a vertical incision in the medial part of the femoral triangle, between the femoral artery and the pubic spine, extending over 10 to 12 cm. The incision is deepened in the space between the adductor magnus and pectineus, and when the latter muscle is retracted the external orifice of the obturator canal is exposed. A large sac is easily freed through this approach, but it may be very difficult to avoid injuring the hernial contents or the vessels, so that Caraven (1941) suggested resecting the iliopubic ramus. However, this would seem to be a most mutilating procedure, best avoided.

The subperitoneal inguinal route described by Milligan uses an incision parallel to the inguinal ligament and two centimeters above it, through which the internal oblique and transversus muscles are detached from the ligament (a better alternative is to incise the floor of the inguinal canal) in order to gain access to the "space of Bogros", and thence to the deep orifice of the obturator canal. It is difficult to close the orifice through this approach, which was modified by Cheatle (1920) and Henry (1936) into a suprapubic horizontal approach, that when enlarged gives better access and allows repair of any coexisting femoral hernia. Our personal preference is for a midline extraperitoneal approach which, when the diagnosis has been made preoperatively, is quick to carry out, and even if the abdomen has been explored for obstruction, can be used following closure of the peritoneum. The literature shows that combined approaches have often been used, which allow successive exposure of the sac and the neck of the hernia, i.e. the superficial and deep orifices of the obturator foramen.

The deep aspect of the obturator canal may be difficult to close, on account of its rigid osseofibrous walls. Various solutions have been suggested. Simple suture of the peritoneal neck via the abdomen carries a risk of recurrence. Suture of the deep orifice of the obturator canal, reinforced by an aponeurotic flap or synthetic patch, taking care to allow room for passage of the neurovascular bundle, is another solution. The obturator canal can be obliterated by omentum, ovary, uterus, or a muscular flap. These methods have nowadays been replaced by the use of a plug of synthetic material. Most present day surgeons prefer, like us, to use a piece of synthetic mesh placed between the peritoneum and the pelvic wall, at the same time exteriorising the obturator neurovascular bundle.

Usually, the operation is carried out for intestinal obstruction via a midline laparotomy. If the obstructed loop proves difficult to reduce, rather than carrying out a supplementary incision in the thigh, it may be better to use sufficient force to withdraw the loop, and then if necessary to resect the bowel. Following resection of the compromised loop, the peritoneum is closed and a prosthetic repair carried out through a clean area, using an appropriately sized patch.

In the elective situation, it is better to use the subperitoneal inguinal approach (Cheatle, Henry, Nyhus) which gives a good view of the obturator foramen which can then be patched. A midline subumbilical approach can also be used, which gives access to both sides and allows the surgeon to insert a large reinforcing prosthesis in front of the peritoneum, as already described in the treatment of groin hernias, and which has proved very satisfactory in our hands.

(2) Results

The 48% mortality described by Watson in 1948 has now come down to 13.2% in the 98 cases described by Gray and Skandalakis in 1974. It is noteworthy that the general state of the patients described by the latter two authors precluded any attempt at repair of the obturator canal. However, there was only one recurrence confirmed at operation, and in one other patient recurrent episodes of intestinal obstruction were in fact due to an obturator hernia on the other side.

References

Bismuth H, Testart J (1971) Les hernies pelviennes. Encycl Med Chir Paris, Techniques chirurgicales, T 1, fasc 40155

Farthouat P, Thouard H, Meusnier F, De Keranga L, Pourrière M, Flandrin P (1996) Hernie obturatrice étranglée. Apport de la TDM abdominale. J Chir (Paris) 133: 284-286

Gray SW, Skandalakis JE (1978) Strangulated obturator hernie. In: Nyhus LM & Condon RE (eds) Hernia, 2nd edn. Lippincott, Philadelphia, p 427

Guivarc'h M, Houssin D (1970) Occlusions du grêle de l'adulte. Encycl Med Chir Paris, Appareil digestif 40430

Howship J (1840) Pratical remarks on the discrimination and appareances of surgical disease. John Churchill, London

Lesurtel M, Barrat C, Champault G (1996) Hernie obturatrice étranglée. Diagnostic préopératoire. J Chir (Paris) 133: 281-283

Marchal F, Parent S, Tortuyaux JM, Bresler L, Boissel P, Regent D (1997) Obturator hernias. Report of seven cases. Hernia 1: 23-26

Romberg MH (1848) Die Operation des eingeklemmten Bruches des eirunden Loches. Operatio herniae foraminis ovalis incarceratae. Dieffenbach JF, Leipzig

Skandalakis LJ, Panagiotis N, Skandalakis SW, et al (1995) In: Nyhus LM, Condon RE (eds) Hernia, 4th edn. Lippincott, Philadelphia, p 425

2. Sciatic Hernias

Protrusion of a sac of the pelvic peritoneum into the buttock, via the greater or lesser sciatic notch, has been given various terms, such as sacrosciatic hernias, buttock hernias and ischioceles. According to Watson (1948), Verdier (1753) was the first to describe these, whereas Bréhant (1960) attributes the first description to Papen (1750).

a) Frequency

Watson reviewed the world literature in 1948 and finding only 35 cases concluded that sciatic hernia was the rarest form of hernia. In 1958 Gaffney and Schanno reported four more cases, including one of their own. Of the 30,000 hernias reported from the Mayo Clinic [Koontz 1978] and in the series of 21,000 hernias reported by Thomas (1964) no single case appeared. It seems that, according to the article by S. Black in the fourth edition of Hernia [Nyhus 1995] the condition predominantly affects women between 20 and 60 years of age, with no predilection for either side.

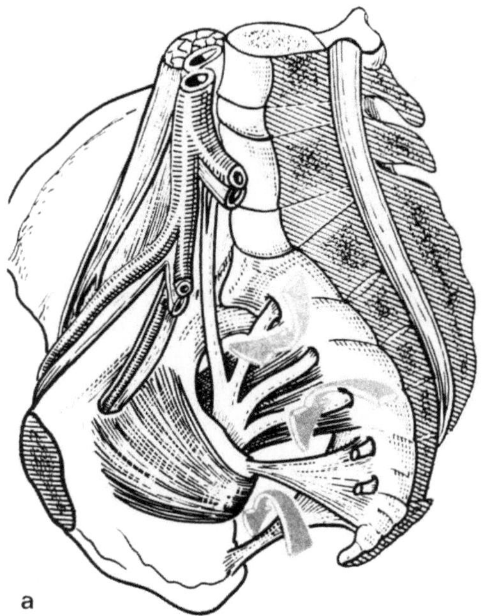

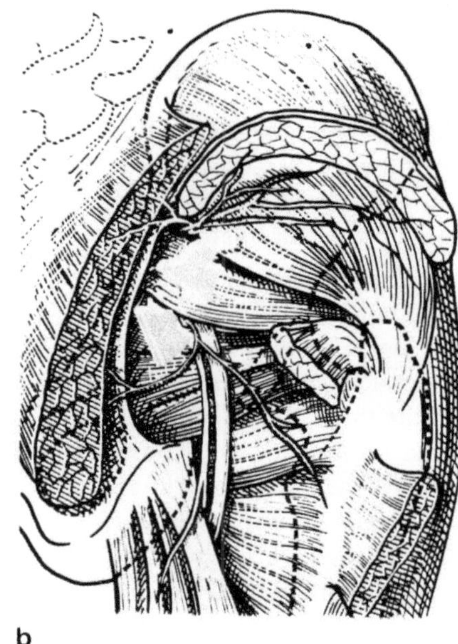

Fig. 9.33. Sciatic hernia. **a** Endopelvic view of the three orifices; *below*, the lesser sciatic notch; *above*, the greater sciatic notch and supra- and subpiriformis canals. **b** Exopelvic view showing the greater sciatic notch with two supra- and subpiriformis hernias [Guivarc'h & Houssin 1970]

b) Pathological Anatomy (Fig. 9.33)

Waldeyer [in Bismuth & Testard 1971] describes three types of sciatic hernia: namely the suprapiriform which emerges through the greater sciatic notch lateral to the gluteal nerves and vessels, and above the piriformis muscle, the infrapiriform, at the lower part of the greater sciatic notch, between the piriformis and the sacrotuberous ligament, medial to the internal pudendal vessels and sciatic nerve, and the infraspinal type which emerges through the lesser sciatic notch between the sacrotuberous and the sacrospinous ligaments, medial to the tendon of obturator internus and the internal pudendal vessels. Thus all the sciatic hernias lie above and lateral to the sacrotuberous ligament, and spread downwards into the buttock, before entering the thigh. In more than 30% of cases the content is small intestine, but bladder, ovary, Fallopian tube, colon, omentum, ureter and Meckel's diverticulum have all been reported.

Sciatic hernias can be congenital, in which case they are usually associated with malformations of the pelvic bones or muscles, or acquired, as a result of increased intra-abdominal pressure or by muscular erosion caused by retroperitoneal tumors invading the buttock.

c) Clinical Picture

Small sciatic hernias cause no symptoms or physical signs. Large ones present as a bulky mass in the buttock region, which increases in size on standing or coughing. Auscultation may reveal bowel sounds. In advanced cases, there may be intestinal obstruction or sciatic neuralgia. Palpation reveals a soft and reducible swelling, though at times the hernia is tense and cystic and reduction may be difficult. It is therefore advisable to examine the buttock region in all cases of intestinal obstruction, as well as examining the usual hernial orifices, as well as in cases of sciatic pain and dysuria. Radiological investigations with contrast medium will identify the contents of the hernia.

d) Treatment

There are two approaches, which can be used separately or in combination. The transabdominal approach is usually required for acute intestinal obstruction. This immediately reveals the diagnosis, as the hernia passes behind the broad ligament and is usually easily reduced by gentle traction. Occasionally it may be necessary to divide the piriformis muscle. The orifice can be repaired either by folding the sac back on itself in order to fill up the defect with the peritoneal plug thus formed, the other method being to use a flap of the piriformis aponeurosis to fill the gap. However, this is a difficult technique and risks injury to the important nerves of the area. Although not yet reported, the use of an extraperitoneal plug or patch of Dacron mesh should prove a useful method.

The posterior route is used in the elective case. The buttock is incised via an oblique incision from the posterior-superior iliac spine as far as the greater trochanter, and this is prolonged by a vertical segment on the lateral side of the thigh. The gluteus maximus is detached and lifted up medially to expose the two spaces above and below the piriformis. The sac is freed and invaginated without opening it. The orifice may be closed by suturing the piriformis to the gluteus medius or to the periosteum of the ilium, being careful to protect the neurovascular pedicles. When a large retroperitoneal tumor herniates into the buttock through one of the sciatic notches (we have seen one such case) a combined approach seems preferable. The abdominal portion of the tumor is resected via the abdomen and the lower part via the buttock. Insertion of a prosthetic mesh is rather easier via the upper approach.

The precise indications and results of these operations are impossible to estimate, given the very small number of published cases, many of which are autopsy studies (of the 35 cases reported by Watson, eight were postmortem).

Reference

Bismuth H, Testart J (1971) Les hernies pelviennes. Encycl Med Chir Ed Paris, Techniques chirurgicales, T 1, fasc 40155

3. Perineal Hernias

We will confine ourselves to spontaneously occurring hernias, excluding those which follow perineal operations. They are also known as pelvic, ischiorectal, pudendal, labial, infrapubic, and vaginal hernias, and also as hernias of the pouch of Douglas. Primary perineal hernias were recognized by de Garangeot (1736). Fewer than 100 cases have been published. The subject was reviewed by R. K. Pearl in the 4th edition of Hernia [Nyhus 1995]. The pelvic floor is formed by the levator ani and ileococcygeus muscles. Two main types of perineal hernia have been described (Fig. 9.34).

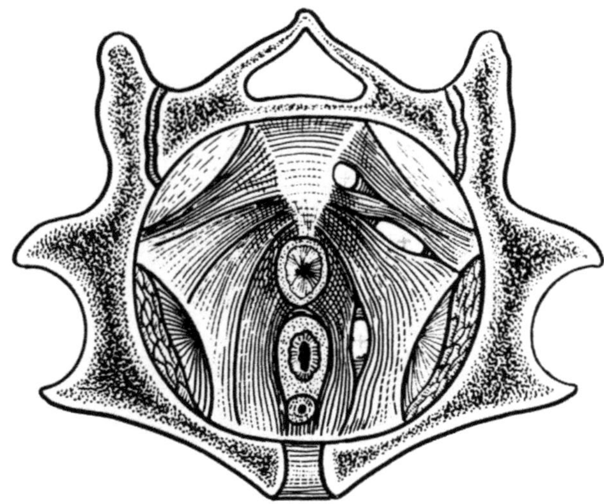

Fig. 9.34. Lateral pelvic hernias emerge through the three orifices shown: anterior to the levator ani, between the levator and coccygeus, posterior to the coccygeus [Guivarc'h & Houssin 1970]

Anterior hernias in women pass in front of the broad ligament and lateral to the bladder, crossing the paravesical fossa and emerging in the perineum in front of the superficial transverse perineal muscle, eventually reaching the labium majus. Posterior hernias pass between the rectum and the bladder in men or between the rectum and the vagina in women, behind the large ligament and lateral to the uterosacral ligament, in the pararectal fossa, and eventually emerge through the ischiococcygeus muscle. Anterior hernias are of equal rarity to sciatic hernias and are three times less common in men than in multiparous women. An abnormally deep pouch of Douglas may explain the predominance of congenital hernias, whereas increased intra-abdominal pressure or an ascitic collection may predispose to the acquired type.

a) Clinical Picture

These symptoms are usually mild. They include some dysuria in anterior hernias and discomfort on standing in large posterior hernias. The crucial physical sign is the finding of a reducible perineal mass with a cough impulse. These features disappear on strangulation, which is a rare event having regard to the breadth of the neck and the degenerate state of the surrounding muscles. These lateral hernias must be distinguished from the various types of vaginal prolapse (rectocele, cystocele or elitrocele) which are the commoner type of midline perineal hernia.

b) Treatment

Surgery is the only treatment. Three approaches may be used.

Laparotomy via a lower midline incision shows the small intestinal colon disappearing into a defect in the pelvic floor. Gentle traction will usually effect reduction, except in large adherent hernias. Pressure on the lower end of the sac will help its emergence into the pelvis. Small defects may be closed by freshening the muscular edges and suturing them with interrupted nonabsorbable stitches. If the defect is large the suture line may be reinforced by a patch of fascia lata or prosthetic material. It is advisable to repair the upper peritoneum following resection or obliteration of the pouch of Douglas [Charrier & Gosset, in Bismuth & Testard 1971].

The perineal approach is more direct and gives good access to the hernial sac, which is easily dissected, opened and resected following reduction of its contents. However it may be difficult to approximate the muscular edges of the hernial defect, using this approach. A combined abdomino-perineal approach is only necessary in those rare cases where a very large hernia is adherent to the soft tissues of the perineum. It is probably better in such a case to excise the distended and redundant perineal skin [Koontz & Kimberly 1959].

The immediate results of operation are usually good, apart from the rare case of strangulation. However, recurrence is common because of the size of the muscular defect and the absence of aponeurotic or tendinous structures which can be used to produce a solid repair. It seems likely therefore that prosthetic materials will come to be used more frequently than in the past, as is the case in many other types of hernia, as already discussed.

References

Bismuth H, Testart J (1971) Les hernies pelviennes. Techniques chirurgicales. Encycl Med Chir Paris T 1, 40155

Pearl KR (1995) Perineal hernia. In: Nyhus LM, Condon RE (eds) Hernia, 4th edn. Lippincott, Philadelphia, p 451

10 Pathology of the Umbilicus

G. Champault

The umbilicus is the cicatrix of the site of implantation of the umbilical cord. This is an area of weakness which gives rise to congenital and acquired hernias. Owing to its connections to certain vestigial structures, the umbilicus is also the site of special pathological processes.

I. Umbilical Hernia

Only acquired hernia in adults will be discussed in this chapter. The reader should consult Chapter 12 (IV) for a discussion of umbilical hernia and omphalocele in children.

Hernia results from dissension of the cicatricial area of the umbilicus. Such hernias account for 6% of all hernias in adults and are most often seen in women in the second half of life [Ajao et al. 1979]. Factors leading to weakness of the umbilical region include pregnancy, obesity, and muscle atrophy [Musca 1967].

A. Pathological Anatomy

Most umbilical hernias are of the direct type. Indirect oblique herniation through Richet's canal is rare (or even contested by certain surgeons). The skin over the hernia is stretched and may show eczematous or ulcerative lesions. The thin, distended peritoneal sac adheres to the integument and to the hernial ring, which resembles a sharp-edged collar. The hernial sac may be subdivided by adhesions or may appear diverticular. The contents of the sac are highly variable and include small bowel or omentum and less often colon, stomach, or even duodenum [Bjorgsvik & Baardsen 1981].

B. Anatomicoclinical Forms

1. Small Hernia

Small umbilical hernia may be asymptomatic. In other cases, tugging or even sharp pain which increases on palpation is encountered. Gastrointestinal disturbances are rare. In thin subjects, the hernia is easily evidenced as a small, round protrusion with unfolding of the umbilical skin at its lower end. The mass can be easily reduced, subsequent to which the rigid outline of the ring is easily palpable. In most cases, the skin appears to be in good condition and the abdominal wall seems tonic.

Small hernia is more difficult to identify in obese patients, since there is no visible protrusion. Careful examination is required to identify the impulsive and more or less reducible mass buried in the fat of the umbilical region.

These hernias tend to increase in size and become irreducible. The major complication is strangulation with sudden onset of acute symptoms associating intestinal occlusion and a hard painful tumefaction which cannot be reduced. Immediate surgical intervention is required. Treatment of small umbilica hernia is simple [Criado 1981; de Medinacelli et al. 1979]. With the patient under general anesthesia, a periumbilical incision is made. The sac is dissected down to its neck, then single-layered closure of the aponeurosis is done. Postoperative course is uneventful, hospitalization is short (3-4 days), and the mortality is nil.

2. Large Hernia

Treatment of large umbilical hernia is problematic. The lesion is evidenced as a very large multilobular tumor covered by thin purplish skin of uneven texture. The mass may be soft or hard and seems to be buried in the fat. Percussion is both sonorous and dull in different parts of the hernia. The force of coughing is more or less transmitted to the hernia. Only very partial reduction can be achieved. This type of hernia is sometimes discovered on hospitalization for various reasons such as abdominal pain with nausea and slight vomiting or interruption of intestinal transit, which regresses either spontaneously after a few days or subsequent to symptomatic treatment.

Large umbilical hernia can lead to various complications.

Skin lesions include eczema, intertrigo, ulceration, lymphangitis, or even abscess or phlegmon. These complications must be treated prior to surgery. Spontaneous rupture [Fischer & Graham-Calkins 1978] is a very rare complication arising subsequent to effort in patients with very severe cutaneous lesions. Hernial peritonitis, also a rare complication, results from episodes of epiploitis; the hernial mass becomes irreducible and shows signs of inflammation with redness, edema, and thickening of the skin. Strangulation is the most important complication. In many cases the onset of strangulation resembles incarceration, but regression does not occur; the patient is often seen at an advanced stage and thus presents with abdominal dissension, arrested intestinal transit, and a voluminous irreducible hernial mass accompanied by dehydration and fever. Emergency surgery is required after preparation for a few hours in the intensive care unit.

Treatment is difficult owing to local, peritoneal, and general risk factors.

Poor patient terrain is the reason for the severity of these large umbilical hernias. Patients are commonly obese women with a flaccid abdominal wall and an enormous hernia, hanging down like an apron over the inferior part of the wall. Cutaneous lesions are almost always present. Diabetes (sometimes undiagnosed) is also rather frequent. Varicose veins or a history of phlebitis further complicate the clinical setting. Many of these patients present with additional hernias (especially femoral) or cardiopulmonary disease (emphysema, chronic bronchitis), conditions which represent a very poor surgical terrain.

Treatment requires surgical intervention, despite the difficulty of repair and the numerous operative risks. Under ideal conditions, surgical repair should be done after thorough local and general preparation, including scrupulous cleansing of the skin, treatment of dermatological lesions, weight loss, cardiovascular and pulmonary evaluation and preparation (respiratory function test, physiotherapy, bronchial mucolytics, antibiotics), and anticoagulants. In some cases of formidable hernia that has "lost the right to reside" in the abdomen, progressive preoperative pneumoperitoneum can be useful.

Surgical repair involves wide omphalectomy [Caravel 1981] with lipectomy via a transverse elliptical incision. The peritoneal cavity is first approached at a distance from the hernia. The herniated viscera are progressively freed from within the sac. The sac is then resected and the viscera are reintroduced into the abdominal cavity. Repair of the abdominal wall is done by transverse fascial suturing or implantation of a prosthesis. Subcutaneous suction drainage is generally required. External reinforcement using adhesive mesh (Contensor) is recommended. The same basic procedures are followed in cases of strangulated hernia. Subsequent to opening of the sac, and according to the lesions observed, the herniated viscera are reintegrated or resection of the involved omentum, small bowel, or colon is done [Wilson 1981]. Postoperative complications include suppuration of the abdominal wall wound dehiscence, and pulmonary and venous disorders. Recurrence is a long-term complication of primary repair. Due to the poor patient terrain, the mortality for these large hernias ranges from 5% to 10%, and up to 15% in cases of strangulation.

3. In Patients with Cirrhosis

Umbilical hernia in patients with cirrhotic ascites results from progressive dissension of the umbilical

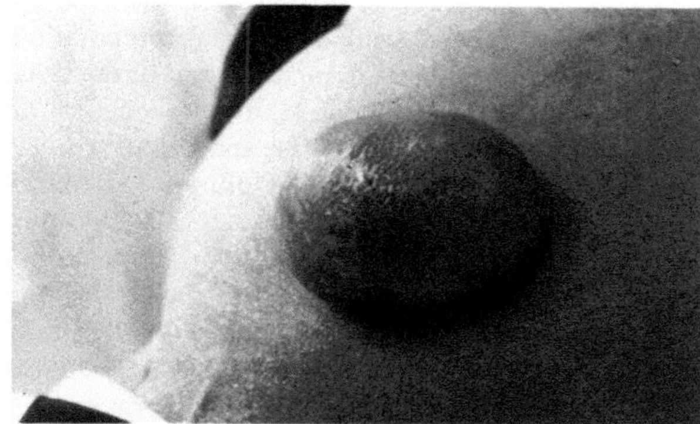
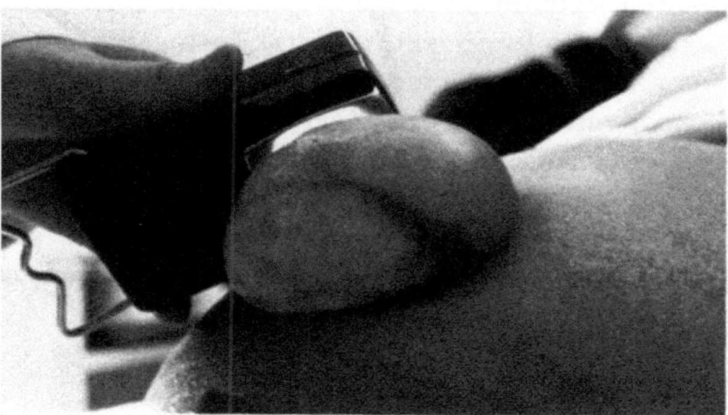

Fig. 10.1. Umbilical hernia. *Above*: trophic lesions; *below*: fluid contents demonstrated by transillumination. (Courtesy of M. Caix)

ring due to the combined effects of increased abdominal pressure, extreme thinning of the abdominal muscles, and chronic malnutrition [Eisenstadt 1979]. The skin of the umbilicus is stretched thin. With the patient standing, the hernia is seen as a cortical or oblong mass, while in the supine position it becomes spherical. The hernia varies in size and may be gigantic in some cases. The herniated area displays numerous veins resulting from the development of the collateral circulation. These hernias are painless. Their size varies with that of the ascites. The contents of the reducible mass are dull on percussion, even though a loop of bowel (generally not adherent) may be found in the sac (Fig. 10.1).

The hernia develops along with the ascites, with episodic complication due to intercurrent disorders, hemorrhage, or nonobservance of dietary restriction. Complications include fissuration with permanent exudasion, and - exceptionally - sudden rupture of the integument on effort. The major risk for these patients is infected ascites. Prognosis is very poor.

Treatment consists of wide omphalectomy, which is done as an emergency procedure in cases of fissuration or rupture. Once again, appropriate preparation is of prime importance and includes care of the skin, evaluation of blood clotting factors, evacuation of ascites by celiocentesis, acid-base and volume equilibration, and administration of diuretics. General anesthesia is preferable to local anesthesia. Rigorous hemostasis is achieved by ligature of the subcutaneous veins distended by the portal hypertension. The ascitic fluid is slowly evacuated. Solid hermetic repair of the abdominal wall is achieved by continuous suturing in order to avoid postoperative leakage. Cicatrization is a slow process in such cases; external reinforcement is helpful. Postoperative care requires scrupulous medical treatment of the ascites. In patients with very poor general health, bandaging of the hernia with evacuation of the ascites is an appropriate temporary risk-free approach to management. The poor prognosis of umbilical rupture in cirrhotic patients is closely correlated to the degree of hepatic insufficiency.

II. Tumors of the Umbilicus

A. Primary Tumors

Tumors of the umbilical region [Blumenthal 1980] are no different from those affecting other parts of the abdominal wall, with the exception of tumor of the embryonic remnants found in this region, i.e., tumor of the urachus, especially cysts and rarely sarcoma, and the exceptional neoplasms of the round ligament or umbilical arteries. Umbilical tumors are usually benign (sebaceous or dermoid cyst, myxoma, fibroma, lipoma, angioma, etc.). Resection of these moderate-sized tumors is not problematic, and repair of the abdominal wall is easily achieved.

B. Secondary Tumors

The umbilicus is a frequent site of metastasis [Galle et al. 1981; Jager & Max 1979]. Generally, umbilical metastasis is seen at the end stage of neoplastic dissemination of primary malignancy of the pancreas, bronchus, kidney, or thyroid gland. In some cases, however, the metastatic lesion of the umbilicus is the first apparent sign of malignancy, and the histological features of the lesion (adenocarcinoma, squamous cell carcinoma, melanosarcoma) obtained from biopsy sampling (which is preferable to needle puncture biopsy) may help to orient the search for the site of the primary tumor.

C. False Tumors

Inflammation leading to profuse granulations may resemble tumor. These granulations can develop in contact with a foreign body, or may be due to recurrent local and chronic infection. In rare cases such tumor-like lesions occur in the umbilical cicatrix resulting from celioscopy [Charles 1981].

Vascular anomalies resulting from portal hypertension may also resemble tumor. The umbilicus, which is the natural site of portosystemic venous shunting, may present a "Medusa-head" venous network in cases of Cruveilhier-Baumgarten syndrome.

A hardened ball of desiccated cells or foreign material can sometimes be found deep in the umbilical skin folds of patients who have poor personal hygiene. *Umbilical endometriosis* [Merrild & Christensen 1982] may also resemble tumor.

III. Fistula and Suppurative Lesions

Suppurative lesions and fistula can be grouped together since they display common symptomatology [Etienne et al. 1982]. The symptoms include pain in the umbilical region (ranging from mild pain or a sensation of local tension to sharp pain on effort) irradiating to the bladder, with a frequent and imperative desire to urinate. At the stage of collected suppuration the pain is exacerbated by contact with clothing, coughing, and sneezing, and it subsides in positions leading to relaxation of the abdominal musculature. Anorexia, nausea, and fever may accompany the pain. On examination, the external umbilical orifice is narrowed by a warm red fluctuant tumefaction, which is very painful to touch. Such a collection will open to the skin. The lesion develops in successive phases of retention and evacuation and eventually becomes a chronic condition. In rare cases, intermittent emission of urine or digestive fluid occurs.

A. Fistula

Umbilical fistula is an abnormal communication between the umbilicus and the digestive or urinary apparatus, or even an embryonic structure.

1. Urinary Fistula

This type of fistula is very rare in adults and results from persistent patency of the urachus. Very rarely, spontaneous or surgical evacuation of an abscess (usually subumbilical) is followed by permanent emission of urine from the umbilicus. Intermittent emission of urine may be seen in patients with urinary retention or increased pressure within the bladder. The presence of recurrent urinary infection should draw attention to the possible existence of this type of fistula. Diagnosis is achieved by opacification of the fistula, by voiding or retrograde cystograms (lateral view), and by the recovery of dye in the urine injected via the fistula.

2. Fistula of the Urachus

This type of fistula is more common than urinary fistula. A cyst of the urachus (usually infected) opens into the umbilicus; the fistula does not communicate with the bladder. Although pollakiuria is often observed, the urine remains sterile. The fistula may manifest as a poorly limited tumefaction deep to the umbilical region. Sonography confirms the midline position of the lesion and its size. Opacification of the fistula is done to confirm the size of the lesion and the absence of communication with the bladder.

3. Fistula of the Digestive Tract

This type of fistulous communication with the umbilicus is more frequent than the above two types and can often be explained on the basis of embryological findings [Mbaku-Nganda et al. 1982]. The more or less long fistula communicates with the ileum, with Meckel's diverticulum, or less frequently with the colon or appendix or even a lesion of Crohn's disease [Philips & Glazer 1981]. Intermittent emission of fecal material or digestive fluid is exceptional. Opacification of the intestinal tract (barium enema, opacification of the ileum) usually does not demonstrate the fistula. Direct opacification of the fistula also gives disappointing results. Fistula resulting from advanced pyostercorous phlegmon, which is the ultimate complication of strangulated hernia, arises via a different mechanism and is accompanied by different symptoms. Diagnosis is based on the patient's history. Such direct fistulas lie in a lateral position and can give off large amounts of fluid.

Mucosal fistula is the most common type of umbilical fistula. It leads to chronic suppuration of the umbilicus. The blind tunnel of the fistula more or less regularly lines the umbilical cavity. The mucosal lining is usually of the digestive rather than the urinary type. The passage of a catheter is rapidly arrested in cases of mucosal fistula. Opacification is either impossible to achieve or difficult to interpret.

4. Treatment

Treatment is relatively standard, regardless of the type of umbilical fistula. Aside from cases where the fistula has been clearly identified on preoperative investigation, the surgical approach should permit correct exploration of the deep layers of the abdominal wall, the subperitoneal space, and even the abdominal cavity. The appropriate approach is therefore via a midline incision centered on the external fistulous orifice (usually a subumbilical incision). Dissection may be difficult owing to the presence of an inflammatory reaction causing fusion of the different structures of the abdominal wall. In such cases, the bowel and omentum often adhere to the deep surface of the peritoneum. Injection of dye allows identification of the often ramified course of the fistula and full resection down to the deep connections of the fistula. According to the case this procedure is completed by resection of a cyst of the urachus, careful suturing of the dome of the bladder with transurethral drainage, or resection of the involved segment of bowel.

B. Suppurative Lesions

1. Secondary Suppuration

The umbilicus is the thinnest part of the abdominal wall, and many suppurative lesions discharge in this region. These secondary lesions include the following: generalized peritonitis due to common pathogens (exceptionally, pneumococcus or tuberculosis); abscess of the appendix or liver, less often periprostatic or ovarian abscess, or intestinal perforation; mesenteric infarction. Diagnosis is usually not achieved due to the rarity of these lesions, which are suggestive of either strangulated hernia with pyostercorous phlegmon or infected cyst of the urachus.

2. Primary Suppuration

Even less frequent than the above secondary lesions, primary suppuration is diagnosed by elimination. Two concomitant factors contribute to the development of primary suppuration: narrowing of the external umbilical orifice (in some cases of pathological origin such as fibroma or myxoma) and poor hygiene. These two factors lead to retention of sebaceous secretion, dead cells, hairs from the umbilical region, or foreign material such as cloth fibers, coal dust, and chalk. Accumulation of these substances causes obstruction of the cutaneous orifice, thereby transforming the umbilicus into a veritable pouch. Infection can result from growth of pathogens found on the skin (*Escherichia coli, Staphylococcus aureus*), and local inflammation will develop. It may either regress or develop into a veritable abscess. Evacuation of the abscess usually occurs spontaneously or subsequent to local treatment. However, in some cases the abscess diffuses to the subcutaneous tissue to form an induration centered around the umbilicus. In rare cases, the abscess extends deep to the linea alba, invading the subperitoneal space via the urachus and round ligament. An exceptional finding is rupture of the abscess into the abdominal cavity. The abscess may be free or sequestered by the anterior surface of the stomach or transverse colon.

The urine is always sterile in these cases. The patient consistently presents with more or less pronounced polymorphonuclear leukocytosis. Bacteriological analysis of the abscess usually reveals the presence of staphylococci, streptococci, or colibacilli. At the stage at which a chronic sinus is present, umbilicography (using hydrosoluble contrast material) can be used to identify the size of the abnormal cavity and to look for extension of the lesion deep to the linea alba. Echography will demonstrate the depth of the abscess (shirt-stud abscess). Such abscess develops as successive retention and evacuation and eventually becomes a chronic condition.

Treatment. At the initial stage, primary uncollected suppuration requires only local treatment: alcohol dressings; evacuation of the concretion after gentle dilatation of the stenotic orifice; local irrigation with antiseptic solutions. Anatomical factors predisposing to suppuration require surgical repair in order to avoid recurrence. In cases of collected suppuration, the abscess should be evacuated followed by excision of the necrotic tissue and opening of the cutaneous orifice. The surgeon should then explore for a possible deep communication. In some cases, partial or total resection of the periumbilical tissue is required.

IV. Conclusion

During embryonic life the umbilicus is a markedly developed zone. In most adults interest is focused on the umbilicus for psychological rather than pathological reasons.

References

Ajao OG, Tolarjejr, Richardson M, Gaventa WC (1979) Umbilical hernia and surgical indication. Trop Doct 9: 176-177

Blumenthal NJ (1980) Umbilical tumors: a case report and review of literature. S Afri Med J 58: 457-458

Bjorgsvik D, Baardsen A (1981) Umbilical hernia with duodenal obstruction. Acta Chir Scand 147: 295

Caravel JB (1981) Plasties abdominales: Technique personnelle de reconstruction ombilicale. Report de la cicatrice au fond de l'ombilic. Ann Chir Plast 3: 289-292

Charles S (1981) Pelvic and umbilical endometriosis presenting with hemorrhagic pleural effusion: a case report. Int Surg 66: 277-278

Chevrel JP (1996) Hernies inguinales, crurales et ombilicales. La Revue du Praticien 46: 1015-1023

Criado FJ (1981) A simplified method of umbilical herniorraphy. Surg Gynecol Obstet 153: 904

de Medinacelli L, Coubret P, Ebrard P (1979) A propos de 180 cas de hernies ombilicales opérées selon un nouveau procédé de réparation. J Chir (Paris) 116: 361-364

Eisenstadt S (1979) Symptomatic umbilical hernias after peritoneo-venous shunt. Arch Surg 114: 1143

Etienne JC, Champault G, Patel JC (1982) Les suppurations primitives de l'ombilic; à propos de 3 cas. Actualités Digestives 4: 119-122

Fisher J, Graham-Calkins W (1978) Spontaneous umbilical hernia rupture. A report of 3 cases. Am J Gastroenterol 69: 689-693

Galle PC, Jobson VW, Homesley HD (1981) Umbilical metastasis from gynecologic malignancies: a primary carcinoma of the fallopian tube. Obstet Gynecol 57: 531-533

Jager RM, Max MH (1979) Umbilical metastasis as the presenting symptom of cecal carcinoma. J Surg Oncol 12: 41-45

Merrild U, Christensen PB (1982) Umbilical endometriosis. Ugeskr Laeger (Den) 144: 159

Mbaku-Nganda W, Wansondela L, Kaya A, Iyethi B (1982) Diverticule de Meckel révélé par une fistule ombilicale chez un garçon de 28 mois. Ann Chir 36: 730-731

Musca AA (1967) Umbilical and ventral herniorraphy: a review of 1000 cases. Int Surg 48: 169-179, 279-285

Phillips RKS, Glazer G (1981) Metastatic Crohn's disease of the umbilicus. Br Med J 283

Rives J, Azoulay C, Nicaise H (1971) Hernies ombilicales de l'adulte. Techniques Chirurgicales, vol 1, fasc 40145, Encycl Med Chir, Paris

Wilson HK (1981) Reconstruction of the umbilicus. Plast Reconstr Surg 67: 564-565

11 Abdominoplasty

D. Marchac

The desire to improve the appearance of an unaesthetic abdomen dates back to antiquity. As described in the Babylonian Talmud (300 BC), Rabbi Eliezer underwent a procedure to resect a considerable amount of abdominal fat [Simon 1966]. Early contemporary publications [see Aston 1980] were also devoted to abdominal lipectomy in obese subjects, as initially proposed in France by Demars and Marx in 1890 [Rees 1980]. In 1905, Gaudet and Morestin presented to the French Congress of Surgery a horizontal technique of cutaneoadipose resection with preservation of the umbilicus [Rees 1980]. In the United States, Kelly [in Rees 1980] proposed transverse resection for purely aesthetic reasons as early as 1910. Since these pioneering studies, a multitude of techniques have been introduced. These can be divided into four groups.

Transverse incision has been proposed by Kelly (1899), Morestin (1911), Thorek (1924) [according to Rees 1980] and by Delbet (1928) [Aston 1980]. More recently, a very low transverse technique has been studied by Vernon (1957), Pitanguy (1967), Callia (1967), Grazer (1973), Regnault (1975), and Vilain (1975) (see Fig. 11.1).

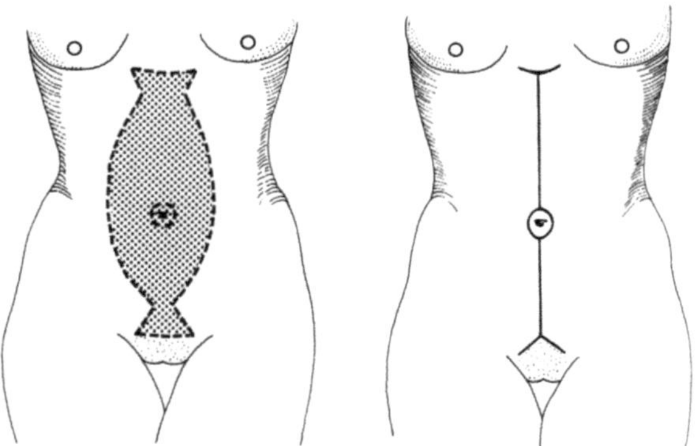

Fig. 11.2. Vertical xiphopubic approach recommended by Fischl (1973) to remove redundant periumbilical skin

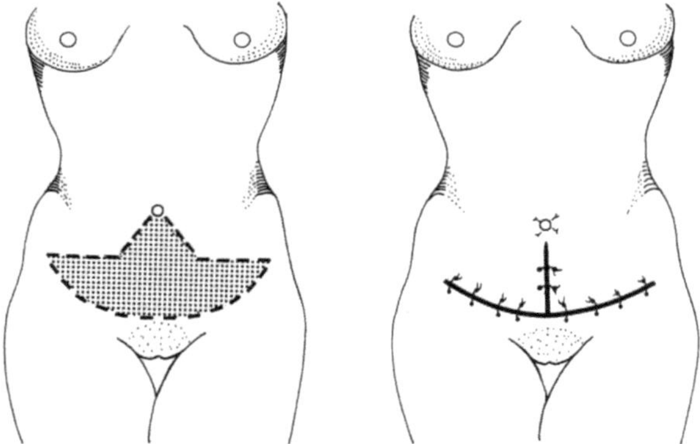

Fig. 11.3. Combined vertical and transverse incision. [Dufourmentel & Mouly 1959]

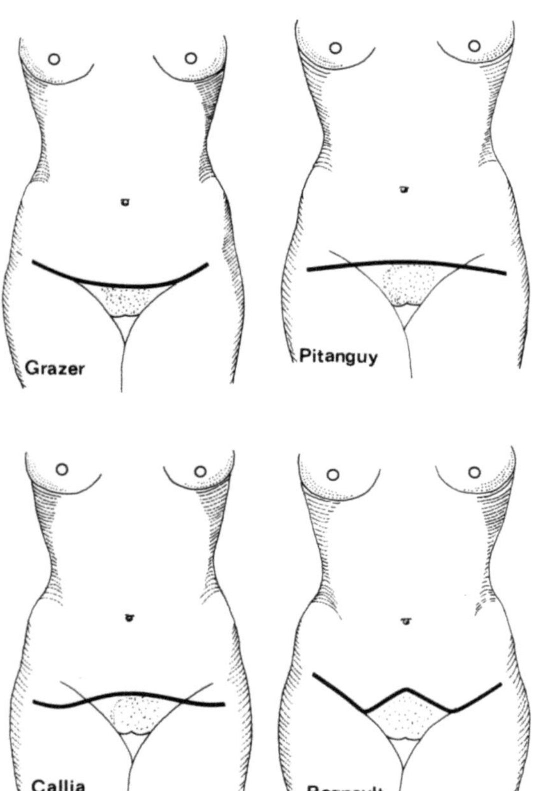

Fig. 11.1. Different types of low transverse incisions

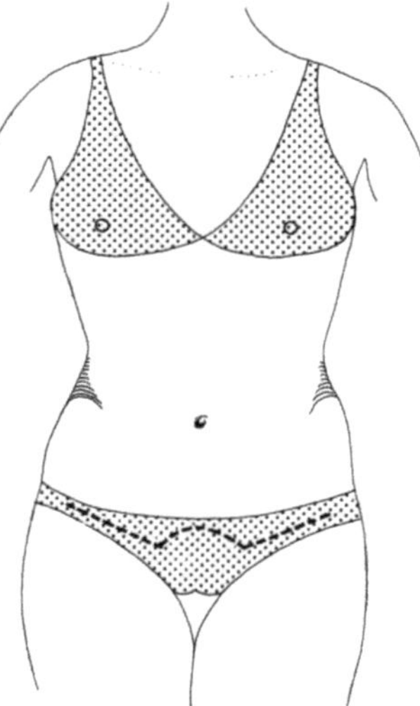

Fig. 11.4. The ideal final scar should lie below the waistline. The umbilicus lies 1 cm above the iliac crests

Vertical xiphopubic incision has been recommended by Desjardins (1911) [Aston 1980], Babcock (1916), Schepelmann (1918) [Aston 1980], and recently by Fischl (1973) in cases of central abdominal adiposity with few striae (see Fig. 11.2).

Combined transverse and vertical resection, leading to a cicatrix in the shape of an inverted T, has been proposed in Germany by Weinhold (1909) [Aston 1980] and in France by Dufourmentel and Mouly (1959) (see Fig. 11.3).

Midabdomen abdominoplasty has been recommended by Passot (1931) [Aston 1980], Galtier (1955), and Stuckey (1979).

In Western countries the goal is to conceal the scar of abdominoplasty below the waistline. Accordingly, low transverse resection has become the most widely used procedure (Fig. 11.4), as outlined by many authors [Lagache & Vandenbussche 1971; Elbaz & Flageul 1977; Jackson & Downie 1978]. However, this procedure is not always possible, and the other techniques thus retain special indications. A patient may request abdominoplasty for many different reasons. The heavy adipose panniculus of obese patients, multiple abdominal scars, and disappearance of the umbilicus raise special problems which will be discussed separately in this chapter. Emphasis will be given to the more common cases of abdominal wall deterioration resulting from pregnancy and variations in body weight.

I. Consultation Prior to Abdominoplasty

Most patients who consult are women, although some men come to seek removal of redundant skin persisting after significant weight loss. The patients complain especially of the disgraceful appearance of their abdomen exposed on summer holiday owing to the presence of pendulous folds and wrinkles. Others request treatment of an abnormally prominent abdomen which can be seen to bulge beneath light clothing. Many patients seen on consultation have tried other measures, especially exercise, which is excellent for improving the strength of the abdominal muscles but obviously cannot suppress diastasis of the recti abdomini or redundant skin.

Examination of the abdominal wall is done to evaluate the quality of the skin, the adipose panniculus,

and the status of the myofascial wall. The patient is examined while standing. The skin is examined for signs of redundancy, which may be general, or may predominate in the supra- or subumbilical region or even the midabdominal area. One should immediately check whether the subumbilical skin can be brought down to the pubis. When this is possible, a low horizontal cicatrix can usually be achieved.

Striae are very common in candidates for abdominoplasty. These markings are secondary to pregnancies or past obesity and may either be disseminated or predominate in one region of the abdomen.

When the striae lie mainly in the subumbilical region they can be removed; supraumbilical or lateral striae are simply lowered.

In some cases, localized cutaneous dissension is accompanied by striae, especially in the periumbilical region; the skin appears fine, plicate, and practically cicatricial. These are the most difficult cases to treat, when overall lowering of the abdominal apron can not be done.

Special attention should be given to the identification of any scars from previous surgery. The presence of transverse or oblique scars in the upper part of the abdominal wall may contraindicate abdominoplasty, since they compromise the vitality of the large superior flap.

The patient's adiposity is next examined. In cases of average adiposity, special precautions must be taken during abdominoplasty to avoid the creation of a step-like appearance of the low horizontal scar with protrusion of the two ends of the scar or insufficient definition of the umbilicus (Fig. 11.7). Where marked adiposity is observed, the patient should be advised to lose weight. Lipolysis or resection without dissection may be required in such cases.

The status of the myofascial wall determines the degree of anterior projection of the abdomen. Diastasis of the recti abdomini is often responsible for a veritable anterior protrusion which is very bothersome to many patients (Fig. 11.6). The quality of the muscles is best assessed with the patient supine. Requesting the patient to elevate the shoulders or legs makes it possible to measure the diastasis, which often predominates in the midabdominal region (just above and below the umbilicus). The muscles are often of good quality, since many patients have tried exercises in an attempt to improve the appearance of their abdomen. The possibilities of subumbilical skin resection are also evaluated by placing the patient in the semi-seated position.

II. Therapy

Abdominoplasty is currently most often done to create an aesthetic abdomen. The goals of therapy include: suppression of redundant skin; possible resection of the subumbilical fatty layer; repair of diastasis of the recti abdomini with renewed tension of the myofascial layer; creation of the best possible cicatrix that can be hidden by clothes below the waistline.

A. Low Transverse Incision

This approach offers the best chances of achieving the above-described goals of abdominoplasty. The procedure consists of resection of the subumbilical part of the abdomen, with the umbilical orifice brought down to the pubis. It is important to ensure that the skin is sufficiently lax. Preoperative measurements should be made with the patient standing (Fig. 11.5a), especially to identify the midline and any possible asymmetry.

We begin by circumscribing the umbilicus with a circular incision. The pedicle of the umbilicus is then freed down to the aponeurotic layer, care being taken to avoid excessive denudation. The next step is to make a modified Grazer's incision (Fig. 11.5a) along the superior edge of the pubic hair, then down toward the inguinal groove, and finally slightly upward along the natural folds of skin. The superficial epigastric and superficial circumflex iliac arteries must be ligated. Beginning at the lowest site of incision, dissection is done upward, flush with the fascial layer. The prefascial areolar tissue is left in place. The blood vessels are carefully coagulated prior to their retraction. Once the umbilicus has been reached, it is convenient to split the middle of the abdominal flap vertically, thereby giving better access to the upper part of the abdomen. The prefascial dissection must be pursued up to the xiphoid process on the midline and out to the costal margin, laterally.

Work can now be started on *the myofascial layer*, after thorough hemostasis has been achieved. The diastasis of the recti abdomini is repaired by a series of buried figure-of-8 sutures (Fig. 11.6e). The laxity of the fascia is assessed by pinching it on the midline. The midline must be carefully identified and the suturing done from the pubis to the xiphoid process. This procedure is almost always indicated to create renewed tension of the myofascial layer. In cases of pronounced diastasis of the recti abdomini it may be preferable to open the rectus sheath in order to perform overlap suturing. We use mersilene (gauge 00) sutures for the myofascial layer.

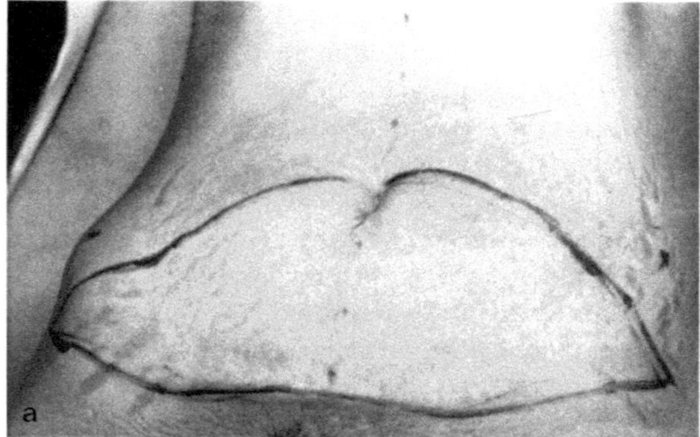

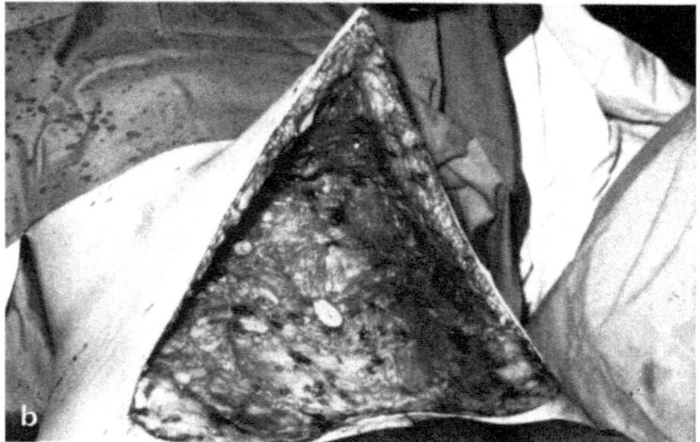

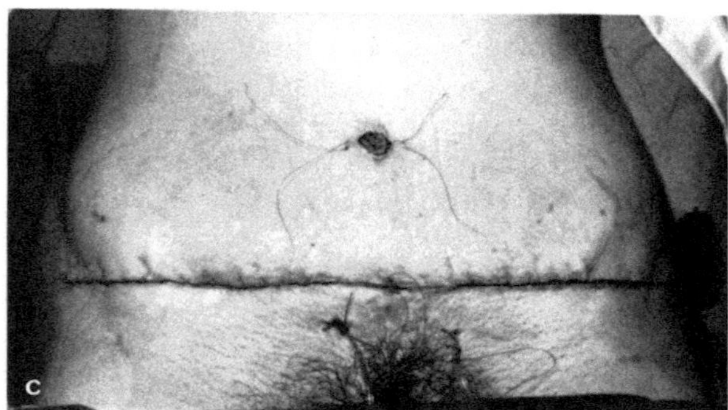

Fig. 11.5a-c. Typical low transverse procedure. **a** The midline and the anterior iliac spines have been identified and a drawing has been made preoperatively. The cutaneous redundancy allows the supraumbilical skin to be easily brought down to the pubis. **b** A circular incision has been made around the umbilicus, which is left in place. Prefascial dissection is done up to the xiphoid process and out to the costal margin. **c** The abdominal flap has been brought down with two-layered suturing including intradermal closure of the skin. The umbilicus is exteriorized. Tension has been renewed on the myofascial layer

The umbilicus is carefully reinserted on the fascia, which is plicated using four cruciform sutures. The umbilical pedicle, which is usually excessively long, can be shortened. Midline plication of the fascia can be complemented by lateral oblique plication in cases where vertical laxity is evidenced.

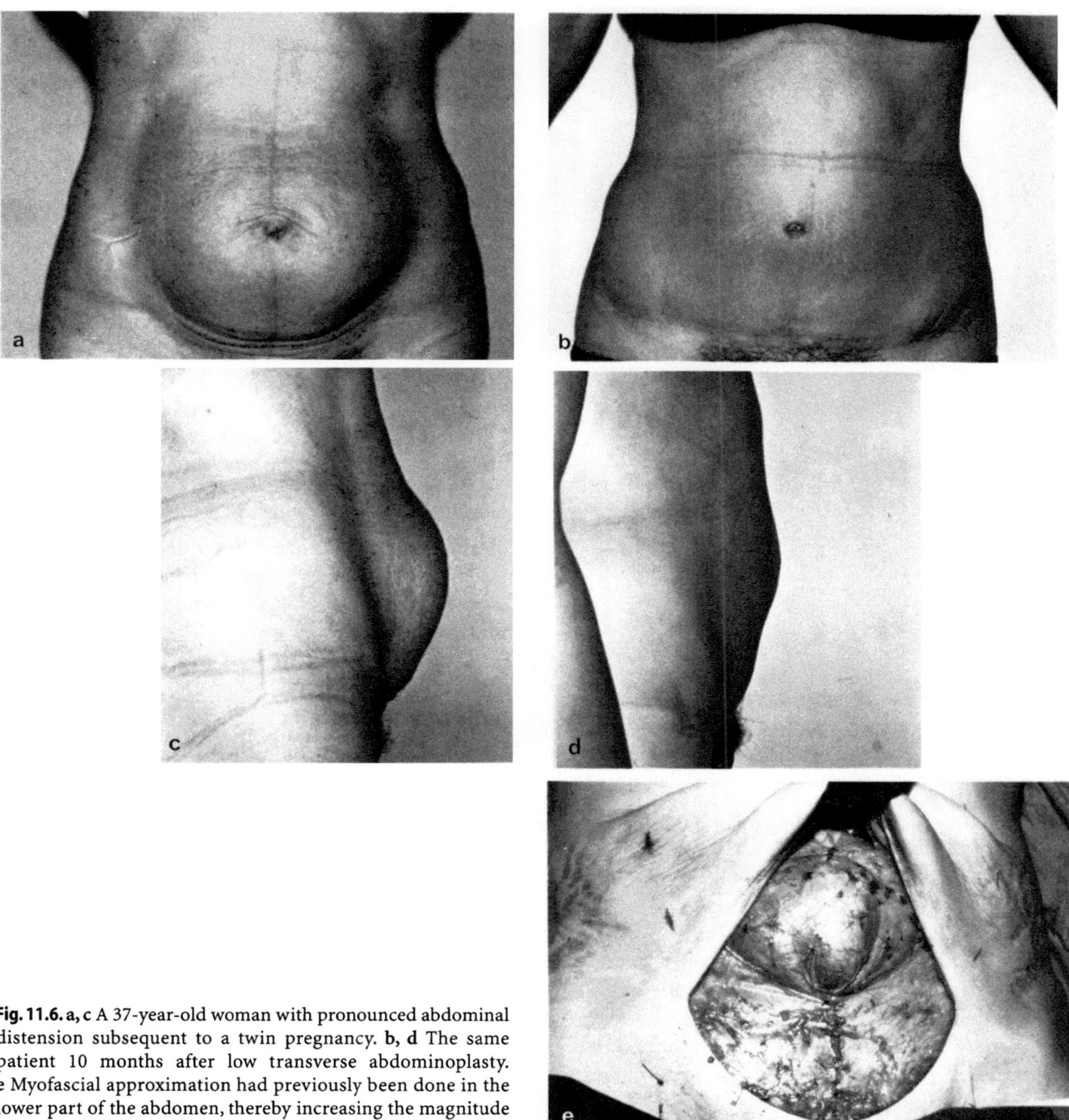

Fig. 11.6. a, c A 37-year-old woman with pronounced abdominal distension subsequent to a twin pregnancy. **b, d** The same patient 10 months after low transverse abdominoplasty. **e** Myofascial approximation had previously been done in the lower part of the abdomen, thereby increasing the magnitude of the diastasis of the recti abdomini

Cutaneoadipose resection is now begun. For this purpose the operating table is tilted slightly and the patient's thighs are elevated (a pillow is slipped under the knees). The first step is to check that the supraumbilical edge of skin can be brought down to the inferior, suprapubic edge. A temporary suture is then made on the midline. Identification of the future umbilical orifice must be made with great care. The surgeon should use the preoperative tracing for identification of the midline. The correct horizontal level is found by palpating the umbilicus beneath the lowered abdominal flap. A transfixing needle can be used to assist identification. A horizontal incision (2 cm long) is made, and the deep fat at the periphery of the incision is very carefully removed.

Cutaneoadipose resection is then begun by pulling the two lowered flaps downward and medially. The incision is made perpendicular to the skin, whereas

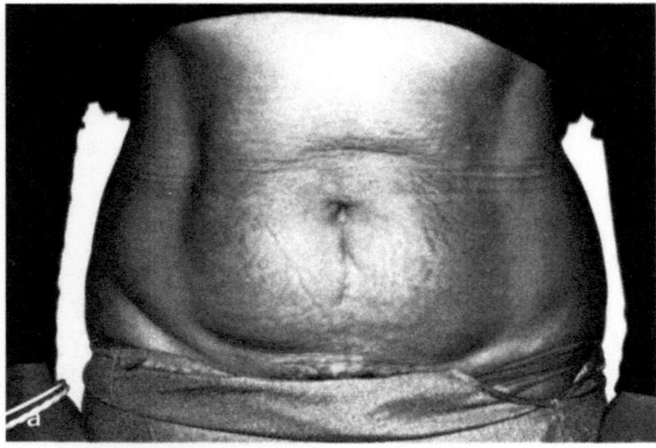

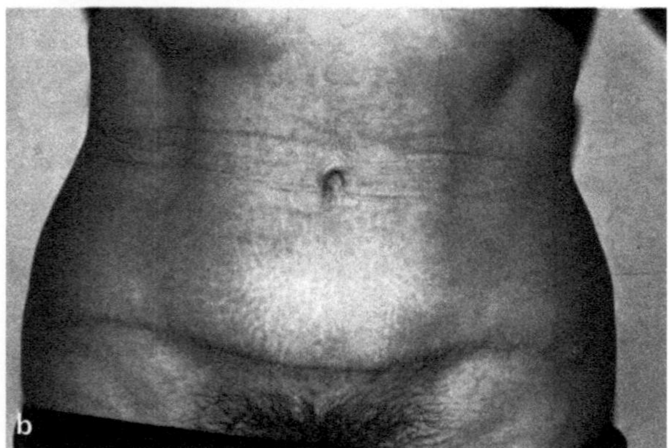

Fig. 11.7. a A 29-year-old woman after two pregnancies and gynecological surgery. **b** The same woman 8 months after low transverse abdominoplasty, which removed the midline subumbilical scar. Since the patient presented marked fatty excess, lipectomy (beveled) was done along the deep surface of the abdominal flap to avoid any shifting effect

beneath it, the incision should be beveled to decrease the thickness of the fatty layer (Fig. 11.7).

Suturing can now be started. We do two-layered suturing. The fatty and deep dermal layer is closed by interrupted inversion sutures (Dexon 3/0), and the skin by a continuous intradermal suture (Prolene 3/0) with adhesive strips added.

The unequal length of the wound edges is corrected by slightly puckering the upper edge. In some cases, the skin removal must be extended laterally beyond the anterior iliac spines; the extension is then made horizontally in the skin creases so that the scar remains below the waistline. The umbilicus is brought out and sutured in two layers with intradermal continuous suturing or interrupted U stitching within the skin (see Fig. 11.14b).

Two suction drains are installed. A plaster shield is made over the dressing. This shield allows even distri-

bution of pressure by a l-kg sand bag and inhibits (for 48 h) excessive movements of torsion or flexion of the abdomen.

The legs are mobilized and the patient is advised to ambulate on the morning after surgery in order to reduce the risk of thromboembolism.

B. Combined Low Transverse and Vertical Incision

This combined procedure may be required in cases where the supraumbilical flap cannot be brought down sufficiently low. In some cases a short vertical incision (4-5 cm long) is sufficient to allow the main transverse incision at the desired inferior level (Figs. 11.3 and 11.8). In other cases the vertical incision runs up to the umbilicus. The combined approach allows transverse resection to diminish the width of the abdominal flap, thereby facilitating the approximation of the upper and lower horizontal skin margins. However, this approach is rarely indicated, since the aim of abdominoplasty is to avoid a visible scar (Fig. 11.1).

C. Indications, Resulting Scar, and Complications

The scar resulting from abdominoplasty merits special emphasis, since this is the prime factor to be evaluated and discussed with the patient before operation. The surgeon must not only deterrnine the most appropriate type of abdominoplasty in a given case, but also clearly explain to the patient the result to be expected regarding the myofascial repair, the suppression of existing striae, and the final scar.

The site of the scar must be indicated to the patient by drawing it on the abdomen. Indeed, many patients think the scar will be much shorter and lower than it really is (Figs. 11.6 and 11.7). The surgeon should also point out that healing of the scar will take a full year and that a transient phase of hypertrophy will render it highly visible. The final appearance of the cicatrix is highly variable, according to the individual case. The scar may be a fine line that is only slightly visible, or it may become distended, pigmented, or discolored. It should be emphasized that an unsightly scar with uneven contours or slight overlapping of the upper margin may justify a second, corrective operation 6-12 months later. When the above features of the scar are explained, some candidates for surgery will prefer to keep their moderate cutaneoadipose excess, and they should not be convinced otherwise.

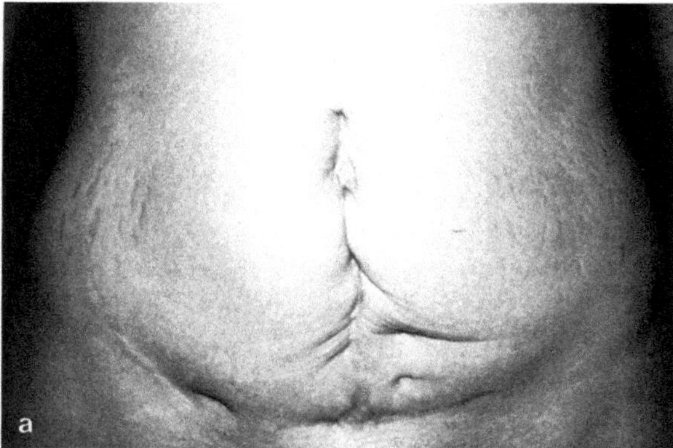

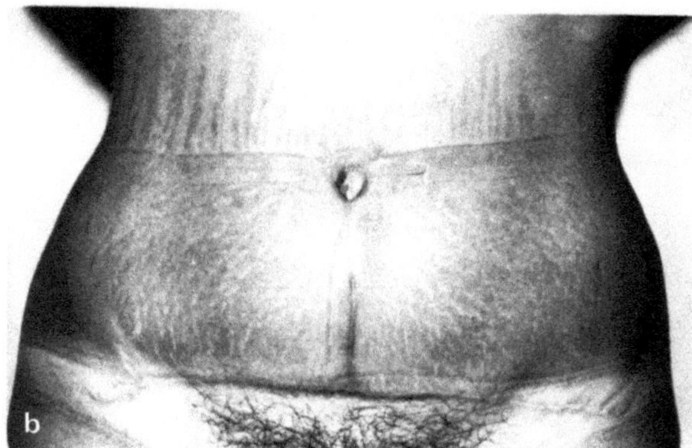

Fig. 11.8. a Patient with abdominal scarring and a midline cicatrix extending above the umbilicus subsequent to tubal pregnancy complicated by hemorrhage. The umbilicus has practically disappeared. **b** The same patient 6 months after abdominoplasty via a low horizontal incision combined with a short vertical incision

With patients who have accepted the facts concerning the scar, the next step is to explain the possible complications of abdominoplasty.

1. Hematoma

This is the most frequent complication of abdominoplasty, owing to the considerable area of surgical dissection. We have not encountered massive hematoma requiring reoperation, although four cases were seen in which partial reopening of the horizontal closure was required to evacuate blood clots. The continuous intradermal suture allows closure to be done without affecting the appearance of the final scar.

2. Lymph Effusion

This complication may arise as a result of the vast prefascial dissection and incision of the upper part of the inguinal lymph channels. Careful preservation of the prefascial areolar sheet and proper ligation may account for our finding of only one case of lymph effusion in 143 abdominoplasties. Repeated puncture and the wearing of an elastic brace are usually sufficient to achieve regression of this complication.

3. Cutaneous Necrosis

This complication is also related to the extensive surgical dissection (Fig. 11.5b). We have seen cases of cutaneous insult only at the site of junction of the flaps in cases of combined T-shaped incision. Significant cutaneous necrosis was reported by Aston (1980) in one patient who smoked 3 packs of cigarettes per day; heavy smoking may have played a role in this case. The surgeon should also identify all old transverse or oblique scars at a higher site, since these may compromise the vascularization of the abdomen.

4. Thromboembolism

The risk of this complication must be thoroughly evaluated by questioning of the patient and clinical examination. We refuse to operate on patients with a history of thromboembolism, since prophylactic anticoagulant therapy carries a high risk of hematoma in the area of vast surgical dissection. Interruption of high-dose oral contraceptives 5 weeks prior to surgery and per- and postoperative infusion of dextran have been advocated. Regardless of these precautions, this complication may occur. Accordingly, it is necessary to monitor the patients closely after surgery.

In a study of 10,490 abdominoplasties reported by Grazer and Goldwyn (1977), the incidence of deep phlebitis was 1.1% and that of pulmonary embolism 0.8%. The latter was the cause of death for six patients (0.1%).

In agreement with most plastic surgeons, we recommend postoperative mobilization of the lower limbs and ambulation on the day after surgery. To date we have seen no cases of significant postoperative phlebitis or embolism.

D. Special Cases

1. Localized or Minor Cases

Cutaneous redundancy essentially involving the subumbilical region with a short supraumbilical segment can sometimes be treated by simple low transverse resection with moderate superior dissection not affecting the umbilicus. A peripubic incision can be used, as proposed by Elbaz (1974) and Glicenstein (1975) (Fig. 11.9). In cases of essentially periumbilical

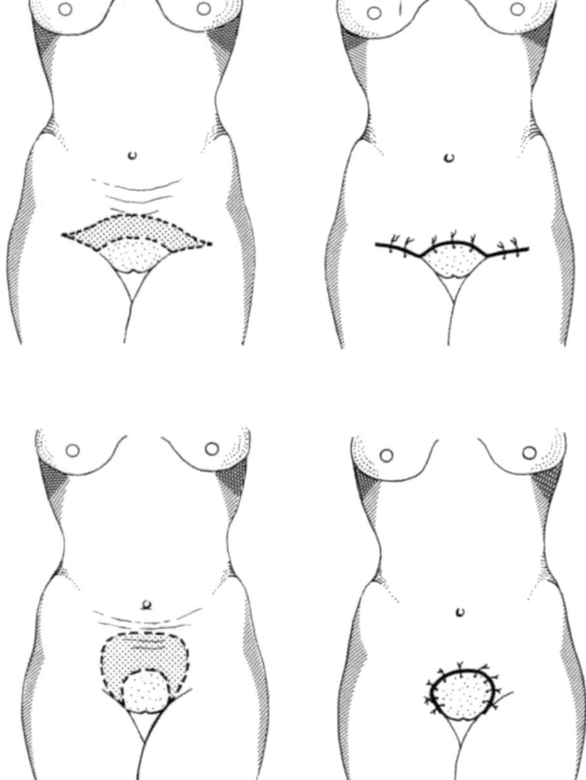

Fig. 11.9. Suprapubic resection [Glicenstein 1975] or peripubic resection [Elbaz 1974] to treat limited dissension of the subumbilical region

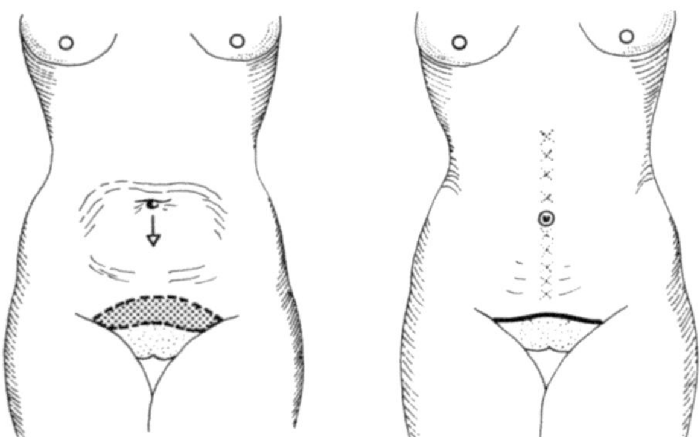

Fig. 11.10. Minor abdominoplasty to correct supraumbilical cutaneous redundancy. The umbilicus is detached and repositioned at a lower site. Correction of diastasis of the recti abdomini and suprapubic resection will then be done

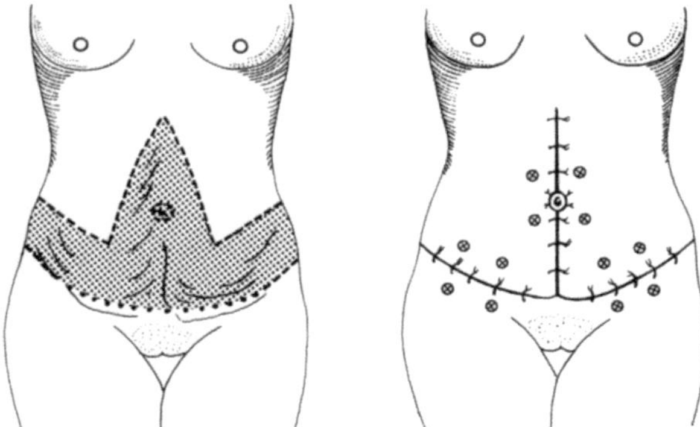

Fig. 11.11. Cutaneoadipose redundancy in a patient with past obesity can be resected by an inverted T incision without dissection [from Castanares & Goethel 1967]

lesions, where the skin shows striae and puckering, direct peripheral or horizontal resection can be done. However, satisfactory results are rarely obtained when this procedure is used.

Cutaneous redundancy essentially involving the supraumbilical region can be corrected by low transverse abdominoplasty with detachment of the umbilicus; it is then repositioned 3-4 cm lower down. A short suprapubic incision can be used to achieve dissection, repair of diastasis of the recti abdomini (frequently associated), repositioning of the umbilicus, and low horizontal resection over a distance of 5-6 cm (Fig. 11.10).

2. Major Cases or Those Accompanying Old Scars

The prominent fat in obese patients can be removed via a large transverse approach without dissection. In cases of transverse redundancy a T-shaped resection is done (Figs. 11.11 and 11.12). Belt lipectomy or circu-

lar lipectomy, as proposed by Gonzalez-Ulloa (1960) and Vilain and Dubousset (1964) may also be appropriate (Fig. 11.13). Once the anterior and lateral resection is done, the patient is placed prone, and posterior resection is preformed. Hematoma, disunion, and delayed cicatrization are more frequently seen in these cases.

In patients with an old vertical xiphopubic midline scar, spindle-like vertical resection can be done (subsequent to circumscription of the umbilicus). Repair of the cutaneomyofascial layer and resection of the excessive skin and fat are thus easily accomplished.

However, the surgeon should be aware that a "dog ear" may appear in the xiphoid area. The procedure is terminated by midline closure, and one of the aims of abdominoplasty is therefore not achieved, i.e., a non-visible abdominal scar (Fig. 11.2).

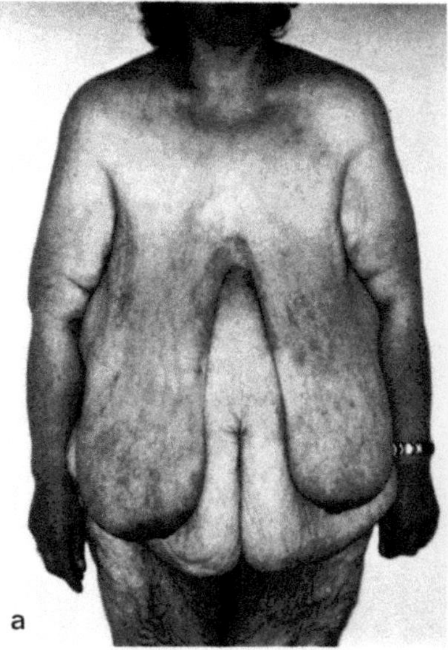 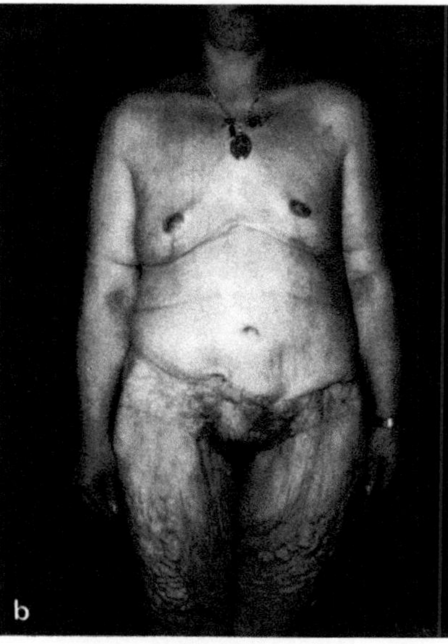

Fig. 11.12. a A 28-year-old patient after weight loss of 85 kg. **b** The same patient 1 year after resection. Mammoplasty with free grafting of the nipples and resection of redundancy along the inner surface of the arm have been done. Improvement of the thigh and abdominal scar can be done

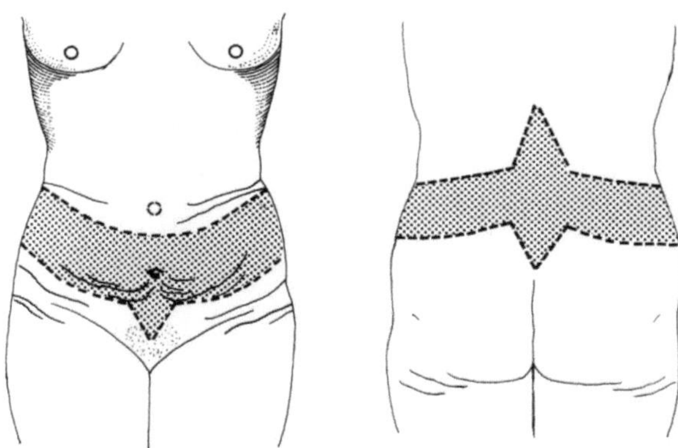

Fig. 11.13. Belt lipectomy may be indicated in cases of redundancy that also involve the flanks and the back [from Gonzalez-Ulloa 1960]

3. Associated Lipolysis

Aspiration of the fatty layer using a blunt cannula [Illouz 1983] allows reduction of the abdominal panniculus practically on request. The aspiration is done via deep subcutaneous tunnel-like channels (parallel or divergent). The fibrous and neurovascular structures are left intact.

This technique may be sufficient to remove limited fatty excess, although it is especially advantageous when combined with abdominoplasty in cases where diffuse fatty excess persists.

Aspiration is rendered easier by a preliminary massive infiltration with cold adrenaline/saline using a pump. A number of small incisions will allow the insertion of cannulae of three to four mm in diameter, which will enable one to restore the fatty layer to the desired thickness. It is necessary to conserve a regular layer of fat to avoid irregularities in outline and adherence to the deeper tissues.

4. Endoscopic Correction

When an abdominal protrusion is due not only to an excess of fatty tissue but also to divarication of the recti, an endoscopic approach achieves a satisfactory correction with a minimal degree of scarring (Fig. 11.14).

Having carried out liposuction of the abdominal wall, a short (5 mm) suprapubic incision is made. The midline area is then freed under endoscopic control, disinserting the umbilicus, as far up as the xiphoid process.

The divarication is then corrected with a running suture of O mersilene, and the umbilicus replaced.

Following liposuction and extensive freeing, the skin usually retracts well (aided by the application of an abdominal support belt), but if there is a significant excess of skin, it is advisable to carry out a short suprapubic resection of a 20 × 5 cm fusiform strip, using the endoscope only for correcting the diastasis in its sub-xiphoid portion.

5. Umbilicoplasty

The umbilicus is an essential component of the normal abdomen; thus, its two main features must be preserved or reconstructed [Baroudi et al. 1974], i.e., the

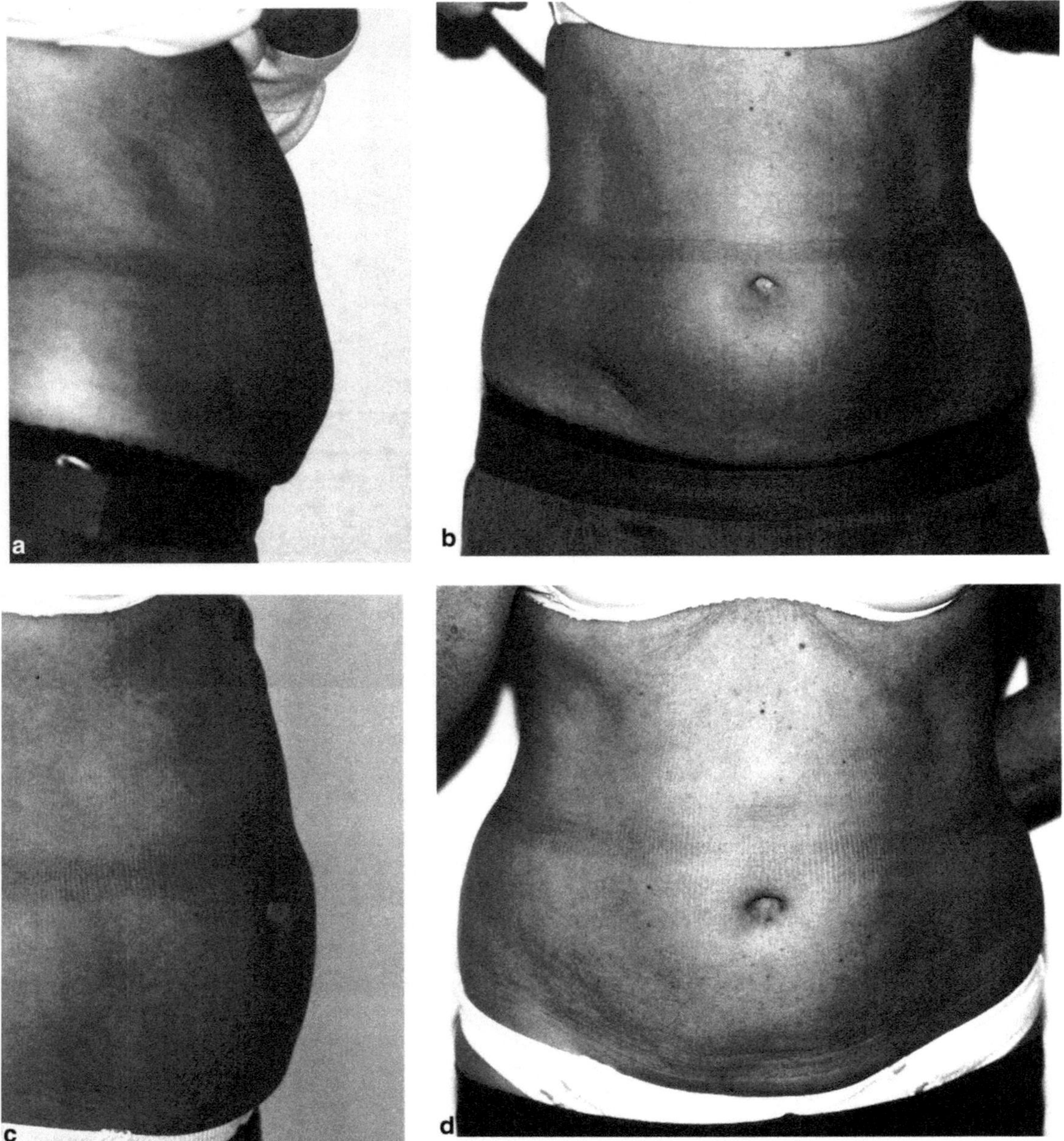

Fig. 11.14. a, b Patient aged 52 presenting with an abdominal protusion together with divarication of the recti and gross excess of subcutaneous fat. **c, d** One year after liposuction and endoscopic correction of the divarication through a short suprapubic incision

ovoid vertical depression of the abdominal wall and the umbilical pit adherent to the fascial layer.

Preservation of the umbilicus in the course of a midline incision requires that a precise incision be made around the umbilicus. To avoid slipping or excessive beveling in the tough skin of this region, tension is applied with two hooks and the edge of the umbilicus is held by multi-toothed forceps. A gauge-15 scalpel can then be used to make the incision precisely at the periphery of the umbilical ring, after which preumbilical cleavage can be started (Fig. 11.15a).

Careful suturing must be done to avoid punctiform scars. We use either a continuous intradermal suture (Fig. 11.15b) or interrupted U-shaped sutures knotted from within. A midline vertical section passing through the fundus of the umbilicus is also sometimes used.

Exteriorization of the umbilicus in the course of abdominoplasty must be done precisely. It is often necessary to shorten the umbilical pedicle and then anchor it to the fascial wall (Fig. 11.16). Identification of the future umbilical orifice is a delicate procedure which must take into account the tension of the abdominal wall. The umbilicus lies at the intersection between the midline and a horizontal line running 1 cm above the iliac crests (see Fig. 11.4). We prefer to make a 2-cm-long horizontal incision slightly concave inferiorly, which will become oval shaped when traction is applied. Deep removal of the fat of the wound margins is helpful to recreate an umbilical depression (Fig. 11.17). Juri et al. (1979) and Delerm (1982) proposed the interpositioning of a small superior pedicle skin flap to prevent stricture of the circular periumbilical cicatrix. However, periumbilical stricture rarely occurs if the orifice is sufficiently large and the sutures have been carefully made. In cases where such stric-

ture occurs, Z-plasty can be used as a corrective procedure.

Detachment of the umbilicus flush with the fascia may be indicated to allow resection of redundant supraumbilical skin (Figs. 11.10 and 11.18), in which case the umbilicus is reinserted lower down. This procedure is also sometimes necessary in the course of secondary correction of an insufficient primary abdominoplasty if the umbilical dimple does not lie over the site of umbilical fascial attachment.

The umbilical pedicle is sectioned flush with the fascia via a suprapubic incision. The fascial wound is carefully closed and the umbilical pedicle reinserted at the desired site, often with plication being done (four cruciform sutures) to shorten the pedicle.

Displacement of the cutaneous umbilical orifice is sometimes required in cases where it was not properly positioned in a previous procedure. A fairly long linear scar can be avoided using the method proposed by Delerm (1982), i.e., closure of the malpositioned orifice by a small flap derived from the newly created orifice.

Creation of a new umbilicus in cases where it has been resected or destroyed is a delicate procedure

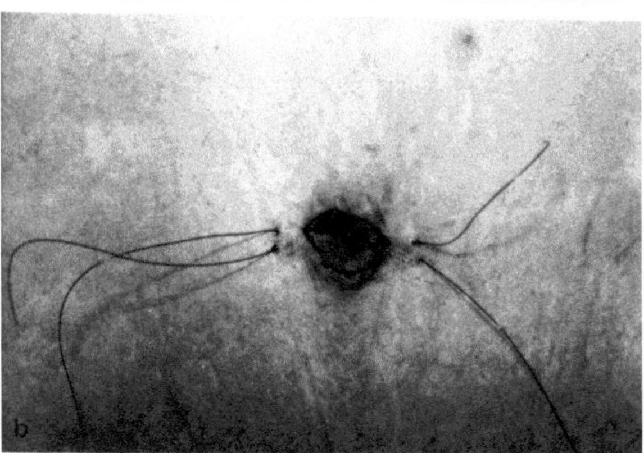

Fig. 11.15. a Precise periumbilical incision is made using two hooks to stretch the skin, while the edge of the umbilical anulus is immobilized by multi-toothed forceps. **b** After exteriorization, the umbilicus is repaired by interrupted absorbable dermal sutures and a continuous intradermal suture

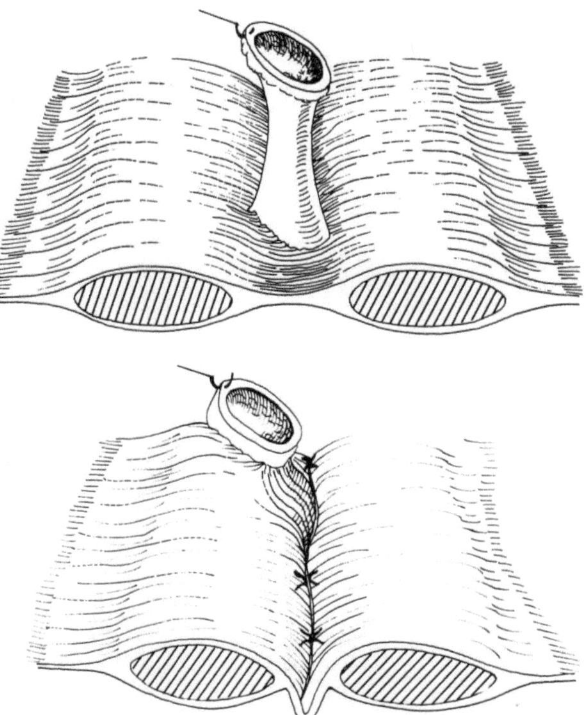

Fig. 11.16. Myofascial plication is done on both sides of the umbilical pedicle [from Aston 1980]

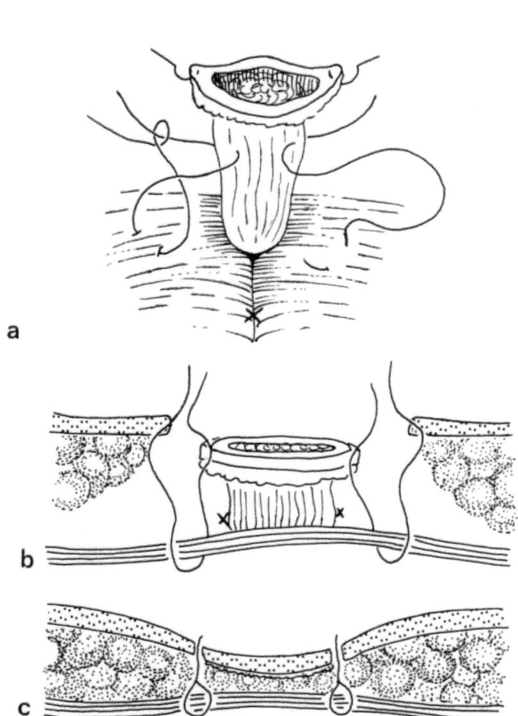

Fig. 11.17a-c. Adjustment of the umbilicus in abdominoplasty. a The umbilical pedicle is shortened by suturing it to the fascia. b The fat is excised from the deep surface of the abdomen in the area around the new umbilical orifice. c Suturing to the fascia to recreate the umbilical dimple [from Aston 1960]

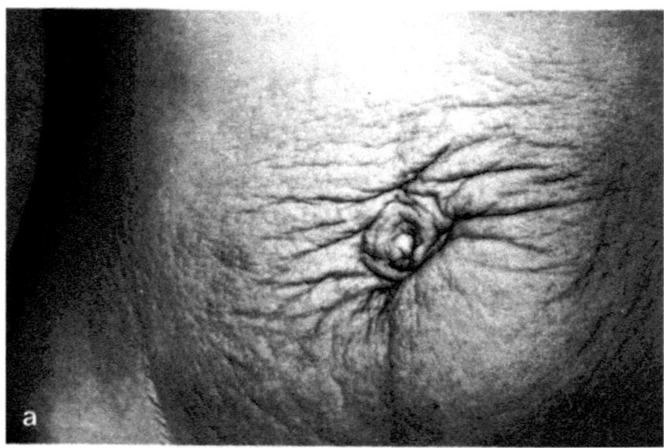

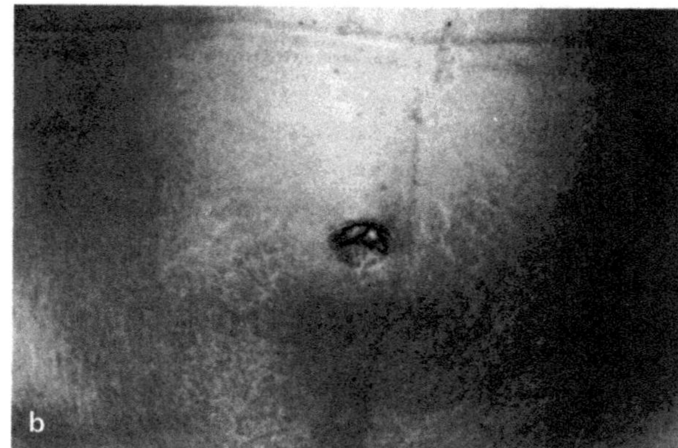

Fig. 11.18. a Periumbilical cutaneous redundancy in a multiparous woman. b The same patient after low transverse abdominoplasty with myofascial plication and shortening of the umbilical pedicle

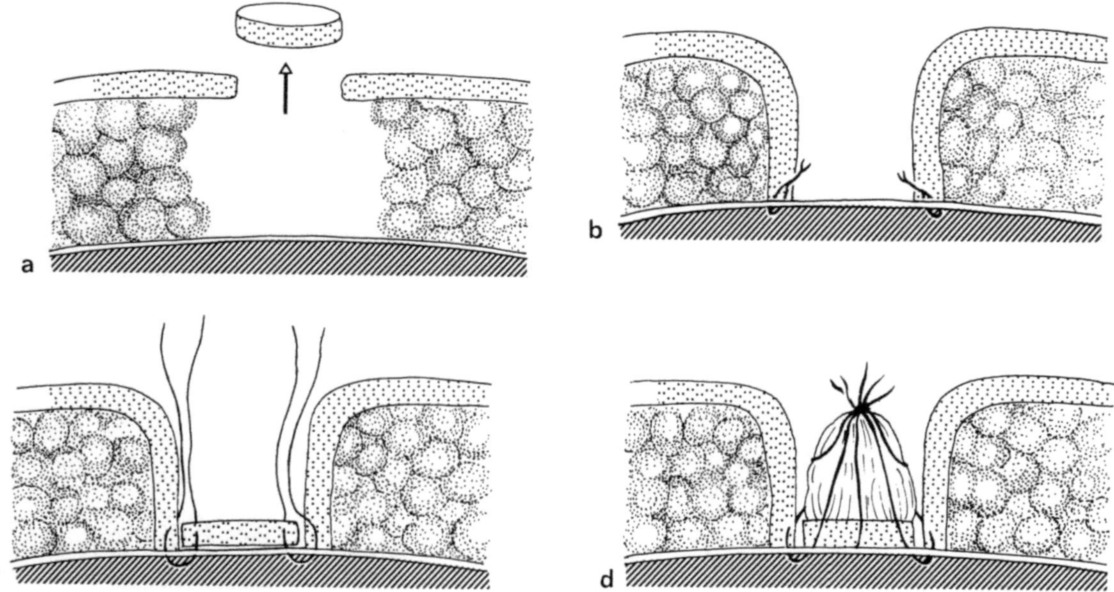

Fig. 11.19a-d. Reconstruction of the umbilicus. a Removal of a cutaneous disc and excision of fat. b Suturing of the skin margins to the fascial layer. c The cutaneous disc is repositioned as a full-thickness free skin graft. d Compression using a pledge

(Fig. 11.8). Simple invagination of the skin is insufficient, since skin must be brought into the fundus of the umbilical dimple.

Once the orifice in the skin has been cut at the desired level, the pediculized islet of skin and its subjacent fat can be preserved [Guererrosantos et al. 1980]. However, such a pedicle is often voluminous and of uncertain quality. We prefer to use this cutaneous disc as a full-thickness free skin graft which is anchored directly to the fascial wall (Fig. 11.19). All fat should be carefully removed around the periphery of the new umbilicus to recreate the umbilical depression and bring the skin in contact with the fascial wall.

References

Aston S (1980) Abdominoplasty in T. Rees. Aesthetic plastic surgery. Saunders, Philadelphia, pp 1007-1038

Babcock WW (1916) The correction of the obese and relaxed abdominal wall with special reference to the use of buried silver chain. Ann J Obstet 74: 596

Baroudi R, Keppke EM, Tozzinetto F (1974) Abdominoplasty. Plast Reconstr Surg 54: 161

Callia WEP (1967) Una plastica para o chirurgiao geral. Med Hosp S Paolo 1: 40-41

Castanares S, Goethel J (1967) Abdominal lipectomy: a modifcation in technique. Plast Reconstr Surg 40: 378

Delerm A (1982) Refinements in abdominoplasty with emphasis on reimplantation of the umbilicus. Plast Reconstr Surg 70: 632

Dufourmentel C, Mouly R (1959) Chirurgie plastique. Flammarion, Paris, pp 381-389

Elbaz JS (1974) Technique du fer à cheval dans les plasties abdominales. Ann Chir Plast 2: 16-22

Elbaz JS, Flageul G (1977) Chirurgie plastique de l'abdomen. Masson, Paris

Fischl RA (1973) Vertical abdominoplasty. Plast Reconstr Surg 51: 139-143

Galtier M (1955) Traitement chirurgical de l'obésité de la paroi abdominale avec ptose. Mens Acad Chir 81: 341

Glicenstein J (1975) Les difficultés du traitement chirurgical des dermodystrophies abdominales. Ann Chir Plast 20: 147

Gonzalez-Ulloa M (1960) Belt lipectomy. Br J Plast Surg 13: 179

Grazer FM (1973) Abdominoplasty. Plast Reconstr Surg 51: 617

Grazer FM, Goldwyn RM (1977) Abdominoplasty assessed by survey with emphasis on complications. Plast Reconstr Surg 59: 513

Guerrosantos J, Dicksheet S, Carrillo C, Sandoval M (1980) Umbilical reconstruction with secondary abdominoplasty. Ann Plast Surg 5: 139

Illouz YG (1983) Body contouring by lipolysis. Plast Reconstr Surg 72: 591-598

Jackson IT, Downie PA (1978) Abdominoplasty. The waistline stitch and other refinements. Plast Reconstr Surg 61: 603

Juri J, Juri C, Raiden G (1979) Reconstruction of the umbilicus in abdominoplasty. Plast Reconstr Surg 63: 580

Kelly HA (1910) Excision of the fat of the abdominal wall. Lipectomy. Surg Gynecol Obstet 10: 299

Lagache G, Vandenbussche F (1961) Indications, contre-indications de la technique de Callia dans le traitement des ptoses cutanées abdominales avec ou sans surcharge graisseuse. Ann Chir Plast 16: 37-50

Lockwood T (1995) High lateral tension abdominoplasty with superficial fascial system suspension. Plast Reconstr Surg 96: 603-615

Marchac D (1975) Plasties abdominales: technique personnelle de reconstruction ombilicale. Report de la cicatrice au fond de l'ombilic. Ann Chir Plast 3: 282-292

Matassaro A (1989) Abdominoplasty. Clin Plast Surg 16: 289

Nahai F, Brown GH, Vasconez LO (1976) Blood supply to the abdominal wall as related to planning abdominal incisions. Am Surg 42: 691

Pitanguy I (1967) Abdominal lipectomy. An approach to it through an analysis of 300 consecutive cases. Plast Reconstr Surg 40: 384

Rees T (1980) Aesthetic plastic surgery. Saunders, Philadelphia

Regnault P (1975) Abdominoplasty by the W-technique. Plast Reconstr Surg 55: 265

Simon I (1966) Qui a pratiqué les premières césariennes sur femmes vivantes? Est-ce les Talmudistes? Compterendu XIX Congr Int Histoire de la Médecine Bâle, 1964. Karger, Basel, pp 276-284

Stuckey JG (1979) Midabdomen abdominoplasty. Plast Reconstr Surg 63: 333

Vernon S (1957) Umbilical transplantation upward and abdominal contouring in lipectomy. Am J Surg 94: 490-492

Vilain R (1975) La technique dite "en soleil couchant" dans les dermodystrophies abdominales. Ann Chir Plast 20: 239-242

Vilain R, Debousset J (1964) Techniques et indications de la lipectomie circulaire. 150 observations. Ann Chir 18: 289

12 The Abdominal Wall in Infants and Children

S. Juskiewenski and Ph. Galinier

I. Omphalocele, Cord Hernia, Laparoschisis

The term "celosomy" [Geoffroy Saint-Hilaire 1832-1837; Wolff 1936, 1948; Morin & Neidhart 1977] signifies defects of closure of the anterior abdominal wall which may extend into that of the thorax. In their major forms, these malformations are mainly combined with complex lesions of the spinal cord and pelvis and sometimes involve the limbs. It is unusual for these infants to arrive at term (Figs. 12.1-12.4).

Most of these major omphaloceles and laparoschises, although having different pathological origins, represent defects of the central part of the abdominal wall. Major omphalocele (Fig. 12.5) is characterized by the presence of the major viscera which have emerged from the abdominal cavity in a pouch of peritoneum corresponding to the amniotic sac. The presence of a loop of intestine at the origin of the umbilical cord is a minor type of this sort of malformation (Fig. 12.6). Laparoschisis or gastroschisis implies an evisceration with no membranous covering, issuing beside the umbilical orifice which occupies its normal place (Fig. 12.7). It must be borne in mind that various abnormalities can result from an aberration of the normal process of development of either the upper or the lower part of the future abdominal wall. The upper type of defect involves not only the abdominal wall but also the anterior part of the diaphragm and the sternum. It prevents the normal separation between pericardium and peritoneum and can affect development of the heart. The most severe form constitutes the rather rare syndrome described by Cantrell et al. (1958) which is a "pentalogy" consisting in an omphalocele, a defect of the anterior diaphragm with a gap in the sternum in "V" or "Y" shape, and a free communication between the peritoneum and pericardium, with downward and forward displacement of a malformed heart (see Figs. 12.11 & 12.12).

Although some therapeutic successes have been reported it is difficult to characterize these because each case poses an individual problem [Jona 1991; Sanchis-Solera et al. 1992]. The Cantrell syndrome [Crittenden et al. 1959; Toyama 1972; Spitz 1975] does not always, however, present with such a major abnormality. An upper celosomy may be limited to a single diaphragmatic defect above an epigastric omphalocele without displacement or abnormality of the heart, as we have observed in three cases [Mahour et al. 1973; Irving & Rickham 1978; Becmeur et al. 1992; Milne et al. 1990].

With lower celosomies, the defect generally extends as far as the cloacal membrane, and may involve the cloaca itself. It comprises therefore a very complex malformation involving cloacal extrophy [Spencer 1965] or a vesico-intestinal fistula [Rickman 1959]. The repair of this type of malformation (Fig. 12.3) can only be done at the cost of very considerable side effects, and seems difficult to support because many of these infants survive for a very limited time, however treated [Boix-Ochoa & Casaja 1970; Fonkalsrud & Lindle 1970; Tank & Lindemayer 1970; Daudet 1971; Hayden et al. 1973; Raffensperger & Ramenofsky 1973; Sukarochana & Sieler 1978; Welch 1979; Howell et al. 1983; Stolar et al. 1990; Lund & Hendren 1993]. There exist however certain intermediate forms as we have seen, which comprise the subumbilical omphalocele and an extrophy of the dome of the bladder (Fig. 12.4), extrophy of a double bladder [Rickwood 1990] or a persistent wide urachal duct which predisposes to bladder prolapse [Suita & Nagasaki 1996].

A. Incidence and Etiological Factors

The global incidence of omphalocele and laparoschisis is difficult to establish. The growing number of interrupted pregnancies before pre-natal diagnosis of these malformations undoubtedly has an influence on their prevalence [Irving 1990]. These vary according to the various fetal and neonatal studies from 1/2,280 to 1/10,000 births [McKeown et al. 1963; McAllister 1977; Schuster 1979; Allen & Wrenn 1969; Irving 1990]. The proportion of these two types of malformation is equally imprecise because of the confusion between the two types which existed for many years. The incidence of laparoschisis is of the order of 1 in 5,000 to 1 in 12,000 births [Colombani & Cunningham 1977; Gierup & Lundkvist 1979; Lindham 1981; Baird & MacDonald 1981]. At the beginning of the 1970s the ratio of laparoschisis to omphalocele appeared to be around 1 in 10 [Daudet & Chappuis 1970; Savage & Davey 1971]. It appears to be much higher today, because of an incontestable rise in the frequency of laparoschisis [Lewis et al. 1973; Wayne & Burrington 1973; Allen 1980; Mayer et al. 1980; King et al. 1980; Lindham 1981; Grosfeld & Weber 1982; Egenaes & Bjerkedal 1982; Irving 1990]. In our experience it is eight to ten.

Simultaneous involvement of twins and familial cases have been reported [Yuzpe & Johnson 1968; Kucera & Goetl 1971; Lowry & Baird 1982; Sarda & Bard 1984; Lurie & Ilyina 1984] but these cases are still rare. Noordjik and Bloemsa-Jonkman (1978) observed that the number of congenital malformations is much higher in the families of patients with

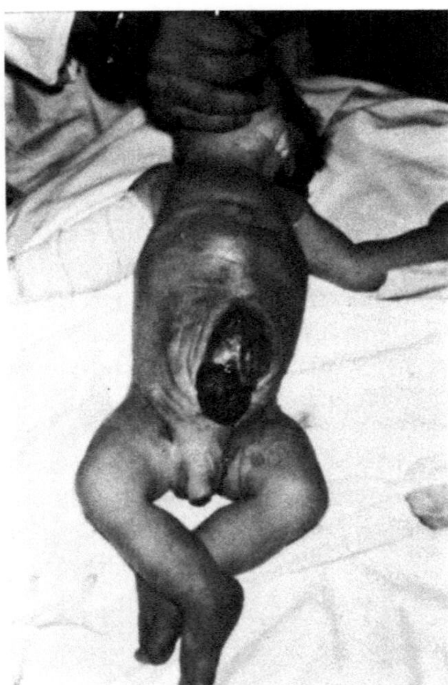

Fig. 12.4. Inferior celosomia with subumbilical omphalocele and partial exstrophy of the bladder

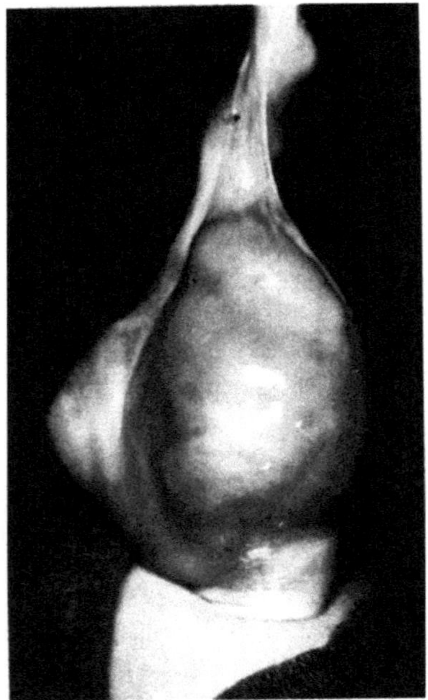

Fig. 12.6. Hernia into the umbilical cord

omphaloceles than with those with laparoschisis. Rott and Truckenbrodt (1974) felt that genetic factors are more important in the etiology of omphaloceles than are exogenic factors, and in cases of laparoschisis the exteriorised gut must be handled with great care so as to avoid any de-peritonisation, or perforation of the lumen. Mahour (1976) takes the opposite view. It is in fact extremely difficult to deduce from these rather scarce observations the relationship between the role of heredity and teratogenic factors. In most cases these malformations are sporadic.

B. Anatomicoclinical Aspects

1. Omphaloceles

The size of the abdominal wall defect is related to the magnitude of the morphogenetic disturbance. In some cases the diameter of the defect is less than 4 cm, while in others it exceeds 10 cm [Schuster 1979; Mayer et al. 1980]. Omphalocele may be a pediculated or a sessile mass. The protrusion is covered by a fine transparent avascular membrane of gelatinous texture, formed by the undifferentiated mucoid mesenchyme of the amnion (Fig. 12.8). The membrane sometimes displays a fine endothelial lining resembling peritoneum. Sometimes a strip of normal skin runs over the

pedicle or base of the omphalocele. The umbilical cord is usually implanted on the inferior wall of the sac, in which case the omphalocele is termed supraumbilical. The opposite case is referred to as subumbilical omphalocele, which is a type of inferior celosomia (Fig. 12.9). The umbilical vein and arteries are separated from one another. The firm but fragile membrane can rupture prior to birth, causing evisceration into the amniotic fluid. In such cases, flaps of the membrane persist on the periphery of the defect. Rupture may also occur on delivery, although this is relatively rare, even in cases of very large omphalocele [Irving & Rickham 1978]. The variable visceral contents of the

Fig. 12.1. Superior celosomia

Fig. 12.2. Superior celosomia: note the presence of the liver and heart in the defect

Fig. 12.3. Inferior celosomia with exstrophy of the cloaca and ileal prolapse

Fig. 12.5. Middle celosomia with supraumbilical omphalocele

Fig. 12.7. Laparoschisis

Fig. 12.13. Four different types of laparoschisis according to intestinal status: note the total necrosis of the eviscereated bowel loop on the *upper right*

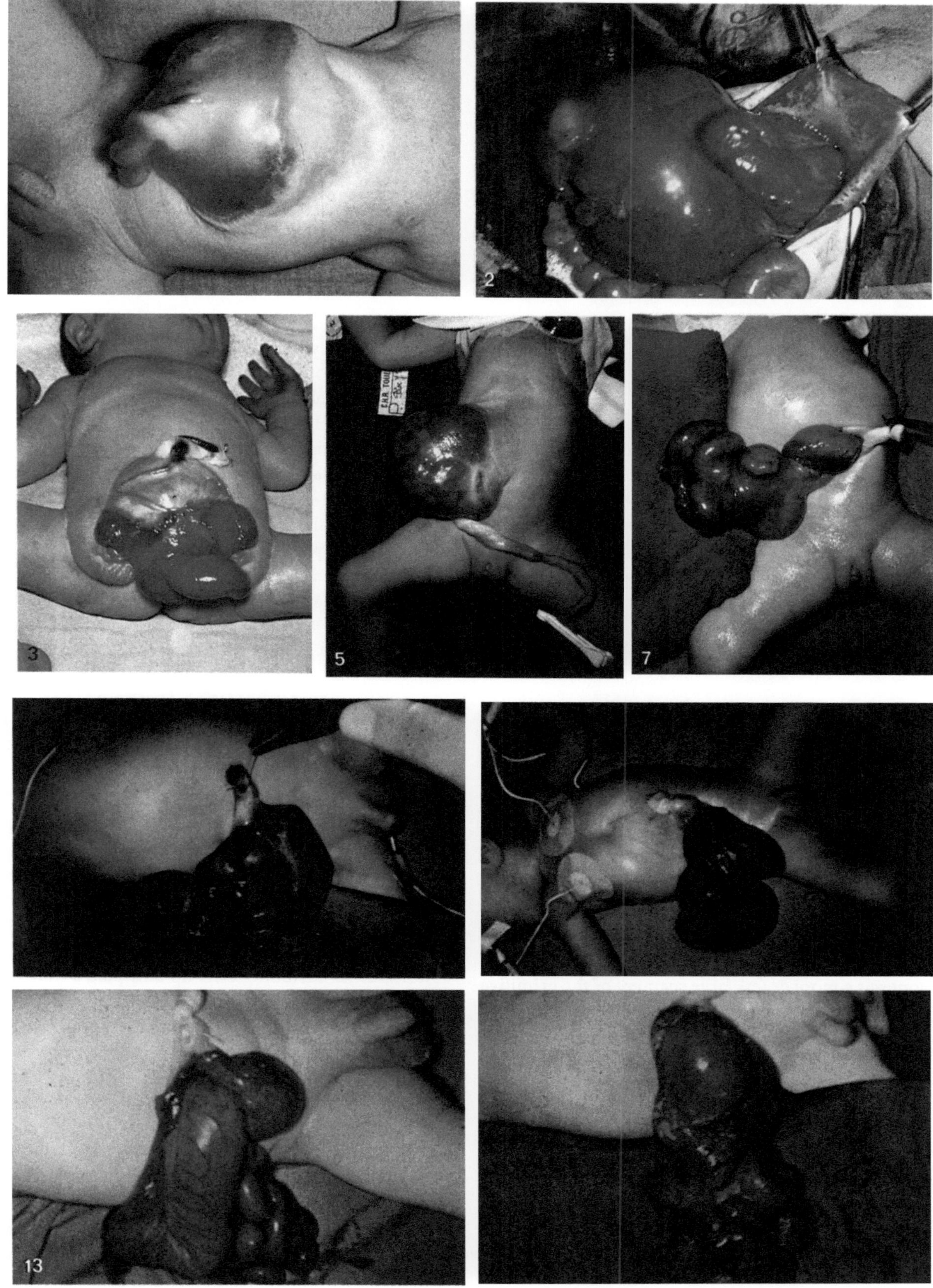

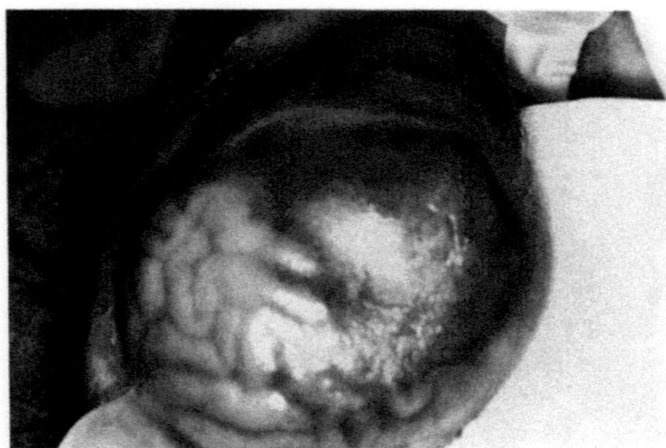

Fig. 12.8. The "pouch" of omphalocele

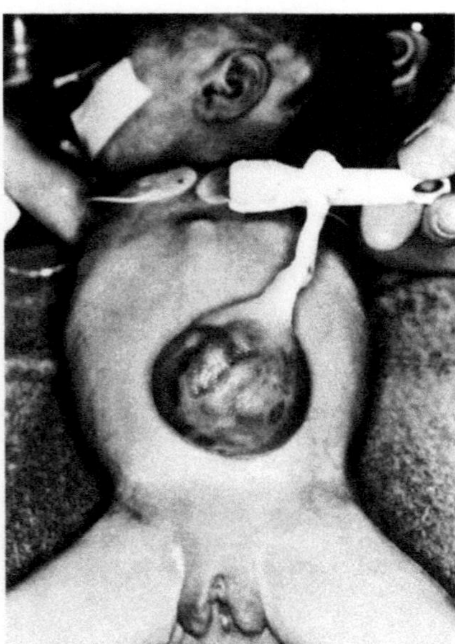

Fig. 12.9. Subumbilical omphalocele without accompanying lesions

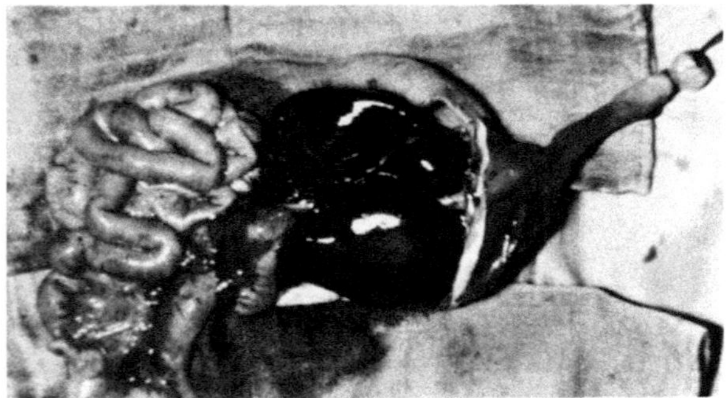

Fig. 12.10. Presence of the liver in the omphalocele

omphalocele can be partially identified by observation through the transparent membrane. The omphalocele contains a more or less large segment of the primitive umbilical loop, whose rotation has stopped at 90° or 120°, with persistance of the common mesentery [Juskiewenski et al. 1981]. Part of the liver may also be found in the sac, especially when the neck of the orifice is large. The liver, modeled to the shape of the defect, is often malformed (Fig. 12.10). Other structures that may be found in the sac are the stomach, spleen, duodenum, pancreas, uterine tubes, ovaries, and bladder. The viscera are generally free within the sac, which is mobile over their surface, although very tight adhesions (especially with the liver) may be seen.

Abnormalities associated with omphaloceles are frequent [Mahour 1976; Moore 1977; Moore & Nur 1986; Mayer et al. 1980; Helardot et al. 1980; Grosfeld & Weber 1982; Hugues et al. 1989] and certainly more frequent given facilities for ante-natal diagnosis (2 out of 3 with 20-30% of chromosomal abnormalities) than in the neonatal series (40-50% with 60% of chromosomal abnormalities), because of the high number of abortions or spontaneous miscarriages. Their frequency is not related to that of omphalocele [Nyburg et al. 1989; Benacerraf et al. 1990; Langer 1996]. The most frequent chromosomal abnormalities are trisomy 13, 18 and 21 [Schuster 1979; Knight et al. 1981; Benacerraf et al. 1990]. The most frequently associated abnormalities are cardiac (15%). These are of variable nature and severity and gravely affect the prognosis [Greenwood et al. 1974]. They include Fallot's tetralogy, interauricular or ventricular defects, aortic coarctation, pulmonary artery stenosis and a single ventricle. Gastro-intestinal abnormalities including atresia, stenosis, duplication, and persistence of the vitello-intestinal duct are less frequent. Intestinal compression occurs in about 10% [Nicolaïdes et al. 1992] at the level of the defect in the wall [Shigemoto et al. 1982] which may produce secondary lesions. Facial abnormalities including cleft lip and palate may be single, or form part of a whole spectrum of chromosomal abnormalities including polydactyly and syndactyly. Urinary malformations have been reported as well as those of the neural tube in some 5% of cases. The presence of an omphalocele also suggests the possibility of a Wiedemann-Beckwith or EMG syndrome associated with exomphalos, macroglossia and gigantism. Umbilical abnormalities are in fact often observed in this complex of malformations which is characterized by a risk of neonatal hypoglycemia due to islet cell hyperplasia [Beckwith 1969; Wiedemann

1973; Irving & Rickham 1978; Sotela-Avila et al. 1980; Waziri et al. 1983].

Several systems of classification of omphalocele have been proposed on the basis of the size of the defect [Jones 1963] or the degree of visceral involvement, especially of the liver [Ingelrans et al. 1964]. Aitken (1963) has defined two types of omphalocele based on these criteria. In type I, the widest part of the defect does not exceed 8 cm in diameter and the sac does not contain the liver. In type II, the largest part of the sac exceeds 8 cm in diameter and/or the liver is present in the sac. Pellerin et al. (1968) added an additional parameter to this classification: the ratio between the size of the omphalocele and the defect, on the one hand, and the perimeter of the base of the thorax, on the other hand. The possibility of reintegration of the herniated viscera into the abdominal cavity is dependent on this parameter. Helardot et al. (1980) proposed a classification similar to that of Aitken but added a third type of omphalocele (widest part of the defect less than or equal to 5 cm).

2. Cord Hernias

These hernias result from the persistence of a wide umbilical ring but in every case are less than 4 cm, so that a loop of intestine may be involved [Benson et al 1949; Schuster 1979]. They may be considered as omphaloceles of small size with a narrow defect. Nonetheless the cord may emerge from the summit of the hernia. Associated malformations are rare. One can sometimes however see a persistent omphalomesenteric duct or the presence of a Meckel's diverticulum more or less fixed to the cord, or an appendix, in the case of failure of rotation of the first intestinal loop [Irving & Rickham 1978].

3. Laparoschisis

This comprises a congenital extrusion of bare viscera. There is no amniotic sac and no vestiges of it except in very rare cases [Rickham 1963; Thomas & Atwell 1976] which allows total distinction from a ruptured omphalocele. The umbilical cord is normal in its site and composition. The wall defect presents as a hole or punched out area, circular or elliptical, the diameter of which lies usually between 15 and 60 mm, although larger defects have been described. It is almost always found to the right side of the cord, although sometimes on the left [Bernstein 1940; Berman 1957; Moore & Stokes 1963; Daudet & Chappuis 1970; Binnington et al. 1974; de Vries 1980] and sometimes at a distance from the umbilicus [Daudet et al. 1968; Pedinelli et al.

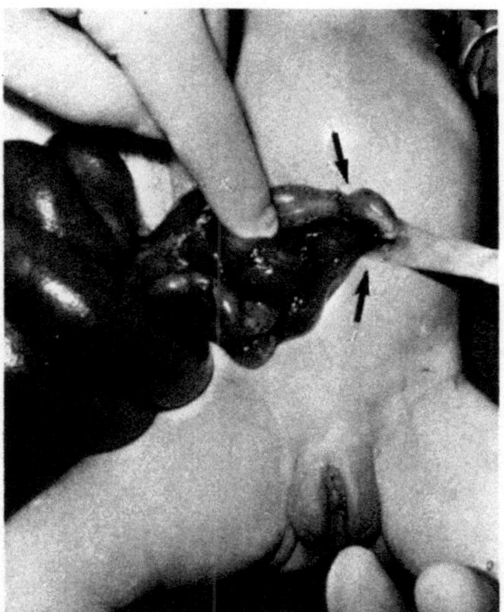

Fig. 12.11. The defect of laparoschisis: note the umbilical cord along the right margin of the defect

1968]. The umbilical cord thus forms the left border of the orifice (see Fig. 12.11) from which it is separated sometimes by a thin cutaneous band [Lotte 1959; Daudet et al. 1968; Allen & Wrenn 1969; Lewis et al. 1973; Thomas & Atwell 1976]. The serous peritoneum continues over the margins of the orifice with no continuity with the skin and Wharton's jelly which normally surrounds the cord. The rectus muscle is intact and its medial border is simply drawn aside. The defect is found at the aponeurotic level as an enlarged umbilical ring, slightly deflected towards the right [Juskievenski et al. 1979]. The sac in every case includes small intestine and a part of the colon, that is to say the primitive umbilicus which represents a failure of rotation and fixation. Other viscera may be present including the stomach, gallbladder, abnormal hepatic lobe, dome of the bladder, uterus and adnexae, and abdominally placed testicles [Cook 1959; Moore & Stokes 1963; Johnston 1965; Pedinelli 1968; Gilbert et al. 1972; Raffensberger & Jona 1974; Juskievenski et al. 1979; Grosfeld & Weber 1982; Moore & Nur 1986; Haddock 1996]. The abnormal viscera are sometimes covered with a sheet of fibrin containing keratin squames and hair (see Fig. 12.12). This serous reaction is caused by maceration of the exteriorised intestine in the amniotic fluid, and the extent of the involvement depends on the stage of maceration [Sherman et al. 1973]. It is possible that fetal urine passed into the amniotic cavity may also have a toxic role [Kluck et al. 1983]. The mesentery is often very thickened. Studies of the abdominal wall are rare and conflicting

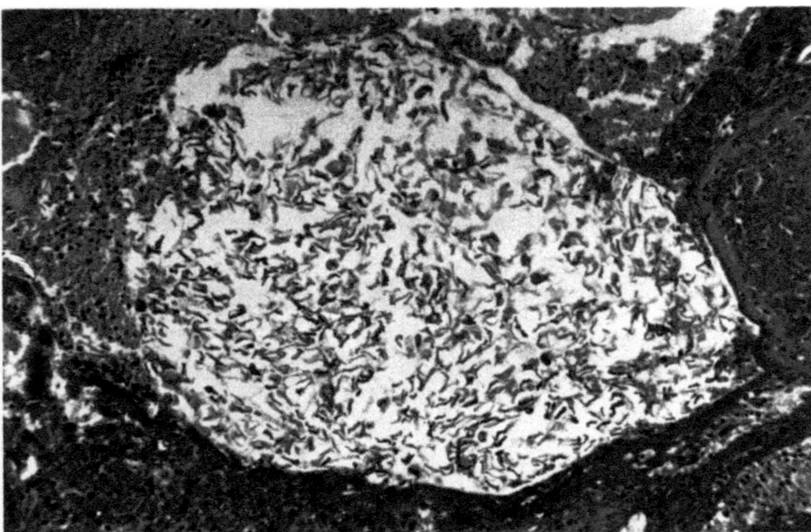

Fig. 12.12. Keratin squamae

[Hegemayer 1955; Haller et al. 1974; Thomas & Atwell 1976; Juskievenski et al. 1979].

Although there may be slight abnormalities of the muscularis and mucosa, there is frequently a hyperplasia of collagen and a diminution in smooth muscle [Langer et al. 1989; Langer et al. 1990; Szinothan 1995], which explains the problems with intestinal motility. Salinas et al. (1979) reported a case of a new-born child with a right-sided umbilical defect, whose evisceration appeared only following the first cry [Aoki et al. 1980; Sherman et al. 1973; Haller et al. 1974].

Associated malformations are much less frequent than is found in cases of omphalocele [Luck et al. 1985]. A persistent Meckel diverticulum has no clinical significance. Duplications are rare [Helmer et al. 1975]. Atresia and stenosis of the small intestine has a frequency of the order of 12-15% [Kiesewetter 1957; Moore & Stokes 1963; Touloukian & Spackman 1971; Lasserre 1972; Hollabaugh & Boles 1973; Raffensberger & Jona 1974; Thomas & Atwell 1976; Noordjik & Bloemsa-Jonkman 1978; Irving & Rickham 1978; Juskievenski et al. 1979; Hrabovsky et al. 1980; Grosfeld & Weber 1982; Di Lorenzo et al. 1987; Brun 1996]. In certain cases these appear as a consequence of compression of the digestive tract which may in extreme cases lead to anecrosis [Van Hoorn et al. 1985]. Most new-born babies with laparoschisis have a birth weight below 2,500 grams and some 60% are premature, perhaps because of retardation of intra-uterine growth which is much more frequent with omphaloceles [Haddock et al. 1996].

In 1963 Moore and Stokes established a *classification* according to the appearance of the intestinal wall which again depends on the length and time of the evisceration. They distinguish between an ante-natal type with gross intestinal changes, a perinatal type where the intestine is nearly normal and an intermediate type. In 1977, Moore suggested a more complex classification into three types according to the diameter of the parietal defect, which varies from 2.5 to 5 to more than 5 cm across, and defined three subgroups in terms of each of those sizes. In 1978 Lefort and Borde put forward another classification into four types based on the state of the prolapsed intestine (type I: little change; type II: changes in the wall; type III: perforation or atresia; type IV: necrosis) (see Fig. 12.13, page 303).

C. Embryological Facts

There has been much debate over the underlying mechanisms leading to omphalocele and laparoschisis. Experimental teratogenesis has not yet provided an answer to all these questions, but both these abnormalities can be reproduced in the experimental laboratory [Lesbre 1927; Gibson & Becker 1968; Barrow & Willis 1972; Miholic et al. 1981; McBride et al. 1982; Baudoin 1982].

According to Duhamel et al. (1966) *ventral embryonic hernias* result from a disturbance in embryonic development and the various malformations of the abdominal wall can be grouped into a continuous series of teratological defects termed "ectroptychies". As regards particularly mid-line omphaloceles, these result from an inhibition of the somato-pleural leaf of the lateral portion of the surrounding folds which eventually determine the constitution of the abdominal wall. The wall continues to gape widely at the level of the umbilicus and the limit of the embryonic rim, circumferential reduction of which is thus blocked, forming, together with the amniotic wall, a hernial sac. De Vries (1980) rejects this hypothesis because of a different concept of the formation of the abdominal wall, according to which differentiation does not take place in situ induced by the action of the para-axial mesoblast, but is rather a result of a ventral extension of the somites from which the myotomes originate. Omphalocele thus results from persistence of the embryonic umbilical pedicle in a region normally occupied by the somatic pleura. Whatever the truth, the abnormality becomes established during embryonic life. More recently Vermeij-Keers (1996) has proposed a new classification of abdominal wall defects, based on the early development of the abdominal wall and the umbilical cord. Omphalocele represents a median form of primary abdominoschisis.

As regards *laparoschisis* which Duhamel et al. (1966) distinguishes completely from omphalocele, this results from the total absence of differentiation of the mesenchyme at a point covered by the somatic pleura, leading to resorption of the epiblast and the formation of a lateral para-umbilical defect. Izant et al. (1966) accepts this hypothesis. According to Muntener (1970) laparoschisis corresponds to a defect in late mesenchyme formation (at around the eighth week) while omphalocele is the consequence of an earlier defect (around the sixth week). Shaw (1975) produces a hypothesis suggesting that laparoschisis is the result of an in-utero rupture of the amniotic membrane at the base of the hernia within the cord, occurring either during the phase of the physiological hernia persisting to the third month of intra-uterine life, or alternatively later on, because of persistence of a weak area at the base of the cord, resulting from the disappearance of the right umbilical vein (Fig. 12.14). The constant presence of a rotation defect of the umbilical loop is for Thomas and Atwell (1976) and for Seashore (1978) an argument against their hypothesis of secondary evisceration. Adhesion of the summit of the umbilical loop in the base of the cord may nonetheless explain the failure of rotation. De Vries (1980) considers that the process of involution of the right umbilical vein, when it is abnormal in its extent or duration, may interfere with the growth and viability of the neighboring mesenchyme leading to a paraumbilical rupture. This author reports two cases of an orifice situated to the left of the umbilical cord in which the left

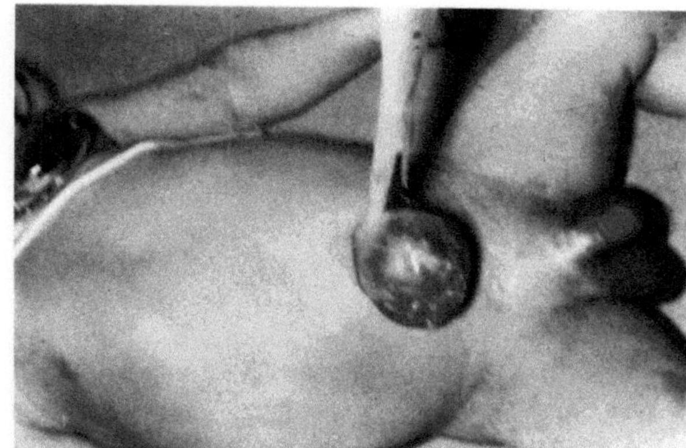

Fig. 12.14. A small juxtaumbilical hernia covered by amniotic membrane

umbilical vein and not the right had become involved. Hoyme et al. (1981) proposes that an interruption of the omphalo-mesenteric artery may lead to necrosis of the base of the cord followed by evisceration through the defect thus created. It is certain that there is a weak area at the right part of the umbilical cord, promoting the appearance of a para-umbilical hernia (Fig. 12.14). We still thus cannot answer the problem as to whether laparoschisis is determined by a mechanical accident or a heritable fault in the development of the abdominal wall, due to a teratogenic action. The fact that it can appear experimentally through the action of teratogenic drugs argues strongly in favor of the second hypothesis, and Vermeij-Keer (1996) considers it to represent a secondary abdominoschisis.

D. Diagnosis

The diagnosis of these malformations is obvious at the moment of birth. There can be no confusion between an omphalocele and a laparoschisis. To overlook a hernia into the umbilical cord may lead to two types of accident. Either a sudden prolapse of viscera may occur in the first few days of life while the cord separates [Irving & Rickham 1978] or an intestinal injury is produced by tying the cord through the hernia, resulting in obstruction or a fistula, as we have seen in three cases [Eckstein 1963; Sandborn & Shafer 1967; Vassey & Boles 1975].

Omphalocele and laparoschisis can almost always been diagnosed in utero. The diagnostic features have become better and better defined, but these do not always determine the prognosis [Cambell 1978; Giulian & Alvear 1978; Cameron et al. 1978; Thoulon et al. 1979; Touloukian & Hobbins 1980; Henrion et al.

1980; Guibaud et al. 1981: Canty et al. 1981; Neilson 1985; Hassan 1986; Sippes 1990; Langer 1993]. The diagnosis of omphalocele can be made from the tenth or eleventh week following the last menstrual period [Curtis & Watson 1988; Ben Achour et al. 1992]. It is characterized by a rounded pre-abdominal mass in continuity with the abdominal contour, limited by a visible membrane above which the cord is implanted, although sometimes it appears at the inferior pole. The contents of the mass are partly fluid but also contain echogenic areas representing herniated viscera. It should be borne in mind that the withdrawal of the primitive umbilical loop only occurs at the twelfth week. At the time it is still exteriorised, its image will be of smaller dimension than that of an omphalocele. If the mass is small and the cord is detached from its apex, it may be confused with a cord hernia. It is very important to deduce some prognostic indicators from these investigations. In particular, associated abnormalities such as neural tube defects, polycystic or agenetic kidneys and congenital cardiac lesions must be carefully sought for. The finding of splenomegaly and a macroglossia may suggest a Wiedeman-Beckwith syndrome. The karyotype should be carefully analyzed. The size of the omphalocele and the presence within it of part of the liver may predict difficulties with vaginal delivery [Hughes et al. 1989] and indicate elective cesarean section [Lewis et al. 1990].

The ultrasound image of laparoschisis is completely different because the intestinal loops float freely within the amniotic liquid. Inspection of these loops gives some idea of the prognosis [Bond et al. 1988; Babcook et al. 1994; Brun et al. 1996]. Dilatation, thickening and hyperechogenicity of the intestinal wall indicate impairment of the digestive tract which sometimes results in delayed intestinal transit following birth. These observations may indicate pre-term delivery in order to prevent them progressing [Langer 1993]. Dilatation to a diameter greater than 17-18 mm suggests atresia particularly if it is asymmetrical, as do the signs of a meconium peritonitis. However, the correlation with post-natal prognosis is not always clear [Brun et al. 1996], and the risks of premature delivery must also be taken into account.

E. Management at the Time of Birth

As the diagnosis will almost always have been made pre-natally, a neonatal surgical team will usually have been alerted. The baby is rapidly transferred in an incubator. Some authors advise immediate operation

for laparoschisis at the place of birth [Goughlin 1993]. The omphalocele or evisceration is handled as little as possible and carefully wrapped in damp sterile towels, covered on the outside by dry protectors in order to limit heat loss. Over this, a waterproof dressing is applied so as to limit loss of fluid. The lower half of the body is enclosed in a sterile plastic bag [Sheldon 1974].

The neonate with laparoschisis should be laid on the right side with thighs flexed, in order to lessen the risk of strangulation at the orifice of the defect. A correctly-applied nasogastric tube aids in compressing the digestive tract. A transfusion is set up immediately in order the correct the loss of fluid and protein which produce a rapid metabolic acidosis. Broad spectrum antibiotics are given. On arrival in the neonatal surgical service an estimation of the serum urea, electrolytes, protein, sugar and blood gases is immediately made. A gentle enema will facilitate evacuation of excess meconium. In the case of a laparoschisis or ruptured omphalocele, the viscera should be replaced as soon as possible, as soon as the infant is in a fit state. When the omphalocele is intact, fluid and calorie losses are of less importance, and time can be taken to assess the total situation and to exclude associated congenital abnormalities, which frequently occur.

F. Treatment

This depends on the ratio between the volume of the prolapsed viscera and that of the peritoneal cavity. Replacement may be immediate, progressive or deferred.

1. Primary Closure

The ideal treatment of omphalocele and laparoschisis consists in immediate replacement of the viscera with closure of the abdominal wall, whilst avoiding an over-elevated abdominal pressure which will interfere with diaphragmatic movement, thus restricting respiration in the newborn and compromising venous return from the vena cava [Lynch 1974]. At the same time, the abdominal viscera may be compressed, leading to obstruction and infarction, and there is the additional risk of rupture of the abdominal sutures. In cord hernias primary repair is often possible as in omphaloceles and laparoschisis, provided that the surgeon is experienced. Haddock et al. (1996) has achieved success in some 80% of cases.

In the *case of omphaloceles* it is sometimes possible to reduce the contents in the un-anesthetised infant, by manual compression of the sac, which allows one to estimate the effects on respiration, and thus to confirm the possible effects of primary closure. The sac is excised at the level of its junction with the abdominal skin and the elements of the cord, vein, artery and urachus are isolated and tied. During dissection of the sac, care must be taken to identify a persistent umbilico-mesenteric duct, or an adhesion to the liver. In either case a portion of the sac may be left behind in contact with the liver parenchyma. The gut should be checked for any possible stenosis or atresia, and the dome of the diaphragm is examined with the finger to exclude anterior retrosternal defects. It is not usually necessary to enlarge the parietal opening in order to reduce the viscera. The intestine is carefully replaced avoiding any rough handling. Gradual manual stretching of the abdominal wall from one part to another of the defect, quadrant by quadrant, greatly facilitates the sutures, which are placed in two layers, namely the peritoneum and aponeurosis, and the skin [Lewis et al. 1973, Raffensberger & Jona 1974]. Free and Tomako (1967) suggested continuous pressure monitoring in the IVC during the reduction of the hernia and the closure of the wall. Wesley et al. (1981) measured the intragastric pressure which seems to correlate well with the peritoneal and caval pressures. [Yaster et al. 1989]. The central venous pressure is simultaneously monitored in the SVC and IVC [Gorenstein et al. 1985] or the intravesicular pressure can be measured [Iberti et al. 1987; Lacey et al. 1993]. Under assisted ventilation, the infant's respiratory tolerance can be estimated by the anesthetist, in terms of the flow volume and insufflation pressure [Bower et al. 1982]. Relaxant drugs may assist in replacing the hernia [Denmark & Georgeson 1983].

In cases of laparoschisis the exteriorised gut must be handled with great care so as to avoid any de-peritonisation, or wounding of the lumen. The cord is removed having ligated its elements. The narrow parietal defect may need to be enlarged in order to effect an atraumatic reduction of the viscera, but this must be carried out with care, as too extensive an enlargement may create difficulties with future closure. As in the preceding case, stretching of the wall allows one to reduce the tension [Ein & Shandling 1980].

The repair is carried out in two lines of sutures. It is sometimes possible to preserve the skin flap at the lower margin of the cord, so as to reconstitute an umbilicus during the skin closure [Lefort et al. 1978]. Due to the recent better understanding of the problems connected with omphalocele and laparoschisis, primary closure is becoming increasingly achievable [Raffensperger & Jona 1974; Tompson & Fonkalsrud 1976; Stringle & Filler 1979; Ho & Reid 1979; Knutrud

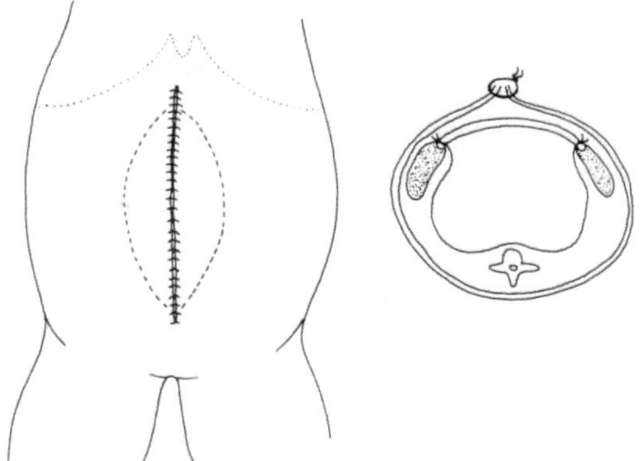

Fig. 12.15. Subcutaneous inert prosthesis

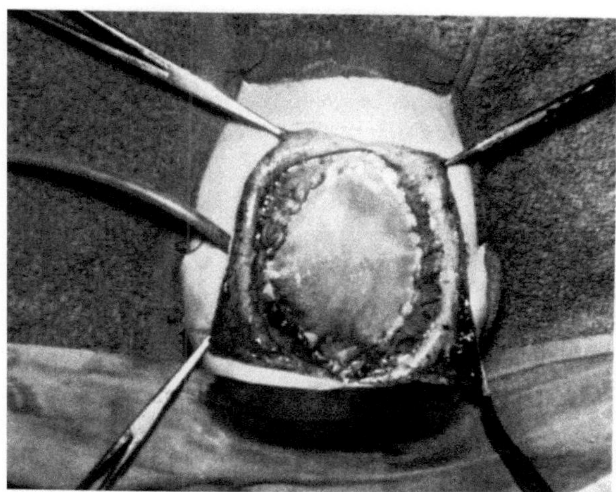

Fig. 12.16. Subcutaneous prosthesis in place

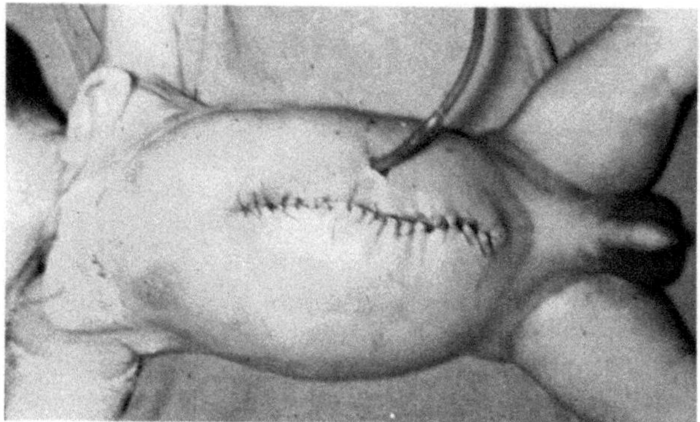

Fig. 12.17. Skin closure over the prosthesis; laparostomy has been done in this case

et al. 1979; Mayer et al. 1980; Ein & Shandling 1980; Fonkalsrud 1980; Grosfeld 1981; Bower et al. 1982; Di Lorenzo et al. 1987; Langer 1996]. When there appears to be excessive tension in the muscular layers leading to an increased abdominal pressure, the closure may be reinforced by a prosthesis cut in hemispheric fashion and closed behind the skin (Fig. 12.15-12.17). We originally used a silicone elastomere patch [Juskievenski 1971] but were discouraged by a case where the patch was extruded leading to a skin dehiscence which may lead to early re-operation. Direct closure is usually possible. Stone (1981) published a series of good results using a similar technique with a sheet of prolene. Gortex [Willis et al. 1995] or resorbable material [Carachi et al. 1995] may still further enhance this technique. The main risk is that of infection.

2. Progressive Replacement

When the disparity between the volume of the abdominal cavity and that of the eviscerated mass renders primary closure impossible or dangerous, recourse must be made to progressive replacement, following the principles laid down by Schuster (1967) which represent important advances in the treatment of omphalocele and laparoschisis.

The Schuster's method consists in the formation of an artificial sac in front of the viscera, in the musculo aponeurotic wall, and obtaining progressive reduction of its contents by repeated increases of pressure in the sac, parallel to enlargement of the abdominal cavity. Following enlargement of the midline defect, two sheets of silastic are sutured to the edges picking up all thicknesses of the wall. These two sheets are then placed over the eviscerated mass and sutured to each other in the midline under moderate tension (Figs. 12.18 & 12.19). The two sheets are approximated every two days by replacement of the midline suture, and eventually it becomes possible to remove them, usually around the tenth or twelfth day [Novotny et al. 1993], or sometimes even earlier [Wesley et al. 1981].

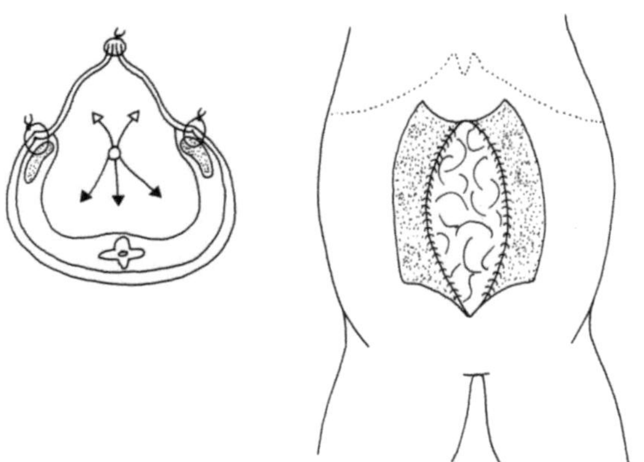

Fig. 12.18. The principle of Schuster's technique

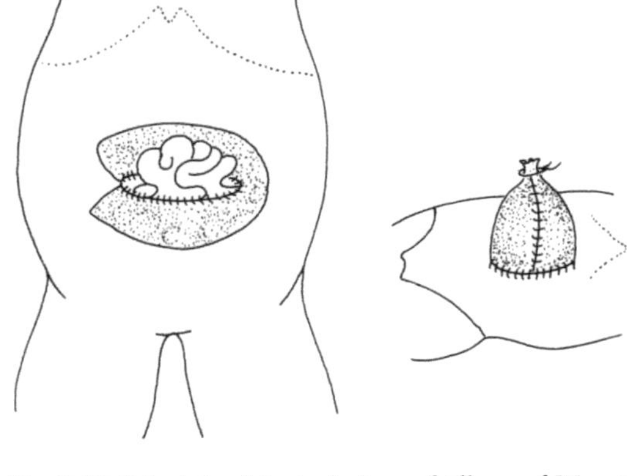

Fig. 12.20. Principle of the technique of Allen and Wrenn

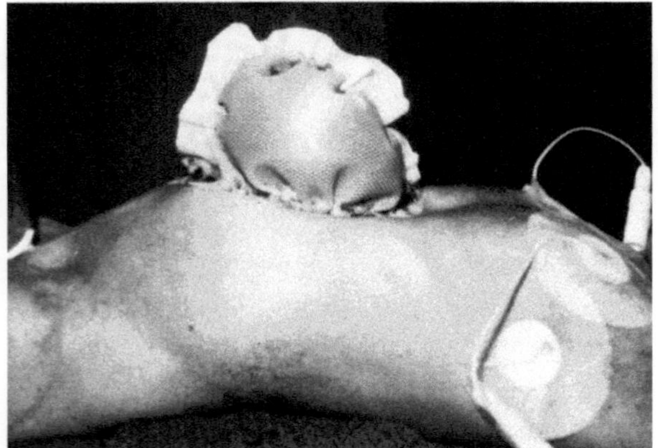

Fig. 12.19. Schuster's technique

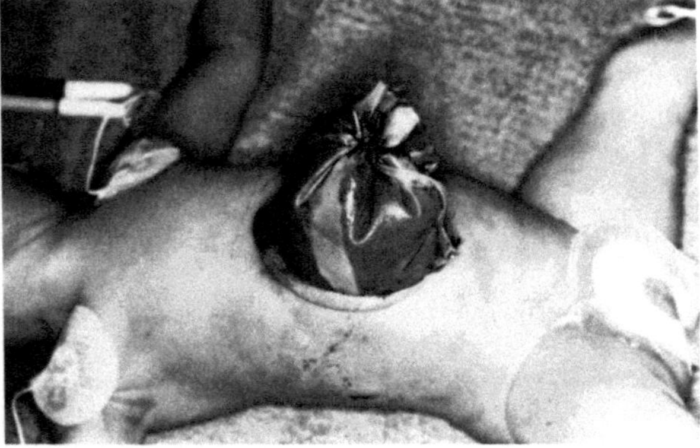

Fig. 12.21. Technique of Allen and Wrenn

The abdominal wall is then closed directly. Alternately, the same result may be achieved by the placement of a single patch between the rectus muscles, in order to avoid undue tension [Krasna 1995]. Many variations on this method have been suggested. Gilbert et al. (1968), Allen and Wrenn (1969) use one single layer arranged as a sac around the extruded visceral mass. The defect is carefully enlarged either vertically or transversely, if it is too narrow. The patch is sutured around the defect in a circular manner, taking up the entire thickness of the wall (Figs. 12.20 & 12.21). The outlet so formed is closed laterally and the operation terminated by placing a ligature at the upper end of the sac thus created: it should always have a large base. When the sac is high it should be fixed by a traction suture at its apex, and kept in place by a dressing, in order to avoid any angulation at its exit from the abdominal wall. Regular gentle pressure on the sac reduces progressive re-entry of the viscera, as described in the preceding methods. Shermata (1976 & 1977) suggested the use of a transparent dressing, permitting observation of the state of the bowel during reduction, replaced later by a preformed sac with a reinforced ring at its base. Othersen and Hargest (1977) introduced an apparatus for pneumatic reduction. It is usually possible to achieve complete reduction allowing direct closure of the abdominal wall, within eight days.

There is a constant risk of infection during the course of progressive reduction, which requires strict supervision of the dressing technique. Separation of the prosthesis through breakdown of the sutures is an extremely severe complication because it abruptly exposes the partially reduced viscera, and may lead to ischemic necrosis and fistula. These complications severely affect the prognosis [Lewis et al. 1973; Hollabaugh & Willis 1973; Zwiren & Andres 1974; Rubin & Ein 1976; King et al. 1980; Mayer et al. 1980; Hrabovsky 1980; Grosfeld et al. 1981] but in most published series the results are very satisfactory. Nonetheless, these methods should be reserved for cases where direct closure does not seem possible. It may sometimes be possible to apply successive ligatures to the apex of the omphalocele sac itself, in order to reduce the bulge [Hong et al. 1994].

3. Deferred Reduction

In 1948 Gross proposed covering large omphaloceles by skin detached from the flanks and sutured over the pouch, in effect creating a large ventral hernia (Fig. 12.22). Alternatively, the skin may be directly closed over the visceral mass [Hutchin & Goldberg 1965;

Pellerin et al. 1968]. More complex cutaneous plasties have been proposed by Kollerman and Schmarzer (1968) as well as division of the rectus muscles at the same time in order to increase the volume of the abdominal cavity [Savage & Davey 1971]. These methods have certain attractions but a large ventral hernia persists (Fig. 12.23) because the volume of the abdominal cavity has little tendency to enlarge and the visceral mass spreads out in a mushroom fashion in front of the musculo-aponeurotic plane [Schuster 1967]. Secondary closure of the defect at the age of 6-15 month is always difficult, whatever technical devices are used [Ravitch 1969; Boles 1971; Thompson & Fonkalsrud 1976; Aoyama 1979; Khope et al. 1989]. It was in order to solve this problem that Schuster (1967) introduced the method of progressive reduction (see Figs. 12.18 & 12.19). However, the technique of skin cover may be useful in certain special cases, as it is

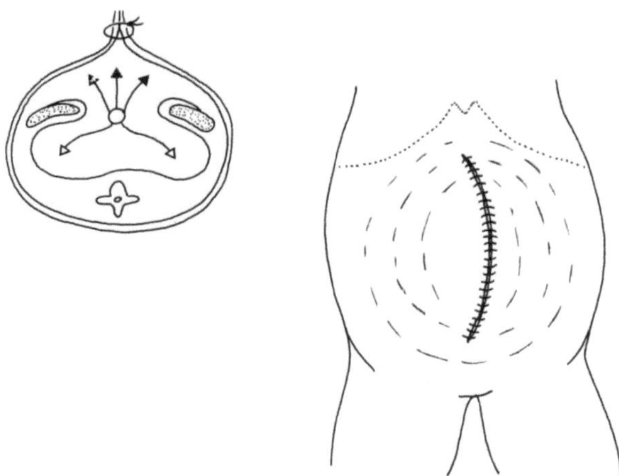

Fig. 12.22. Principle of Gross' technique

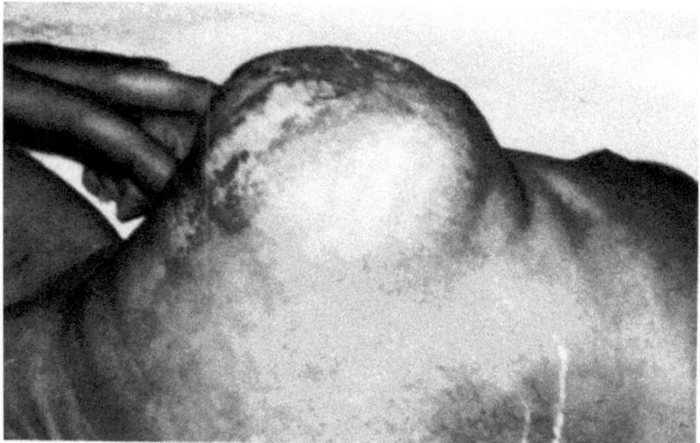

Fig. 12.23. Gross' technique with residual eventration

sometimes necessary to remove synthetic material during the course of progressive reduction, because of disruption or infection.

4. Conservative Treatment

In 1963 Grob advised the application of mercurochrome to large omphalocele pouches in order to obtain a dry eschar. When this eschar is removed it reveals a layer of granulation tissue which becomes secondarily epithelialised from the edges (Fig. 12.24). The resulting herniation needs secondary closure. This method has allowed survival of several omphaloceles [Soave 1968; Firor 1971; Adam et al. 1991]. Various antiseptic solutions have been used to diminish the toxic risk which the repeated use of mercurochrome inevitably poses [Stanley-Brown & Frank 1971; Fagan et al. 1977]: these include zephiran and silver nitrate. The main disadvantage of these methods is that it takes some time to produce the eschar, during which the patient is at risk. Also the resulting eventration is difficult to control. They are nonetheless still indicated in certain special cases (Fig. 12.24) such as high risk premature infants, severe cardiac defects or hyaline membrane disease [Pompino & Kröling 1974; Venugopal et al. 1976; Stringel & Filler 1979; Allen 1980]. Ein & Shandling (1978) suggested covering major omphaloceles with "Opsite" plastic membrane, beneath which epithelialisation gradually occurs. Lyophilized dura has also been used [Reid & Cummins 1977; Currie et al. 1979; Nüllen et al. 1980], as have amniotic membrane [Gharib 1978; Seashore et al. 1975], and pigskin. These biological dressings can be of use in the management of postoperative complications.

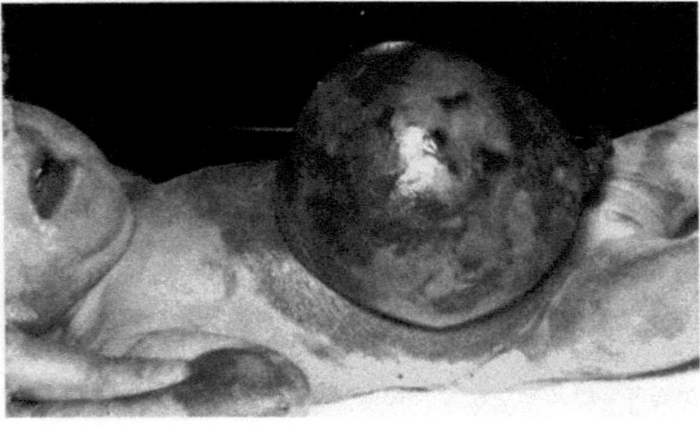

Fig. 12.24. Grob's technique

5. Special Problems Resulting from GI Tract Abnormalities

Stenosis and atresia pose difficult problems and gravely affect the prognosis. However management of the gastroschisis or omphalocele should not be affected by the presence of an intestinal malformation. Three policies are available: resection and primary anastomosis, resection with exteriorisation, and delayed treatment by secondary operation when the abdominal wall problem is resolved. Primary resection and anastomosis has given good results even in cases of anti-natal laparoschisis as we have personally observed [Raffensberger & Jona 1974; Amoury et al. 1977; Graisfield 1981], but in some cases the anastomosis has had to be revised [Grosfeld et al. 1981; Hrabovsky et al. 1980]. The fact that the intestine rapidly resumes an almost normal aspect after reduction may encourage one to carry out such primary anastomoses [Pokorny et al. 1981]. Temporary exteriorisation is possible even if one uses a method of progressive reduction, and the enterostomy does not seem to increase the risk of sepsis [Hollabaugh & Boles 1973; Hrabovski et al. 1980; King et al. 1980; Gornall 1989]. Intestinal resection may be deferred provided that the GI tract is decompressed and parenteral nutrition maintained until surgery. It is difficult to define precisely the indications for these various options, which must be adapted to each individual case, and they remain controversial [Van Horn et al. 1985; Shaw 1991].

When there is a pre-existing perforation without atresia or stenosis it seems preferable to treat it by suture or resection at the time of the parietal repair [Grosfeld & Weber 1982]. The appearance of a fistula or peritonitis during the course of progressive reduction requires immediate re-operation and bypass. In certain cases however intestinal decompression and parenteral nutrition have allowed the fistula to heal [Schuster 1979; Allen 1980; Fonkalsrud 1980].

6. Postoperative Management

Ventilation is often required during the first hours or days following surgery, when closure of the abdominal wall has increased the intra-abdominal pressure, besides which some of these children have a degree of pulmonary hypoplasia [Hershenson et al. 1985]. This should not be considered as a contraindication to primary closure [Ein & Rubin 1980; Bower et al. 1982]. Prolonged ventilation may also be required during progressive reduction and postoperative ileus may severely limit respiration. The degree of respiratory support needs to be adapted to circumstances. In many cases of omphalocele with an intact membrane fluid and electrolyte losses are not very great and can be controlled along the standard lines used in neonatal abdominal surgery [Grosfeld & Weber 1982]. In cases of evisceration and laparoschisis, the losses and needs for replacement are far greater, particularly during the first 24 h [Philippart et al. 1972; Mollitt et al. 1978; Bower et al. 1982]. Correcting these losses reduces the postoperative morbidity and early deaths from shock, renal failure or diminished gut blood flow [Knutrud et al. 1979]. Care should be taken to avoid over-transfusion by careful monitoring of the venous return and of hepatic renal and intestinal blood flow [Masey et al. 1985]. Necrotising enterocolitis is a constant risk [Oldham et al. 1988]. The choice of antibiotics is disputed because of the risk of resistance [Ein & Rubin 1980; Stringel & Filler 1979]. However, hypogammaglobulinemia [Guttenberger et al. 1973] is a particular problem with cases of ruptured omphalocele or laparoschisis so that they should always be used particularly when progressive reduction is contemplated. Antibiotics are withdrawn 48 h after removal of the prosthesis.

Whereas some cases of intact omphalocele rapidly regain intestinal function postoperatively, prolonged ileus, which may last for several weeks or months, is frequently seen with ruptured omphalocele or laparoschisis. This requires parenteral nutrition, which has been responsible for the great improvement in clinical results over the course of the last 15 years [Stringel & Filler 1979; Fonkalsrud 1980; Bower et al. 1982]. The central lines need to be supervised by a skilled team, in order to prevent infection. As soon as intestinal function appears to be re-established, enteral nutrition is resumed, at first using continuous flow and then introducing fractionation and variety. Milk intolerance is often seen [Thomas et al. 1982]. Delay in resumption of intestinal transit may prolong hospital stay for over two months.

G. Results

The last 20 years have seen a considerable reduction in the mortality of omphalocele and laparoschisis. The reasons for this include improvement in the immediate postnatal care following ante-natal diagnosis, prevention of hypothermia, accurate replacement of blood and fluid losses, improved surgical technique, prevention of infection and prolonged parenteral nutrition [Gierup et al. 1982; Krasna 1992]. However, *mortality figures* remain high at around 15-25%, including all types of lesion [Hasse & Mahlo 1979; Knutrud

et al. 1979; Stringel & Filler 1979; Mayer et al. 1980; Allen 1980; Grosfeld et al. 1981; Knight et al. 1981; Canty & Collins 1983; Yazbeck et al. 1986; Yokomori et al. 1992; Krasna 1995]. Associated abnormalities, predominantly cardiac, mean that the mortality rate remains high in spite of advances in treatment. Isolated midline omphaloceles without other chromosomal problems and severe malformations carry a much better prognosis, with a mortality below 16% [Mayer et al. 1980; Knight et al. 1981; Grosfeld et al. 1981; Grosfeld & Weber 1982]. A study of eight North American centers between 1979 and 1981 illustrates the high *survival rate* of laparoschisis, showing the success rate of 316 out of 361 infants (87.5%) [Grosfeld & Weber 1982]. Other series [Fonkalsrud 1980; King et al. 1980; Grosfeld et al. 1981; Hrabovsky et al. 1980; Bond et al. 1988; Cianino et al. 1990; Novotny et al. 1993; Babcook et al. 1994; Haddock et al. 1996] have survival rates of over 90%. The *long-term prognosis* is essentially that of the associated cardiac abnormality [Swartz et al. 1986; Larsson & Kullendorf 1990; Tunell et al. 1995]. In the absence of such lesions it is excellent. Intestinal function usually becomes normal at around the sixth month [Touloukian & Spackman 1971; Hollabaugh & Boles 1973; O'Neill et al. 1974]. Gastro-esophageal reflux may appear during the months following repair of the abdominal wall, but rarely requires surgery [Stringel & Filler 1979; Grosfeld et al. 1981]. Inguinal hernias often appear, but the relation between cause and effect is difficult to establish. There is always a risk of obstruction through bands or adhesions [Tunell et al. 1995]. The growth curve is normal.

In utero exploration may allow earlier diagnosis of omphalocele and laparoschisis, so that treatment can be planned accordingly. The generally good prognosis of midline omphalocele without a major associated abnormality, and particularly a laparoschisis, deserves to be better known, when decisions regarding interruption of pregnancy are taken.

References

Adam AS, Corbally MT, Fitzgerald RJ (1991) Evaluation of conservation therapy for exomphalos. Surg Gynecol Obstet 172: 394-396

Aitken J (1963) Exomphalos. Arch Dis Child 38: 126-132

Allen RG (1980) Omphalocele and laparoschisis. In: Holder TM, Ashcraft KW (eds) Pediatric surgery. WB Saunders, Philadelphia, pp 572-588

Allen RG, Wrenn EL (1969) Silon as a sac in the treatment of omphalocele and gastroschisis, J Pediatr Surg 4: 3-8

Amoury RA, Ashcraft KW, Holder TM (1977) Gastroschisis complicated by intestinal atresia. Surgery 82: 373-381

Angerpointer Th, Radtke W, Marken JD (1981) Catamnestir investigations in children with malformations of the gastro intestinal tract and the abdominal wall. Z Kinderchir 32: 129-144

Aoki Y, Ohshio T, Komi N (1980) An experimental study of gastroschisis using fetal surgery. J Pediatr Surg 15: 252-256

Aoyama K (1979) A new operation for repair of large ventral hernias following giant omphalocele and gastroschisis. J Pediatr Surg 14: 172-176

Babcook K, Hedrick MH, Goldstein RB, Callen PW, et al (1994) Gastroschisis: can sonography of the fetal bowel accurataly predict post-natal outcome? J Ultrasound Med 13: 701-706

Baird PA, Mc Donald EC (1981) An epidemiologic study of congenital malformations of the anterior abdominal wall in more than half a million consecutive live births. Am J Hum Genet 33: 470-478

Barrow MV, Willis LS (1972) Ectopia cordis and gastroschisis induced in rats by maternal administration of lathyrogen beta-amino propionitrile. Am Heart J 83: 518-526

Baudoin AR (1982) Teratogenic action of platinum thymine blue. Life Sci 31: 757-762

Becmeur F, Livolsi A, Heintz C, Sauvage P (1992) Le Syndrome de Cantrell ou la pentalogie "peau de chagrin" - A propos de trois observations. Ann Pediatr 39: 578-581

Beckwith JB (1969) Macroglossia, omphalocele, adrenal cytomegaly, gigantism and hyperplastic visceromegaly. Birth Defects 5: 188

Benaceraff BR, Saltzman DH, Estroff JA, Frigoletto Jr FD (1990) Abnormal karyotype of fetuses with omphalocele: prediction based on omphalocele contents. Obstet Gynecol 75: 317-319

Ben Achour D, Daghfons MH, Rachdi R. Bourhmai T, Koudja H (1992) Le diagnostic échographique précoce de l'omphalocèle. A propose de deux cas et revue de la littérature. Rev Fr Gynecol Obstet 87: 45-48

Berman EJ (1957) Gastroschisis with comments on embryological development and surgical treatment. Arch Surg 75: 788-791

Bernstein P (1940) Gatroschisis, a rare teratological condition in the new-born. Arch Pediatr 57: 503-505

Bertin P, Anglade G (1973) Omphalocèles et gastroschisis. Cahiers Anesthésie 21: 59-65

Binnington HF, Keatine JP, Ternberg JL (1974) Gastroschisis. Arch Surg 108: 455-459

Boix-Ochoa J, Casaja JM (1970) La fissure vésico-intestinale, différentes formes anatomocliniques. Ann Chir Inf 11: 225-234

Bond SJ, Harrison MR, Filly RA, Callen PW, Anderson RA, Golbus MS (1988) Severity of intestinal damage in gastroschisis: correlation with prenatal sonographia findings. J Pediatr Surg 23: 520-525

Bower RJ, Bell MJ, Ternberg JL, Cobb ML (1982) Ventilatory support and primary closure of gastroschisis. Surgery 91: 52-55

Brock DJH (1976) Mechanism by which amniotic-fluid alpha-foeto protein may be increased in fetal abnormalities. Lancet 2: 345-346

Brun M, Grignon A, Guibaud L, Garel L, Sain-Vil D (1996) Gastroschisis: are prenatal ultrasonographic findings useful for assessing the prognosis. Pediatr Radiol 26: 723-726

Cambell S (1978) Early diagnosis of exomphalos. Lancet 1: 1098-1099

Cameron GM, Mc Quown DS, Modanlou HD, Zemlyn S, Pillsbury SC Jr (1978) Intrauterine diagnosis of an omphalocele by diagnostic ultra sonography. Am J Obstet Gynecol 131: 821-822

Cantrell JR, Haller JA, Ravich MM (1958) A syndrome of congenital defects involving the anterior abdominal wall, sternum, diaphragme, pericardium and heart. Surg Gynecol Obstet 107: 602-611

Canty TG, Leopold GR, Wolf DA (1981) Maternal ultrasonography for the antenatal diagnosis of surgically neonatal anomalies. Am Surg 194: 353-365

Canty TG, Collins DL (1983) Primary fascial closure with gastroschisis and omphalocele. A superior apporach. J Pediatr Surg 18: 707-712

Carachi R, Audry G, Ranke A, et al (1995) Collagen-coated vicryl mesh; A new bioprothesis in pediatric surgical practice. J Pediatr Surg 30: 1302-1305

Cianino DA, Ginnpease ME, Brokan B (1990) An individualized approach to the management of gastroschisis. J Pediatr Surg 25: 297-300

Colombani PM, Cunningham D (1977) Perinatal aspects of omphalocele and gastroschisis. Am J Dis Child 131: 1386-1388

Cook TD (1959) Gastroschisis, a method of treatment. Surgery 46: 618-622

Coughlin JP, Drucker DEM, Jewell MR et al. (1993) Delivery room repair of gastroschisis. Surgery 114: 822-827

Crittenden IH, Adams FH, Mulder DG (1959) A syndrome featuring defects of the heart sternum, diaphragm and anterior abdominal wall. Circulation 20: 396-401

Currie ABM, Doraiswany NV, Durbin GM (1979) Gastroschisis: lyodura repair. J R Coll Surg Edinb 24: 288-292

Curtis JA, Watson I (1988) Sonographic diagnosis of omphalocele in the first trimester of fetal gestation. J Ultrasound Med 7: 97-100

Daudet M, Chappuis JP, Carron JJ, Chavrier Y (1968) Le laparoschisis: réflexion à propos de différents aspects anatomiques et de malformations intestinales associées. Ann Chir Infant 9: 303-316

Daudet M, Chappuis JP (1970) Omphalocèles et autres malformations curables de la région. Rev Prat 20: 1159-1179

Daudet M (1971) Exstrophie du cloaque ou formes chirurgicales de la celosomie inférieure. Ann Chir Infant 12: 497-507

Denmark SM, Georgeson KE (1983) Primary closure of gastroschisis, facilitation with postoperative muscle paralysis. Arch Surg 118: 66-68

De Vries PA (1980) The pathogenesis of gastroschisis and omphalocele. J Pediatr Surg 15: 245-251

Di Lorenzo M, Yazbeck S, Ducharme JC (1987) Gastroschisis: a 15 years experience. J Pediatr Surg 22: 710-712

Duhamel B, Haegel P, Pages R (1966) Morphogénèse pathologique. Des monstruosités aux malformations. Masson, Paris

Duhamel JF, Coupris L, Revillon Y, Bondeux D, Briard ML, Nihoul-Fekete C, Ricour C (1979) Laparoschisis: étude d'une série de 50 cas de 1960 à 1976 et indications thérapeutiques. Arch Fr Pediatr 36-40-48

Eckstein HB (1963) Exomphalos. Br J Surg 50: 405-411

Egenaes J, Bjerkedal T (1982) Occurence of gastroschisis and omphalocele in Norway, 1967, 1979. Tidsskr Nor Laegeforen 102: 172-176

Ein SH, Shandling B (1978) A new nonoperative treatment of large omphaloceles with a polymer membrane. J Pediatr Sur 13: 255-257

Ein SH, Shandling G (1980) Polymer membrane covering of eviscerated bowell in neonate. Arch Surg 15: 549-552

Ein SH, Rubin SR (1980) Gastroschisis primiary closure on silon pouch. J Pediatr Surg 15: 549-552

Fagan DG, Ptrichard JS, Clarkson TW (1977) Organ mercury levels in infants with omphalocele treated with organic mercurial antiseptic. Arch Dis Child 52: 962-967

Firor HV (1971) Omphalocele: an appraisal of therapeutic approches. Surgery 69: 208-212

Fonkalsrud EW (1980) Selective repair of neonatal gastroschisis based on degree of viscero-abdominal disproportion. Ann Surg 191: 139-144

Fonkalsrud EW, Lindle LM (1970) Successful management of vesicointestinal fissure. Report of two cases. J Pediatr Surg 5: 309-314

Free EA, Takamoto R (1967) Measurement of inferior vena cava pressure at the time of closure of omphalocele. Z Kinderchir 5: 279-284

Gaillard D, Morville P, Birembaud P, Mourah H, Quereux C, Leroux B, Daoud S (1981) La célosomie supérieure. Ann Pediatr 28: 51-54

Geoffroy Saint Hilaire G (1832-1837) Histoire Générale et particulière des anomalies de l'organisation chez l'homme et chez les animaux (Traité de Tératologie). Baillière JB, Paris

Gharib M (1978) Operative Versorgung der Gastroschisis mit geburtseigener Eihnant. Z Kinderchir 25: 81-85

Gibson JE, Becker B (1968) Modification of cyclophophamide teratogenicity by phenobarbital and SKF-525-A in mice. Teratology 1: 224-229

Gierup J, Lundkivst K (1979) Gastroschisis: a pilot study of its incidence and the possible influence of teratogenic factors. Z Kinderchir Grenzberg 28: 39-42

Gierup J, Olsen L, Lundkvist K (1982) Aspects of the treatment of omphalocele and gastroschisis. Twenty year's clinical experience. Z Kinderchir 35: 3-6

Gilbert MG, Mencia LF, Bronnw T, Linn BS (1968) Staged surgical repair of large omphalocele and gastroschisis. J Pediatr Surg 3: 702-709

Gilbert MG, Mencia LF, Puranik SR, Litt RE, Altmann DH (1972) Management of gastroschisis and short bowel: report of 17 cases. J Pediatr Surg 7: 598-607

Giulian BB, Alvear DT (1978) Prenatal ultra sonographic diagnosis of fetal gastroschisis. Radiology 129: 473-475

Gorenstein A, Goiten K, Schiller M (1985) Simultaneous superior and inferior vena cava pressure recording in giant omphalocele repair. A possible guide of postoperative circulatory complications. Z Kinderchir 40: 329-332

Gornall P (1989) Management of intestinal atresia complicating gastroschisis. J Pediatr Surg 24: 522-524

Greenwood RD, Rosenthal A, Nadas AS (1974) Cardiovascular malformations associated with omphaloceles. J Pediatr 85: 818-826

Grob M (1963) Conservative treatment of exomphalos. Arch Dis Child 67: 519-523

Grosfeld JL, Dawes L, Weber TR (1981) Congenital abdominal wall defects; current management and survival. Surg Clin North Am 61: 1037-1049

Grosfeld JL, Weber TR (1982) Congenital abdominal wall defects: gastroschisis et omphalocele. Current Problems in Surgery 19: 159-213

Gross RE (1948) A new method for surgical treatment of large omphaloceles. Surgery 24: 277-282

Guibaud S, Bonnet M, Coicaud C, Thoulon JM, Dumont M, Guibaud P, Robert JM (1981) Problèmes posés par le diagnostic anténatal des malformations de la paroi abdominale. J Genet Hum 29: 93-101

Guttenberger JE, Miller DL, Dibbins AW (1973) Hypogammaglobulinemie and hypoalbuminemie in neonates with ruptured omphaloceles and laparoschisis. J Pediatr Surg 8: 263-267

Haddock G, Davis CF, Raine PAM (1996) Gastroschisis in the decade of prenatal diagnosis: 1983-1993. Eur J Pediatr Surg 6: 18-22

Halavad S, Noblett H, Speidel D (1979) Familial occurence of omphalocele suggesting sex-linked inheritance. Arch Dis Child 54: 142-143

Haller AJ, Kehrer BH, Shaker IJ, Shermeta DW, Wyllie RG (1974) Studies of the physiopathology of gastroschisis in fetal sheep. J Pediatr Surg 9: 627-632

Hasse W, Mahlo P (1979) Omphalocele and gastroschisis. Prog Pediatr Surg 13: 71-86

Hayden PW, Chapman WH, Stevenson JK (1973) Exstrophy of the cloaca. Am J Dis Child 125: 879-883

Hegemayer FW (1955) Über eine Gastroschisis. Zentralbl Chir 80: 1987-1991

Helardot P, Foucard C, Bienayme J (1980) L'omphalocèle: une malformation curable. Etude rétrospective de 86 cas. J Gynecol Obstet Biol Reprod 9: 267-272

Helmer F, Howanietz L, Krejci A, Lachmann D (1975) Zur Klinik und Therapie der Gastroschisis. Wien Klin Wochenschr 87: 536-540

Henrion R, Aubry JP, Aubry MG, Wagernier MG, Dubuisson JB, Dumez Y (1980) Echographie et conseil génétique. J Genet Hum 28: 49-72

Hershenson MB, Brouillette RT, Klemkal, et al (1985) Respiratory insufficiency in newborns with abdominal wall defects. J Pediatr Surg 20: 348-353

Ho ST, Reid IS (1979) The management of gastroschisis. Aust N Z J Surg 49: 470-472

Hollabaugh RS, Boles ET (1973) The management of gastroschisis. J Pediatr Surg 8: 263-270

Hong AR, Sigalet DR, Guttman FM, et al (1994) Sequential sac ligation for giant omphalocele. J Pediatr Surg 24: 413-415

Howell C, Caldamone A, Snyder H, Ziegler M, Duckett J (1983) Optimal management of cloacal exstrophy. J Pediatr Surg 18: 365-369

Hoyme HE, Higginbottom MC, Jones KL (1981) The vascular pathogenesis of gastroschisis; intrauterine interruption of the omphalomesenteric artery. J Pediatr 98: 228-231

Hrabovsky EE, Boyd JB, Savrin RA, Boles ET (1980) Advances in the management of gastroschisis. Ann Surg 192: 244-251

Hughes MD, Nyberg DA, Mack LA, Pretorius DH (1989) Fetal omphalocele: prenatal US detection of concurrent anomalies and other predictors of outcome. Radiology 173: 371-376

Hutchin P, Goldberg JS (1965) Surgical Treatment of omphalocele and gastroschisis. Arch Surg 101: 598-602

Iberti TH, Kelly KM, Gentili DR, et al (1987) A simple technique to accurataly determine intra-abdominal pressure. Crit Care Med 15: 1140-1142

Irving IM (1990) Umbilical abnormalities. In: Lister J, Irving I (ed) Neonatal surgery. Butteworth, London, pp 376-402

Izant R, Brown F, Rothmann BF (1966) Current embryology and treatment of gastroschisis and omphalocele. Arch Surg 93: 49-53

Johnston G (1965) Accessory lobe of liver through a congenital deficiency of anterior abdominal wall. Arch Dis Child 40: 541-543

Jona JZ (1991) The surgical approach for reconstruction of the sternal and epigastric defects in children with Cantrell's deformity. J Pediatr Surg 26: 702-706

Jones PG (1963) Exomphalos. Arch Dis Child 38: 180-186

Juskiewenski S, Petel B, Pasquie M (1971) Le laparoschisis: à propos de 6 observations. Arch Fr Pediatr 28: 346-349

Juskiewenski S, Vaysse Ph, Guitard J, Moscovici J, Fourtanier G (1979) Etude anatomique du laparoschisis (gastroschisis). Anat Clin 2: 111-122

Juskiewenski S, Guitard J, Vaysse Ph, Fourtanier G, Moscovici J (1981) Troubles de rotation et de fixation de l'anse ombilicale primitive (intestin moyen). Anat Clin 3: 107-125

Khope S, Paik A, Rao PL (1989) Omphalocèle: secondary repair of ventral hernia: a new operative technic. J Pediatr Surg 24: 1142-1143

Kiesewetter WB (1957) Gastroschisis: report of a case. Arch Surg 75: 28-30

King DR, Savrin R, Boles ET Jr (1980) Gastroschisis update. J Pediatr Surg 15: 553-557

Kluck P, Tiroel D, van der Kamp AWM, Molenaar JC (1983) The effect of fetal urine on the development of the bowel in gastroschisis. J Pediatr Surg 15: 47-50

Knight PJ, Buckner D, Vassy LE (1981) Omphalocele: treatment options. Surgery 89: 332-336

Knutrud O, Bjordal RI, Ro J, Bo G (1979) Gastroschisis and omphalocele. Prog Pediatr Surg 13: 51-62

Krasna IH (1995) Is early fascial closure necessary for omphalocele and gastroschisis? J Pediatr Surg 30: 23-28

Kucera J, Goetl P (1971) Exomphalos in four consecutive pregnancies. Human Genet 13: 58-62

Lacey SR, Carris LA, Beyer AL, et al (1993) Bladder pressure monitoring significantly enhances care of infants with abdominal wall defects. A prospective clinical study. J Pediatr Surg 28: 1370-1375

Langer JC, Longaker MT, Comblehome TM, et al (1989) Etiology of bowel damage in gastroschisis I: effects of amniotic fluid exposure and constriction in a fetal lamb model. J Pediatr Surg 24: 992-997

Langer JC, Bell JG, Castillo RO, et al (1990) Etiology of intestinal damage in gastroschisis II: timing and reversibility of histologic changes mucosal function and contractibility. J Pediatr Surg 25: 1122-1126

Langer JC, Khanna J, Caco C, et al (1993) Prenatal diagnosis of gastroschisis. Development of objective sonographic criteria for predicting outcome. Obstet Gynecol 81: 53-56

Langer JC (1993) Fetal abdominal wall defects. Seminars Pediatr Surg 2: 121-128

Langer JC (1996) Gastroschisis and omphalocele. Seminars Pediatr Surg 5: 124-128

Larsson LT, Kullendorf CM (1990) Late surgical problems in children born with abdominal wall defects. Ann Chir Gynaecol 79: 23-25

Lasserre J, Saint Supery G, Bondonny JM, Legroux PH (1972) Laparoschisis, affection pas forcément mortelle. Bordeaux Med 10: 1179-1180

Lefort J, Borde J, Mitrofanoff P, Ewsel J (1978) Laparoschisis: analyse d'une série de 19 cas. Chir Pediatr 19: 77-82

Lesbre FX (1927) Traité de tératologie de l'homme et des animaux domestiques. Vigot, Paris

Lewis JE, Kraeger RR, Danis RK (1973) Gastroschisis. Ten year review. Arch Surg 107: 218-222

Lewis DF, Towers CV, Garite TJ, Jackson DN, Nagoette MP, Major CD (1990) Fetal gastroschisis and omphalocele: is cesarean section the best mode of delivery. Am J Obstet Gynecol 163: 773-775

Lindham S (1981) Omphalocele and gastroschisis in Sweden 1965-1976. Acta Paediatr Scand 70: 55-60

Lotte J (1959) Une malformation rarissime: le para-omphalocèle. Ann Chir Plast 4: 156-157

Lowry RB, Baird PA (1982) Familial gastroschisis and omphalocele. Am J Hum Genet 34: 517-518

Luck SR, Sherman JO, Raffensperger JG, et al (1985) Gastroschisis in 106 consecutive newborn infants. Surgery 98: 677-683

Lund DP, Hendren WH (1993) Cloacal exstrophy: experience with 20 cases. J Pediatr Surg 28: 1360-1369

Lurie IW, Ilyina HG (1984) Familial omphalocele and recurrence risk. Am J Med Genet 17: 541-543

Lynch FP, Tomoshige O, Scully JM, Williamson ML, Dudgeon DL (1974) Cardiovascular effects of increased intra-abdominal pressure in newborn piglets. J Pediatr Surg 9: 621-626

Mc Allister ET (1977) Cité par Irving IM, Rickham PP, Mc Bride WG, Vazoy PH, FRENCH J (1982) Effects of scopolamine hydrobromide on the development of the chick and rabbit embryo. Anesth J Biol Sci 35: 173-178

Mc Keown T, Mc Mahon B, Record BG (1963) An investigation of sixty-nine cases of exomphalos. Am J Hum Genet 5: 168-172

Mahour GH (1976) Omphalocele. Surg Gynecol Obstet 143: 821-828

Mahour GH, Weitzman JJ, Rosenkrantz JG (1973) Omphaloceles and laparoschisis. Ann Surg 177: 478-482

Masey SA, Koehler RC, Buck JR, et al (1985) Effect of abdominal distension on central and regional hemmodynamics in neonatal lambs. Pediatr Res 19: 1244-1249

Mayer T, Black R, Matlak ME, Jonhston DG (1980) Gastroschisis omphalocele. Ann Surg 192: 783-787

Miholic J, Wurnig P, Hopfgartner L (1981) Gastroschisis and omphalocele: factors affecting prognosis. Z Kinderchir 34: 235-240

Milne LW, Morosin AM, Campbell JR, Harrison MW (1990) Pars sternalis diaphragmatic hernia with omphalocele: a report of two cases. J Pediatr Surg 25: 726-730

Mollit LD, Ballantyne TVN, Grosfeld JL, Quinter D (1978) A critical assessement of fluid requirement in gastroschisis. J Pediatr Surg 13: 217-220

Moore TC (1963) Gastroschisis with antenatal evisceration of intestine and urinary bladder. Ann Surg 158: 263-269

Moore TC (1977) Gastroschisis and omphalocele: clinical differences. Surgery 82: 561-568

Moore TC, Stokes GE (1963) Gastroschisis: report of two cases treated by modification of gross operation for omphaloceles. Surgery 33: 112-120

Moore TC, Nur K (1986) An international survey of gastroschisis and omphaloceles (490 cases) in nature and distribution of additional malformations. Pediatr Surg Int 1: 46-50

Morin A, Neidhart JH (1977) Les célosomies humaines. Bulletin Association des Anatomistes 82: 605-651

Muntener M (1970) Zur Genese der Omphalozele und "Gastroschisis" (paraumbilikaler Bauchwanddefekt). Z Kinderchir 8: 380-390

Nicolaïdes KH, Snijders RJM, Cheng HH, et al (1992) Fetal gastro-intestinal and abdominal wall defects. Associated malformations and chromosomal abnormalities. Fetal Diagn Ther 7: 102-115

Noordjik JA, Bloemsa-Jonkman F (1978) Gastroschisis no myth. J Pediatr Surg 13: 47-49

Novotny DA, Klein RL, Boeckman CR (1993) Gastroschisis: an 18 years review. J Pediatr Surg 28: 650-652

Nüllen J, Müller E, Schütter FW (1980) Komplikationen und Überlebensrate bei operativ versorgten Omphalozelen und Gastroschisis. Z Kinderchir 30: 41-45

Nyberg DA, Fitzsimmons J, Mack LA et al (1989) Chromosomal abnormalities in fetuses with omphalocele. The significance of omphalocele contents. J Ultrasound Med 8: 299-308

Oldham KT, Coran AG, Drongowski RA et al (1988) The development of necrotizing enterocolitiss of survivors of gastroschisis and omphalocele. A surprisingly high incidence. J Pediatr Surg 23: 945-949

O'Neill JA, Grosfeld JL, Boles ET (1974) Intestinal malformation after antenatal exposure of viscera. Am J Surg 127-129

Osuna A. Lindham S (1976) Four cases of omphalocele in two generations of the same family. Clin Genet 9: 354-356

Othersen MB, Hargest TS (1977) A pneumatic reduction device for gastroschisis and omphalocele. Surg Gynecol Obstet 144: 243-248

Pedinelli L, Ponthieu A, Masson L, Pott P (1968) A propos d'un cas particulier de laparoschisis avec éviscération de l'appareil digestif et de l'appareil génital plus atrésie du grêle. Ann Chir Infant 9: 205-207

Pellerin D, Bertin P, Nihoul-Fekete CL (1968) Omphalocèles et laparoschisis (100 cas d'ectroptychies). Chirurgie 94: 707-716

Philippart AI, Canty TG, Filler RM (1972) Acute fluid volume requirements in infants with anterior abdominal wall defects. J Pediatr Surg 7: 553-558

Pokorny WJ, Harberg FJ, McGill CW (1981) Gastroschisis complicated by intestinal atresia. J Pediatr Surg 16: 261-263

Pompino HJ, Kröling P (1974) Vergleichende Prognose Neugeborener mit geschlossener Omphalocele nach operativer und konservativer Behandlung. Z Kinderchir 15: 338-344

Raffensperger JG, Ramenofsky ML (1973) The management of cloaca. J Pediatr Surg 8: 647-657

Ravitch MM (1969) Omphalocele: secondary repair with the aid of pneumoperitoneum. Arch Surg 99: 166-171

Reid JS, Cummmins G (1977) Gastroschisis treated with lyophilized dura. Arch Dis Child 52: 593-594

Rickham PP (1959) Vesico-intestinal fissure. Arch Diss Child 34: 14-21

Rickham RP (1963) Rupture of exomphalos and gastroschisis. Arch Dis Child 38: 138-141

Rickwood AMK (1990) Exstrophic anomalies. In: Lister J, Irving IM (eds) Neonatal Surgery. Butterworth, London, pp 709-717

Rott HD, Truckenbrodt H (1974) Familial occurence of omphalocele. Humangenetik 24: 259-265

Rowe MI, Taylor M (1981) Transepidermal water loss in the infant surgical patient. J Pediatr Surg 16: 878-882

Rubin SZ, Ein SH (1976) Experience with 55 silon pouches. J Pediatr Surg 11: 803-807

Salinas CF, Barthoshesky L, Othersen HB Jr (1979) Familial occurence of gastroschisis. Four new cases and review of literature. Am J Dis Child 133: 514-517

Sanchis-Solera L, Beltra-Pico R, Castro-Sanchez M, Serrano-Gonzalez A, et al (1992) Cantrell's pentalogy: complete treatment step by step. Chir Pediatr 5: 101-104

Sandborn WD, Shafer AD (1967) Appendiceal-umbilical fistula. J Pediatr Surg 2: 461-463

Sarda P, Bard H (1984) Gastroschisis in a case of dizygotic twins: the possible role of maternal alcohol consumption. Pediatrics 74: 94-96

Savage JP, Davey RB (1971) The treatment of gastroschisis. J Pediatr Surg 6: 148-152

Schuster SR (1967) A new method for the staged repair of large omphalocele. Surg Gynecol Obstet 125: 837-850

Schuster SR (1979) Omphalocele, hernia of the umbilical cord and gastroschisis. In: Ravitch Hm, Benson CD, Welah KJ, Randolph JG, Aberdeen EO (eds) Pediatric surgery, 3rd edn. Year Book, Chicago, pp 778-801

Seashore JH (1978) Congenital abdominal wall defects. Clin Perinatol 5: 61-77

Seashore JH, Mac Naughton RJ, Talbert JL (1975) Treatment of gastroschisis and omphalocele with biological dressings. J Pediatr Surg 10: 9-17

Shah R, Woolley MM (1991) Gastroschisis and intestinal atresia. J Pediatr Surg 26: 787-789

Shaw A (1975) The myth of gastroschisis. J Pediatr Surg 10: 235-244

Sheldon RE (1974) The bowel bag: a sterile transportable method for warming infants with skin defects. Pediatrics 53: 267-271

Sherman NJ, Asch MJ, Isaacs H, Rosenkrantz JG (1973) Experimental gastroschisis in fetal rabbits. J Pediatr Surg 8: 165-169

Shermata DW (1977) Simplified treatment of large congenital ventral wall defects. Am J Surg 13: 78-80

Shermata DW, Haller JA Jr (1976) A new performed silo for the management of gastroschsis. J Pediatr Surg 10: 973-975

Shigemoto H, Horiya Y, Isomuto T, Yamamoto Y, Sano K, Saito M (1982) Duodenal atresia secondary to intrauterine midgut strangulation by an omphalocele. J Pediatr Surg 17: 420-421

Soave F (1968) Conservation treatment of giant omphalocele. Arch Dis Child 38: 130-136

Sotelo-Avila, Gonzalez-Crussi, Fowler JW (1980) Complete and incomplete forms of Beckwith-Wiedeman syndrome: their oncogenic potential. J Pediatr 96: 47-50

Spencer RW (1965) Exstrophia splanchnica (Exstrophy of the cloaca). Surgery 57: 751-766

Spitz L (1975) Combined anterior abdominal wall, diaphragmatic, pericardial an intra-cardic defects: a report of 5 cases and their management. J Pediatr Surg 10: 491-496

Srinathan SK, Langer JC, Blenner Hasset MR, Harrison GJ, et al (1995) Etiology of intestinal damage in gastroschisis III: Morphometric analyses of the smooth muscle and submucosa. J Pediatr Surg 30: 379-383

Stanley-Brown EB, Frank JE (1971) Mercury poisoning from application to omphalocele. JAMA 216: 2144-2146

Stolar CH, Randolph JG, Flanigan LP (1990) Cloacal exstrophy: individualized management trough a staged surgical approach. J Pediatr Surg 25: 505-507

Stone HH (1981) Immediate permanent fascial prothesis for gastroschisis and massive omphalocele. Surg Gynecol Obstet 153: 221-224

Stringel G, Filler RM (1979) Prognostic factors in Omphalocele and Gastroschisis. J Pediatr Surg 14: 515-519

Sukarochana K, Sieler WK (1978) Vesico-Intestinal fissure revisited. J Pediatr 13: 713-719

Suita S, Nagasaki A (1996) Urachal remnants. Seminars in Pediatr Surg 5: 107-115

Swartz KR, Harrison MW, Campbell JR, et al (1986) Long term follow up of patients with gastroschisis. Am J Surg 151: 546-549

Tank ES, Lindemayer SM (1970) Principles of management of exstrophy of the cloaca. Am J Surg 119: 95-98

Thomas DF, Atwell JD (1976) The embryology and surgical management of gastroschisis. Br J Surg 63: 893-897

Thomas DW, Sinatra FR, Swanson VL, Hanson G (1982) Milk hypersensitivity in an infant with gastroschisis. J Pediatr Surg 17: 309-310

Thompson J, Fonkalsrud EW (1976) Reappraisal of skin flaps closure of neonatal gastroschisis. Arch Surg 111: 684-687

Thoulon JM, Combet A, Coicaud C, Guibaud S, Bonnet M, Vitrey D, Dumont M (1979) Diagnostic anténatal avant 20 semaines d'une omphalocèle et d'une laparoschisis. J Gynecol Obstet Biol Reprod 8: 415-417

Touloukian RJ, Hobbins JC (1980) Maternal ultra sonography in the antenatal diagnosis of surgically correctable fetal abnormalities. J Pediatr Surg 15: 573-577

Toyama WM (1972) Combined congenital defects of the anterior abdominal wall, sternum, diaphragm, pericardum and heart: a case report and review of the syndrom. Pediatrics 50: 778-792

Tunell WP, Puffinbarger NK, Tuggle DW, et al (1995) Abdominal wall defects in infants: survival and implications for adult life. Ann Surg 221: 525-530

Van Horn WA, Hazebroek FWJ, Molenaar JC (1985) Gastroschisis associated with atresia. A plea for delay in resection. Z Kinderchir 40: 368-370

Vassey LE, Boles ET Jr (1975) Iatrogenic ileal atresia secondary to clamping of an occult omphalocele. J Pediatr Surg 10: 797-802

Venugopal S, Zachary RB, Spitz L (1976) Exomphalos and gastroschisis. A 10 year review. Br J Surg 63: 523-525

Wayne ER, Burrington ED (1973) Gastroschisis. Am J Dis Child 125: 218-221

Waziri M, Patil SR, Hanson JW, Bartley JA (1983) Abnormality of chromosoma 11 in patients with features of Beckwith-Wiedeman syndrome. J Pediatr 102: 837-836

Welch KJ (1979) Cloacal exstrophy (vesico intestinal fissure). In: Ravitch MM, Benson CD, Welch JK, Randolph JG, Aberdeen EO (eds) Pediatric surgery 3rd rdn. Year Book, Chicago

Wesley JR, Drongowski R, Coran AG (1981) Intragastric pressure measurement: a guide for reduction and closure of the silastic chimney in omphalocele and gastroschisis. J Pediatr Surg 26: 264-270

Wiedemann HR (1973) EMG Syndrome. Lancet 2; 626-630

Willis PH, Albanese CT, Rowe MI, et al (1995) Long termal results following repair of neonatal abdominal wall defects with Gore tex. Pediatr Surg Int 10: 95-96

Wolff E (1936) Les bases de la térétogenèse expérimentale des vertèbres amniotes. Arch Anat Histol Embryol 22: 1-375

Wolff E (1948) La science des monstres. Gallimard, Paris

Yaster M, Sherer TLR, Stone MM, et al (1989) Prediction of successful primary closure of congenital abdominal wall defects using intra-operative measurements. J Pediatr Surg 24: 1217-1220

Yazbeck S, Ndoye M, Khan AH (1986) Omphalocele: a 25 year experience. J Pediatr Surg 21: 761-763

Yokomori K, Ohkura M, Kitano Y, et al (1992) Advantages and pitfalls of amnion inversion repair for the treatment of large unrupted omphalocele: results of 22 cases. J Pediatr Surg 27: 882-884

Yuzpe AA, Johnson HD (1968) Omphalocele affecting both members of a twin pregnancy. Can Med Assoc J 99: 374-377

Zwiren GT, Andres HG (1974) Progress in the management of gastroschisis. Am Surg 40: 45-53

II. Pathology of the Umbilicus Due to Defective Involution of the Omphalomesenteric Duct and Urachus

The umbilical pedicle contains, as well as the placental vessels, the allantoic sac and the vitelline pouch, communicating with the intestine via the vitello-intestinal duct (Fig. 12.25). From the fifth week of embryonic life there is a rapid involution of these structures leading to a total disappearance of the vitelline duc, vitello-intestinal duct and their accompaning vessels. At the same time, the allantoic sac becomes progressively obliterated, and forms the urachus. The only structures remaining within the umbilical cord are now the umbilical vessel surrounding by Wharton's jelly, which represents the remnants of the extra-embryonic mesenchyme. Any interruption of this double process of involution causes persistence of abnormal structures, which, if they maintain a connection with the umbilicus, lead to abnormalities of this area.

A. Defective Involution of the Omphalomesenteric Duct

Pasquie et al. (1971) classified these problems into four types, in order of severity.

- The duct persists in its entirety, as a broad but short tube, connecting the small intestine directly to the umbilicus (Fig. 12.26a).

- A failure of involution leads to narrowing of the canal or obliteration of its lumen. There thus persists

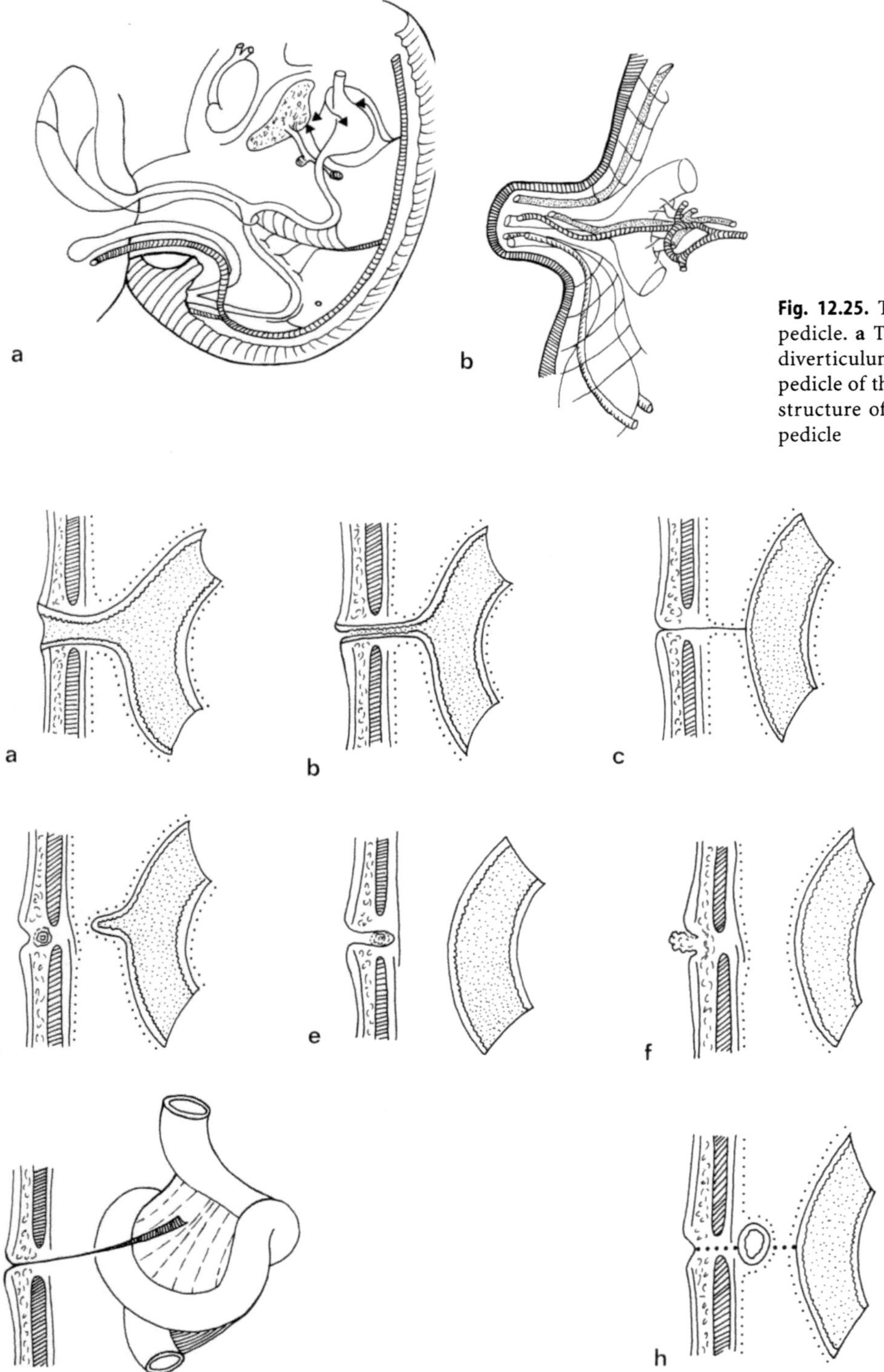

Fig. 12.25. The embryonic umbilical pedicle. **a** The yolk sac and allantoic diverticulum form the umbilical pedicle of the embryo. **b** Details of the structure of the embryonic umbilical pedicle

Fig. 12.26. Defective involution of the omphalomesenteric duct. **a** Full persistence of the duct. **b** Persistence of the duct with a narrow lumen. **c** Persistence of the duct where the lumen has given way to a fibrous band. **d** Persistence of the deep part of the duct, leading to formation of Meckel's diverticulum. **e** Persistence of the superficial part of the duct, leading to formation of urachal sinus. **f** Persistence of the superficial part of the duct, leading to formation of an umbilical remnant of digestive mucosa. **g** Persistence of the middle part of the duct, leading to formation of a vitelline cyst. **h** Persistence of the vitelline vessels

a narrow fistula or fibrous band uniting the ileum to the umbilical scar (Fig. 12.26b, c).

- The involution only involves one portion of the canal, leaving its inner part as a Meckel's diverticulum (Fig. 12.26d) which its external part remains as an umbilical sinus or a small rest of intestinal mucosa at the umbilicus (Fig. 12.26e, f), while its middle portion forms a vitelline cyst, lying along the line of the primitive duct (Fig. 12.26g).

The vitelline vessels, which normally involute at the same time as the duct, may persist in isolation [Kleinhaus et al. 1974] and form a band, taking origin from the mesentery in contact with the ileum and running as far as the umbilicus, to which it is fixed (Fig. 12.26h).

There are various varieties of these abnormalities. Thus a Meckel's diverticulum may be connected to the umbilicus by a fibrous band or a vascular adhesion along the line of the diverticular artery. Otherwise an umbilical sinus may be prolonged into a fibrous band running as far as the intestine or its mesentery (Fig. 12.27a, b). Total persistence, fistulae and mucosal remnants are only one expression of abnormalities at the umbilicus. They may be associated with defective involution of the urachus. Overall, these defects of involution are commoner in boys than girls [Moore 1996].

1. Total Persistence of the Omphalomesenteric Duct

The broad passage which connects the intestine to the umbilicus is identical in structure to that of the ileum from which it arises. There may be some persistence of heterotopic gastric or pancreatic mucosa, as is often seen in a Meckel's diverticulum. This aberrant mucosa may give rise to ulceration and hemorrhage [Chiang 1982; Moore 1996]. It is usually covered by a peritoneal serosa and vascularised by a single vitelline artery. The length varies from 3 to 5 cm. Areas of atresia may be found immediately above or below the lesion [Petrikovsky et al. 1988; MacMullin et al. 1987; Moore 1996]. Total persistence presents during the first few days of life. The diagnosis can be made at birth by the finding of an enlarged and reddened umbilical cord. Very soon a fistula appears at the base of the cord or at one of its aspects. Separation of the cord is followed by a large red raspberry-like tumor, bleeding on contact and usually accurately delimited. It emits a greenish material which is clearly ileal in origin, and increases in the postprandial period. Sometimes the discharge is chyme, as occurred in one of our cases where the afferent upper loop was connected to the caecum (Fig. 12.28) and this may lead to obstruction

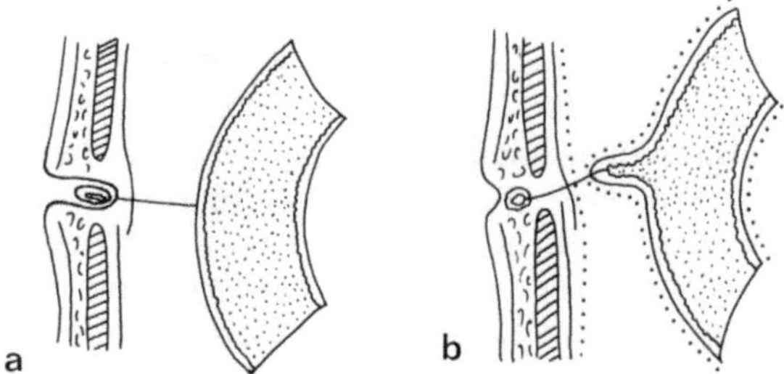

Fig. 12.27. Transitional anomalies. **a** Umbilical sinus connected to the ileum by a fibrous band. **b** Meckel's diverticulum connected to the umbilicus by a fibrous or vascular band

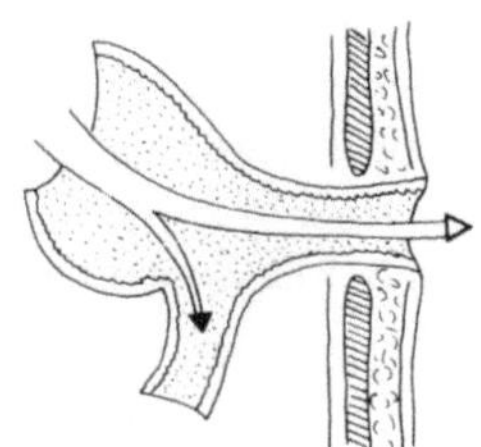

Fig. 12.28. Full patency of the omphalomesenteric duct

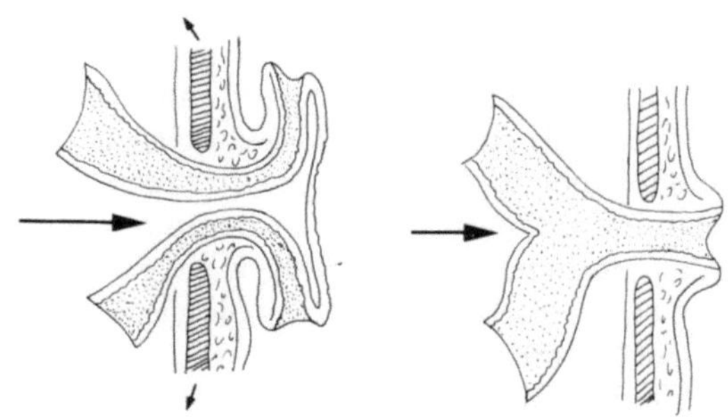

Fig. 12.29. Bicornate intestinal prolapse complicating a persistent patent omphalomesenteric duct

[Zachary 1971]. The surrounding skin rapidly becomes ulcerated by the action of digestive juice.

The canal is large enough to allow an intestinal prolapse at any time, as one sometimes sees at the stoma of an enterostomy. If only the mucosa is involved the result is to render the umbilical rosette more prominent, but more often it is the junction of the duct and the involved loop which is involved so that both the efferent and afferent loops become invaginated forming a double T-shaped prolapse [Moore 1956 & 1996] transversely aligned and perpendicularly attached to a sagittal cylinder emerging from the umbilicus (Fig. 12.29). Sometimes the prolapse originates from the intestine itself so that it is only the afferent loop which becomes exteriorised, in the form of a cylindrical tumor which, in contrast to the above, forms a prolapse shaped like a vertical letter I [Moore 1956]. Rarely, double evaginations may be seen [Mustafa 1973]. Whatever the type, the prolapse develops rapidly, as the infant cries, and a large length of intestine will become exteriorised in this way, within a very short time. Increasing oedema of the wall may lead to intestinal ischemia. Once recognized, this situation requires immediate surgery in order to avoid the risk of further prolapse and ischemia [Ingelrans et al. 1967; Kling 1968; Mustafa 1973]. Removal of the persistent duct with resection of the loop from which it originates, carried out via a paraumbilical route, is quite straightforward; it is sometimes possible to reduce the prolapse at the beginning but quite often this reduction can only be achieved at the time of surgery, and extensive resection of the small intestine may be necessary.

2. Entero-umbilical Fistula

The caliber of the fistula is much narrower than that of the loop of intestine from which it arises. The outer end shows a small umbilical mass corresponding to the inverted mucosa. The discharge is more mucous than fecal, sometimes blood stained and with a fetid odor. It may only emerge intermittently. Persistence of an entero-umbilical fistula may remain hidden beneath an umbilical hernia, or beneath a normal umbilical scar and present purely by an area of swelling, or a GI hemorrhage, if heterotopic gastric mucosa is present [Moore 1996].

With such a minor lesion, the diagnosis of fistula is by no means always obvious. It may be confirmed by a fistulogram, but the orifice may be difficult to catheterize. If the mucosal bud is overlooked, the lesion may present as a severe complication such as intestinal obstruction [Pellerin et al. 1976] or hemorrhage from heterotopic gastric mucosa at the site of the fistula [Pasquie et al. 1971; Moore 1996].

The fistula is approached from the site of the umbilicus. According to the site of origin it may be treated by simple excision or, better, by a wedge resection of the ileum, which will take care of the possibility of heterotopic mucosa at the base of the fistula.

3. Umbilical Remnants

Remnants of the omphalo-mesenteric duct present in two ways. There may be a purely mucosal remnant either as a very short sinus although in some cases there may be a segment of intestine attached to the umbilicus [Michalland et al. 1972]. These lesions present as a small velvety red excrescence, secreting mucus and bleeding on contact [Chiang 1982]. Moore (1996) has recorded a case of profuse hemorrhage emerging from a long sinus containing heterotopic gastric mucosa. This may be seen as a simple granuloma as often persists following separation of the cord, but these granulomata disappear very quickly after a brief application of silver nitrate or the cryocautery [Sheth & Macpani 1990]. However there exists in the middle of the bud a small orifice which is catheterisable by a stylet over a short distance. Examination with an otoscope confirms that there is indeed a blind sinus [Shaw 1979]. Fistulography is often difficult because of the narrow breadth of the lumen. One can usually exclude the possibility of entero-umbilical fistula but it is difficult to determine the vitelline or allantoic origin of the lesion. Additionally, in a certain number of cases, a fibrous band prolongs the blind sinus or mucosal remnant, and may lead to secondary obstruction [Kutin et al. 1979]. Ultrasound gives excellent information, but its interpretation is difficult and may at times lead to false positives.

Excision of the tumor is a minor procedure. The sole problem appears through the possible existence of a deep prolongation. Some authors have suggested carrying out frozen section of the mucosa in order to confirm its ileal character and to exclude the unusual gastric or pancreatic hetaropathy. [Harris & Wenzl 1963]. If its character is confirmed it is wise to expose the deep aspect of the umbilicus in order to exclude the presence of a band [Pellerin et al. 1976]. It is our practice to carry out such an exploration routinely, in every excision of an umbilical bud.

B. Defective Involution of the Urachus

There are four recognizable types, in which patency is preserved either of the whole of the urachus or of its outer, middle or internal portions [Hector 1961; Blichert-Toft & Nielsen 1971; Kontogeorgos & Kokotas 1977; Bauer & Retik 1978; Shaw 1979; Suita & Nagasaki 1996]. Persisted of the entire urachal lumen leads to a fistula between the bladder and the umbilicus. It may be regular in outline or show segmental cystic dilatations (Fig. 12.30a, b). Partial persistence may, according to its level, present as a blind umbilical sinus, a retroparietal cyst or a diverticulum of the dome of the bladder with no umbilical connection (Fig. 12.30c, e). These abnormalities may be combined with abnormal

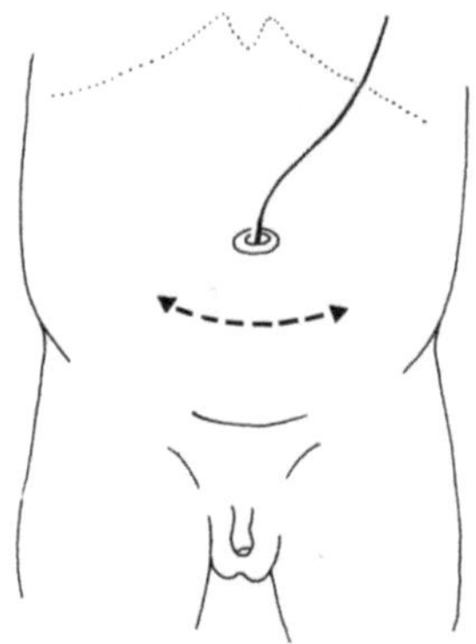

Fig. 12.31. Transverse subumbilical incision used in the treatment of urachal fistula

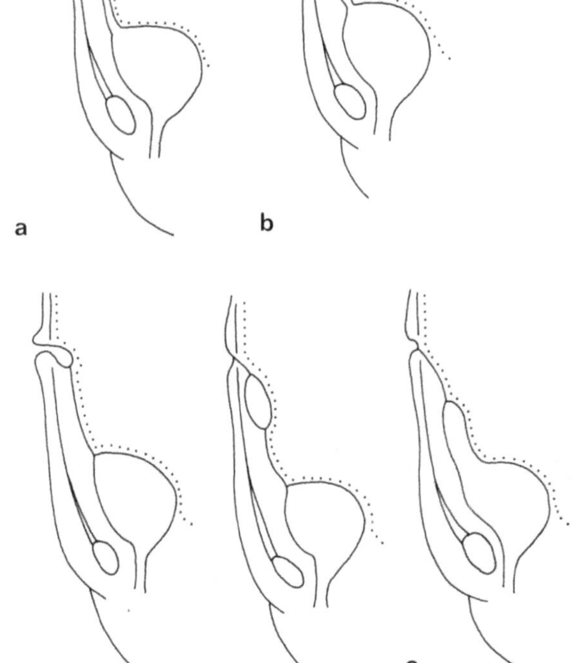

Fig. 12.30. Defective involution of the urachus. **a** Fully patent urachus. **b** Patent urachus with urachal cyst. **c** Partially patent urachus (outer segment) leading to formation of umbilical sinus. **d** Partially patent urachus (middle segment) leading to formation of a retroparietal cyst. **e** Partial patency leading to diverticulum of the dome of the bladder

involution of the omphalo-mesenteric duct [Griffith et al. 1982] and are seen more frequently in boys than girls. Other abnormalities are often found, in particular involving the urinary tract, such as vesico-urethral reflux, or of the GI tract such as a rectal atresia [Rich et al. 1983]. Total and partial persistence of the urachus is seen in about 25 cases of the congenital muscular abnormality known as the "prune belly syndrome".

Urachal remnants are prone to give rise to septic complications such as peritoneal abscess [Savanelli et al. 1984; MacNeily et al. 1992]. Cases of actinomycosis have been reported [Van Wisk & Lodder 1991]. One has also seen the appearance of malignant tumors such as adenocarcinoma [Sheldon et al. 1984; Shaw 1986] which may appear in adolescence [Cornil et al. 1967; Rankin et al. 1993]. Yoke sac tumors have been reported [d'Alessio 1994] as well as benign tumors such as adenoma, fibroma and fibroadema [Dawson et al. 1994].

1. Urachal Fistula

The umbilical cord is often very large at the time of birth, because of oedema of Wharton's jelly arising from hypotonic fetal urine [Tsuchida & Ishida 1969; Ente et al. 1970]. In other cases, it appears normal, but its base is swollen and seems to contain a fleshy mass. Several cases have been reported in which the caliber of the fistula is such that it allows evagination of the urachus or even of the dome of the bladder [Suita & Nagasaki 1996]. When the cord separates, urine begins to emerge. At first coming drop by drop, a jet may be produced by pressure on the lower abdomen. A fistulogram or an injection of indigo-carmine will confirm the communication with the bladder. Intravenous methylene blue may produce blue-colored urine at the umbilicus. The best information is given by ultrasound, provided that there is skilled interpretation. Nowadays, the diagnosis is frequently made before birth by the observation of a cystic mass at the base of the umbilical cord, closely related to the fetal abdominal wall. Differential diagnosis includes a small omphalocele, a persistent omphalo-mesenteric duct or cystic degeneration of Wharton's jelly [Persutte et al. 1988; Persutte & Lenke 1990; Frazier et al. 1995; Sepulveda et al. 1995]. IVU is mandatory, in order to exclude other abnormalities, including lower urinary tract obstruction, although this does not seem to be a potent cause of fistula formation. The urachus can be resected by a peri-umbilical incision which may need to be prolonged downwards, in order to gain access to the dome of the bladder and excise the communication, which should be closed by an absorbable suture. A short transverse subumbilical incision (Fig. 12.31) gives good access to the posterior aspect of the umbilicus, as well as to the urachus [Eckstein 1977].

2. Urachal Sinus

A blind urachal sinus presents as a mucosal button at the umbilicus, with a chronic purulent discharge. This may lead to a surrounding cellulitis, which may in turn be followed by severe septic complications [Kosloske et al. 1981].

3. Urachal Cyst

This is often discovered late [Rich et al. 1983]. It usually lies beneath the abdominal wall and appears as a swelling immediately below the umbilicus, though it may appear at the umbilicus itself [Irving & Rickham 1978]. Ultrasound reveals the diagnosis [Kenigsberg 1975; Goodman et al. 1980]. Often infected, it may present as an abscess opening at the umbilicus, into the peritoneal cavity or on to the abdominal wall [Mac Millan et al. 1973]. It can be completely excised via a transverse subumbilical incision. In the case of an abscess it may be necessary to precede this by incision and drainage, delaying resection until the infection has subsided. Urachal cysts have been excised in the adult laparoscopically [Trondsen et al. 1993; Redmond et al. 1994]. This technique will certainly be applied to neonates and children, provided that there is no infection.

References

Bauer SR, Retik AB (1978) Urachal anomalies and related umbilical disorders. Urol Clin North Am 5: 195-211

Blichert-Toft M, Nielsen OV (1971) Congenital patent urachus and acquired variants diagnosis and treatment; review of the literature and report of five cases. Acta Chir Scand 137: 807-814

Chiang LS (1982) Vitelline duct remnant appearing as an hemorragic umbilical mass. JAMA 247: 2812-2813

Cornil C, Reynolds CT, Kickman DJE (1967) Carcinoma of the urachus. J Urol 98: 93.

d'Alessio A, Verdelli G, Bernadi M, et al (1994) Endodermal sinus (Yolk sac) tumor of the urachus. Eur J Ped Surg 4: 180-181

Dawson JS, Crisp AJ, Boyd SM, et al. (1994). Case report: begnin urachal neoplasm. Br J Radiol 67: 370-372

Eckstein HB (1977) Abnormalities of the urachus. In: Eckstein HG, Hohenfellner R. Williams DJ (eds) Surgical pediatric urology. Georg Thieme, Stuttgart.

Ente G, Penler PH, Kenigsberg K (1970). Giant umbilical cord associated with patent urachus. Am J Dis Child 120: 82-83

Frazier HA, Guerrieri JP, Thomas RL, et al (1995). The detection of a patent urachus and allantoic cyst of the umbilical cord on prenatal ultrasonography. J Ultrasound Med, 14: 47-51

Gangopadhyay AN, Kulsheshtha S (1991) A newer surgical approach for patent vitello-intestinal duct anomalies. Surg Gynecol Obstet 173: 69-70

Goodman JD, Schneider M, Haller JO (1980) Ultrasound demonstration of on infected urachal cyst. Urol Radiol 1: 245-246

Griffith GL, Mulcahy JJ, Mc Roberts JW (1982) Patent urachus associated with completaly patent omphalomesenteric duct. South Med J 75: 252-256

Harris LE, Wenzl JE (1963) Heterotopic pancreatic tissue and intestinal mucosa in the umbilical cord. N England Med 268: 721-722

Hector A (1961) Les vesiges de l'ouraque et leur pathologie. J Chir 8: 449-464

Ingelrans P, Saint Aubert P, Lejeune M (1967) La persistance totale du canal omphalomésentérique. Ann Chir Inf 8: 169-175

Irving JM, Rickham PP (1978) Umbilical abnormalities. In: Richam PP, Lister J, Irving JM (eds) Neonatal surgery, 2nd edn. Butterworth, London, pp 309-333

Kenigsberg K (1975) Infection of umbilical artery simulating patent urachus. J Pediatr 86: 151-152

Kleinhaus S, Cohen MJ, Boley SJ (1974) Vitelline artery and vein remnants as a cause of intestinal obstruction. J Pediatr Surg 9: 295-299

Kling S (1968) Patent omphalomesenteric duct - a surgical emergency. Arch Surg 96: 545-548

Kontogeorgos I, Kokotas N (1977) Congenital abnomalities of the urachus. Int Urol Nephrol 9: 309-312

Kosloske AM, Custing AH, Borden TA, Woodside JR, Klein MD, Kulasinghe HP, Bailey WC (1981) Cellulitis and necrotizing fascitis of the abdominal wall in pediatric patient. J Ped Surg 16: 246-251

Kutin ND, Allen JE, Jewett TC (1979) The umbilical polyp. J Ped Surg 14: 741-744

Mac Millan R, Schullinger JN, Santulli TV (1973) Pyourachus, an unusual surgical problem. J Pediatr Surg 8: 387-389

Mac Mullin N, Beasley SW, Kelly JH (1987) Prenatal intersusception of a vitello-intestinal direct in association with ileal atresia. Pediatr Surg Int 2: 122-123

Mac Neily AE, Koleilat N, Kiruluta HG, et al (1992) Urachal abscesses: protean manifestations, their recognition and management. Urology 40: 530-535

Michalland G, Bensahel H, Bourreau M (1972) Un cas exceptionnel d'ombilic suintant. Ann Chir Inf 13: 183-186

Moore TC (1956) Omphalomesenteric duc anomalies. Surg Gynececol Obstet 103: 159-163

Moore TC (1996) Omphalomesenteric duc malformations. Seminars in Pediatr Surg 5: 116-123

Mustafa R (1973) Double interssuception of the small bowel through a patent vitello-intestinal duct. Br J Surg 63: 452-455

Pasquie M, Juskiewenski S, Petel B, Vaysse Ph (1971) Les défauts d'involution du canal omphalo-mésentérique et leur pathologie chez l'enfant. Sciences Médicales 2: 703-710

Pellerin D, Harouchi BE, Filler RM (1983) Surgery for anomalies or the urachus. J Pediatr Surg 18: 370-372

Persutte WH, Lenke RR (1990) Disappearing fetal umbilical cord masses. Are these findings suggestive of urachal anomalies? J Ultrasound Med 9: 547-551

Persutte WH, Lenke RR, Krop K, et al (1988) Antenatal diagnosis of fetal patent urachus. J Ultrasound Med 7: 399-403

Petrikovsky BM, Nochimson DJ, Campbell WA, et al (1988) Fetal jejunoileal atresic with persistant omphalomesenteric duct. Am J Obstet Gynecol 158: 173-175

Rankin LF, Allen GD, Yuppa FR, et al (1993) Carcinome of the urachus in a adolescent. A case report. J Urol 140: 1472-1473

Redmond HP, Ahmed JM, Watson RGK, et al (1994) Laparoscopic excision of a patent urachus. Surg Laparos Endos 4: 384-385

Rich RH, Hardy BE, Filler RM (1983) Surgery for anomalies or the urachus. J Pediatr Surg 18: 370-372

Savanelli A, Cigliano B, Esposito G (1984) Infected and ruptured cyst causing peritonitis. Z Kinderchir 39: 267-268

Sepulveda W, Bower S, Dhillion HK, et al (1995) Prenatal diagnosis of congenital patent urachus and allantoic cyst: the value of color flow imaging. J Ultrasound Med 14: 47-51

Shaw A (1986) Disorders in the umbilicus. In: Welch KJ, Randolph JG, Ravitch HM, et al (eds) Pediatric surgery. Year Book, Chicago, pp 731-739

Scheye TH, Vanneuville G, Francannet P, et al (1994) Anatomic bases of pathology of the urachus. Surg Radiol Anat 16: 135-141

Sheldon CA, Clayman RV, Gonzalez R, et al (1984) Malignant urachal lesions. J Urol 131: 1-8

Sheth S, Macpani A (1990) The management of umbilical granulomas by cryocautery. Am J Dis Child 144: 146-147

Suita S, Nagasaki A (1996) Urachal remnants. Seminar in Pediatr Surg 5: 107-115

Trondsen E, Reiertsen O, Rosseland AR (1993) Laparoscopic excision of urachal sinus. Eur J Sug 159: 127-128

Tsuchida Y, Ischida M (1969) Osmolar relationships between enlarged umbilical cord and patent urachus. J Pediatr Surg 4: 465-467

Van Wisk FJ, Lodder JV (1991) Actinomycosis of urachal remnants. Eur Urol 19: 339-340

Vane DW, West KW, Grosfeld JL (1987) Vitelline duct anomalies: exterience with 217 childhood cases. Arch Surg 122: 542-547

Wheatlhey JM, Stephens FD, Hutson JM (1996) Prune Belly syndrome: on going controversies regarding pathogenesis and management. Seminars in Pediatr Surg 5: 95-106

Zachary RB (1971) Intestinal obstruction. Prog Pediatr Surg 2: 57-72

III. Groin Hernias in Children

In almost every case, inguinal hernias in children are the result of an abnormal persistence of the processus vaginalis, and are thus oblique hernias passing through a healthy and muscular abdominal wall. Direct inguinal hernias and femoral hernias are exceedingly rare.

A. The Processus Vaginalis

This diverticulum of the peritoneal cavity follows the inguinal canal of the fetus to reach either the scrotum or the labium majus, and remains open up to the time of birth. In boys, it becomes progressively obliterated in its proximal portion, eventually forming a fibrous tract within the spermatic cord. Its distal, intra-scrotal portion becomes the tunica vaginalis of the testicle (Fig. 12.32). In girls, the processus which is known as the Canal of Nück, becomes completely obliterated, leaving only a thin fibrous remnant.

The processus vaginalis remains open in 80-90% of neonates. At the end of the first year it is still present in 50%, especially girls [Sachs 1885; Hrabovsky & Pinter 1994]. The process of obliteration continues up to the age of 2 [Rowe et al. 1969]. In the adult, a patent duct is found in 15-23% of subjects examined [Ramonede 1883; Hessert 1910; Morgan & Anson 1942]. This persistence does not imply the presence of a hernia, but simply a potentiality for hernia formation [Surana & Puri 1993; Fonkalsrud 1995; Ulman et al. 1995]. Failure of the processus to close may be total, allowing the appearance of an inguinal scrotal hernia, or partial, giving rise to a funicular hernia (Fig. 12.33) or rarely an interstitial hernia [Maish et al. 1972; Festen 1974]. Incomplete occlusion may result in a canal too small to allow passage of viscera but which leads to the development of a hydrocele or a cyst in the cord, through accumulation of peritoneal fluid (Fig. 12.34). Persistent processus vaginalis is commoner on the

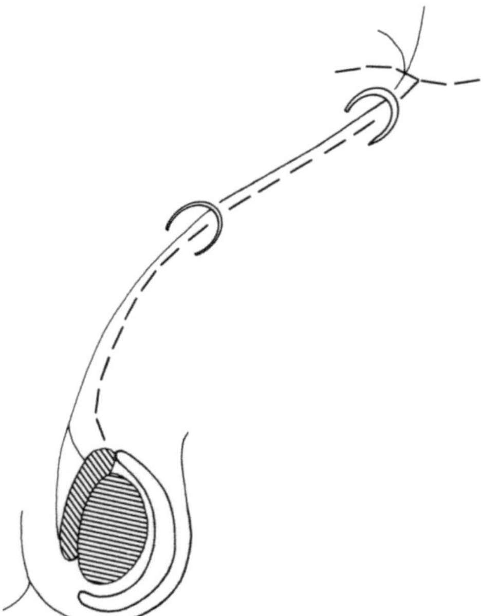

Fig. 12.32. Development of the processus vaginalis with formation of the tunica testis and subjacent fibrous involution

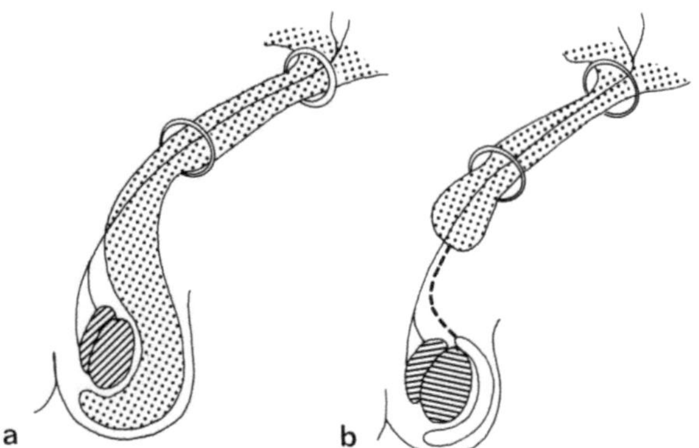

Fig. 12.33. Mechanism leading to congenital inguinal hernia. **a** Full patency of the processus vaginalis. **b** Partial patency of the processus vaginalis

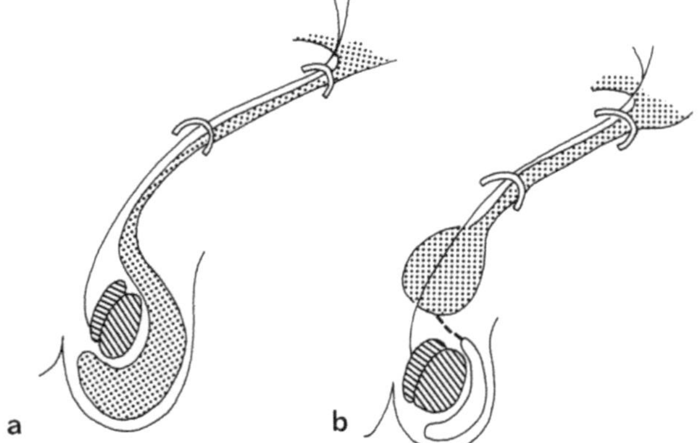

Fig. 12.34. Mechanism of formation of hydrocele (**a**) or cyst of the umbilical cord (**b**) by incomplete occlusion of the processus vaginalis

right, so that right-sided hernias are more frequently seen than left-sided. In our experience of more than 4,000 groin hernias in children, 60% are on the right, 32% on the left and 8% were bilateral. The right/left ratio is 3:1 in boys, but rather less in girls [Scorer & Farrington 1971], in whom bilateral forms are commoner (15%). The duct may remain patent on both sides: this seems to be commoner in girls than boys. The percentage of frequency of a persistent contralateral duct during exploration of a hernia varies from 6-60%, according to the author. Both the age and the sex of the child must be borne in mind [Holcomb 1965; Gunnlaugsson et al. 1967; Kiesewetter & Oh 1980; Given & Rubin 1989]. This percentage falls off sharply after the age of 6 [Lynn & Johnson 1961; Laufer & Eyal 1962; Spackman 1962]. A contralateral hernia is thus more prone to develop when the first hernia presents at an early age [Rickham 1965; Rowe et al. 1969]. This possibility is higher in the case of a left than a right-sided hernia. Generally speaking, a contralateral hernia develops in from 6-60% of cases [Hamrich & Williams 1962; Struve-Christensen & Jensen 1970; Rickham 1978; Given & Rubin 1989]. In our experience, the later appearance of a contralateral hernia occurs in only 2% of left-sided repairs and 10% on the right side. We carry out a bilateral repair in every case where there is the slightest suspicion of a patent processus vaginalis.

B. Incidence

The frequency of inguinal hernias leads to this operation being one of the commonest to be carried out in children. It is particularly high during the first few years of life. Wooley (1979) found 38% of hernias occurring in the first six months and 59% during the first year. In our experience, 39% of cases occur in children less than one year. The frequency is particularly high with premature infants [Walsh 1962]. The incidence falls off sharply after the age of six. Hernias are much more frequent in boys (71.6% in our series), but in the younger age groups the female incidence is significantly higher [Bronsther et al. 1972; Wooley 1979]. It seems that the frequency is slightly higher in black than in white races [Rowe & Clatworthy 1970].

C. Diagnosis

The diagnosis immediately comes to mind in the presence of an *inguinal or inguino-scrotal swelling*. The clinical signs are clear, which include an elongated swelling with a cough and cry impulse, opaque to translumination and reducible, sometimes with a gurgling sensation, while the testicle is clearly felt at the bottom of the scrotum. The diagnosis is more difficult particularly in the small child when the hernia does not emerge on crying or on manual pressure on the abdomen. The description given by the mother is nonetheless highly suggestive. The small diameter of the external inguinal ring means that the usual diagnostic maneuver of inserting a finger into the neck of the scrotum to assess the size of the ring and search for a cough impulse, is of no value. However, by palpating the cord against the pubic tubercle with one or two fingers one can spread out the components of the spermatic cord and identify the neck of the sac which rolls under the finger and enlarges the breadth of the elements of the cord.

The distinction between a *hernia* and a *hydrocele* does not usually give rise to problems. A hydrocele presents as a firm ovoid or pear-shaped elastic structure at the neck of the scrotum, which rarely ascends above the superficial inguinal ring. Large ones distend the scrotum and give it a bluish appearance. They may attain quite a large size in the new-born, and bilateral lesions are not uncommon. The volume may vary because of the persistent communication with the peritoneal cavity, and the family may notice that the swelling becomes smaller in the morning than the evening, as fluid runs back into the peritoneal cavity while the infant is sleeping. Transillumination confirms the diagnosis.

Cysts of the cord share the same features. They are generally found midway between the upper pole of the testis and the superficial inguinal ring, with an easily felt upper pole, but on occasion the cyst passes through the ring and enters the inguinal canal. Transillumination is helpful but is more difficult than with a hydrocele and requires a pointed light source. Occasionally there is a funicular hernia above a hydrocele, giving rise to a scrotal swelling with an inguinal cough impulse on crying (Fig. 12.35). We have seen three cases in which a very large hydrocele presented as a double sac, both inguinal and scrotal [Ahmed 1971; Saharia et al. 1979; Burgues 1986; Booth 1987; Kahn 1987; Squire & Gough 1988; Spier et al. 1995].

Persistent processus vaginalis is common in cases of undescended testis, particularly if the testicle is highly

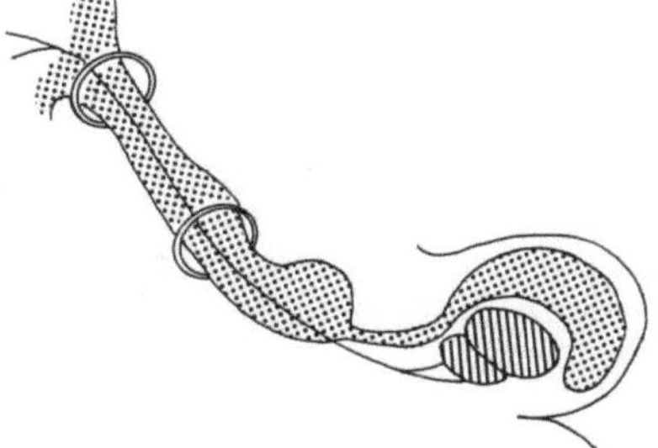

Fig. 12.35. Association of funicular hernia and hydrocele

placed [Hutchinson & Koop 1956; Scorer & Farrington 1971]. *Combined hernia and ectopia* is thus quite often seen. The hernia has the same features as described above but the testicle is not present in the scrotum. Following reduction of the hernia it may or not become palpable depending on its relationship to the external oblique aponeurosis.

Hernias have the same clinical features in girls as in boys, and frequently contain an ovary (419 out of 110 cases in our experience). This may lie freely within the sac or may draw down part of the Fallopian tube with it. It presents as a firm mass which may or may not be reducible, but the ovary may be adherent to the sac. This type of ectopic ovary occurs through sliding of the peritoneum of the broad ligament in the development of the canal of Nück. The hernia appears as a firm irreducible swelling but is non-tender and produces no functional disturbance.

An inguinal hernia may at any time become irreducible and this may be the presenting feature, particularly in early infancy. In our experience of 256 strangulated hernias, 70% were in infants of less than six months. *Incarceration* or *strangulation* leads to severe pain and often early reflex vomiting. Signs of obstruction appear later. The diagnosis is made by the finding of a tender irreducible inguinal swelling which later becomes inflamed. This diagnosis usually presents no problem except in the case of a previously unsuspected hernia in a small infant, which should be carefully sought for if there is any sign of obstruction. In the new-born there may be scrotal oedema and sometimes an increase in the volume of the testis, suggesting a torsion. Plain abdominal X-ray may disclose air in the inguino-scrotal region, which is diagnostic [Currarino 1974]. Ultrasound resolves the situation. Injection of contrast medium into the peritoneal cavity will disclose the hernia and show up a patent processus on the other side. This technique described by Ducharme et al. (1967), Guttman et al. (1972), Braun et al. (1975) has been widely used in order to resolve the problem posed by a bilaterally patent processus [White et al. 1968; James & Hunsicker 1972; Thompson et al. 1972; Blan et al. 1973; Gallegos et al. 1974; Broutin et al. 1975; Jewett et al. 1976; Kiesevetter & Oh 1980; Vanneuville et al. 1983]. Although in experienced hands this technique presents few problems, it seems to us to be somewhat disproportionate to the situation. Other techniques, such as pneumoperitoneum, have been suggested [Christenberry & Powell 1987; Bulow 1974; Powell 1985; Timberlake et al. 1989]. Ultrasound, however, is a straightforward test, the reliability of which increases with experience, and may serve to reveal an unsuspected contralateral hernia or a persistent processus [Erez et al. 1996].

D. Treatment

1. Uncomplicated Hernias

It is justifiable to adopt a waiting policy during the first few months of life, as spontaneous obliteration of the canal may occur. This may be assisted by the use of a bandage including a double truss, adjusted to the size of the infant and kept in place with thigh straps. Such a truss is contra-indicated in large hernias, which are difficult to reduce, or by an undescended testis. It may irritate the skin and restrict movement, so that it should be reserved for special cases. There is no reason to delay treatment in the full term infant [Rowe 1995; Wiener et al. 1996] bearing in mind that the risk of incarceration during the first few months of life is higher than is commonly thought (14-30%) [Puri et al. 1984; Moss & Hatch 1991; Stylianos et al. 1993]. Surgery may be deferred in the premature baby, but many surgeons operate regardless of the age or weight of the patient. The operation is perfectly safe at any age, provided that the surgeon is experienced in treating infants and children. Simple closure of the processus is all that is required, and repair of the abdominal wall is unnecessary, though with large hernias the transversalis fascia must be carefully reconstituted at the deep inguinal ring. The inguinal canal in the infant is short so that it is possible to reach the origin of the patent processus through the superficial ring, without incising the external oblique [Banks 1884]. Although this method has been widely used [Boureau 1978; Rickman 1978] it seems to us better to open the inguinal canal in order to expose the cord and the peritoneal sac, which is often very delicate. We have needed to re-operate five times for hernias treated by this method, as inadequate excision of the processus has led to a recurrence. We do not routinely explore the other side unless there is clinical or ultrasound evidence [Rothenberg & Barnett 1955; Hamrich & Williams 1962; Laufer & Eyal 1962; Kiesewetter & Oh 1980]. Such a policy gives widely varying results according to the author and the age of the patient [Weber & Tracy 1993; Rowe 1995]. Routine exploration carries a definite risk to the vas deferens and the testicular vessels [Homonnai et al. 1980; Shandling & Janik 1981; Janik & Shandling 1982; Rathauser 1985]. Routine preoperative herniorraphy [Hecker et al. 1973] or needle aspiration of the contralateral side [Kramer & Davis 1967; Levy 1972] is probably not indicated. Recently a number of authors [Lobe & Schropp 1992; Holcomb et al. 1996; Wolf & Hopkins 1994] have advocated laparoscopy, which may be carried out via the hernial sac during repair [Groner et al. 1995; Grosman et al. 1995; Wulkan 1996], or better with a fine 70° endoscope [Liu 1995]. However this technique adds to the time of operation and is probably useless in most cases.

The inguinal canal is approached by a transverse incision in the lower groin fold (Fig. 12.36). Oblique incisions such as they are used in the adult leave an unsightly and often retracted scar. The aponeurosis of external oblique is incised from the superficial inguinal ring or above it. The ilio-inguinal nerve, often accompanied by a fine vascular bundle, is easily seen and left in contact with the aponeurosis. Clearing of the fibers of the cremaster isolates the peritoneal sac which lies in front of the elements of the cord. It is not usually necessary to mobilize the cord in order to free up the sac, which may injure the vas deferens or testicular vessels. When the sac is large it is often necessary to open it in order to free it completely (Fig. 12.37). If the sac is long, which is often the case, its distal part is left behind as dissection in this area increases the risk to the testicular vessels. The sac is closed at its neck by a single stitch, or, if it is broad, it can be overrun (Fig. 12.38). The technique of twisting the sac to make sure that it is empty and then ligating it without previously opening it [Duhamel 1957], can only be done with very small sacs. The ligature should be applied as high as possible, at the level of the epigastric vessels. When the deep inguinal ring is broadened, the transversalis fascia should be reconstituted above the point of exit of the cord, by two or three sutures. It is usually not necessary to fix the internal oblique and conjoint tendon in front of the cord, unless the abdominal wall is greatly distended (Fig. 12.39). The spermatic fascia and cremaster muscle should be closed in every case. Before closing the abdominal wall the position of the

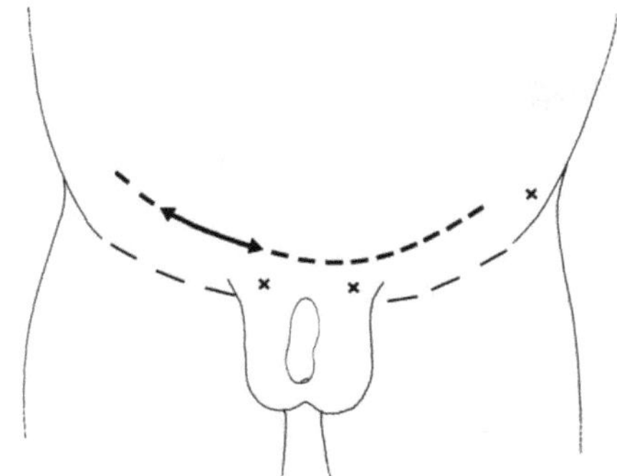

Fig. 12.36. Transverse incision through the inferior inguinal fold in the treatment of uncomplicated inguinal hernia

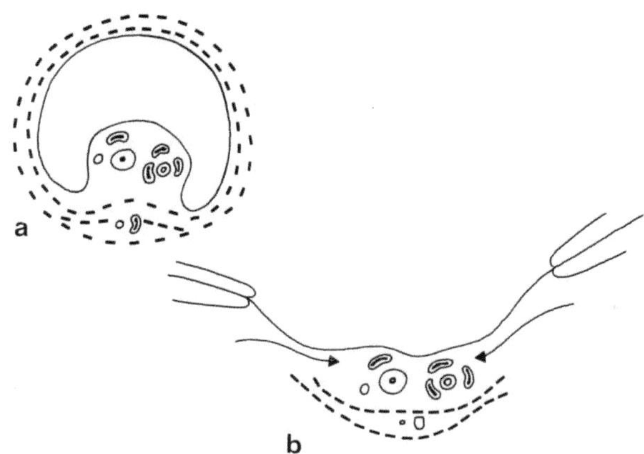

Fig. 12.37. Repair of the hernial sac. **a** The unopened sac is freed. **b** Opening of the sac allows it to be more easily separated from the spermatic cord

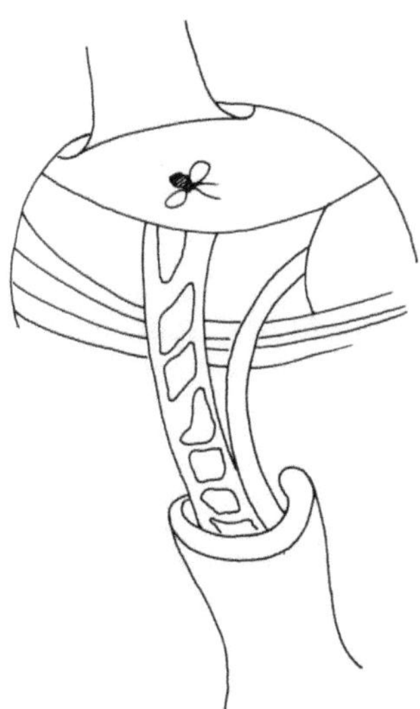

Fig. 12.38. Closure of the base of the hernial sac using a Meunier suture

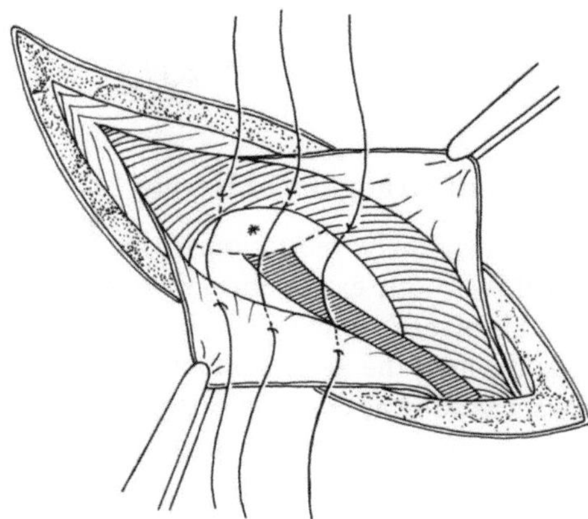

Fig. 12.39. Lowering of the conjoint tendon down to the inguinal ligament in front of the spermatic cord

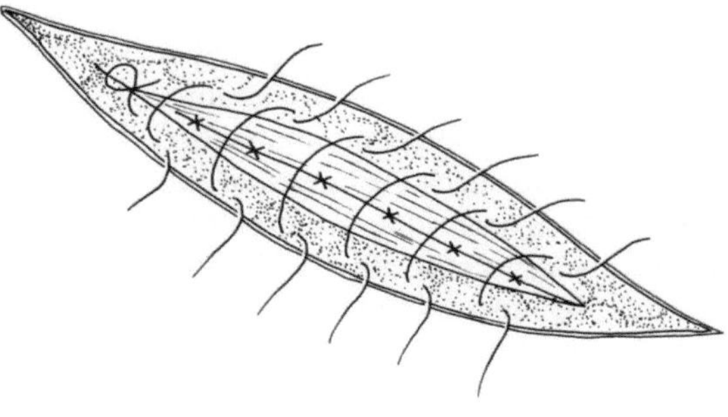

Fig. 12.40. Suturing of the aponeurosis of the external oblique and subcutaneous closure

testicle within the scrotum should be checked, in order to prevent any postoperative fixation by fibrous tissue. The external oblique aponeurosis is closed by a running suture of absorbable material and the subcutaneous tissue and skin approximated with a running suture or intradermal stitches (Fig. 12.40). The preperitoneal approach recommended by Duhamel (1957), Boley and Kleinhaus (1966) and Fowler (1973 & 1975) has no particular advantage over the above technique in the repair of an uncomplicated hernia, but facilitates the operation in the small infant.

The postoperative course is usually uneventful. We have only seen complications such as hematoma or abscess in 0.7% of cases [Audry et al. 1994]. This benign course means that the operation can quite safely be performed on a day case basis [Cohen et al. 1980]. Theoretically, repair of an inguinal hernia should represent a good indication for laparoscopic surgery, since the essential step is ligation of the processus vaginalis with no repair of the abdominal wall, and this approach allows inspection of the opposite side, and any necessary treatment. However, information is at present lacking, especially in the case of small children.

2. Obstructed and Strangulated Hernia

If the child is seen early, reduction of the hernia is usually possible, in our experience. Following sedation, the child is placed supine, with the bed or cot tilted upwards towards the head. Reduction may occur spontaneously as soon as crying has stopped. If, when maximum sedation has been reached, this does not occur, gentle pressure may be applied along the axis of the inguinal canal. It is customary to attempt this reduction in a hot bath in order to ensure that the child is relaxed, but this is awkward and often ineffective. Reduction is obtained in a great number of cases. A truss should be applied immediately in order to avoid recurrence, and operation carried out as soon as local oedema has dispersed [Rickham 1978; Palmer 1978]. The child is carefully monitored over the next 48 hours, in order to check for intestinal damage.

If the child is seen late, no attempt at reduction should be made, because of possible interference with bowel viability. Loss of fluid and electrolyte may be quite severe in the new born, for whom a strangulated hernia is always a severe accident [Rickham 1978], and may even lead to death, as we have ourselves unfortunately seen in two late cases. Furthermore, strangulation may lead to testicular infarction through compression of the vascular pedicle [Hill et al. 1962; Sloman & Mylius 1963; Sauer & Menardi 1975]. A very conservative attitude is indicated in these cases, because there is a very real possibility of recovery, which is difficult to estimate but it is considerably greater than following torsion, although secondary atrophy may occur. The technique of repair is no different from that described above; however, in certain cases it is possible to approach the deep inguinal ring via a preperitoneal route [Jones & Towns 1983] or to close it following reduction of the herniated viscera, transperitoneally [Misra 1995].

3. Inguinal Hernia with Undescended Testis

This combination completely contraindicates treatment with a truss. Operation is required whatever the age of the child and should include correction of the maldescent at the same time [Swenson 1964; Scorer 1967; Boureau 1978]. In fact the fibrosis caused by dissection of the sac in contact with the spermatic cord and the testicle makes later orchidopexy much more difficult. Using a conventional technique, the testicle is

placed in the scrotum between the skin and the fibrous layers, via a small counter incision (Fig. 12.41). A strangulated hernia may be difficult to distinguish from torsion of an ectopic testis, but in either case immediate operation is mandatory.

4. Inguinal Hernia in Girls

When an ovary is present in the hernia, whether by prolapse or by sliding (Fig. 12.42) its vitality is always threatened by a possible strangulation. Operation is therefore always indicated, at whatever age, particularly as dissection of the sac is safe and easy [Boley et al. 1991]. If the ovary is adherent, it is not possible to resect the sac and ligate it at its origin, but it should be inverted with two or three purse string sutures, as in other sliding hernias [Boureau 1978; Wooley 1979] (Fig. 12.43). Exploration of the other side [Wright 1982] is less of a problem than in boys. It is generally carried out before the age of three or four, particularly in cases of left-sided hernia [Wiener et al. 1996].

It is very important when one operates on an inguinal hernia in a girl to examine the ovary carefully and to check that a tube is present. Occasionally one discovers in a child who is phenotypically female a gonad of which the morphology and connections are those of a testicle. In these cases of the syndrome of "testicular feminisation" the Müllerian system has not developed and there is neither tube nor uterus. The gonad should be biopsied, and the nature of the inter-sexuality determined by a karyotype. The psychological approach to the family following this discovery requires great tact and prudence. The relative frequency of this situation indicates a careful examination of the genital tract by anorectal palpation at the preoperative examination, and certain authors [Rickham 1975] routinely examine the buccal chromatin in all girls presenting with inguinal hernia.

E. Particular Problems

The surgeon should be aware of certain problems which may occur during treatment of inguinal hernia in children.

1. Hernial Appendix

Appendicitis in a hernia giving rise to symptoms of strangulation is unusual [Alvear 1976; Srouji & Buck 1978; Bar Moar & Zeltzer 1978]. One may nonetheless on occasion find an appendix on opening the processus vaginalis, either lying free or fixed to the sac by its mesentery. The latter case represents a true sliding

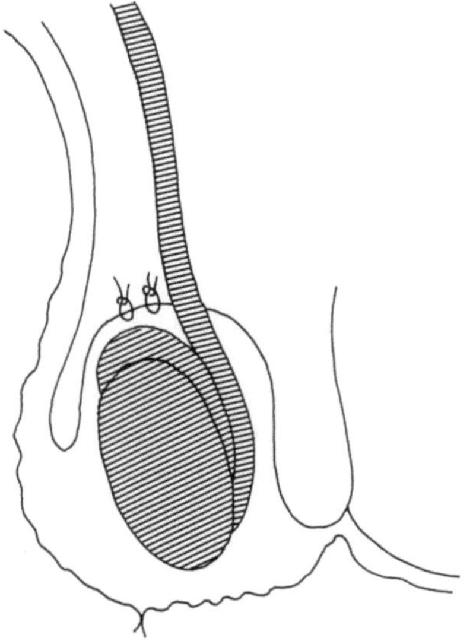

Fig. 12.41. Inguinal hernia with testicular ectopy. The testis is positioned in the scrotum between the skin and fibrous layer

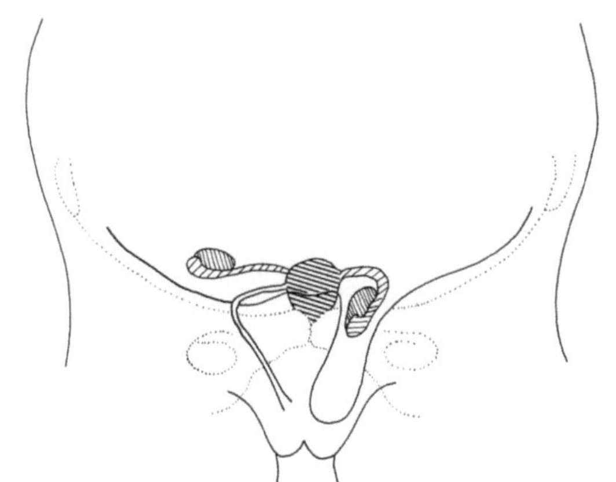

Fig. 12.42. Inguinal hernia in a girl. Herniation of the ovary caries a risk of strangulation

hernia [Rose & Santulli 1978] and appendicectomy is necessary in order to close the sac at its origin. On the other hand, routine appendicectomy during operations for right-sided hernia, which has been recommended in the past [Duhamel 1957] is a septic procedure which may lead to contamination of the wound, and is inadvisable.

2. Meckel's Diverticulum

The presence of a Meckel's diverticulum within the hernial sac constitutes the well-described but very rare hernia of Littré. For the same reasons which apply to the appendix it is not advisable to carry out routine excision of the diverticulum during repair of the hernia.

3. Splenogonadal Fusion and Aberrant Splenic Nodules

It is occasionally found during operation on a left-sided hernia that there is a band of splenic fibrous tissue between the gonad and the spleen [Putscher & Mannion 1956; Peruchio et al. 1957; Sieber 1969; Mizutani et al. 1974; Given & Guiney 1978]. Alternatively there may be isolated nodule of splenic tissue [Putscher & Mannion 1956; Stowens 1959]. Resection of the splenic tissue and replacement of the testicle in the scrotum usually presents no difficulty.

4. Adrenal Nodules

In the same way, there may be some heterotopic tissue which on histological examination proves to be of adrenal origin, as seen in one of our patients [Roosen-Tunge & Lund 1972; Berry & Lynch 1972]. Removal of such a nodule again presents no problem.

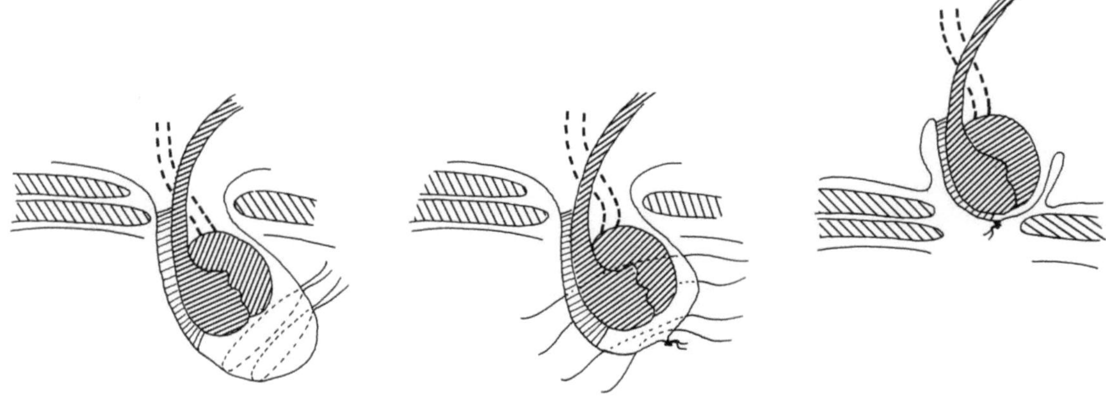

Fig. 12.43. Treatment of a herniated ovary. The hernial sac is invaginated by two or three purse-string sutures, allowing reduction of the ovary

5. Anomalies of Testicle and Vas Deferens

Operation for hernia may reveal certain abnormalities of the male genital structures. There may be a duplex testicle [Scorer & Farrington 1971; Adams & Jordan 1972]. Removal of the supernumary testicle may be indicated after careful dissection and identification of all the abnormal structures. The vas deferens may be abnormal in certain cases of cryptorchidism and present a free lower end. This does not strongly suggest testicular agenesis because again it may be found in an iliac position, totally separated from its duct [Scorer & Farrington 1971; Mourot et al. 1975]. If possible, the testicle should be replaced in the scrotum. Again, absence of the vas deferens with a normally present testicle may be seen in cases of renal agenesis [Ochsner et al. 1972; Lukash et al. 1975], or in mucoviscidosis [Gracey et al. 1969; Klotz 1973; Lukash et al. 1975]. Ultrasound examination and a sweat test [Rickmann 1978] are indicated in this cases.

6. Mullerian Structures in Boys

Vestigial Mullerian structures may be found in contact with the vas deferens [Stallings et al. 1976; Sloan & Walsh 1976; Pappis et al. 1979]. They should be resected although it is sometimes difficult to preserve the vas deferens.

7. Herniation of the Bladder

In children the bladder and the deep inguinal ring lie very close together, and one quite often observes "inguinal horns" of the bladder, on cystography. Operation discloses prevesical fat at the base of the hernial sac. However, true hernias of the bladder and rare [Shaw & Santulli 1967; Colodny & Lebowitz 1979].

8. Cystic Hygroma

Prolongation of a subperitoneal cystic hygroma may extend into the inguinal canal towards the scrotum or labium majus, and present as an irreducible hernia [Hoffman 1965; Kafka & Novak 1970]. In two personal cases the finding of iliac tumor in continuity with the inguinal swelling allowed us to make the diagnosis. Excision of the hygroma requires a larger incision than for a simple herniotomy.

9. Hernias and General Congenital Abnormalities

Wooley et al. (1967) have drawn attention to the surgical and anesthetic problems posed by inguinal hernias associated with other abnormalities such as the Hurler syndrome [Coran & Eraklis 1967] or Ehlers-Danlos disease, and the frequency of recurrence in these circumstances [McEntyre & Raffensperger 1977].

F. Direct Inguinal Hernias

Direct hernias are rarely seen in childhood or adolescence [De Boer 1957; Packard & McLaughin 1953; Fonkalsrud et al. 1965]. They may occur following repair of an indirect hernia, as we have seen and has been reported in various publications [Fonkalsrud 1965; Viidik & Marshall 1980; Wright 1994]. It occurs exclusively in boys. It is possible that the transversalis fascia is weakened at the first operation. The direct recurrence usually occurs quite early. A broad-necked sac which enlarges the deep inguinal ring may also give rise to a direct hernia. When the hernia is "primary" it may suggest an inherent weakness of the fascia. One can also occasionally see a combination of a direct and indirect hernia forming a "pantaloon" hernia. Surgical repair presents no particular problem. The transversalis fascia must be carefully reconstituted and the conjoint tendon of the internal oblique and transversus fixed to the arcade.

G. Recurrences

Recurrence of an inguinal hernia may be the result of incomplete removal of the sac or, as has just been described, the secondary appearance of a direct hernia [Wright 1994].

H. Femoral Hernia

Femoral hernias are equally rare in children [Fosburg & Mahin 1965; Lavina et al. 1966; Wright 1994], and especially so in small infants. We have seen only seven cases, none of which had followed a previous repair of an inguinal hernia, as has been reported elsewhere [Immordino 1972]. The hernia may be confused with an inguinal hernia although it quite clearly presents below Malgaigne's line.

The hernia can be approached through the inguinal canal by opening the transversalis fascia sufficiently high to leave enough of the fascia below the incision to allow sound reconstruction. The dissection is extended in the subperitoneal fatty plane towards the femoral canal from which the sac can usually be freed totally. There is often a fair-sized lipoma lying in front of the sac. Simple ligation at the base of the sac is usually all that is required, but it may be preferred to narrow the femoral ring [Marshall 1983] by a few sutures passed between Cooper's ligament and the femoral arch, which may take up the transversus. The transversalis fascia must be carefully repaired. Marshall and Jellie (1981) have drawn attention to the possibility of pre-femoral hernias, in which the sac is spread out in front of the femoral vessels rather than medial to them, while its neck lies lateral to the epigastric vessels rather than medial.

References

Adams JR, Jordan WP (1972) Polyorachism. South Med. 65: 594

Ahmed SI (1971) Abdominoscrotal hydrocele in an infant. Surgery 70: 136

Alvear DI (1976) Acuta appendicitis presenting as a scrotal mass. J Pediatr Surg 13: 181-182

Audry G, Johanet S, Achrafi H, Lupold M, Gruner M (1994) The risk of wound infection after inguinal incision in pediatric out patient surgery. Eur J Pediatr Surg 4: 87-89

Bar Moar JA, Zeltzer M (1978) Acuta appendicitis located in a scrotal hernia of a premature infant. J Pediatr Surg 13: 181-182

Banks WM (1884) Note on radical cure of hernia. Harisson and Sons, London

Berry BE, Lynch RC (1972) Aberrant adrenal cortical tissue with inguinal hernia: a case report. J La State Med Soc 124: 153

Boley SJ, Kleinhaus S (1966) A place for the Cheatle-Henry approach in pediatric surgery? J Pediatr Surg 1: 394-397

Boley SJ, Cahn D, Laueur T, et al (1991) The irreductible ovary: a true emergency. J Pediatr Surg 26: 1035-1038

Booth J (1987) Abdominoscrotal hydrocele. J Pediatr Surg 22: 177-178

Boureau M (1978) Reliquats du canal péritonéo-vaginal et insuffisance de migration testiculaire. In: Pellerin D, Bertin P (eds) Technique chirurgicale pédiatrique. Masson, Paris, pp 526-536

Blan JS, Keating TH, Stockinger FS (1973) Radiological diagnosis of inguinal hernia in children. Surg Gynecol Obstet 131: 401

Braun P, Lopez-Ruiz P. Bensoussan AL, Durcharme JE (1975) Inguinale Herniographie beim Kind. Z Kinderchir 16: 294

Bronsther B, Abrahms MW, Elboim C (1972) Inguinal hernia in children. A study of 1,000 cases and review of the litterature. JAMA 27: 552

Broutin M, Gruner M, Faure C (1975) La péritonéographie dans les hernies de l'enfant. Entretiens de Bichat: Chirurgie et Spécialités Chirurgicales, p 29-34

Bulow S (1974) Artificial pneumoperitoneum during inguinal herniotomy in children. Acta Chir Scand 140: 127-130

Burgues P (1986) Abdominoscrotal hydrocele. J Pediatr Surg 21: 987-988

Christenberry DP, Powell RW (1987) Intra-operative pneumoperitoneum (Goldstein test) in the infant and child with unilateral inguinal hernia. Am J Surg 154: 628-630

Cohen D, Keneally J, Black A, Gaffney S, Johnson A (1980) Experience with day-stay surgery. J Pediatr Surg 15: 21-25

Colodny AH, Lebowitz RL (1979) Abnormalities of the bladder and prostate. In: Ravitch MM, Welche KJ, Benson CD, Aberdeen E, Randolph JG (eds) Pediatric surgery, 3rd edn. Year Book, Chicago, pp 1306-1314

Coran AG, Eraklis AJ (1967) Inguinal hernia in the Hurler-Hunter syndrome. Surgery 61: 302

Currarino G (1974) Incarcerated inguinal hernia in infants. Pediatr Radiol 2: 247-250

De Boer A (1957) Inguinal hernia in infants and children. Arch Surg 75: 920

Ducharme JC, Bertrand R, Chacar R (1967) Is it possible to diagnose inguinal hernia by X-ray? A preliminary report of herniography. J Assoc Can Radiol 18: 448

Duhamel B (1957) Technique Chirurgicale Infantile. Masson, Paris, pp 56-67

Erez J, Rathaus V, Werner M, Narsesyants I, Lazar L, Katl S (1996) Preoperative sonography of the inguinal canal prevents a necessary controlateral exploration. Pediatr Surg Int 11: 487-489

Festen C (1974) Der interstitielle Leistenbruch bei Säuglingen. Z Kinderchir 14: 230

Fonkalsrud EW, de Lorimier AA, Clatworthy HW Jr (1965) Femoral and direct inguinal hernias in infants and children. J Am Med Assoc 192: 597

Fonkalsrud EW (1995) Is routine controlateral exploration advisable for children with unilateral inguinal hernias? Am J Surg 169: 285

Fosburg RG, Mahin HP (1965) Femoral hernia in children. Am J Surg 109: 470

Fowler R (1973) Preperitoneal repair of inguinal hernias in infancy and childhood. Aust Paediat J 9: 83

Fowler R (1975) The applied surgical anatomy of the peritoneal fascia of the groin and the "secondary" internal inguinal ring. Aust N Z J Surg 45: 8

Gallegos F, Glass HG, Lynch RH (1974) Inguinal herniography in cases of unilateral hernia to detect controlateral hernia. Int Surg 59: 279

Ger R, Monroe K, Duvivier R, et al (1990) Management of indirect inguinal hernia by laparoscopic closure of the neck of sac. Am J Surg 159: 370-373

Given HF, Guiney EJ (1978) Splenic gonadal fusion. J Pediatr Surg 13: 341

Given JP, Rubin SZ (1989) Occurence of controlateral inguinal hernia following unilateral repair in pediatric hospital. J Pediatr Surg 24: 963-965

Gracey M, Campbell P, Noblett H (1969) Atretic vas deferens in cystic fibrosis. N Engl J Med 280: 276

Groner JL, Marlow J, Teich S (1995) Groin Laparoscopy. A new technique for controlateral groin evaluation in pediatric inguinal hernia repair. J Am Coll Surg 181: 168-170

Grosman PA, Wolf SA, Hopkins JW, et al (1995) The efficacy of laparoscopic examination of the internal ring in children. J Pediatr Surg 30: 214-217

Gunnlaugsson GH, Dawson B, Lynn HB (1967) Treatment of inguinal hernia in infants and children: experience with controlateral exploration. Mayo Clin Proc 42: 129

Guttman FM, Bertrand R, Ducharme JC (1972) Herniography and the pediatric controlateral inguinal hernia. Surg Gynecol Obstet 135: 551

Hamrich LC, Williams JO (1962) Is controlateral exploration indicated in children with unilateral inguinal hernia? Am J Surg 104: 52

Harrison CB, Kaplan GW, Scherz H, et al (1990) Diagnostic prenumoperitoneum for the detection of the clinically occult controlateral hernia in children. J Urol 114: 510-511

Hecker WCh, Waag KL, Fendel H (1973) Intraoperative herniographie beim Säugling. Z Kinderchir 12: 273

Hessert W (1910) The frequency of congenital sac in oblique inguinal hernia. Surg Gynecol Obstet 10: 252

Hill RH Jr, Pollock WF, Sprong DH Jr (1962) Testicular infarction and incarcerated inguinal hernia. Anat Surg 85: 351

Hoffman E (1965) Multicystic retroperitoneal lymphangioma presenting as an indirect inguinal hernia in a newborn. Am Surg 31: 515

Holcomb GW Jr (1965) Routine bilateral inguinal hernia repair in infants and children. Am J Dis Child 109: 114

Holcomb GW, Brock JW, Morgan WN (1994) Laparoscopic evaluation for controlateral processus vaginalis. J Pediatr Surg 20: 970-973

Holcomb GW, Morgan WN, Brock JW (1996) Laparoscopic evaluation for controlateral processus vaginalis: part II. J Pediatr Surg 31: 1170-1173

Homonnai ZI, Fainman N, Paz GF, et al (1980) Testicular function after herniotomy. Andrologia 12: 115-120

Hrabovszky Z, Pinter AB (1994) Routine bilateral exploration for inguinal hernia in infancy and childhood. Eur J Pediatr Surg 5: 152-155

Hutchinson C, Koop CE (1956) The relastionship of the testis and processus vaginalis testis in the infant. Anat Rec 124: 310

Immordino PA (1972) Femoral hernia in infancy and childhood. J Pediatr Surg 7: 40-43

James PM, Hunsicker R (1972) Is herniogram the answer to routine bilateral hernia repair? Am Surg 38: 43

Janik JS, Shandling B (1982) The vulnerability of the vas deferens (II). The case against routine bilateral inguinal exploration. J Pediatr Surg 17: 585-588

Jewett TC, Kuhn JP, Allen JE (1976) Herniography in children. J Pediatr Surg 11: 451

Jones PF, Towns GM (1983) An abdominal extraperitoneal approach for the incarcerated inguinal hernia of infancy. Br J Surg 70: 719-720

Kafka V, Novak K (1970) Multicystic retroperitoneal lymphangioma in infant appearing as an inguinal hernia. J Pediatr Surg 5: 173

Kahn A (1987) Abdominoscrotal hydrocele: a cause of abdominal mass in children. A case report and review of the litterature. J Pediatr Surg 22: 809-810

Kiesewetter WB, Oh KS (1980) Unilateral inguinal hernias in children. What about the opposite side? Arch Surg 115: 1443-1445

Klotz PG (1973) Congenital absence of the vas deferens. J Urol 109: 662-663

Kramer SG, Davis SE (1967) Transperitoneal detection of occult inguinal hernia. Milit Med 132: 512-514

Laufer A, Eyal Z (1962) Controlateral exploration in a child with unilateral hernia. Arch Surg 85: 521

Lavina H, Lickley A, Trubler GA (1966) Femoral hernia in children. J Pediatr Surg 1: 338-341

Levy JL (1972) Evaluation of transperitoneal probing for detecting controleateral inguinal hernia in infants. Surgery 71: 412

Liu C, Chin T, Jan SE, Wei C (1995) Intraoperative laparoscopic diagnosis of controlateral patent processus vaginalis in children with unilateral inguinal hernia. Br J Surg 82: 106-108

Lobe TE, Schropp KP (1992) Inguinal hernias in pediatrics: initial experience with laparoscopic exploration on the controlateral side. J Laparoendosc Surg 2: 135-140

Lukash F, Zwiren GT, Andrews HG (1975) Significance of absent vas deferens at hernia repair in infants and children. J Pediatr Surg 10: 765-769

Lynn HB, Johnson WW (1961) Inguinal herniorrhaphy in children: a critical analysis of 1,000 cases. Arch Surg 83: 573

Mc Gregor DB, Halverson K, McVay CB (1980) The unilateral pediatric inguinal hernia: should the controlateral side be explored? J Pediatr Surg 15: 313-317

Maish B, Swarmy, Altman B (1972) Bilateral interstitial hernia in the newborn infant. Surgery 69: 557

Marshall DG, Jellie H (1981) Prevascular femoral hernia with ectopic testis in an infant. J Ped Surg 16: 519-520

Marshall DG (1983) Femoral hernias in children. J Pediatr Surg 18: 160-162

McEntyre RL, Raffensperger JG (1977) Surgical complications of Ehler-Danlos syndrome in children. J Pediatr Surg 12: 531-534

Misra D, Hewitt G, Potts SR, Boston VE (1995) Transperitoneal closure of internal ring in incarcerated infantile inguinal hernias. J Pediatr Surg 30: 95-96

Mizutani S, Kiyohara H, Sonoda T (1974) Splenic-gonadal fusion in a Japanese boy. J Urol 112: 528-529

Morgan EH, Anson BJ (1942) Anatomy of region of inguinal hernia. IV The internal surface of the parietal layers. W Bull Northwestern Univ Med School 16: 20

Moss RL, Hatch EI (1991) Inguinal hernia repair in early infancy. Am J Surg 161: 596-599

Mourot M, Aubert D, Sava P, Gille P (1975) L'indépendance épididymo-testiculaire totale. A propos de deux observations. Ann Chir Infant 16: 189-191

Ochsner HG, Brannan W, Goodier E (1972) Absent vas deferens associated with renal agenesis. JAMA 222: 1055

Packard GB, McLaughlin CH (1953) Treatment of inguinal hernia in infancy and childhood. Surg Gynecol Obstet 97: 603

Palmer BV (1978) Incarcerated inguinal hernia in children. Ann R Coll Surg Engl 60: 121-124

Pappis C, Constantinides C, Chiotis D, Dacou Voutetakis C (1979) Persistant müllerien duct structures in cryptorchid male infant: surgical dilemnas. J Pediatr Surg 14: 128-131

Peruchio P, Soutoul J, Mollaret L, Dejussieu (1957) Cordon spléno-testiculaire et hernie inguinale. Presse Med 65: 138-140

Powell RW (1985) Intraoperative diagnostic pneumoperitoneum in pediatric patients with unilateral inguinal hernias: the Goldstein test. J Pediatr Surg 20: 418-421

Puri P, Guiney EJ, O'Donnell B (1984) Inguinal hernia in infants: the fate of the testis following in carceration. J Pediatr Surg 19: 44-46

Putscher WCJ, Mannion WC (1956) Splenic-gonada fusion. Am J Pathol 32: 15

Ramonede L (1883) Le canal péritonéo-vaginal et la hernie péritonéo-vaginale étranglée chez l'adulte. Thèse Médecine, Paris

Rathauser F (1985) Historical owerview of the bilateral approach to pediatric inguinal hernias. Am J Surg 150: 527-532

Rickham PP, Soper RT, Stauffer UG (1975) Synopsis of pediatric surgery. Georg Thieme, Stuttgart, pp 258-262

Rickham PP (1975) Incarcerated inguinal hernia. In: Rickham PP, Lister J, Irving IM (eds) Neonatal surgery, 2nd edn. Butterworths, London, pp 301-307

Roosen-Tunge EC, Lund J (1972) Abnormal sex cord formation and an intratesticular adrenal cortical nodule in a human foetus. Anat Rec 173: 57

Rose E, Santulli TV (1978) Sliding appendiceal inguinal hernia. Surg Gynecol Obstet 146: 626-627

Rothenberg RE, Barnett T (1955) Bilateral herniotomy in infants and children. Surgery 37: 947

Rowe WI, Copelson LW and Clatworthy HW (1969) The patent processus vaginalis and the inguinal hernia. J Pediatr Surg 4: 102

Rowe WI, Clatworthy HW (1970) Incarcerated and strangulated hernias in children. Arch Surg 101: 136

Rowe WI, Marchildon MB (1981) Inguinal hernia and hydrocele in infants and children. Surg Clin North Am 61: 1137-1145

Rowe WI (1995) Inguinal and scrotal disorders. In: Rowes, O'Neill, Grosfeld, et al. (eds) Essentials in pediatric surgery. Mosby Year Book, St Louis, pp 446-461

Sachs H (1885) Untersuchungen über den Processus Vaginalis peritonei als Prädisponierendes Moment für die aussere Leisthenhernie. Inaugural Dissertation, Dorpot

Saharia PC, Bronsther B, Abrams MW (1979) Abdominoscrotal hydrocele case presentation and review of the literature. J Pediatr Surg 14: 713-714

Sauer H, Menardi G (1975) Hodengangrän als Komplikation der Inkarzeration der Säuglingshernia. Z Kinderchir 16: 421

Scorer CG (1967) Early operation for the undescended testis. Br J Surg 54: 694

Scorer CG, Farrington GH (1971) Congenital deformities of the testis and epidiymis. Butterworths, London, pp 157-174

Shandling B, Janik JS (1981) The vulnerability of the vas deferens. J Pediatr Surg 16: 461-464

Shaw A, Santulli TV (1967) Management of sliding hernias of the urinary bladder in infants. Surg Gynecol Obstet 124: 1314

Sieber WK (1969) Splenotesticular cord (splenogonadal fusion) associated with inguinal hernia. J Pediatr Surg 4: 208

Slim MS, Mishalany HG (1971) Outpatient inguinal herniorraphy in childhood. Br J Clin Pract 25: 223

Sloan WR, Walsh CR (1976) Familial persistent müllerian duct syndrome. J Urol 115: 456-461

Sloman JG, Mylius RE (1963) Testicular infarction in infancy: its association with irreductible inguinal hernia. In: Stephens FD, Webster R (eds) Congenital malformations of the rectum, anus and genito-urinary tracts. Livingstone, London, pp 321-324

Spackman RS (1962) Bilateral exploration in inguinal hernia in juvenile patients. Surgery 51: 393

Spier LN, Cohen H, Kenigsberg K (1995) Bilateral abdominoscrotal hydrocele: a case report. J Pediatr Surg 30: 1382-1383

Squire R, Gough DC (1988) Abdominoscrotal hydrocele in infancy. Br J Urol 61: 347-349

Srouji M, Buck BE (1978) Neonatal appendicitis: ischemic infarction incarcerated inguinal hernia. J Pediatr Surg 13: 177-179

Stallings MW, Rose AH, Auman GL (1976) Persistant müllerian structures in male neonate. Pediatrics 57: 568-569

Stowens D (1959) Pediatric pathology. Williams & Wilkins, Baltimore

Struve-Christensen E, Jensen LE (1970) Inguinal herniotomy in children. Z Kinderchir 8: 245

Stylianos S, Jacir NN, Harris BH (1993) Incarceration of inguinal hernia in infants prior to elective repair. J Pediatr Surg 28: 582-585

Surana R, Puri P (1993) Fate of patent processus vaginalis: a case against routine controlateral exploration for unilateral inguinal hernia in children. Pediatr Surg Int 8: 412-414

Swenson O (1964) Diagnostic and treatment of inguinal hernia. Pediatrics 34: 412

Thompson W, Lomgerbeam JK, Reeves C (1972) Herniograms - An aid to the diagnosis and treatment of groin hernias in infants and children. Anat Surg 105: 71

Timberlake CA, Ochsner MG, Powell RW (1989) Diagnostic pneumoperitoneum in the pediatric patient with a unilateral inguinal hernia. Arch Surg 124: 721-723

Ulman I, Demircan M, Arikan A, et al (1995) Unilateral inguinal hernia in girls. Is routine controlateral exploration justified? J Pediatr Surg 30: 1684-1686

Vanneuville G, Fabre JL, Merle P, Dalens B, Tanguy A (1983) Intérêt de la herniographie dans la conduite thérapeutique des hernies inguinales de la fille. A propos de 148 observations. Chir Pediatr 24: 95-99

Viidik T, Marshall DG (1980) Direct inguinal hernias in infancy and early childhood. J Pediatr Surg 15: 646-647

Walsh SZ (1962) The incidence of external hernia in premature infants. Acta Pediatr Scand 51: 161

Weber TR, Tracy TF Jr (1993) Groin hernias and hydroceles. In: Asheraft KW, Holder TM (eds) Pediatric Surgery. Sannders, Philadelphia, pp 562-570

White JJ, Parks LL, Haller JA (1968) The inguinal herniogram. Surgery 63: 991

Wiener ES, Touloukian RJ, Rodgers BM, Grosfeld JL, Smith ES, Ziegler MM, Coran AG (1996) Hernia survey of the section on surgery of the American Academy of Pediatrics. J Pediatr Surg 31: 1166-1168

Wolf SA, Hopkins JW (1994) Laparoscopic incidence of controlateral patent processus vaginalis in boys with clinical unilateral hernias. J Pediatr Surg 29: 1118-1120

Wooley NM (1979) Inguinal hernia. In: Ravitch MH, Welch KJ, Benson CD, Aberdeen E, Randolph JG (eds) Pediatric Surgery, 3rd edn. Year Book, Chicago, pp 815-826

Wooley NM, Morgan S, Hays DM (1967) Heritable disorders of connective tissue. Surgical and anesthesic problems. J Pediatr Surg 2: 325-331

Wright JE (1994) Direct inguinal hernia in infancy and childhood. Pediatr Surg Int 9: 161-163

Wright JE (1994) Recurrent inguinal hernia in infancy and childhood. Pediatr Surg Int 9: 164-166

Wright JE (1994) Fermoral hernia in childhood. Pediatr Surg Int 9: 167-169

Wright JE (1982) Inguinal hernia in girls: desirability and dangers of bilateral exploration. Aust Paediat J 18: 55-57

Wulkan ML, Wiener ES, Van Balen N, Vescio P (1996) Laparoscopie through the open ipsilateral sac to evaluate presence of controlateral hernia. J Pediatr Surg 31: 1174-1177

IV. Umbilical Hernias in Children

Umbilical hernias are very frequently seen in infants and young children. Most of them resolve spontaneously and complications are rare. However, a considerable number of children are brought to the surgeon for consultation.

A. Incidence

The incidence of umbilical hernia is high during the first few months of life, particularly in premature babies or those who exhibit delayed intrauterine growth [Moore 1977]. Certain congenital abnormalities such as trisomy 18 and 21, the Wiederman-Beckwith syndrome, the Hurler syndrome, and thyroid insufficiency, are associated with an increased incidence. Girls and boys are equally affected (51% and 49% in our experience). It is customarily recognized that the incidence is six to ten times more frequent in the black as against the white population [Evans 1941; Crump 1952]. A study by Blumberg (1980) led to a reconsideration of this idea because in a comparative study of 1,106 white as against 709 black children, the overall incidence of umbilical hernia was respectively 19 and 23%. When the two groups were followed up it was found that the incidence at birth was 40% in white and 30% in black children and at the age of two it was 15% in white and 30% in black children and the respective figures at the age of three were 9 and 10%. There seems therefore to be a difference in the speed of spontaneous closure of the umbilical ring, which occurs earlier in whites than blacks. Spontaneous closure is thus seen in most cases, and usually occurs during the first three years, though it may be delayed. It is customarily said that the larger the defect, the slower its closure [Heifetz et al. 1963; Walker 1967] but this is not absolutely true [Blumberg 1980]. Persistence of a congenital hernia into adult life is possible, although most adult hernias seem to be of the acquired type and a direct relationship is difficult to establish [Haller 1971]. The hernia emerges through the umbilical scar and becomes more obvious when the child coughs or cries. Large hernias may completely unfold the umbilicus and the skin becomes very thin. The size of the defect can be assessed with the finger. Sometimes the gap is very symmetrical being larger at the top, or may lie immediately above the umbilicus. This is a paraumbilical hernia which displaces the scar downwards (Fig. 12.44). Divarication of the rectus muscles, or epigastric hernia, may occur separately from an umbilical hernia.

B. Diagnosis

The child is usually brought for consultation because of the unsightly aspect of the navel. Although there may be complaints of abdominal pain, often following food, it is difficult to connect these with an umbilical hernia particularly as at that age recurrent abdominal pain is frequent and usually unimportant. Whatever the character of the pain, small children almost always point to the umbilicus as its site. Complications are exceptional, though rupture and acute evisceration has been described by some authors [Shaw 1979]. Incarceration or strangulation of omentum or intestine is very rarely seen [Benson 1962] and the risk seems to be less than 1 in 1,000.

C. Treatment

The use of a truss with a flat plate, or a small coin wrapped in gauze or cotton, placed over the umbilicus in an attempt to hasten spontaneous closure, has been suggested but is of little proven value and may damage the skin. Once the parents have been clearly informed of the usual natural course of events, their anxiety subsides.

Surgery is almost never indicated below the age of one year, and rarely so up to three. It may be necessary if there is a very large swelling presenting on crying, covered with thin and translucent skin. A large hernia which persists up to school age may require surgery, especially if painful, but each case must be decided on its merits. The operation is carried out under general anesthesia and usually requires a very brief stay in hospital, or may be done as a day case. The hernia is approached by a semicircular incision to the left of or below the umbilical scar (o). The peritoneal sac is freed up and the ring defined. One can then resect the sac and close the defect in one layer with a nonabsorbable stitch [Daudet 1978] or free it from the skin and invaginate it. The sutures pick up the aponeurotic

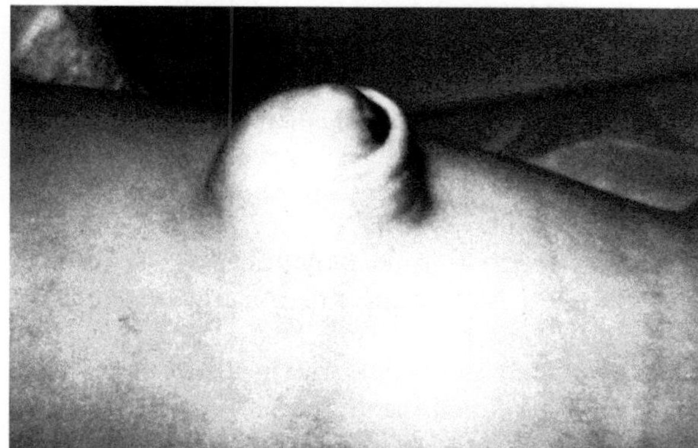

Fig. 12.44. Adumbilical hernia in a child

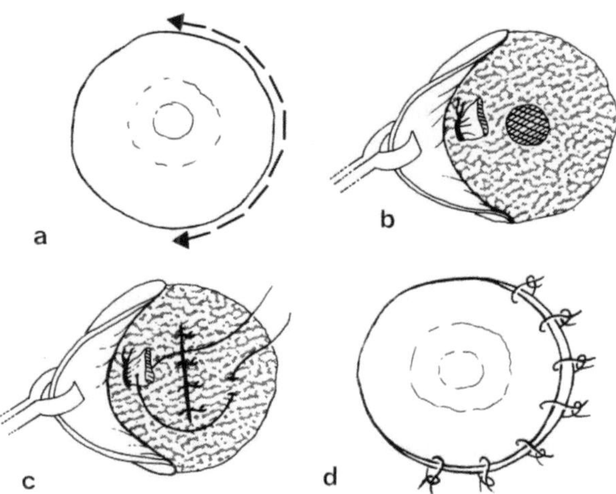

Fig. 12.45. Surgical treatment of umbilical hernia in children. **a** Skin incision. **b** Freeing of the aponeurotic ring and resection of the hernial sac. **c** Single-layered repair. **d** Cutaneous closure via interrupted intradermal sutures

layer [Miller & Shaw 1978]. The umbilical scar is replaced and stitched to the deeper layer so as to avoid redundancy (Fig. 12.45c). The skin is closed by a few absorbable intradermal sutures. Any excess skin can be cut away. A small gauze dressing is fixed with adhesive under low pressure, so as to avoid the formation of a hematoma. Complications are rare and recurrence should not be seen. The umbilical scar is sometimes a little prominent, but becomes normal in the course of growth.

References

Benson CO (1962) Umbilical hernia. In: Benson CB, Mustard WT, Ravitch MM, Snyder WH, Welch KJ (eds) Pediatric Surgery. Year Book, Chicago, pp 598-600

Blumberg NA (1980) Infantile umbilical hernia. Surg Gynecol Obstet. 150: 187-191

Cone JB and Golladay EJ (1983) Purse-skin closure of umbilical hernia repair. J Pediatr Surg 18: 297-298

Crump EP (1952) Umbilical hernia occurence of the infantile type in negro infants and children. J Pediatr 40: 214-220

Daudet M (1978) Hernies ombilicales. In: Pellerin D, Bertin P (eds) Technique de chirurgie pediatrique. Masson, Paris, pp 228-230

Evants AG (1941) The comparative incidence of umbilical hernias in colored anc white infants. J Nat Med Assoc 33: 158

Haller JA (1971) Repair of umbilical hernia in childhood to prevent adult incarceration. Am Surg 37: 245-248

Heifetz CJ, Bilsel ZJ, Gans WW (1963) Observations on the desappearance of umbilical hernia in infancy and childhood. Surg Gynecol Obstet 116: 469-473

Moore TC (1977) Gastroschisis and omphalocele: clinical differences. Surgery 82: 561-568

Shaw A (1979) The umbilicus. In: Ravitch MM, Welch KJ, Benson CB, Aberdeen E, Randolph JG (eds). Pediatric Surgery. Year Book, Chicago, pp 771-778

Vohr BR, Rosenfield AG, Oh W (1977) Umbilical hernia in the low birth weight infant. J Pediatr 90: 807-811

Walker SH (1967) The natural history of umbilical hernia. Clin Pediatr 6: 29-32

V. Epigastric Hernias in Children

Small midline epigastric hernias may occur between the xiphoid process and the umbilicus, the defect in the linea alba seldom exceeding 1 or 2 cm. It usually contains a small mass of extraperitoneal fat in the form of a lipoma, or a peritoneal sac in which there may be a fringe of omentum.

The child or its parents will generally notice a small nodule, but sometimes the hernia may be painful, particularly on pressure, which is an indication for surgery. Although these hernias are difficult to reduce, strangulation is very rare.

Surgical correction is simple. The site of the hernia is identified under general anesthesia and approached directly by a short vertical or (better) horizontal incision. The sac is freed from the margins of the defect and opened having checked the omental contents. The defect is closed by a suture that takes up the peritoneum and the aponeurosis, depending on the site of the defect, either longitudinal or transversely. The subcutaneous tissues and skin are closed with absorbable material.

VI. Divarication of the Recti in Children

The rectus muscles are quite often divaricated in children, giving rise to a longitudinal midline swelling from the xiphoid to the umbilicus, in which the abdominal wall consists only of the aponeurotic layer. Upon straining a painless and easily reducible elongated swelling appears. This condition is not in the least dangerous and often improves with growth. The great majority require no surgical treatment.

VII. Spigelian Hernia in Children

The appearance of a Spigelian hernia at the lateral border of the rectus muscle below the umbilicus is exceptional in children [Graivier et al. 1988]. We have seen three cases. The fact that certain of these are noted shortly after birth [Wright 1994] suggests a local abnormality in development of the aponeurosis of transversus, particularly as bilateral cases have been reported [Antony & Medlery 1972]. There may be an associated maldescent of the testis [Silberstein et al. 1996] but the connection between these two problems is not clear.

The diagnosis is difficult if the swelling, as occurs in the majority of cases, is only occasionally seen, or presents on coughing. One then has to rely on the description given by the parents. Ultrasound and tomodensitometry are of uncertain value. The exact location should be checked accurately before the operation, to ensure a repair of the abdominal wall which is problem free. A few cases of strangulation have been reported [Podkamener et al. 1986; Bar Moar & Sweed 1989].

References

Antony J, Medlery AV (1972) Congenital bilateral Spigelian hernia. Int Surg 57: 580-582

Bar Moar JA, Sweed Y (1989) Spigelian hernia in children, two cases of unusual etiology. Pediatr Surg Int 4: 357-359

Graivier L, Bronsther B, Feins NR, Mestel AL (1988) Pediatric lateral ventral (Spigelian) hernias. South Med J 81: 325-326

Silberstein PA, Kern IB, Shi ECP (1996) Congenital Spigelian hernia with cryptochidism. J Pediatr Surg 31: 1208-1210

Podkamenev VV, Uman NV, Moroz VN (1986) Strangulated Spigelian hernia in a child. Klin Khir 6: 72

Wright JE (1994) Spigelian hernia in childhood. Pediatr Surg Int 9: 170-171

Subject Index

Imprimé en France, à Niort, par Soulisse et Cassegrain en septembre 1997 — Dépôt légal : octobre 1997 — N° d'impression : 3637.

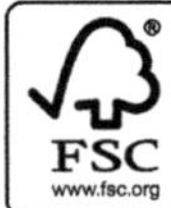

MIX
Papier aus verantwortungsvollen Quellen
Paper from responsible sources
FSC® C105338

If you have any concerns about our products,
you can contact us on
ProductSafety@springernature.com

In case Publisher is established outside the EU,
the EU authorized representative is:
**Springer Nature Customer Service Center GmbH
Europaplatz 3, 69115 Heidelberg, Germany**

Printed by Libri Plureos GmbH
in Hamburg, Germany